# The Endothelium
# in Clinical Practice

# FUNDAMENTAL AND CLINICAL CARDIOLOGY

*Editor-in-Chief*

**Samuel Z. Goldhaber, M.D.**

*Harvard Medical School*
*and Brigham and Women's Hospital*
*Boston, Massachusetts*

*Associate Editor, Europe*

**Henri Bounameaux, M.D.**

*University Hospital of Geneva*
*Geneva, Switzerland*

**ADDITIONAL VOLUMES IN PREPARATION**

# The Endothelium in Clinical Practice

## Source and Target of Novel Therapies

edited by

## Gabor M. Rubanyi

*Berlex Biosciences, Inc.*
*Richmond, California*

## Victor J. Dzau

*Brigham and Women's Hospital*
*and Harvard Medical School*
*Boston, Massachusetts*

MARCEL DEKKER, INC.          NEW YORK • BASEL • HONG KONG

**ISBN: 0-8247-9809-0**

The publisher offers discounts on this book when ordered in bulk quantities. For more information, write to Special Sales/Professional Marketing at the address below.

This book is printed on acid-free paper.

MARCEL DEKKER, INC.
270 Madison Avenue, New York, New York  10016

Current printing (last digit):
10  9  8  7  6  5  4  3  2  1

**PRINTED IN THE UNITED STATES OF AMERICA**

# Series Introduction

Marcel Dekker, Inc., has focused on developing beautifully produced books that facilitate the integration of rapidly advancing information for both the clinical specialist and the researcher. As editor of the Fundamental and Clinical Cardiology series, I have had the privilege of working with world-renowned individuals whose talents have permitted the exploration of virtually every facet of cardiovascular medicine.

The current monograph, *The Endothelium in Clinical Practice: Source and Target of Novel Therapies*, is the 29th book in our series. It is very special because it summarizes key findings that, until now, have required extensive reading from a wide array of texts. The editors, Gabor M. Rubanyi and Victor J. Dzau, are to be congratulated for their successful integration of basic science and clinical applications related to the endothelial cell. The efforts of the editors and their invited authors demonstrate that, when properly planned, technology can be successfully transferred from the "wet laboratory" to the "bedside." This exquisitely written book also serves as a model for mutually beneficial collaboration among leading scientists in industry and academia.

On a personal note, I have had the pleasure of knowing Dr. Dzau for almost 20 years. I am certain that in his role as Chairman of the Department of Medicine at Brigham and Women's Hospital he will carry forth the principles of collaboration and technology transfer that are so nicely epitomized in this monograph.

*Samuel Z. Goldhaber*

# Preface

Key discoveries in past decades have proven that the vascular endothelium is more than just a passive barrier between blood and tissue, and have contributed to significant progress in our understanding of basic mechanisms in vascular biology and pathophysiology. Endothelial cells play an important role in many aspects of animal and human physiology and pathophysiology. They contribute to cardiovascular homeostasis by maintaining the fluidity of the blood and by adjusting the caliber of blood vessels to the ever-changing hemodynamic and hormonal environment. The vascular endothelium performs these functions primarily by the production of biologically active substances that include pro- and anticoagulant factors; proliferative and antiproliferative substances; and molecules that modulate the tone of underlying vascular smooth muscle and contribute to angiogenesis, tissue remodeling, inflammation, and immune reactions.

In certain diseases the endothelium cannot perform its physiological functions. Activation of endothelial cells by various noxious stimuli (e.g., viruses, oxidized lipoproteins, and hemodynamic forces) leads to dysfunction of the endothelium that can be defined as an imbalance between physiological and pathophysiological factors and processes. This imbalance can lead to serious pathophysiological consequences, including localized (vasospasm) or generalized (hypertension) increase in vascular tone, vessel wall proliferation associated with chronic inflammation (e.g., atherosclerosis), and thrombosis. Endothelial dysfunction (as either a cause or a consequence) has been identified for numerous diseases, including thrombosis, atherosclerosis, restenosis, hypertension, diabetes, and inflammatory/ immune diseases involving the vascular wall.

Based on the accumulated knowledge and progress in basic sciences, there has been a transition from these laboratory observations to the clinic in recent years. This book is based on the realization that the endothelium is both the source and the target of novel therapeutic concepts and approaches. The former can be illustrated by both existing therapies (i.e., stable analogs of prostacyclin) and emerging novel therapeutic principles (e.g., selective inhibition of inducible nitric oxide synthase and blockade of endothelin production). The latter includes exciting novel therapies and therapeutic concepts based on inhibition (cancer) or stimulation (chronic ischemia) of angiogenesis; prevention of thrombosis; targeting of inflammatory and immune mediators involved in arteriosclerosis; and exploration of innovative approaches aimed at preventing or reversing endothelial cell dysfunction in hypertension, diabetes, and restenosis. Better understanding of the molecular basis of gene expression, and the fact that the endothelium is in direct contact with the circulating blood, has made the vascular endothelium an important target of gene therapy.

Several excellent monographs have reviewed the progress of basic research in various fields of endothelial cell biology and pathobiology. This book attempts to summarize the transition from basic research findings to therapeutic principles and concepts already used or to be introduced in the clinic. The book's primary goal is to demonstrate this quantum leap.

The book is divided into three parts. The first part describes existing and emerging therapies based on endothelial factors and molecules. These approaches include substituting deficient protective factors (e.g., prostacyclin) and inhibiting the excessive production (e.g., endothelin) or blocking the function (e.g., inflammatory mediators and procoagulant factors) of pathological substances. The second part summarizes novel therapeutic approaches targeting pathophysiological processes associated with the vascular endothelium, including the complement system and conditions such as rupture of atherosclerotic plaques, restenosis, hypertension, diabetes, and hyperlipoproteinemia. The involvement of the endothelium in the remarkable cardiovascular protection by the ovarian sex hormone estrogen is also described. The last part provides examples of the role of endothelium in gene therapy by describing animal and human studies of the endothelial cell–specific angiogenic growth factor VEGF and of the use of nitric oxide synthase gene transfer to prevent restenosis following angioplasty.

With its focus on the transition from basic research to clinical applications, this book is recommended for basic scientists and clinicians from a variety of disciplines, including molecular and cell biology, biochemistry, physiology, pharmacology, pathology, angiology, vascular surgery, organ transplantation, and cardiology. It will also appeal to those involved in research in lipoprotein disorders, atherosclerosis, diabetes, and coagulopathies.

We wish to thank the leading scholars whose excellent contributions made this book possible, and the staff of Marcel Dekker, Inc., for their very efficient handling and timely publication of this volume.

*Gabor M. Rubanyi*
*Victor J. Dzau*

# Contents

## III.  Gene Therapy

# Contributors

**Juan J. Badimon, Ph.D.**   Associate Professor of Medicine, Cardiovascular Institute, Mount Sinai Medical Center, New York, New York

**Lina Badimon, Ph.D.**   Professor, Cardiovascular Research Center, Barcelona, Spain

**Glyn Belcher, M.A., Ph.D., M.B., M.F.P.M.**   Cardiovascular Clinical Research, Schering AG, Berlin, Germany

**James H. Chesebro, M.D.**   Professor of Medicine, Cardiovascular Institute, Mount Sinai Medical Center, New York, New York

**John A. Dormandy, F.R.C.S.(Eng), F.R.C.S.(Ed), D.Sc.**   Professor, Department of Vascular Surgery, St. George's Hospital and Medical School, London, England

**Victor J. Dzau, M.D.\***   Chairman, Department of Medicine, and Chief, Division of Cardiovascular Medicine, Stanford University School of Medicine, Stanford, California

---

*Current affiliation:* Professor and Chairman, Department of Medicine, Brigham and Women's Hospital and Harvard Medical School, Boston, Massachusetts.

**Jack O. Egan, Ph.D.**  Postdoctoral Associate, Department of Biochemistry, College of Medicine, University of Vermont, Burlington, Vermont

**Garret A. FitzGerald, M.D.**  Robinette Foundation Professor of Cardiovascular Medicine and Chairman, Department of Pharmacology, The University of Pennsylvania, Philadelphia, Pennsylvania

**Valentin Fuster, M.D., Ph.D.**  Director, Cardiovascular Institute, Department of Cardiology, Mount Sinai Medical Center, New York, New York

**Richard Gallo, M.D.**  Research Associate, Cardiovascular Institute, Mount Sinai Medical Center, New York, New York

**J. Gamble, M.Sc., Ph.D.**  Vascular Biology Laboratory, Division of Human Immunology, Hanson Centre for Cancer Research, Institute of Medical and Veterinary Science, Adelaide, South Australia, Australia

**Katsutoshi Goto, Ph.D.**  Professor, Department of Pharmacology, Institute of Basic Medical Sciences, The University of Tsukuba, Tsukuba, Ibaraki, Japan

**David J. Grainger, M.A., Ph.D.**  Doctor, Department of Biochemistry, University of Cambridge, Cambridge, England

**Osamu Hori, M.D.**  Postdoctoral Research Scientist, Department of Physiology, Columbia University College of Physicians and Surgeons, New York, New York

**Steven D. Hughes, Ph.D.**  Postdoctoral Fellow, Life Science Division, Lawrence Berkeley National Laboratory, University of California at Berkeley, Berkeley, California

**Jeffrey M. Isner, M.D.**  Professor of Medicine and Pathology, Tufts University School of Medicine, and Chief, Cardiovascular Research, St. Elizabeth's Medical Center, Boston, Massachusetts

**Michael Kalafatis, Ph.D.**  Assistant Professor, Department of Biochemistry, College of Medicine, University of Vermont, Burlington, Vermont

**Katalin Kauser, M.D., Ph.D.**  Scientist, Cardiovascular Department, Berlex Biosciences, Inc., Richmond, California

**Yeesim Khew-Goodall, Ph.D.**  Division of Human Immunology, Hanson Centre for Cancer Research, Institute of Medical and Veterinary Science, Adelaide, South Australia, Australia

**Thomas F. Lüscher, M.D.**  Professor of Medicine, Cardiology, and Cardiovascular Research, University Hospital, Bern, Switzerland

**Kenneth G. Mann, Ph.D.** Chairman, Department of Biochemistry, College of Medicine, University of Vermont, Burlington, Vermont

**Emma A. Meagher, M.D.** Assistant Professor of Medicine, Center for Experimental Therapeutics, The University of Pennsylvania, Philadelphia, Pennsylvania

**Jawahar L. Mehta, M.D., Ph.D.** Professor of Medicine, Department of Medicine, University of Florida, Gainesville, Florida

**James C. Metcalfe, M.A., Ph.D.** Professor, Department of Biochemistry, University of Cambridge, Cambridge, England

**Pierre Moreau, Ph.D.** Postdoctoral Fellow, Molecular Medicine, Hôtel-Dieu de Montreal Research Center, Montreal, Quebec, Canada

**John F. Parkinson, Ph.D.** Senior Scientist, Department of Immunology, Berlex Biosciences, Inc., Richmond, California

**Louis P. Perrault, M.D., F.R.C.S.(C)** Clinician-Scientist Program of the Medical Research Council of Canada, and Fellow, Institut de Recherches Servier, Suresnes, France

**Gary B. Phillips, Ph.D.** New Lead Discovery, Berlex Biosciences, Inc., Richmond, California

**Michael A. Reidy, Ph.D.** Professor, Department of Pathology, University of Washington, Seattle, Washington

**Gabor M. Rubanyi, M.D., Ph.D.** Director, Vascular and Endothelial Research, Cardiovascular Department, Berlex Biosciences, Inc., Richmond, California

**Edward M. Rubin, M.D., Ph.D.** Senior Scientist, Associate Professor, and Group Leader, Human Genome Center, Lawrence Berkeley National Laboratory, University of California at Berkeley, Berkeley, California

**Una S. Ryan, Ph.D.** President, Chief Operating Officer, and Chief Scientific Officer, T Cell Sciences, Inc., Needham, Massachusetts

**Ann Marie Schmidt, M.D.** Assistant Professor, Department of Medicine and Surgery, Columbia University College of Physicians and Surgeons, New York, New York

**Karsten Schrör, M.D.** Professor of Pharmacology, Director, and Head, Institut für Pharmakologie, Heinrich-Heine-Universität Düsseldorf, Düsseldorf, Germany

**Stephen M. Schwartz, M.D., Ph.D.** Professor, Department of Pathology, University of Washington, Seattle, Washington

**Brian Stein, M.B., B.S., F.R.A.C.P.** Division of Human Immunology, Hanson Centre for Cancer Research, Institute of Medical and Veterinary Science, Adelaide, South Australia, Australia

**Matthew A. Vadas, B.Sc.(Med), M.B.B.S., Ph.D., F.R.A.C.P., F.R.C.P.A.** Professor/Director, Division of Human Immunology, Hanson Centre for Cancer Research, Institute of Medical and Veterinary Science, Adelaide, South Australia, Australia

**Paul M. Vanhoutte, M.D., Ph.D.** Vice President, Research and Development, Institut de Recherches Internationales Servier, Courbevoie, France

**Jean Paul Vilaine, M.D.** Chief, Division of Cardiovascular Pharmacology, Institut de Recherches Servier, Suresnes, France

**Heiko E. von der Leyen, M.D.** Instructor in Medicine, Division of Cardiovascular Medicine, Department of Medicine, Stanford University School of Medicine, Stanford, California

**Shi Du Yan, M.D.** Assistant Professor of Clinical Pathology, Department of Pathology, Columbia University College of Physicians and Surgeons, New York, New York

**Baichun C. Yang, M.D., Ph.D.** Assistant Scientist, Department of Medicine, University of Florida, Gainesville, Florida

# 1

# Prostacyclin (Prostaglandin I$_2$) and Atherosclerosis

**Karsten Schrör**

*Institut für Pharmakologie, Heinrich-Heine-Universität Düsseldorf,
Düsseldorf, Germany*

## I. INTRODUCTION: WHY PROSTACYCLIN?

Shortly after the detection of prostacyclin (prostaglandin I$_2$ [PGI$_2$]), a lipid mediator of the eicosanoid superfamily (1), it became evident that the compound was not only a vasodilator and the most potent endogenous inhibitor of platelet aggregation but also exerted a number of other remarkable effects on vascular cells, circulating blood elements, and soluble macromolecules. This included inhibition of white cell function, modulation of cell proliferation and immune reactions, as well as multiple interferences with lipid metabolism, most notably with that of cholesterol (2). The vascular endothelium is the major site of PGI$_2$ biosynthesis (3), and endothelium-dependent PGI$_2$ generation can be evoked by almost any kind of stimulus (2). This led to defining PGI$_2$ as a unique endothelium-derived lipid mediator that is generated continuously in physiological conditions but without major effects of its own. If, however, an imbalance of vascular control is impeding, PGI$_2$ formation becomes stimulated and acts to keep the system in a stable condition. Thus, inhibition of vascular PGI$_2$ formation in healthy individuals does not cause functional disturbances. Functional disturbances, such as an increase in vascular resistance, may however occur if endogenous PGI$_2$ production becomes a limiting factor of homoeostasis; for example, control of regional perfusion (4).

*1*

The first finding that showed a connection between $PGI_2$ and atherosclerosis was the detection in animals, who were fed a cholesterol-rich diet, of reduced $PGI_2$ generation in vessel pieces prepared from atherosclerotic arteries (5–7). A diminished $PGI_2$ production was also found in human atherosclerotic vascular tissue (8–9). The reduced $PGI_2$ generation was obviously associated with morphological alterations in the vessel wall; that is, with the fibroproliferative tissue reaction and lipid deposition, both of which are typical for plaque formation in early atherogenesis (10). As endothelial dysfunction is considered to be a general denominator of atherosclerotic vessel disease (11–12), it was concluded that the incidence and progression of atherosclerosis may be related to insufficient $PGI_2$ production by the endothelium (2,13). Experimental studies showing that exogenous $PGI_2$ or more stable $PGI_2$-mimetics, including $PGE_1$, may retard the progression of atherosclerotic lesions and inhibit smooth muscle cell proliferation after stimulation by growth factors (10,14) also supported this view. Although the situation turned out to be more complex, especially after the detection of additional endothelium-derived mediators, such as "endothelium-derived relaxing factor" (nitric oxide, NO) and endothelin (15), there is little doubt that most, if not all, biological activities of $PGI_2$ are antiatherosclerotic in nature. They are part of the vascular control by endothelial cells of the regulation of hemostasis, regional perfusion, and vascular remodeling.

The loss of the functional integrity of the vascular endothelium is accompanied by transformation of the endothelium from a nonthrombogenic surface which generates vasodilatory, anticoagulant, profibrinolytic, platelet- and leukocyte-repellent, and growth-modulating substances into a prothrombotic, growth-promoting, and platelet- and leukocyte-adhesive surface (16). Presumably of particular significance is the loss of endothelial control of vascular smooth muscle cells, eventually resulting in loss of their contractile function and conversion into a secretory phenotype (17). These nonadaptive changes in endothelial structure and function, provoked by pathophysiological stimuli, affect *all* types of mediators that are released and processed by endothelial cells. Although this chapter focuses on the role of $PGI_2$, the unique activities of this compound can only be appreciated in the context of overall changes in vascular control.

## II.  PRINCIPLES OF $PGI_2$ GENERATION AND ACTION

Local levels of eicosanoids are determined by local biosynthesis. This is also valid for $PGI_2$, which is the main, if not the only, cyclooxygenase product in endothelial and smooth muscle cells of large arteries (18); that is, the primary sites of atherosclerotic lesions. $PGI_2$ biosynthesis in the vessel wall occurs preferentially in the endothelium. This is due to its mass (comparable to the size of the liver) (19) as well as the high level of cyclooxygenase-protein expression as opposed to that of vascular smooth muscle cells (20). Interestingly, there is an approximately 12-fold higher $PGI_2$ synthase protein content in smooth muscle cells as compared with endothelium (21). This suggests that vascular smooth muscle may become an important source of $PGI_2$ production in the vessel wall if sufficient prostaglandin endoperoxide precursor is available from adjacent cells, such as platelets or macrophages, by transcellular metabolism (see Section II.A.3).

## A. $PGI_2$ Production by Endothelial Cells

Two principally different mechanisms determine $PGI_2$ formation: (1) availability of substrate and (2) mass and activity of synthesis-controlling enzymes.

### 1. Biosynthetic Pathways of $PGI_2$ Generation

$PGI_2$ is generated from free arachidonic acid by the sequential action of a phospholipase $A_2$ ($PLA_2$), cyclooxygenase(s) (COX) with peroxidase activity, and a cytochrome P-450–type isomerase ($PGI_2$ synthase) (Fig. 1).

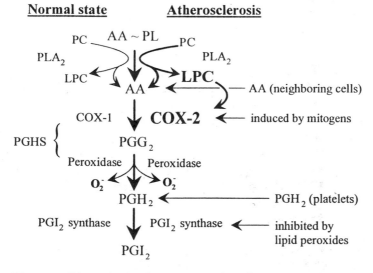

**Figure 1**   Biosynthesis of prostacyclin ($PGI_2$) in vascular cells under physiological conditions (left) and in atherosclerosis (right). PL, phospholipid; $PLA_2$ phospholipase $A_2$; AA, arachidonic acid; PC, phosphatidylcholine; LPC, lyso-phosphatidylcholine; COX, cyclooxygenase. (See text for further explanations.)

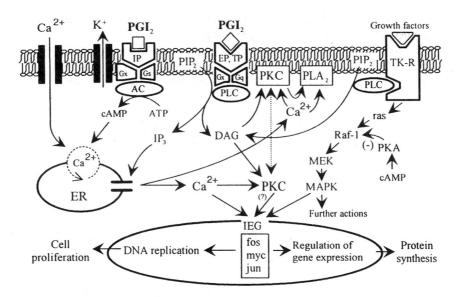

**Figure 2** Signal transduction pathways of PGI$_2$ in vascular cells. AC, adenylate cyclase; PLC, phospholipase C; PLA$_2$, phospholipase A$_2$; IP$_3$, inositoltrisphosphate; DAG, diacyglycerol; PKC, protein kinase C; MEK, mitogen-activated protein kinase kinase; MAPK, mitogen-activated protein kinase; IEG, immediate early genes; TK-R, tyrosine receptor kinase. (See text for further explanations.)

Cyclooxygenase and the inherent peroxidase activity are frequently summarized as PGH-synthase (PGHS). Of these three enzymes involved in PGI$_2$ production, PLA$_2$ is considered to initiate prostaglandin synthesis, whereas COX is thought to control the amount and duration of prostaglandin production (22). Thus, COX activity is critical for product formation.

*Arachidonic Acid and Phospholipases.*   Arachidonic acid is a major constituent of cell membranes and is esterified at the *sn*-2 position of phospholipids. The cellular stores may be refilled by arachidonic acid derived from high-density lipoprotein (HDL)–cholesteryl esters (23). In agreement with this observation, HDL but not low-density lipoprotein (LDL) cholesterol was found to stimulate PGI$_2$ production in cultured endothelial cells (24).

Arachidonic acid release by PLA$_2$ is initiated by phospholipase C (PLC)–dependent cleavage of membrane phospholipids, resulting in the activation of the phosphatidylinositol cycle and generation of the intracellular messengers inositol trisphosphate (IP$_3$) and diacylglycerol (DAG) (Fig. 2). PLC-coupled arachidonic acid release is a consequence of receptor stimulation and phospholipid breakdown, respectively. This explains why all kinds of physiological or noxious stimuli cause tissue-specific eicosanoid release as a consequence of the concerted actions of PLC and $PLA_2$ (25–26).

Weksler and colleagues (27) originally demonstrated that $Ca^{2+}$ iono-phores stimulate $PGI_2$ formation in endothelial cells, pointing to a role of elevated cytosolic $Ca^{2+}$ levels for $PGI_2$ biosynthesis. Later studies showed that agonist-induced $PGI_2$ release in endothelial cells is quantitatively linked to $Ca^{2+}_i$ (28–30), possibly by a $Ca^{2+}$-dependent activation of in-tracellular $PLA_2$ (31) (Fig. 2). The contributions of further cellular signal transduction pathways to $PGI_2$ biosynthesis are only incompletely under-stood. Some data suggest involvement of protein kinase C (PKC) (32). However, others have shown that phorbol esters with a longer duration of action than the physiological agonist DAG potentiate agonist-induced $PGI_2$ production by a leftward shift of the $Ca^{2+}$ activation dose-response curve for $PGI_2$ release and not by stimulation of PI turnover (33). These acute effects of PKC on $PGI_2$ formation have to be separated from long-term effects which require several hours and are probably due to upregulation of COX-2 protein synthesis (34) (see Section III.A.2). There is also evidence in vascular smooth muscle cells that conversion from the contractile to the secretory phenotype (see Section III.B.5) may funda-mentally alter the mechanisms controlling $PGI_2$ biosynthesis (35).

A compound very similar to $PGI_2$ in several aspects and also a major product of endothelial cells is nitric oxide (NO). It has been postulated that release of $PGI_2$ and NO are coupled during receptor-stimulated activation of PLC-dependent pathways in endothelial cells (36). However, there are important differences in the release kinetics, mechanism, and site of action of these two mediators, suggesting that they are serving different purposes. The time course of agonist-induced $PGI_2$ release and the velocity of the development of tachyphylaxis is more rapid and more pronounced than that for NO. There is a strict dependency on extracellular $Ca^{2+}$ of NO, but not of $PGI_2$, formation after activation of the constitutive enzymes in endothelial cells. PKC stimulates $PGI_2$ release but blocks NO generation (29–30). There are no receptors in the classic sense for NO and only one target enzyme, the soluble guanylate cyclase which stimulates cellular cGMP levels, as second messenger. In the case of $PGI_2$, the situation is more complex. Specifically, membrane-bound receptors are coupled to different intracellular signaling pathways, including adenylate cyclase, phospholipase C, and $K^+$ channels (see Section II.B).

*Cyclooxygenases.* In physiological conditions, the amount of COX-derived products is controlled both by the availability of nonesterified arachidonic acid (substrate) and lipid peroxide (activator) (37).

In the presence of free substrate, COX activity determines the amount of product formation. There are two isoforms of the enzyme: COX-1 and COX-2. COX-1 is purportedly constitutive, developmentally regulated (38), and may be upregulated with a subsequent increase in $PGI_2$ production by hypoxia in pulmonary artery endothelial cells (39) but not by growth factors (40). Overexpression of the COX-1 gene in virally transformed endothelial cells resulted in an about 20-fold higher mRNA and protein levels which were associated with corresponding increases in agonist-induced $PGI_2$ production (41). COX-1 and COX-2 as well as $PGI_2$ synthase in cultured vascular endothelial and smooth muscle cells are localized within the nuclear membrane and the endoplasmatic reticulum, suggesting direct effects of the eicosanoid on the nucleus (18,42). Because of this colocalization of the enzymes, it has been suggested that the mechanisms of prostanoid transport from the inside to the outside of the cell are the same for both isoenzymes (43). COX-1 determines vascular $PGI_2$ production in physiological conditions. The principal enzyme for $PGI_2$ production in atherosclerotic vessels and vascular lesions is COX-2 (see Fig. 2). COX-2 is present but not upregulated in endothelial cells in the absence of growth factors or cytokines (see Section III.A.2).

*$PGI_2$ Synthase.* The $PGI_2$ synthase is an isomerase that converts the PG endoperoxide $PGH_2$ into $PGI_2$. The enzyme has been cloned and sequenced and was found to belong to the P-450 family (44). The half-life of the mRNA encoding for $PGI_2$ synthase in endothelial cells is 24 hr; that is the message is four times more stable than the mRNA for COX-2 in the same preparation. Bovine aortic endothelial cells in culture are capable of increasing their $PGI_2$ production via induction of $PGI_2$ synthase protein. This was combined with a long-lasting half-life of its mRNA (21). Although others could not confirm that $PGI_2$ synthase protein is induced by cytokines in human endothelial cells (45), it is an interesting hypothesis that endothelial cells are capable of increasing their $PGI_2$ production at the level of transcription; that is, gene regulation (21).

## 2. Metabolism of $PGI_2$

The half-life of $PGI_2$ in the circulation is short and amounts to about 6 min in whole blood (46). This half-life can be considerably prolonged (five-fold) by binding to ApoA-I, which is a major apoprotein in HDL (47). The relationship between HDL and "$PGI_2$-stimulating" factor, which was found in endothelial and smooth muscle cells (48), is unknown. The shortened half-life of $PGI_2$ in atherosclerotic diseases may be related to reduced amounts of HDL or increased levels of (ox)-LDL, respectively (49).

## 3.  Control of Cellular $PGI_2$ Generation

$PGI_2$ is an intercellular signal molecule. Therefore, the $PGI_2$-synthesizing machinery in endothelial cells needs to be controlled by extracellular mechanical, chemical, or hormonal signals that are dispatched from other sources and adapt cellular $PGI_2$ production to the level necessary for appropriate signal transmission. Two principal types of control can be separated: paracrine and autocrine.

*Paracrine Control.*  Generation of $PGI_2$ as a messenger of intercellular signal transduction is involved in the cross talk between different cell types in two ways: (1) generation in response to any agonist with subsequent modulation of the activity of cells in the neighborhood and (2) generation from precursors taken up from cells in the vicinity by transcellular metabolism. In the latter case, the donor cell (e.g., platelets) needs activation in order to release unstable intermediates to a recipient cell (endothelial cell, smooth muscle cell) that requires no activation to produce new eicosanoids. Platelet/ endothelial cell interactions are an example where PG endoperoxides of platelets are used for vascular $PGI_2$ biosynthesis (50). Although this transcellular metabolism cannot always be demonstrated in vitro (51), it definitely operates in vivo; for example, between platelets and vascular cells at a site of vessel injury (52). This transcellular metabolism with generation of new signal molecules is actually the end result of agonist stimulation of the donor cell (53) and plays an important role in intercellular communication in atherosclerosis (see Section III.A.2).

Another type of paracrine control is exerted by chemical agonists that induce $PGI_2$ biosynthesis which in turn modifies their actions. $PGI_2$ production in response to PLC-coupled chemical agonists (ATP, $\alpha$-thrombin, bradykinin) is transient in nature and stops within a few minutes. Elevation of cyclic AMP levels in endothelial cells attenuates thrombin or $Ca^{2+}$ ionophore–induced $PGI_2$ release (54–55). Similar results were obtained with synthetic cAMP analogues and phosphodiesterase inhibitors, suggesting that the release of $PGI_2$ is strictly controlled by a cAMP-mediated negative feedback loop (54,56). Possible reasons are a rapid downregulation of receptor number or affinity (57), uncoupling of the receptor from PLC, resulting in a reduced production of $IP_3$, or exhaustion of available intracellular $Ca^{2+}$ stores. This may not allow the intracellular $Ca^{2+}$ to become elevated to the threshold level of $PLA_2$ stimulation; that is, 0.8–1.0 $\mu M$ (30,58), which is necessary for phospholipid breakdown and subsequent release of arachidonic acid.

*Autocrine Control.*  Autocrine control of $PGI_2$ synthesis is exerted by $PGI_2$ on the cell which synthesizes it. This control appears to be mediated via $PGI_2$-induced downregulation of its own $PGI_2$ receptor–mediated signaling. In several studies $PGI_2$ did not stimulate the cAMP response in the same endothelial cells where it was synthesized (54,56). This was explained by an agonist-induced desensitization of $PGI_2$ receptors, because a cAMP response was seen after inhibition of endogenous $PGI_2$ production by COX inhibitors (57). It was concluded that biological effects of endogenous $PGI_2$ are entirely paracrine in nature (59). The autocrine desensitization of the cAMP response by a receptor down-regulation may allow for a higher release rate of this autacoid. Evidence for a homologous desensitization of $PGI_2$ receptors was also found with respect to antimitogenic effects of $PGI_2$ in vascular smooth muscle cells (60) (see Section III.B.5).

## B.  $PGI_2$ Receptors and Second Messengers

### 1.  $PGI_2$ Receptors

The actions of $PGI_2$ are receptor mediated. High-affinity ligand binding sites, which are coupled to intracellular signal transduction pathways (IP receptors), have been detected in several vascular cells, including endothelial and smooth muscle cells (61–62). A human IP receptor has recently been cloned and sequenced and was found to belong to the superfamily of G protein–coupled receptors with seven transmembrane domains (63–64). The IP receptor mRNA is widely expressed in the cardiovascular system; most abundantly in the aorta. Interestingly, there was no potential consensus site for phosphorylation by cAMP-dependent protein kinases (63). No subtypes of IP receptors or splicing variants have been published so far (65). There is practically no information on regulation of IP receptors in vascular cells. This is a severe limitation for the design and targeting of new $PGI_2$-mimetics for clinical use.

### 2.  Second Messengers

The IP receptor appears to be coupled to at least two different cellular signal transduction pathways: $G_s$ protein–coupled stimulation of adenylate cyclase and $G_{(o?,p?,q?)}$ protein–coupled stimulation of PLC (64,66–67). It has been shown that vasocontractile actions of $PGI_2$ at higher concentrations may be mediated via the thromboxane (TP) receptor (68) (see Fig. 2). It is currently unknown whether this finding is also of relevance for growth control by $PGI_2$ (see Section III.B.5). The vasorelaxing action of $PGI_2$ is probably due to opening of ATP-dependent $K^+$ channels (69). Thus, the cellular signals generated after IP receptor stimulation may modify the atherosclerotic process in different ways and may origin from receptor(s) that are coupled to different second messengers (70).

## III. PGI$_2$ GENERATION AND ACTIONS IN ATHEROSCLEROSIS

Vascular PGI$_2$ formation in atherosclerosis is determined by mechanisms different from those under physiological conditions and, in general, is much more variable. In addition, species differences and assay conditions may modify PGI$_2$ synthesis (71). Endothelial injury with the expression of adhesion molecules allows for close and sustained interactions between the vessel wall and blood constituents such as platelets and monocytes/macrophages. This facilitates transcellular metabolism, specifically in the presence of hyperreactive platelets. There is induction of the inducible COX-2 isoform in almost all cell types involved, except platelets, under the action of cytokines and growth factors.

On the other hand, endothelial injury results in generation of products, such as oxygen-centered free radicals, which enhance lipid peroxidation, eventually resulting in inhibition of PGI$_2$ synthase, and enhanced degradation of endothelial messengers, such as NO (72). Vascular smooth muscle cells synthesize PGI$_2$ as a major product and will become a significant source of PGI$_2$ production after endothelial injury (73) or cell stimulation by growth factors (74). Vascular cyclooxygenases are much more resistant against aspirin than those of the platelet (51,73), probably because of the expression of COX-2 and the high level of PGI$_2$ synthase protein (21). Cholesterol feeding reduces PGI$_2$ production by cultured vascular smooth muscle cells (75–76), whereas aortas from cholesterol-fed rabbits subjected to pulsatile flow (i.e., shear-stress) ex vivo exhibit a more stable PGI$_2$ release than perfused aortas from nonhypercholesterolemic controls (77). These data underline the complexity of PGI$_2$-synthesizing pathways in atherosclerosis as well as the bifunctional role of neointimal smooth muscle cells, being both generators and recipients of the PGI$_2$ signal.

### A. Changes in PGI$_2$ Formation in Atherosclerosis

#### 1. Time-Dependent Changes of PGI$_2$ Generation

Initial animal experiments indicated that PGI$_2$ production was reduced in rabbits and pigs made atherosclerotic by feeding a cholesterol-enriched diet (5–7,9). PGI$_2$ production in the aorta of cholesterol-fed rabbits tended to become normal after some months (78). Others found PGI$_2$ generation by aortic tissue unchanged in vitro under carefully controlled conditions at 4–8 months of cholesterol feeding despite the presence of severe atherosclerotic lesions (79–80). Voss et al. (81) even found an enhanced PGI$_2$ formation in atherosclerotic plaques at 9 months of cholesterol feeding. Endothelial injury by angioplasty reduced the amount of PGI$_2$ released in atherosclerotic rabbits (82), suggesting that the endothelium contributed significantly to PGI$_2$ formation. Accordingly, generation of proliferative, foam cell–containing lesions in the rabbit aorta by placing a Silastic collar around the vessel for 1 week without direct endothelial injury was not associated with reduced vascular PGI$_2$ synthesis (83–84). These data suggest a time-dependent variation in vascular PGI$_2$ production after endothelial injury by mechanical disruption or cholesterol overloading.

More detailed studies on the time course of alterations in vascular PGI$_2$ production in animal experiments have demonstrated a triphasic response (85): An initial fall shortly after starting cholesterol feeding (2 weeks) which preceded the morphological appearance of plaques. This was followed by a marked increase. In a third stage, PGI$_2$ production fell again, indicating the replacement of normal endothelium by atherosclerotic plaques (86). Accordingly, there is no strong correlation between the severity of hypercholesterolemia, endothelial dysfunction, and PGI$_2$ synthesis. Norman and Miller (87) have studied the correlation between cholesterol feeding–induced coronary atherosclerosis and plasma 6-oxo-PGF$_{1\alpha}$ (a stable degradation product of PGI$_2$) levels in the pig. At 6 months, hypercholesterolemia was positively correlated with the development of coronary atherosclerosis but 6-oxo-PGF$_{1\alpha}$ was not. Clearly, the situation might be quite different at longer lasting endothelial injury as it occurs in humans. An age-dependent reduction in PGI$_2$ biosynthesis by vascular endothelial cells was found by several groups (71,88). Similar findings have been reported for vascular smooth muscle cells (71). This was accompanied by an increased sensitivity of smooth muscle cells to mitogens, including platelet-derived growth factor (PDGF) (89). These findings might have an impact to the advanced aging process in atherosclerosis and endothelial dysfunction in humans.

## 2. Cell-Dependent Features of Endogenous PGI$_2$ Production

*Additional Sources for PGI$_2$ Precursors in Atherosclerosis.*   Basal PGI$_2$ production by vascular cells prepared from atherosclerotic tissue tends to be unchanged or reduced (75–76) but is stimulated at least to the same extent as in nonatherosclerotic cells by appropriate agonists. For example, PDGF stimulates vascular PGI$_2$ production and acts synergistically with serotonin (90). This is probably related to the degradation of membrane phospholipids with enhanced availability of arachidonic acid and lysophospholipids that stimulate PGI$_2$ production (91) and generation of Ca$^{2+}$ signals induced by growth factors (see Fig. 1). In situ, the situation differs from that in isolated cell cultures because of the presence of nonvascular cells, such as platelets or macrophages, with a significant constitutive (platelets) or inducible (macrophages) cyclooxygenase activity. Thus, with the progression of atherosclerosis, the transcellular exchange of precursors, such as prostaglandin endoperoxides from these cells, may become important, and is facilitated by the expression of appropriate adhesion molecules at the vessel surface. $PGI_2$ generation within the circulation is enhanced in advanced atherosclerosis in parallel with platelet hyperreactivity in both animal experiments (92) and in men (93–94). Utilization of platelet-derived PG endoperoxides by vascular cells will explain the failure of aspirin even at low doses (e.g., 50 mg/day) selectively to block platelet thromboxane production in patients with severe atherosclerosis without simultaneous inhibition of $PGI_2$ formation (95–97).

*Induction of COX-2.* The main difference between normal and atherosclerotic vascular tissue is the change in the structure and composition of the vessel wall. This includes endothelial dysfunction, the appearance of new cells, such as monocyte-derived macrophages within the vessel wall, as well as the transformation of vascular smooth muscle cells from a contractile to a secretory phenotype (16). In atherosclerosis, there is gene activation and expression of the inducible form of the cyclooxygenase (COX-2) by macrophages (98), fibroblasts (99), vascular endothelial cells (100–102), and smooth muscle cells (40,101,103). Gene induction is due to cell-specific extracellular signals such as cytokines, hormones, and growth factors (104). In vascular cells, it is only COX-2 which becomes expressed at the level of transcription. This causes a marked increase in $PGI_2$ production by endothelial cells (91). Stimulation by growth factors of vascular smooth muscle cells resulted in an about 100-fold stimulation of $PGI_2$ and $PGE_2$ release due to COX-2 induction (40). There is no or only very limited activation of COX-1 (21,40,91). This suggests an important role of COX-2–derived $PGI_2$ for tissue protection under the transforming "pressure" of cytokines and growth factors; for example, in the restoration of thromboresistance of the neointima after endothelial injury (105). There is also enhanced generation of 15-HETE (hydroxy-eicosatetraenoic [acid]) by atherosclerotic vessels (106). Interestingly, 15-(R)HETE is a major cyclooxygenase metabolite of COX-2 but not of COX-1 (107).

Recent studies on thrombin-stimulated vascular smooth muscle cells have shown that both COX-1 and COX-2 coexist in the same cell line but are differentially regulated. After exposure to growth factors, the constitutive isoform remained coupled to the thrombin receptor, whereas the serum-inducible isoform did not (108). This suggests that the coupling of receptors to intracellular signal transduction pathways may be changed in growth factor–exposed vascular tissue.

Interestingly, the expression of the COX-2 message and protein in endothelial cells was markedly stimulated by lysophosphatidylcholine

(91). This lysophospholipid is well known to be involved in the development of atherosclerosis (109). In vivo, lysophosphatidylcholine is elevated in parallel with an increasing severity of coronary atherosclerosis, probably resulting from an elevated lecithin cholesterol acyltransferase (LCAT) activity (110) (see Section III.B.4). Thus, induction of COX-2 may be an important vasoprotective mechanism that tends to limit the progression of atherosclerotic lesions and to promote their regression (91).

The upregulation of COX-2 by cytokines and growth factors suggests that vascular $PGI_2$ formation is under genetic control. Children whose parents had early coronary heart disease had reduced $PGI_2$ levels and decreased HDL cholesterol (111–112). However, sons of earlier infarcted patients showed an about two-fold elevated plasma $PGI_2$ and thromboxane level (113).

### 3. Inhibition of $PGI_2$ Synthase

Endothelial $PGI_2$ formation is sensitive to lipid peroxides which are present in human atherosclerotic tissue. Oxidized metabolites of polyunsaturated fatty acids have been shown to rather selectively block $PGI_2$ formation both in fresh (114) and cultured (115) endothelial cells. Incubation of human umbilical vein endothelial cells with several oxidized cholesterol derivatives but not cholesterol itself was found to reduce $PGI_2$ production and to enhance the platelet adherence to endothelial cells (116).

The conversion of arachidonic acid to $PGI_2$ in tissue samples of human atherosclerotic lesions was reduced with the severity of the disease (9). This points to a selective inhibition of $PGI_2$ synthase by lipid peroxides, generated, for example, by oxygen-centered free radicals released from endothelial cells (72). Interestingly, $PGE_2$ generation in the same material was enhanced with the progression of the disease. An increase in aortic $PGE_2$ generation reaching a peak after 1 month was also found in rabbits fed an atherogenic diet (117). As an explanation, COX-2 expression by growth factors and cytokines could cause an overall increase of COX products but depressed $PGI_2$ synthesis because of specific inhibition of $PGI_2$ synthase.

### B. Actions of $PGI_2$ in Atherosclerosis

Putative important actions of $PGI_2$ in atherosclerosis are actions on vascular endothelium, smooth muscle cells, and all kinds of blood components. Another significant issue is the interference of $PGI_2$ with the cholesterol metabolism. Prostaglandins might also be considered differentiation signals that keep vascular smooth muscle in the quiescent, contractile state. An overview on the mutually important antiatherosclerotic actions of $PGI_2$ is shown in Table 1.

**Table 1**  Antiatherosclerotic Effects of Prostacyclin in
Vascular Cells and Platelets

| Target | Effect |
|---|---|
| Endothelial cells | Inhibition of tissue factor expression |
| | Preservation of endothelium-dependent relaxation |
| | Preservation of barrier function for macromolecules |
| | Inhibition of monocyte/macrophage adhesion |
| Smooth muscle cells | Inhibition (modulation) of proliferation |
| | Maintenance of contractile phenotype |
| Cholesterol metabolism | Stimulation of neutral and acid cholesterylester hydrolases |
| | Inhibition of ACAT ($PGE_2$) |
| Platelets | Inhibition of mitogen release (PDGF) |
| | Inhibition of vasoconstrictor generation ($TXA_2$) and release (5-HT) |
| | Inhibition of aggregation |

## 1. Endothelial Cells

Integrity of the vascular endothelium is a key event in vascular control. As already discussed, most of the pathological alterations in atherosclerosis can be interpreted as a consequence of endothelial dysfunction. In addition to generating and receiving chemical messages, endothelial cells have also an important barrier function for cells and various macromolecules. An increase in endothelial permeability for macromolecules is one of the earliest events in atherosclerosis and may allow for the accumulation and oxidation of lipoproteins (19,118). Furthermore, an increase in endothelial permeability in addition to disturbed blood flow allows local accumulation of agents that can further injure the endothelium (119).

Despite of the significant changes in endothelium-dependent product formation in atherosclerosis (see Section III.A), there is only little information on the modulation by $PGI_2$ of endothelial functions. $PGI_2$ at nanomolar concentrations inhibits the transcellular transport of macromolecules through arterial endothelial cells. This action is probably cAMP mediated (120). Shirotani and colleagues (121) have compared the action of the $PGI_2$-mimetic ciprostene on growth factor–stimulated endothelial and smooth muscle cells of the bovine aorta. There was no inhibition of DNA synthesis in endothelial cells up to concentrations of the compound (30 $\mu$M) which blocked the DNA synthesis of smooth muscle cells by about 60%. Studies in cholesterol-fed rabbits have shown that treatment with $PGI_2$-mimetics preserves endothelium-dependent relaxation (122). This suggests endothelium-protective actions of $PGI_2$. The mechanism of this action remains unknown. Gryglewski et al. (123) suggested that vessel intima in vivo may release $PGI_2$ intraluminally, whereas NO is secreted abluminally, and thus these two mediators may act independently: Endogenous $PGI_2$ maintains endothelial thromboresistance, whereas NO controls the tone of arterial myocytes and perfusion of the microcirculation.

2.   Platelets

Platelet hyperreactivity is a typical feature of experimental and clinical atherosclerosis. In addition to their role in forming a hemostatic plug, platelets generate and release vasocontractile and growth-promoting factors, such as thromboxane $A_2$ and serotonin, PDGF, and other mitogens (124). In addition, platelets are the most important source of thrombin generation in vivo. Experimental studies have shown that continuous removal of platelets will prevent or retard the development of atherosclerotic lesions (125–126), whereas destruction of circulating platelets had the opposite effect and accelerated the development of atherosclerotic lesions in cholesterol-fed rabbits (127). Although platelets may not play the key role in initial smooth muscle cell proliferation after traumatic endothelial injury as originally believed (11), they may contribute to later events; for example, the formation of a neointima by stimulation of migration of smooth muscle cells from the media into the intima (128).

PGI_2 is the most potent inhibitor of platelet/platelet interactions; that is, platelet aggregation. $PGI_2$ stimulates platelet cAMP at low nanomolar concentrations and inhibits all aspects of platelet function except platelet adhesion to the subendothelium. This platelet adhesion still amounts to 45% at 1 $\mu$M $PGI_2$ (129) and brings platelets in close contact to vascular smooth muscle cells. This will facilitate transcellular metabolism by precursor exchange (see Section III.A.2). The situation may be different in atherosclerotic plaques where $PGI_2$ was found to inhibit platelet deposition (130). In vitro studies suggested that it is the $PGI_2$ production by endothelial cells that accounts for their overall platelet-inhibitory potency (131). Zmuda et al. (6) have originally reported that platelets of cholesterol-fed rabbits are more sensitive to $PGI_2$. Human studies have reported opposite results,

**Table 2** Iloprost-Binding Capacities and Affinity Constants of Platelet Membranes in Simvastatin (SIM)-Treated Hypercholesterolemic (HC) Patients, Untreated HC Patients, and Healthy Controls.

| Group | $B_{max}$ (fmol/mg prot) | $K_d$ (nM) | cAMP (nM) | Collagen-induced platelet secretion (AU) | Collagen-induced thromboxane formation (nM) |
|---|---|---|---|---|---|
| Controls | 121 ± 6 | 38 ± 3 | 136 ± 7 | 100 ± 9 | 76 ± 8 |
| HC | 56 ± 7[a] | 31 ± 2 | 78 ± 6[a] | 150 ± 10[a] | 135 ± 16[a] |
| HC + SIM | 84 ± 3[b] | 24 ± 4 | 131 ± 17[b] | 119 ± 15 | 86 ± 8 |

Platelet ATP secretion and thromboxane formation after stimulation with 0.6 μg/ml collagen, and cAMP levels were measured after stimulation with 30 nM iloprost.
The data are means ± SEM of three to five pooled samples in each group: [a]$P < .05$ (HC vs control); [b]$P < .05$ (HC + SIM vs HC).
*Source:* Modified from ref. 136.

mostly a reduced sensitivity to $PGI_2$ (132,133). This is probably associated with a reduced number of $PGI_2$ receptors and a diminished affinity of the receptor sites. Jaschonek and Muller (134) have shown that incubation of human platelets with cholesterol-hemisuccinate resulted in an apparent loss of $PGI_2$ binding sites. Colli et al. (135) demonstrated that LDL and very low-density lipoprotein (VLDL) in vitro stimulated platelet aggregation without affecting the $PGI_2$-mediated elevation of platelet cAMP and inhibition of platelet function. We have studied the number of platelet $PGI_2$ receptors in relation to platelet function in hypercholesterolemic subjects and found a marked reduction of $PGI_2$ receptors which could be corrected by appropriate treatment of hypercholesterolemia (133,136) (Table 2).

Treatment with aspirin, that is, inhibition of platelet-dependent thromboxane formation, did not retard (137–140) but even tended to aggravate the progression of atherosclerotic lesions (141), whereas removal of platelets by antiplatelet serum had rather a protective effect (125–127). Contradictory findings have been reported in cynomolgus monkeys (142–143). In the human, high-dose aspirin (900 mg/day) was found to reduce the progression of carotid atherosclerosis more significantly than 50 mg aspirin/day (144). Non–thromboxane-related actions of aspirin may explain this interesting observation.

According to current understanding, platelets are not responsible for the initial intimal proliferative response, but they may play a critical role in later stages of neointimal formation, specifically in its migration stage (128,145). Inhibition of platelet-dependent PDGF release has been considered in a number of studies to contribute to or even to explain the antimitogenic actions of PGI$_2$ and its analogues (146–148). In addition, platelet-dependent thrombus formation is the key event in acute thromboembolic complications of the disease; that is, myocardial infarction and stroke. Thus, the antiplatelet effects of prostacyclins may well contribute to the overall antiatherosclerotic actions of the compounds.

### 3.  Coagulation and Fibrinolysis

Part of endothelial dysfunction in atherosclerosis is the conversion of the endothelial lining from an anticoagulant into a procoagulant surface. This is a complex response which involves both downregulation of anticoagulant properties as well as the expression of procoagulant mechanisms; in particular tissue factor. Epidemiological data indicate a close relationship between increased levels of fibrinogen, enhanced blood coagulant activity, and the severity of atherosclerosis. This led to the conclusion that atherosclerosis is a disease of the coagulation and fibrinolysis systems (149).

Tissue factor (thromboplastin) is a cell membrane–associated glycoprotein that initiates the extrinsic coagulation pathway, acting as receptor for the activated serin protease factor VIIa. Tissue factor activity is not present in blood, the vascular intima, or endothelium under physiological conditions but becomes expressed in atherosclerosis and arterial injury in monocytes/macrophages and the vessel wall (150–151). Tissue factor mediates the procoagulant activity of the neointima and endothelial cells. Expression of tissue factor by cells in atherosclerotic lesions may also mediate plaque rupture (152) and acute coronary syndroms (153).

Prostacyclins inhibit monocyte chemotaxis and adherence to endothelial cells (154) and tissue factor expression (155). This includes also inhibition of tissue factor expression in endothelial cells exposed to transforming stimuli such as cytokines or endotoxin. Probably these effects are cAMP mediated, because they are enhanced in the presence of phosphodiesterase inhibitors (156). PGI$_2$ does not directly inhibit tissue factor expression by endothelial cells because of its inability to elevate their cyclic AMP levels (156). As noted above, endogenous PGI$_2$ generation will prevent the cAMP response, most likely by an autocrine downregulation of PGI$_2$ receptors (see Section II.A.3).

### 4.  Cholesterol Metabolism

Cholesterol deposition in the arterial wall, specifically in atherosclerotic vessel lesions, is a long-known stimulus of the progression and severity of the disease (157). Cholesterol is a major constituent of cell membranes and, therefore, essential for tissue proliferation. Vascular cells take up cholesterol mostly as cholesteryl esters via the LDL receptor. Consequently, LDL receptors are upregulated by growth factors (PDGF) and downregulated by free cytoplasmic cholesterol. LDL is contained in coated vesicles that fuse with a lysosome. Within the lysosome, acid cholesterol ester hydrolase (ACEH) frees cholesterol, which enters the cytosolic compartment. This free cholesterol can be reesterified by the cytoplasmic acyl-CoA–acyltransferase (ACAT) and stored in the cell-forming insoluble lipid droplets characteristic of fatty streak lesions. The normal means of escape of cholesterol from these lipid droplets is cleavage of the ester by the cytoplasmic neutral cholesteryl ester hydrolase (NCEH). Free cholesterol leaves the cell by a chemical gradient and becomes bound to the HDL phospholipid surface. The facilitation of cholesterol efflux by HDL is a protective mechanism against excess accumulation of cholesterol and the formation of atherosclerotic foam cells. The plasma enzyme LCAT splits fatty acids from the phosphatidylcholine of the HDL phospholipid envelope. The extracellular cholesteryl esters, because of their hydrophobic nature, then become internalized into the core of the particle. As a consequence, there are new binding sites for cholesterol at the surface of the lipoprotein, a process catalyzed by ApoA-1, the major apoprotein of HDL (10,14) (Fig. 3).

Endogenous $PGI_2$ and $PGE_2$ maintain the cellular cholesterol content at a

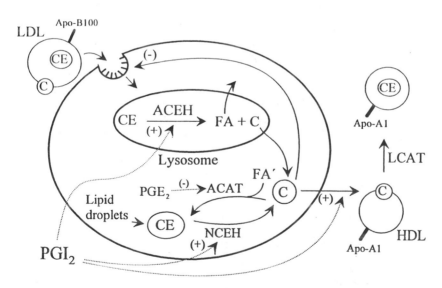

**Figure 3** Cholesterol metabolism in vascular cells. C, cholesterol; CE, cholesteryl ester; FA, fatty acid; ACAT, acyl-CoA-cholesteryl-acyltransferase; ACEH, acidic cholesteryl ester hydrolase; NCEH, neutral cholesteryl ester hydrolase; LCAT, lecithin cholesteryl-acyltransferase; (+), stimulation by $PGI_2$. (See text for further explanations.)

low level. $PGI_2$ and in some studies $PGE_1$ increase the activity of both acid and neutral cholesteryl ester hydrolases (158–161). This results in increased cytosolic cholesterol which inhibits the generation of LDL receptors and facilitates the escape of free cholesterol from the cell. Experiments in cocultured bovine vascular smooth muscle and endothelial cells have shown that endothelial cell–derived $PGI_2$, but not $PGE_2$ or $PGE_1$, stimulates lysosomal ACEH and acts synergistically in this respect with PDGF. The action of $PGI_2$ was prevented by aspirin treatment, whereas that of PDGF was not, suggesting that endothelial cell–derived $PGI_2$ controls cholesterol metabolism of smooth muscle cells (162). These actions of $PGI_2$ are cAMP mediated and result in a net loss of free cholesterol from vascular cells (163) as long as the acceptor capacity of HDL for cholesterol binding is sufficient (10). $PGE_2$ inhibits the enhanced ACAT activity (117), which is typical for animal models of atherosclerosis as well as the human disease. This causes reduced cholesteryl ester synthesis and accumulation, enhanced cholesteryl ester degradation, and reduced LDL cholesterol uptake (164–165). HDL also stimulates endothelial cell $PGI_2$ synthesis (24). There is a potentiation of the hydrolytic activity of $PGI_2$ in the presence of HDL or ApoA-I respectively (166). Thus, any reduced local $PGI_2$ generation in atherosclerotic lesions of the vessel wall (see Section III.A) facilitates an increase in vascular cholesteryl ester content and promotes the progression of the disease (53). It is, however, also possible that downregulation of $PGI_2$ receptors occurs because of increased $PGI_2$ levels at sites of transcellular metabolism (60). Both events will produce the same result; namely, a reduced $PGI_2$-mediated signaling.

Chemically stable prostacyclins did not modify the cholesteryl ester content or DNA synthesis of normal human arterial smooth muscle cells but reduced both parameters in fatty streak and plaque tissue (163,167). The opposite effect was seen with thromboxane mimetics (168). The actions of prostacyclins appeared to be cAMP-mediated (167,169). Interestingly, there was a marked (by 50%) suppression of DNA synthesis by synthetic prostacyclins (carbacyclin) at unchanged (low) cholesteryl ester content of intimal smooth muscle cells of human aorta (Table 3). Taken together, these findings demonstrate multiple cholesterol-lowering actions of $PGI_2$ and other vasodilating eicosanoids in vascular tissue that may be an integral part of the overall antiatherosclerotic action of the compounds.

## 5. Growth Promotion and Control

The formation of a neointima, that is, intimal thickening subsequent to migration and proliferation of vascular smooth muscle cells, is part of the healing process after endothelial injury. Similar alterations occur in atherosclerotic lesion formation (11). However, the phenotypic state of vascular

**Table 3** [$^3$H]Thymidine Uptake and Cholesteryl Ester Content of Cultured Intimal Smooth Muscle Cells of Human Aorta Under Effect of Carbacyclin

| Treatment/injury | [$^3$H]Thymidine uptake (cpm/10$^5$ cells in 24 hr) | | | Cholesteryl ester content ($\mu$g/10$^5$ cells) | | |
|---|---|---|---|---|---|---|
| | none | fatty streak | plaque | none | fatty streak | plaque |
| Control | 3.4 ± 0.2 | 7.2 ± 0.4 | 4.1 ± 0.4 | 6.8 ± 0.9 | 29.3 ± 3.1 | 42.4 ± 2.7 |
| Carbacyclin (100 ng/ml) | 1.7 ± 0.1[a] | 2.7 ± 0.4[a] | 2.1 ± 0.3[a] | 6.8 ± 0.6 | 16.4 ± 1.9[a] | 24.8 ± 1.9[a] |
| % change (none = 100) | −50 | −62 | −49 | 0 | −44 | −42 |

Data are × ± SEM of n = three independent experiments: [a]$P < .05$ (injury vs no injury = none).
*Source:* Modified from ref. 163.

smooth muscle cells within atherosclerotic lesions changes. There is transformation from a differentiated "contractile" cell type into a less differentiated "synthetic" type which looses contractile filaments, produces extracellular matrix, and reacts to mitogens with cell division. Since growth-promoting factors in many cases are vasoconstrictors, the mechanisms of signal transduction may be similar. For example, peptidergic growth factors activate PLC and generate $IP_3$ and DAG with a subsequent elevation of cytosolic $Ca^{2+}$ (170). There might also be changes in the involved second-messenger systems after stimulation of receptor tyrosin kinases (R-TK) by growth factors (171–173) (see Fig. 2). Endothelial cells secrete positive and negative differentiation signals. However, little is known regarding the regulation of the balance between these two opposing activities (17).

*Endogenous Prostaglandins.* There are several additional sources of vascular $PGI_2$ generation in atherosclerosis, specifically an upregulated COX-2 (see Section III.A.2). Thus, proliferating vascular cells in the presence of platelets synthesize more $PGI_2$ than quiescent cells (174). Additionally, upregulation of vascular LDL receptors after stimulation with PDGF may provide free arachidonic acid for $PGI_2$ synthesis (175). Cytokines, such as interleukin 1 (176), and growth factors (177) not only induce proliferation of vascular smooth muscle cells but also require endogenous prostaglandin for this effect. Their mitogenic actions are largely inhibited after blockade of endogenous prostaglandin formation. This suggests a growth-modulating function of endogenous prostaglandins and leads to the question of why in most studies endogenous prostaglandins do not block pathological smooth muscle cell proliferation; for example, subsequent to angioplasty.

One explanation is that the amount of endogenous $PGI_2$ is insufficient. This would explain the antiproliferative actions of exogenous $PGI_2$- and $PGI_2$-mimetics discussed below (see Section IV.A) in terms of a supplementation therapy. Another could be that generation and action of endogenous $PGI_2$ are dependent on the cell cycle. Mitogenic agonists, such as arginine vasopressin, have been shown to inhibit DNA synthesis in vascular smooth muscle by inhibiting progression of the $G_1$ to S phase but not at later time points of the cycle. This inhibitory action was mediated by prostaglandin synthesis (178). Finally, $PGI_2$ receptors at the cell membrane may be downregulated. This has been originally shown for thromboxane receptors in PDGF-stimulated vascular smooth muscle cells (179) but has not been studied so far for endogenous $PGI_2$. In this respect, it is an interesting question of whether or not antimitogenic actions of iloprost and other $PGI_2$-mimetics are mediated by receptors at the cell membrane or by direct growth-modulating effects on the cell nucleus (14). A cDNA encoding for an endogenous prostaglandin transporter was recently cloned and sequenced and showed extremely low, if any, binding affinity to iloprost, whereas the binding activity for $PGE_1$ was high (in the nanomolar range) (180). This suggests that the sites of action of PGE-type compounds and of prostacyclins might be different.

Endogenous vessel–derived $PGI_2$ may exert a bimodal function in the control of mitogenesis and the differentiation state of vascular smooth muscle cells. One is to facilitate tissue repair by stimulating more vascular cells to enter the cell cycle and to proliferate. The other is to keep the cell in the differentiated state. Thus, vessel wall–derived eicosanoids serve to maintain the cell in the contractile, quiescent phenotype, which is responsive to vasoactive stimuli and not responsive to mitogens (14).

*Exogenous $PGI_2$ and $PGI_2$-Mimetics.* The first direct evidence for a growth-inhibitory action of prostaglandins in vascular smooth muscle cells of the guinea pig aorta was published in 1977 (181). This antiproliferative effect of vasodilator prostaglandins, mainly $PGE_1$ and $PGI_2$, was confirmed in numerous later trials, mainly tissue culture studies of vascular smooth muscle cells of human and animal origin (146,161,182–186). Synthetic, chemically more stable $PGI_2$-mimetics (carbacylin, iloprost, ciprostene, beraprost) also inhibit the proliferation of vascular smooth muscle cells (121,178,187).

*Role of cAMP in growth control by $PGI_2$.* Since many of the receptor-mediated actions of $PGI_2$ are due to $G_s$-coupled adenylate cyclase stimulation, cAMP was thought in some (187–189), but not all (190) studies to be also a messenger of its growth-modulating effects. In addition, $PGI_2$ and NO may act in concert to suppress continuously smooth muscle cell proliferation in arteries in vivo via cAMP and cGMP, respectively (188). The antimitogenic effect of cAMP or cAMP analogues was considered to be stronger than that of cGMP-elevating agents or analogues such as 8-Br-cGMP (187). The inhibition of DNA synthesis by cAMP elevation (189) may result from phosphorylation of raf-1 by protein kinase A and subsequent interruption of the MAP-kinase pathway (191–193) (see Fig. 2). Preliminary data suggest that the $PGI_2$-mimetic iloprost also inhibits PDGF-induced MAP-kinase activation at concentrations that block DNA synthesis (194).

Intracellular cAMP is regulated by adenylate cyclase activity and serves different functions during the cell cycle (195). Franks and colleagues (196) have shown that adenylate cyclase activity and DNA synthesis are stimulated in parallel by growth factors in vascular smooth muscle cells. Cycloheximide blocked DNA synthesis but not the increase in adenylate cyclase activity, suggesting that DNA replication required de novo protein synthesis. In other studies, $PGE_1$ inhibited PDGF-induced DNA synthesis when added during $G_1$ or at the beginning of S phase but not when added at later time points (197). Similar results were obtained by Owen (184). She showed that a (transient) increase in cAMP formation was necessary to start the cell cycle, whereas increased cAMP during the S phase had the opposite effect and inhibited DNA synthesis.

These data allow the conclusion that a rise in intracellular cAMP during $G_0$ or $G_1$ is necessary for entering and progression of the cell cycle, respectively, whereas elevations of cAMP in late $G_1$ or early S phase will inhibit proliferation. The first event may be important for wound healing, including stimulation of cell division, and the second event for the role of prostacyclins as antiproliferative agents in atherosclerotic plaque formation (184,196).

*Regulation of PGI$_2$ receptors.* The extent and duration of a receptor-mediated event is critically dependent on the number of accessible binding sites that are coupled to cellular signal transduction pathways. We have previously shown that the PGI$_2$ receptor on endothelial cells undergoes an agonist-induced downregulation after prolonged exposure to PGI$_2$ (57). We have, therefore, studied the possibility that PGI$_2$ receptors on vascular smooth muscle cells may behave similarly. Studies were carried out in bovine coronary artery smooth muscle cells (60,194). Endogenous PGI$_2$ production of these cells was abolished by indomethacin treatment. There was a marked suppression of PDGF-induced mitogenesis by both iloprost and cicaprost if the compound was added during the S phase of the cell cycle. However, the antiproliferative effects of the PGI$_2$-mimetics disappeared if the substances were added to quiescent cells, that is, at the same time as the mitogens, indicating that the cells became tolerant to PGI$_2$. In contrast, PGE$_1$ at an equieffective antimitogenic concentration did not show any tolerance development and there was also no cross desensitization as seen from an unchanged antimitogenic effect of PGE$_1$ in PGI$_2$-tolerant smooth muscle cells (60). This is different from the situation in nonvascular cells (NG108-15) where PGE$_1$ pretreatment produced a 75–80% decrease in IP receptor number (198). Furthermore, forskolin suppressed DNA synthesis in both tolerant and nontolerant tissue for the same extent (Fig. 4), suggesting that elevation of cAMP was involved in these antiproliferative actions of prostacyclins and that tolerance development occured at the receptor-coupling or receptor-G protein–coupling level, respectively.

These data provide a possible explanation of the failure of other investigators to detect inhibition of growth responses in several types of vascular smooth muscle cells which were treated with PGI$_2$ for 1–4 days (10). In one study with exogenous PGI$_2$, it was found that only the addition of the compound at 10–16 hr after growth stimulation of quiescent cells inhibited

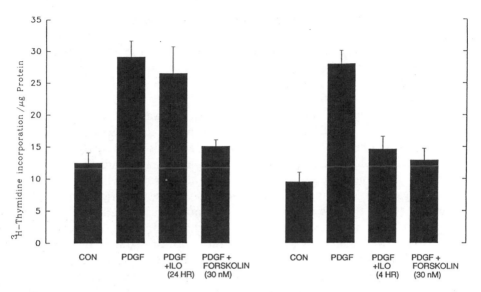

**Figure 4** Desensitization of iloprost-induced inhibition of PDGF-stimulated DNA synthesis. Bovine coronary artery smooth muscle cells were cultured and passaged. Cells of passage 5 were stimulated for 24 hr with PDGF (20 ng/ml) and showed a significant increase in DNA synthesis as assessed from the incorporation rate of [$^3$H]thymidine. This stimulation of DNA synthesis by PDGF was prevented after addition of iloprost (100 nM) during the synthesis phase of the cell cycle; that is, the last 4 hr of incubation. The inhibition disappeared if iloprost was present in the medium for the total time of PDGF stimulation; that is, for 24 hr. Direct stimulation of cAMP formation by forskolin caused also a complete inhibition of DNA synthesis which was cell cycle independent. The data suggest downregulation of IP receptors in these smooth muscle cells as a possible explanation of this loss of antimitogenic action of iloprost. (From Großer et al., unpublished data.)

DNA synthesis (177). This could have been due to the instability of the compound, because a stable $PGI_2$ analogue was more effective. Another study demonstrated an inhibition of growth factor–stimulated DNA synthesis in bovine aorta smooth muscle cells by ciprostene. There was a maximum inhibition of DNA synthesis (by 50%) and increase in cAMP when the compound was added during the first 3 hr of growth factor stimulation of previously quiescent cells (121).

Species variations, different experimental protocols, specifically the presence or absence of (defined) growth factors to stimulate DNA synthesis (172), the use of fresh or cultured cells with changes in activities of important enzymes (199), as well as unknown modulatory effects by endogenous eicosanoids, in particular $PGI_2$, may explain these controversial findings.

Specifically, the function of the second-messenger cAMP depends on the amount and activity of cyclic nucleotide–degrading phosphodiesterases. In some studies, phosphodiesterase inhibitors did not cause cAMP accumulation or inhibition of DNA synthesis (177), whereas in others they did (146). In any case, more information is necessary about $PGI_2$ receptors, their structural organization, and regulation.

*Other messengers and mediators.* The pathways of cellular signal transduction of growth responses are only partly understood, and a detailed discussion of them is beyond the scope of this chapter. By comparison with the physiological actions of $PGI_2$, one may argue that in addition to cAMP-mediated responses, there is also a role for PLC-associated pathways; that is, changes in free cytosolic $Ca^{2+}$ concentration and PKC activity (200). Studies in rabbit aortic smooth muscle cells have shown that PDGF at a mitogenic concentration did not elevate cytosolic $Ca^{2+}$ nor did cAMP analogues inhibit $Ca^{2+}$ mobilization induced by serum at concentrations which inhibited DNA synthesis (188). From these data, it was concluded that cyclic nucleotides exert their antiproliferative actions via mechanisms other than inhibition of $Ca^{2+}$ exchange. This might be related to the loss of receptor-mediated $Ca^{2+}$ mobilization after transformation of the cells from the quiescent to the proliferative phenotype (188) which is associated with a loss of contractility (171). As noted above, exposure of vascular smooth muscle cells to growth-promoting factors resulted in an uncoupling of the thrombin receptor to some intracellular signal transduction pathways under conditions when serum-stimulated responses were maintained (108). The mitogenic actions of thrombin involve PDGF release from vascular endothelial and smooth muscle cells (201–203). Thus, inhibition of PGDF release by $PGI_2$ and stable $PGI_2$-mimetics is another explanation for the antimitogenic actions of these compounds (10,146,148). In that case, the antiproliferative effects of $PGI_2$ are indirect in nature and a consequence of suppression of mitogen release from vascular and nonvascular sources (203), including secretory vascular smooth muscle cells (204).

PKC(s) have been shown to exert both proliferative and antiproliferative effects on cultured vascular smooth muscle cells (200). In addition, the involvement of $Ca^{2+}$-activated PKC(s) in proliferation depends on the type of mitogen. Therefore, no conclusion with respect to possible mediation of antiproliferative actions of $PGI_2$ by PKC can be drawn.

*Matrix production.* One important property that distinguishes contractile from secretory vascular smooth muscle cells is the generation of an extracellular matrix. Similar to cell migration and proliferation, the synthesis of extracellular matrix is equally important for wound healing and tissue repair as well as for the initiation and progression of acquired diseases, including atherosclerosis (205). The increased thrombogenicity of atherosclerotic lesions was documented by increased platelet deposition and attributed to changes in quantity and nature of matrix proteins above all collagens (206).

Kato and colleagues (207) have shown that $PGE_2$ and iloprost inhibit PDGF-induced DNA synthesis and the production of a precursor of matrix metalloproteinase 1 in cultured human aortic smooth muscle cells, suggesting that these compounds are negative regulators of PDGF-induced matrix production. Similar results were obtained with the synthetic $PGI_2$-mimetic, beraprost, which was found to inhibit glycosaminoglycan synthesis but not protein synthesis, that is, cell hypertrophy, at concentrations which inhibited DNA synthesis (208). Thus, prostacyclins may inhibit matrix generation eventually in relation to their modulating effect on the phenotype expression of vascular smooth muscle cells. The interesting observation that $PGE_1$ has a dual effect on the transition of vascular smooth muscle cells from the contractile to the secretory state (209) requires further studies.

## IV. PHARMACOLOGICAL MANIPULATION OF ATHEROSCLEROSIS VIA $PGI_2$-RELATED MECHANISMS

As discussed above, endothelium-derived $PGI_2$ will inhibit proliferation of vascular smooth muscle cells, will help to maintain anticoagulant properties of the endothelium, and will also prevent excessive cholesterol accumulation within the vessel wall. Since disturbed generation and action of $PGI_2$ is a generalized feature of endothelial dysfunction, a restoration of this physiological control by administration of $PGI_2$ appears to be a most useful means to retard the progression of atherosclerosis and to prevent its acute thromboembolic complications. In fact, numerous experimental studies confirm the concept of a reduced progression of atherosclerosis by $PGI_2$, $PGE_1$, and other $PGI_2$-mimetics. However, clinical experience is mainly focused on already existent, mostly advanced stages of atherosclerosis, specifically peripheral arterial occlusive disease. Thus, animal data and clinical findings may not be directly comparable. Moreover, atherosclerosis is typically accompanied by enhanced circulating $PGI_2$ levels (92,93). Thus, the question arises whether the $PGI_2$-related disturbance of vascular hemostasis is really due to insufficient $PGI_2$ formation or an insufficient $PGI_2$ action; for example, after downregulation of $PGI_2$ receptor–dependent signaling. However, the kind and regulation of $PGI_2$ receptors is still a largely unsolved issue (see Section III.B.V). Clearly, high circulating levels of any active $PGI_2$ and/or analogue will tend to further downregulate $PGI_2$ receptors.

## A.  PGI$_2$-Mimetics as Antiatherosclerotic Agents in Vivo

### 1.  Animal Studies

The oral treatment of cholesterol-fed rabbits with cicaprost at a nonhypotensive dose was found to reduce aortic plaque formation and to improve endothelium-dependent vasodilation in both aortic tissue and coronary arteries (122). These beneficial effects, therefore, also included some improvement of endothelial dysfunction. TFC-132, a synthetic PGI$_2$ analogue, not only inhibited DNA synthesis of human aortic cultured SMC but also inhibited neointimal thickening after oral administration to rabbits (147). Beraprost given subcutaneously to cholesterol-fed rabbits inhibited restenosis after balloon injury of the femoral artery (210). It is interesting to note that these beneficial effects in cholesterol-fed animals occurred in the absence of any reduction of the markedly (about 10- to 20-fold) elevated plasma cholesterol levels.

In contrast, the administration of the PGI$_2$ agonists octimibate and BMY 42393 to cholesterol-fed hamsters reduced foam cell formation and fatty streaks in vivo which was related to suppressed monocyte/macrophage atherogenic activity and cytokine production as well as reduced plasma total cholesterol and triglyceride levels (165). Levitt et al. (211) showed that a 2-week infusion of iloprost did not prevent experimental intimal hyperplasia in the rat after endothelial injury. Recently, gene transfer of the COX-1 gene was found to prevent arterial thrombosis after carotid angioplasty in pigs and to enhance PGI$_2$ synthesis fourfold (212). Whether this approach results in prevention of restenosis and will be applicable and effective in man remains to be shown.

Taken together, the majority of available findings in animal studies confirm the cell culture and in vitro data; namely, a functional PGI$_2$ deficiency. If this is overcome by exogenous administration, then prostacyclins exert antiatherosclerotic effects, specifically an inhibition of smooth muscle cell growth and preservation of endothelial function. Interestingly, these actions can be demonstrated in the absence of any significant fall in blood pressure (122).

### 2.  Clinical Trials

Because of the potent antiplatelet, antineutrophil, cholesterol-lowering, and vasodilatory actions of PGI$_2$, there was much enthusiasm to use this compound for the treatment of the advanced stages of atherosclerosis; that is, stroke, myocardial infarction, and peripheral arterial occlusive diseases. Initially, preliminary results from uncontrolled trials in small numbers of patients were rather enthusiastic (213). However, later double-blind trials under more carefully controlled conditions could not always confirm beneficial results of $PGI_2$, $PGI_2$-mimetics, and $PGE_1$ (214), leading to the conclusion in the European Consensus Document on Critical Limb Ischemia that treatment with these compounds should be considered in patients unsuitable for reconstructive surgery or PTA (percutaneous transluminal angioplasty) except those who require immediate amputation (215). In contrast to peripheral arterial disease, exogenous $PGI_2$-mimetics appear not to be useful in the prevention or treatment of acute myocardial ischemia but might even introduce or aggravate ischemia owing to their vasodilatory action (216–217). The new $PGI_2$ analogue, beraprost also reduced exercise tolerance in patients with stable angina pectoris despite significant improvements of several laboratory parameters of hemostasis (218). There are several possible explanations for these unsatisfactory results: the short duration of action of the natural agonist and the blood pressure–lowering activity of all natural and synthetic prostacyclins which limits their dosage in humans in vivo. For example, on a weight basis, anti-ischemic doses of $PGI_2$ and iloprost, which can be administered to laboratory animals without significant change in blood pressure, are 50- to 100-fold higher than those which can be given safely to the human. This is of particular relevance at advanced stages of atherosclerosis, where the perfusion pressure becomes a critical determinant for regional perfusion of important organs, such as heart and brain. In addition, there may be downregulation of $PGI_2$ receptors in some tissues, for example, platelets (134), which limits the anti-ischemic efficacy of the compounds. Thus, the generation of a circulating level of active $PGI_2$ by exogenous administration appears to be the general denominator of these complications.

There is only very limited information on the action of $PGI_2$ on smooth muscle cell proliferation. Sinzinger and colleagues (148) measured the number of activated smooth muscle cells in the plaque and media of femoral and popliteal arteries of patients prior to surgery (amputation) because of end-stage peripheral arterial occlusive disease. The percentage of "activated" smooth muscle cells, as determined from the microscopic appearance, tended to be reduced in patients who were treated with $PGI_2$ infusions for 6 hr during 5 days prior to amputation. In patients with carotid atheromatous lesions, short-term administration of the orally active $PGI_2$-mimetic TRK-100 for 4 weeks resulted in a significant reduction of ADP-induced platelet aggregation and platelet accumulation in carotid atheromas but no significant change in plaque size (219).

## B. Agents that Modulate Endogenous $PGI_2$ Formation

An alternative approach to benefit from the antiatherosclerotic actions of $PGI_2$ is to enhance its effectivity by stimulating endogenous biosynthesis or by improving its action. Stimulation of endogenous $PGI_2$ occurs in atherosclerotic patients subsequent to treatment with ACE inhibitors and is possibly caused by accumulation of endogenous bradykinin (220). Restored $PGI_2$ generation may also be involved in the antiatherosclerotic effects of calcium antagonists (221) and the antiatherosclerotic actions of lipid-lowering drugs, such as simvastatin and cholestyramine (133,136). Similar results, that is, a significant increase in endothelial $PGI_2$ formation in the presence of activated platelets and an antiatherosclerotic action in vivo, was found with defibrotide, a single-stranded DNA preparation (222–223). More information is necessary to establish the role of $PGI_2$ of these multiple-site active compounds in the clinical outcome.

## V.  SUMMARY AND CONCLUSIONS

$PGI_2$ is the major eicosanoid synthesized via the COX pathway in vascular endothelial and smooth muscle cells. Biosynthesis under physiological conditions is initiated via activation of $Ca^{2+}$-dependent phospholipases C and $A_2$, whereas the extent of product formation is determined by the activity of cyclooxygenases, mainly the constitutive isoform COX-1.

$PGI_2$ biosynthesis in atherosclerosis is changed. There is expression of the inducible isoform COX-2 by cytokines and growth factors, possibly also stimulated by lysophospholipids which results in enhanced vascular generation of PG endoperoxides. The local levels of $PGI_2$ in atherosclerotic plaques are reduced. This may be due to selective inhibition of $PGI_2$ synthase by lipid peroxides and/or enhanced degradation of $PGI_2$ by oxygen-centered free radicals. In addition, adherent platelets and macrophages may provide additional $PGI_2$ precursors by transcellular metabolism. The total cardiovascular $PGI_2$ formation, as assessed from the measurement of urinary excretion of index metabolites, is enhanced, possibly reflecting the degree of platelet activation.

$PGI_2$ exerts numerous effects on vascular and nonvascular cells which are generally antiatherosclerotic in nature. This involves vasodilatory, anticoagulant, profibrinolytic, and platelet- and leukocyte-repellent actions. In addition, $PGI_2$ in concert with $PGE_2$ tends to lower vascular cholesteryl-ester accumulation by modification of several enzymes in cholesterol metabolism. Most, if not all, of these activities are mediated via specific $PGI_2$-(IP) receptors at the cell membrane and involve stimulation of cellular cAMP as a second messenger.

$PGI_2$, $PGE_1$, and several synthetic analogues were found to prevent the progression of atherosclerotic vessel diseases in most, but not all, animal experiments. Regarding the profile of pharmacological activities, it was probably the modulation of growth responses in relation to neointima formation combined with platelet- and leukocyte-inhibitory actions which explained these results. In men, $PGI_2$ mimetics and $PGE_1$ have been extensively studied in the advanced stages of peripheral arterial occlusive diseases and have now become established drugs in these diseases. There is no benefit with prostacyclins in the prevention or treatment of stroke or myocardial infarction but rather an aggravation or even induction of the disease. Very little is known about possible beneficial effects of these compounds in early atherosclerosis and restenosis prevention.

Several aspects of mutual clinical importance appear to be insufficiently studied in the past and require further consideration. This includes studies on the type(s) and regulation of IP-receptors in different tissues; the signal transduction pathways via IP-receptors; specifically, the modulation of pathological (restenosis) versus physiological (wound healing and scar formation) cell proliferation and the design and development of new $PGI_2$-related compounds. There is a definite need for high-affinity IP-receptor antagonists which, as seen with many other hormones and autacoids, are still the most reliable way to detect receptor subtypes and, possibly, to design more potent and more specific antiatherosclerotic compounds on $PGI_2$ basis than known so far.

## ACKNOWLEDGMENTS

The work was supported by the Deutsche Forschungsgemeinschaft, SFB 351 Hormonresistenz - Biochemie und Klinik Teilprojekt D7 (Düsseldorf) and the Forschungsgruppe Herz-Kreislauf (Düsseldorf). The author is most grateful to Erika Lohmann for excellent secretarial assistance.

## REFERENCES

1. Moncada S. Gryglewski R, Bunting S, Vane JR. An enzyme isolated from arteries transforms prostaglandin endoperoxides to an unstable substance that inhibits platelet aggregation. Nature 1976; 263:663–665.
2. Moncada S, Palmer RMJ, Higgs EA. Prostacyclin and endothelium-derived relaxing factor: biological interactions and significance In: Verstraete M, Vermylen J, Lijnen HR, Arnout J, eds. Thrombosis and Hemostasis, Leuven: University Press, 1987:597–618.
3. Weksler BB, Marcus AJ, Jaffe EA. Synthesis of prostaglandin $I_2$ (prostacyclin) by cultured human and bovine endothelial cells. Proc Natl Acad Sci USA 1977; 74:3922–3928.
4. Klockenbusch W, Braun M, Schröder H, Heckenberger RE, Strobach H, Schrör K. Prostacyclin rather than nitric oxide lowers umbilical artery tone in vitro. Eur J Obstet Gynecol Reprod Biol 1992; 47:109–115.
5. Dembinska-Kiec A, Gryglewska T, Zmuda A, Gryglewski RJ. The generation

of prostacyclin by arteries and by the coronary vascular bed is reduced in experimental atherosclerosis in rabbits. Prostaglandins 1977; 14:1025–1034.

6. Zmuda A, Dembinska-Kiec A, Chytkowski A, Gryglewski RJ. Experimental atherosclerosis in rabbits: platelet aggregation, thromboxane $A_2$ generation and antiaggregatory potency of prostacyclin. Prostaglandins 1977; 14:1035–1042.

7. Sinzinger H, Silberbauer K, Winter M. Effects of experimental atherosclerosis on prostacyclin ($PGI_2$) generation in arteries of miniature swine. Artery 1979; 5:448–462.

8. Silberbauer K, Sinzinger H, Winter M. Prostacyclin production by vascular smooth muscle cells. Lancet 1978; 1:1356–1357.

9. Rolland PH, Jouve R, Pellegrin E, Mercier C, Serradimigni A. Alteration in prostacyclin and prostaglandin $E_2$ production. Correlation with changes in human aortic atherosclerotic disease. Arteriosclerosis 1984; 4:70–78.

10. Willis AL, Smith DL, Vigo C. Suppression of principal atherosclerotic mechanisms by prostacyclins and other eicosanoids. Prog Lipid Res 1986; 25:645–666.

11. Ross R. The pathogenesis of atherosclerosis— an update. New Engl J Med 1986; 314:488–500.

12. Ross R, Fuster V. The pathogenesis of atherosclerosis. In: Fuster V, Ross R, Topol EJ, eds. Atherosclerosis and Coronary Artery Disease. Philadelphia: Lippincott-Raven 1996:411–460.

13. D'Angelo Y, Villa S, Mysliewic M, Donati MB, de Gaetano G. Defective fibrinolytic and prostacyclin-like activity in human atheromatous plaques. Thromb Haemost 1978; 39:535–536.

14. Pomerantz KB, Hajjar DP. Eicosanoids in regulation of arterial smooth muscle cell phenotype, proliferative capacity, and cholesterol metabolism. Arteriosclerosis 1989; 9:413–429.

15. Vane JR, Änggard EE, Botting RM. Regulatory functions of the vascular endothelium. New Engl J Med 1990; 323:27–36.

16. DiCorleto PE, Gimbrone MA Jr. Vascular endothelium. In: Fuster V, Ross R, Topol EJ, eds. Atherosclerosis and Coronary Artery Disease. Philadelphia: Lippincott-Raven, 1996:387–399.

17. Owens GK. Role of alterations in the differentiated state of vascular smooth muscle cells in atherogenesis. In: Fuster V, Ross R, Topol EJ, eds. Atherosclerosis and Coronary Artery Disease. Philadelphia: Lippincott-Raven, 1996:401–420.

18. Smith WL. Prostaglandin biosynthesis and its compartimentation in vascular smooth muscle and endothelial cells. Ann Rev Physiol 1986; 48:251–262.

19. Simionescu N, Simionescu M. Endothelial Cell Dysfunction. New York: Plenum Press, 1992.

20. DeWitt DL, Day JS, Sonnenburg WK, Smith WL. Concentrations of prostaglandin endoperoxide synthase and prostaglandin $I_2$ synthase in the endothelium and smooth muscle of bovine aorta. J Clin Invest 1983; 72:1882–1888.

21. Nüsing RM, Klein T, Siegle I, Brugger R, Ullrich V. Regulation of prostanoid synthesis in the cardiovascular system. In: Schrör K, Pace-Asciak CR, eds. Mediators in the Cardiovascular System: Regional Ischemia, Agents Actions Suppl 45. Basel: Birkhäuser 1995:1–10.

22. Smith WL, Lands WEM. Oxygenation of polyunsaturated fatty acids during prostaglandin biosynthesis by sheep vesicle gland. Biochemistry 1972; 11: 3276–3285.

23. Vollet X, Perret B, Chollet F, Hullin F, Chap H, Douste-Blazy L. Uptake of HDL unesterified and esterified cholesterol by human endothelial cells. Modulation by HDL phospholipolysis and cell cholesterol content. Biochim Biophys Acta 1988; 958:81–92.

24. Fleisher LN, Tall AR, Witte LD, Miller RW, Cannon PJ. Stimulation of arterial endothelial cell prostacyclin synthesis by high density lipoproteins. J Biol Chem 1982; 257:6653–6655.

25. Gryglewski RJ, Moncada S, Palmer RMJ. Bioassay of prostacyclin and endothelium-derived relaxing factor (EDRF) from porcine aortic endothelial cells. Br J Pharmacol 1986; 87:685–694.

26. Pirotton S, Raspe E, Demolle D, Erneux C, Boeynaems JM. Involvement of inositol 1,4,5-trisphosphate and calcium in the action of adenosine nucleotides on aortic endothelial cells. J Biol Chem 1987; 262:17461–17466.

27. Weksler BB, Ley CW, Jaffe EA. Stimulation of endothelial cell prostacyclin production by thrombin, trypsin and the ionophore A23187. J Clin Invest 1978; 68:923–930.

28. Jaffe EA, Grulich J, Weksler BB, Hampel G, Watanabe K. Correlation between thrombin-induced prostayclin production and inositol triphosphate and cytosolic free calcium levels in cultured human endothelial cells. J Biol Chem 1987; 262:8557–8565.

29. Lückhoff A. Release of prostacyclin and EDRF from endothelial cells is differentially controlled by extra- and intracellular calcium (review). Eicosanoids 1988; 1:5–11.

30. Carter TD, Pearson JD. Regulation of prostacyclin synthesis in endothelial cells. NIPS 1992; 7:64–69.

31. Bosch van den H. Intracellular phospholipase A. Biochim Biophys Acta 1980; 504:191–196.

32. Demolle D, Boeynaems JM. Role of protein kinase C in the control of vascular prostacyclin: study of phorbol esters effect in bovine aortic endothelium and smooth muscle. Prostaglandins 1988; 35:243–257.

33. Carter TD, Hallam TJ, Pearson JD. Protein kinase C activation alters the sensitivity of agonist-stimulated endothelial cell prostacyclin production to intracellular ionised calcium. Biochem J 1989; 262:431–437.

34. Wu KK, Hatzakis H, Lo SS, Seong DC, Sanduja SK, Tai HH. Stimulation of de novo synthesis of prostaglandin G/H synthase in human endothelial cells by phorbol esters. J Biol Chem 1988; 263:19043–19047.

35. Demolle D, Boeynaems JM. Cholera and pertussis toxins amplify prostacyclin synthesis in aortic smooth muscle cells. Br J Pharmacol 1989; 98:717–720.

36. deNucci G, Gryglewski RJ, Warner TD, Vane JR. Receptor-mediated release of endothelium-derived relaxing factor and prostacyclin from bovine aortic endothelial cells is coupled. Proc Natl Acad Sci USA 1988; 85:2334–2338.

37. Warso MA, Lands WEM. Lipid peroxidation in relation to prostacyclin and thromboxane physiology and pharmacology. Br Med Bull 1983; 39:277–280.
38. Brannon TS, North AJ, Wells LB, Shaul PW. Prostacyclin synthesis in bovine pulmonary artery is developmentally regulated by changes in cyclooxygenase-1 gene expression. J Clin Invest 1994; 93:2230–2235.
39. North AJ, Brannon TS, Wells LB, Campbell WB, Shaul PW. Hypoxia stimulates prostacyclin synthesis in newborn pulmonary artery endothelium by increasing cyclooxygenase-1 protein. Circ Res 1994; 75:33–40.
40. Rimarachin JA, Jacobson JA, Szabo P, Maclouf J, Creminon C, Weksler BB. Regulation of cyclooxygenase-2-expression in aortic smooth muscle cells. Arterioscler Thromb 1994; 14:1021–1031.
41. Xu X-M, Ohashi K, Sanduja SK, Ruan K-H, Wang L-H, Wu KK. Enhanced prostacyclin synthesis in endothelial cells by retrovirus-mediated transfer of prostaglandin H synthase cDNA. J Clin Invest 1993; 91:1843–1849.
42. Smith W, DeWitt D, Allen M. Bimodal distribution of the prostaglandin $I_2$ synthase antigen in smooth muscle cells. J Biol Chem 1983; 258:5922–5926.
43. Regier MK, DeWitt DL, Schindler MS, Smith WL. Subcellular localization of prostaglandin endoperodixe synthase-2 in murine 3T3 cells. Arch Biochem Biophys 1993; 301:439–444.
44. Pereira B, Wu KK, Wang L-H. Molecular cloning and characterization of bovine prostacyclin synthase. Biochem Biophys Res Commun 1994; 203:59–66.
45. Spisni E, Bartolini G, Orlandi M, Belletti B, Santi S, Tomasi V. Prostacyclin ($PGI_2$) synthase is a constitutively expressed enzyme in human endothelial cells. Exp Cell Res 1995; 219:507–513.
46. Orchard MA, Robinson C. Stability of prostacyclin in human plasma and whole blood: studies on the protective effect of albumin. Thromb Haemost 1981; 46:645–647.
47. Yui Y, Aoyama T, Morishita H, Takahashi M, Takatsu Y, Kawai C. Serum prostacyclin stabilizing factor is identical to apoprotein A-I (Apo A-I). A novel function of Apo A-1. J Clin Invest 1988; 82:803–807.
48. Ono Y, Hashimoto T, Umeda F, Masakado M, Yamauchi T, Mizushima S, Isaji M, Nawata H. Expression of prostacyclin-stimulating factor, a novel protein, in tissues of Wistar rats and in cultured cells. Biochem Biophys Res Commun 1994; 202:1490–1496.
49. Pirich C, Banyai M, Efthimiou Y, Sinzinger H. Lipoproteins and prostacyclin stability. Semin Thromb Hemost 1993; 19:138–143.
50. Marcus AJ, Weksler BB, Jaffe EA, Broekman MJ. Synthesis of prostacyclin from platelet-derived endoperoxides by cultured human endothelial cells. J Clin Invest 1980; 66:979–986.
51. Baenziger NL, Becherer PR, Majerus PW. Characterization of prostacyclin synthesis in cultured human arterial smooth muscle cells, venous endothelial cells and skin fibroblasts. Cell 1979; 16:967–974.
52. Nowak J, FitzGerald GA. Redirection of prostaglandin endoperoxide metabolism at the platelet-vascular interface in man. J Clin Invest 1989; 3:380–385.

53. Marcus AJ, Hajjar DP. Vascular transcellular signaling. J Lipid Res 1993; 34:2017–2031.
54. Adler B, Gimbrone MA, Schafer AI, Handin RI. Prostacyclin and $\beta$-adrenergic catecholamines inhibit arachidonate release and PGI$_2$ synthesis by vascular endothelium. Blood 1981; 58:514–517.
55. Lückhoff A, Mülsch A, Busse R. cAMP attenuates autacoid release from endothelial cells: Relation to internal calcium. Am J Physiol 1990; 258:H960–H966.
56. Brotherton AFA, Hoak JC. Role of Ca$^{++}$ and cyclic AMP in the regulation of the production of PGI$_2$ by the vascular endothelium. Proc Natl Acad Sci USA 1982; 79:495–499.
57. Schröder H, Schrör K. Prostacyclin-dependent cyclic AMP formation in endothelial cells. Naunyn-Schmiedebergs Arch Pharmacol 1993; 347:101–104.
58. Hallam TJ, Pearson JD, Newedham LA. Thrombin-stimulated elevation of human endothelial cell cytoplasmic free calcium concentration causes prostacyclin production. Biochem J 1988; 251:243–249.
59. Schröder H, Strobach H, Schrör K. Nitric oxide but not prostacyclin is a autocrine endothelial mediators. Biochem Pharmacol 1992; 43:533–537.
60. Großer T, Bönisch D, Zucker T-P, Schrör K. The inhibition of growth factor-stimulated mitogenesis of coronary artery smooth muscle cells by prostacyclin is attenuated by homologous receptor desensitization. Circulation 1994; 90:I-636.
61. Town MH, Schillinger E, Speckenbach A, Prior G. Identification and characterization of a prostacyclin-like receptor in bovine coronary arteries using a specific and stable prostacyclin analog, iloprost, as a radioactive ligand. Prostaglandins 1982; 24:61–72.
62. Rücker W, Schrör K. Evidence for high affinity prostacyclin binding sites in vascular tissue: radioligand studies with a chemically stable analogue. Biochem Pharmacol 1983; 32:2405–2410.
63. Nakagawa O, Tanaka I, Usui T, Harada M, Sasaki Y, Itoh H, Yoshimasa T, Namba T, Narumiya S, Nakao K. Molecular cloning of human prostacyclin receptor cDNA and its gene expression in the cardiovascular system. Circulation 1994; 90:1643–1647.
64. Katsuyama M, Sugimoto Y, Namba T, Irie A, Negishi M, Narumiya S, Ichikawa A. Cloning and expression of a cDNA for the human prostacyclin receptor. FEBS Lett 1994; 344:74–78.
65. Pierce KL, Gil DW, Woodward DF, Regan JW. Cloning of human prostanoid receptors. Trends Pharmacol Sci 1995; 16:253–256.
66. Watanabe T, Yatomi Y, Sunaga S, Miki I, Ishii A, Nakao A, Higashihara M, Seyama Y, Ogura M, Saito H, Kurokawa K, Shimizu T. Characterization of prostaglandin and thromboxane receptors expressed on a megakaryoblastic leukoemia cell line, MEH-01s. Blood 1991; 78:2228–2236.
67. Schwaner I, Seifert R, Schultz G. The prostacyclin analogues, cicaprost and iloprost, increase cytosolic Ca$^{++}$-concentration in the human erythroleukemia cell line, HEL, via pertussis toxin-insensitive G-proteins. Eicosanoids 1992; 5:S10–S12.

68. Williams SP, Dorn GW, Rapoport RM. Prostaglandin $I_2$ mediates contraction and relaxation of vascular smooth muscle. Am J Physiol 1994; 267:H796–H803.

69. Siegel G, Carl A, Adler A, Stock G. Effect of the prostacyclin analogue iloprost on $K^+$-permeability in the smooth muscle cells of the canine carotid artery. Eicosanoids 1988; 2:213–222.

70. Oka M, Negishi M, Nishigaki N, Ichikawa A. Two types of prostacyclin receptor coupling to phosphatidylinositol hydrolysis in a cultured mast cell line, Bnu-2c13 cells. Cell Signalling 1993; 5:643–650.

71. Ager A, Gordon J, Moncada S, Pearson J, Salmon J, Trevethick M. Effects of isolation and culture on prostaglandin synthesis by porcine aortic endothelial and smooth muscle cells. J Cell Physiol 1982; 110:9–16.

72. Ohara Y. Peterson TE, Harrison DG. Hypercholesterolemia increases endothelial superoxide anion production. J Clin Invest 1993; 91:2546–2551.

73. Baenziger NL, Dillender MJ, Majerus PW. Cultured human skin fibroblasts and arterial cells produce a labile platelet-inhibitory prostaglandin. Biochem Biophys Res Commun 1977; 78:294–301.

74. Larrue J, Rigaud M, Daret D, Demond J, Durand J, Bricaud H. Prostacyclin production by cultured smooth muscle cells from atherosclerotic rabbit aorta. Nature 1980; 285:480–482.

75. Whiting J, Salata K, Bailey JM. Aspirin: An unexpected side effect of prostacyclin synthesis in cultured vascular smooth muscle cells. Science 1980; 210:663–665.

76. Larrue J, Leroux C, Bricaud H. Decreased prostaglandin production in cultured smooth muscle cells from atherosclerotic rabbit aorta. Biochim Biophys Acta 1982; 710:257–263.

77. Brunkwall J, Mattsson E, Bergqvist D. Diet induced atherosclerosis in rabbits alters vascular prostacyclin release. Eicosanoids 1992; 5:197–202.

78. Gryglewski RJ, Dembinska-Kiec A, Zmuda A, Gryglewska T. Prostacyclin and thromboxane biosynthesis capacities of heart, arteries and platelets at various stages of experimental atherosclerosis in rabbits. Atherosclerosis 1978; 31:385–394.

79. Schrör K, Latta G, Seidel H, Smith EF III, Palmer M. Thromboxane and prostacyclin generation in hearts, platelets and aorta of cholesterol-fed rabbits in relation to platelet function. Naunyn-Schmiedebergs Arch Pharmacol 1986; 332: R 35.

80. Wang T, Falardeau P, Powell WS. Synthesis of prostaglandins and thromboxane $B_2$ by cholesterol fed rabbits. Arterioscler Thromb 1991; 11:501–508.

81. Voss R, Don JA, Ten Hoor F. Prostacyclin formation by the rabbit aorta: Relation to atherosclerosis. Prostagl Leukotr Med 1983; 11:451–456.

82. Mattsson E, Brunkwall J, Falt K, Bergqvist D. Prostanoid release immediately after balloon angioplasty in three models of atherosclerosis in rabbits. Eur J Surg 1993; 159:15–21.

83. Booth RFG, Martin JF, Honey AC, Hassall DG, Beesley JE, Moncada S. Rapid development of atherosclerotic lesions in the rabbit carotid artery induced by perivascular manipulation. Atherosclerosis 1989; 75:257–268.

84. Martin JF, Hassall DG. The endothelium and atherosclerosis. In: Warren JW, ed. The Endothelium: An Introduction into Current Research. New York: Wiley-Liss, 1990:95–105.

85. Beetens JR, Coene M-C, Verheyen A, Zonnekeyn L, Herman AG. Biphasic response of intimal prostacyclin production during the development of atherosclerosis. Prostaglandins 1986; 32:319–334.

86. Myers SI, Russell DH, Parks L, Reed MK. Triphasic response of prostacyclin production in rabbit thoracic aorta in early atherosclerosis. Prostagl Leukotr Essent Fatty Acids 1991; 44:31–36.

87. Norman JF, Miller CW. Prostacyclin, thromboxane $A_2$, and atherosclerosis in young hypercholesterolemic swine. Prostagl Leukotr Essent Fatty Acids 1994; 51:293–298.

88. Tokunaga O, Yamada T, Fan JL, Watanabe T. Age related decline in prostacyclin synthesis by human aortic endothelial cells. Qualitative and quantitative analysis. Am J Pathol 1991; 138:941–949.

89. McCaffrey T, Nicholson A, Szabo P, Weksler M, Weksler B. Aging and atherosclerosis. The increased proliferation of arterial smooth muscle cells isolated from old rats is associated with increased platelet-derived growth factor–like activity. J Exp Med 1988; 167:163–174.

90. Coughlin S, Moskowitz M, Antoniades H, Levine L. Serotonin receptor-mediated stimulation of bovine smooth muscle cell prostacyclin synthesis and its modulation by platelet-derived growth factor. Proc Natl Acad Sci USA 1981; 78:7134–7138.

91. Zembowicz A, Jones SL, Wu KK. Induction of cyclooxygenase-2 in human umbilical vein endothelial cells by lysophosphatidylcholine. J Clin Invest 1995; 96:1688–1692.

92. Tremoli E, Socini A, Petroni A, Galli C. Increased platelet aggregability is associated with increased prostacyclin production by vessel walls in hypercholesterolemic rabbits. Prostaglandins 1982; 24:397–404.

93. FitzGerald GA, Smith B, Pedersen AK, Brash AR. Increased prostacyclin biosynthesis in patients with severe atherosclerosis and platelet activation. New Engl J Med 1984; 310:1065–1068.

94. Seigneur M, Dufourcq P, Conri C, Constans J, Mercie P, Pruvost A, Amiral J, Midy D, Baste JC, Boisseau MR. Levels of plasma thrombomodulin are increased in atheromatous arterial disease. Thromb Res 1993; 71:423–431.

95. Weksler BB, Pett SB, Alonso D, Richter RC, Stelzer P, Subramanian V, Tack-Goldman K, Gay WA. Differential inhibition by aspirin of vascular and platelet prostaglandin synthesis in atherosclerotic patients. New Engl J Med 1983; 308:800–805.

96. Carlsson I, Benthin G, Petersson AS, Wennmalm A. Differential inhibition of thromboxane $A_2$ and prostacyclin synthesis by low dose acetylsalicylic acid in atherosclerotic patients. Thromb Res 1990; 57:437–444.

97. Force T, Milani R, Hibberd P, Lorenz R, Uedelhoven W, Leaf A, Weber P. Aspirin-induced decline in prostacyclin production in patients with coronary

artery disease is due to decreased endoperoxide shift. Circulation 1991; 84: 2286–2293.

98. Lee SH, Soyoola E, Chanmugam P, Hart S, Sun W, Zhong H, liou S, Simmons D, Hwang D. Selective expression of mitogen-inducible cyclooxygenase in macrophages stimulated with lipopolysaccharide. J Biol Chem 1992; 267: 25934–25938.

99. Habenicht AJR, Goerig M, Grulich J, Rothe D, Gronwald R, Loth U, Schettler G, Kommerel B, Ross R. Human platelet-derived growth factor stimulates prostaglandin synthesis by activation and by rapid de novo synthesis of cyclooxygenase. J Clin Invest 1985; 75:1381–1387.

100. Hla T, Neilson K. Human cyclooxygenase-2 cDNA. Proc Natl Acad Sci USA 1992; 89:73–84.

101. Jones DA, Carlton DP, McIntyre TM, Zimmerman GA, Prescott SM. Molecular cloning of human prostaglandin endoperoxide synthase type II and demonstration of expression in response to cytokines. J Biol Chem 1993; 268:9049–9054.

102. Habib A, Créminon C, Frobert Y, Grassi J, Pradelles P, Maclouf J. Demonstration of an inducible cyclooxygenase in human endothelial cells using antibodies raised against the carboxy-terminal region of the cyclooxygenase-2. J Biol Chem 1993; 268:23448–23454.

103. Pritchard KA, O'Banion MK, Miano JM, Vlasic N, Bhatia UG, Young DA, Stemerman MB. Induction of cyclooxygenase-2 in rat vascular smooth muscle cells in vitro and in vivo. J Biol Chem 1994; 269:8504–8509.

104. Herschman HR. Regulation of prostaglandin synthase-1 and prostaglandin synthase-2. Cancer Metastasis Rev 1994; 13:241–256.

105. Eldor E, Falcone DJ, Hajjar DP, Minick CR, Weksler BB. Recovery of prostacyclin production by deendothelialized rabbit aorta: critical role of neointimal smooth muscle cells. J Clin Invest 1981; 67:735–741.

106. Simon TC, Makheja AN, Bailey JM. Relationship of vascular 15 lipoxygenase induction to atherosclerotic plaque formation in rabbits. Prostagl Leukotr Essent Fatty Acids 1990; 41:273–278.

107. Lecomte M, Laneuville O, Jo C, De Witt DL, Smith WL. Acetylation of human prostaglandin endoperoxide synthase-2 (cyclooxygenase-2) by aspirin. J Biol Chem 1994; 269:13207–13215.

108. Bailey JM, Salata K, Makheja AN: Dysfunction recovery of prostacyclin synthase in aspirin-treated vascular cells: implications for prophylaxis of cardiovascular disease. Biochem Soc Trans 1994; 22:168S.

109. Vidaver GA, Ting A, Lee JW. Evidence that lysolecithin is an important causal agent of atherosclerosis. J Theoret Biol 1985; 115:27–41.

110. Wells IC, Peitzmeier G, Vincent JK. Lecithin: Cholesterol acyltransferase and lysolecithin in coronary atherosclerosis. Exp Mol Pathol 1986; 45:303–310.

111. Peto J, Mihai K, Makary A. Low level of prostacyclin as a risk of ischaemic heart disease. Int J Cardiol 1991; 30:237–239.

112. Szamosi T, Mihai K, Peto J, Makary A, Kramer J. Potential markers of the atherosclerotic process in high risk children. Clin Biochem 1991; 24:185–187.

113. Akimova EV. Prostacyclin and thromboxane $A_2$ levels in children and adolescents with an inherited predisposition to coronary heart disease: a family study. Coron Artery Dis 1994; 5:761–765.
114. Mayer B, Moser R, Gleispach H, Kukovetz WR. Possible inhibitory function of endogenous 15-hydroperoxyeicosatetraenoic acid on prostacyclin formation in bovine aortic endothelial cells. Biochim Biophys Acta 1986; 875: 641–653.
115. Hadjiagapiou C, Spector AA. 12-hydroxyeicosatetraenoic acid reduces prostacyclin production by endothelial cells. Prostaglandins 1986; 31:1135–1144.
116. Peng SK, Hu B, Peng AY, Morin RJ. Effect of cholesterol oxides on prostacyclin production and platelet adhesion. Artery 1993; 20:122–134.
117. Berberian P, Ziboh V, Hsia S. Prostaglandin $E_2$ biosynthesis: changes in rabbit aorta and skin during experimental atherogenesis. J Lipid Res 1976; 17:46–52.
118. Ross R. Cell biology of atherosclerosis. Annu Rev Physiol 1995; 57:791–804.
119. Packham MAS, Mustard JF. The role of platelets in the development and complications of atherosclerosis. Semin Hematol 1986; 23:8–26.
120. Mizuno-Yagyu Y, Hashida R, Mineo R, Ikegami S, Ohkumo S, Takano T. Effect of $PGI_2$ on transcellular transport of fluorescein dextran through an arterial endothelial monolayer. Biochem Pharmacol 1987; 36:3809–3813.
121. Shirotani M, Yui Y, Hattori R, Kawai C. U 61,431F, a stable prostacyclin analogue, inhibits the proliferation of bovine vascular smooth muscle cells with little antiproliferative effect on endothelial cells. Prostaglandins 1991; 41:97–110.
122. Braun M, Hohlfeld T, Kienbaum P, Weber AA, Sarbia M, Schrör K. Antiatherosclerotic effects of oral cicaprost in experimental hypercholesterolemia in rabbits. Atherosclerosis 1993; 103:93–105.
123. Gryglewski RJ, Choopicki S, Swies J, Niezabitowski P. Prostacyclin, nitric oxide, and atherosclerosis. Ann NY Acad Sci 1995; 748:194–206.
124. Shattil SJ, Anaya-Galindo R, Bennett J, Colman RW, Cooper RA. Platelet hypersensitivity induced by cholesterol incorporation. J Clin Invest 1975; 55:636–643.
125. Moore S, Friedman RJ, Singal DP, Gauldie J, Blajchman MA, Roberts RS. Inhibition of injury-induced thromboatherosclerotic lesions by antiplatelet serum in rabbits. Thromb Haemost 1976; 35:70–81.
126. Friedman RJ, Stemerman MB, Wenz B, Moore S, Gauldie J, Gent M, Tiell ML, Spaet TH. The effect of thrombocytopenia on experimental atherosclerotic lesion formation in rabbits. J Clin Invest 1977; 60:1191–1201.
127. Kristensen SD, Roberts KM, Kishk YT, Martin JF. Accelerated atherogenesis occurs following platelet destruction and increases in megakaryocyte size and DNA content. Eur J Clin Invest 1990; 20:239–247.
128. Fingerle J, Johnson R, Clowes AW, Majesky MW, Reidy MA. Role of platelets in smooth muscle cell proliferation and migration after vascular injury in rat carotid artery. Proc Natl Acad Sci USA 1989; 86:8412–8416.
129. Weiss HJ, Turitto VT. Prostacyclin (Prostaglandin $I_2$, $PGI_2$) inhibits platelet adhesion and thrombus formation on subendothelium. Blood 1979; 53:244–250.

130. Sinzinger H, Fitscha P. Epoprostenol and platelet deposition in atherosclerosis (letter). Lancet 1984; 1:905–906.
131. Benistant C, Achard F, Marcelon G, Lagarde M. Platelet inhibitory functions of aortic endothelial cells. Effects of eicosapentaenoic and docosahexaenoic acids. Atherosclerosis 1993; 104:27–35.
132. Aviram M, Brook JG. Platelet activation by plasma lipoproteins. Prog Cardiovasc Dis 1987; 30:61–72.
133. Löbel P, Steinhagen-Thiessen E, Schrör K. Cholestyramine treatment of type IIa hypercholesterolemia normalizes platelet reactivity against prostacyclin. Eur J Clin Invest 1988; 18:256–260.
134. Jaschonek K, Muller CP. Platelet and vessel associated prostacyclin and thromboxane $A_2$/prostaglandin endoperoxide receptors. Eur J Clin Invest 1988; 18:1–8.
135. Colli S, Maderna P, Tremoli E, Baraldi A, Rovati GE, Gianfranceschi G, Nicosia S. Prostacyclin-lipoprotein interactions. Studies on human platelet aggregation and adenylate cyclase. Biochem Pharmacol 1985; 34:2451–2457.
136. Schrör K, Löbel P, Steinhagen-Thiessen E. Simvastatin reduces platelet thromboxane formation and restores normal platelet sensitivity against prostacyclin in type IIa hypercholesterolemia. Eicosanoids 1989; 2:39–46.
137. Bailey JM, Makheja AN, Butler J, Salata K. Antiinflammatory drugs in experimental atherosclerosis. Atherosclerosis 1979; 32:195–203.
138. Jouve R, Juhan-Vague I, Aillaud M-F, Serment-Jouve M-P, Payan H. Comparison of the effects of aspirin and indomethacin on aortic atherogenesis induced in rabbits. Atherosclerosis 1982; 42:319–322.
139. Chyatte D, Chen TL. Patterns of failure of aspirin treatment in symptomatic atherosclerotic carotid artery disease. Neurosurgery 1990; 26:565–569.
140. Sun Y-P, Zhu B-Q, Sievers RE, Isenberg WM, Parmley WW. Aspirin inhibits platelet activity but does not attenuate experimental atherosclerosis. Am Heart J 1993; 125:79–86.
141. Debons AF, Fani K, Jimenez FA. Enhancement of experimental atherosclerosis by aspirin. J Toxicol Environ Health 1981; 8:899–906.
142. Hollander W, Kirkpatrick B, Paddock J, Columbo M, Nagraj S, Prusty S. Studies on the progression and regression of coronary and peripheral atherosclerosis in the cynomolgus monkey. I. Effects of dipyridamole and aspirin. Exp Mol Pathol 1979; 30:55–73.
143. Pick R, Chediak J, Glick G. Aspirin inhibits development of coronary atherosclerosis in cynomolgus monkeys (macaca fascicularis) fed an atherogenic diet. J Clin Invest 1979; 63:158–162.
144. Ranke C, Hecker H, Creutzig A, Alexander K. Dose-dependent effect of aspirin on carotid atherosclerosis. Circulation 1993; 87:1873–1879.
145. Schwartz SM. How vessels narrow. Z Kardiol 1995; 84(suppl 4):129–135.
146. Nilsson J, Olsson AG. Prostaglandin $E_1$ inhibits DNA synthesis in arterial smooth muscle cells stimulated with platelet-derived growth factor. Atherosclerosis 1984; 53:77–82.
147. Asada Y, Kisanuki A, Hatakeyama K, Takahama S, Koyama T, Kurozumi S,

Sumiyoshi A. Inhibitory effects of prostacyclin analogue, TFC 132, on aortic neointimal thickening in vivo and smooth muscle cell proliferation in vitro. Prostagl Leukotr Essent Fatty Acids 1994; 51:245–248.

148. Sinzinger H, Steurer G, Kaliman J, Ettl K. Interaction between the platelet derived growth factor and prostaglandin $I_2$ is important for atherosclerosis. Adv Prostagl Thromb Leukotr Res 1987; 17:216–218.

149. Tanaka K, Sueishi K. Biology of Disease. The coagulation and fibrinolysis systems and atherosclerosis. Lab Invest 1993; 69:5–18.

150. Drake TA, Morrisey JH, Edgington TS. Selective cellular expression of tissue factor in human tissues: implications of disorders of hemostasis and thrombosis. Am J Pathol 1989; 134:1087–1097.

151. Wilcox JN, Smith KM, Schwartz SM, Gordon D. Localization of tissue factor in the normal vessel wall and in the atherosclerotic plaque. Proc Natl Acad Sci USA 1989; 86:2839–2843.

152. Martin DMA, Boys WG, Ruf W. Tissue factor: molecular recognition and cofactor function. FASEB J 1995; 9:852–859.

153. Annex BH, Denning SM, Channon KM, Sketch MH, Stack RS, Morrisey JH, Peters KG. Differential expression of tissue factor protein in directional atherectomy specimens from patients with stable and unstable coronary syndroms. Circulation 1995; 91:619–622.

154. Hassall DG, Ward J, Moncada S, Martin JF, Booth RFG. Monocyte adherence and chemotaxis are inhibited by carbacyclin. In: Suckling KE, Groot PHE, eds. Hyperlipidaemia and Atherosclerosis. San Diego: Academic Press 1988:212–213.

155. Crutchley DJ, Hirsh MJ. The stable prostacyclin analog, iloprost, and prostaglandin $E_1$ inhibit monocyte procoagulant activity in vitro. Blood 1991; 78:382–386.

156. Crutchley DJ, Conanan LB, Toledo AW, Solomon DE, Que BG. Effects of prostacyclin analogues on human endothelial cell tissue factor expression. Arteriosclosis Thromb 1993; 13:1082–1089.

157. Anitschkow N. Über die Veränderungen der Kaninchenaorta bei experimenteller Cholesterinsteatose. Beitr Path Anat Allg Pathol 1913; 56:379–404.

158. Subbiah MTR, Dicke B. Effects of prostaglandins $E_1$ and $F_1\alpha$ on the activities of cholesteryl ester synthetase and cholesteryl ester hydrolase of pigeon aorta in vitro. Atherosclerosis 1977; 27:107–111.

159. Hajjar DP, Weksler BB, Falcone DJ, Hefton JM, Tack-Goldman K, Minick CR. Prostacyclin modulates cholesteryl ester hydrolytic activity by its effect on cyclic adenosine monophosphate in rabbit aortic smooth muscle cells. J Clin Invest 1982; 70:479–488.

160. Hajjar DP, Weksler BB. Metabolic activity of cholesteryl esters in aortic smooth muscle cells is altered by prostaglandins $I_2$ and $E_2$. J Lipid Res 1983;24:1176–1185.

161. Hajjar DP, Weksler BB. Modulation of arterial cholesteryl ester metabolism by prostacyclin and prostaglandin $E_2$. Adv Prostagl Thrombox Leukotr Res 1985; 15:249–252.

162. Hajjar DP, Marcus AJ, Hajjar KA. Interactions of arterial cells. Studies on the mechanisms of endothelial cell modulation of cholesterol metabolism in co-cultured smooth muscle cells. J Biol Chem 1987; 262:6976–6981.

163. Orekhov A, Tertov VV, Smirnov VN. Prostacyclin analogues as anti-atherosclerotic drugs. Lancet 1983; II:521.

164. Makary A, Kolthay E, Pataki M, Peto J, Kovacs G, Lusztig G. Inhibition of ACAT activity after 7 oxo $PGI_2$ treatment in cholesterol fed rabbits. Exp Toxicol Pathol 1992; 44:105–107.

165. Kowala MC, Mazzucco CE, Hartl KS, Seiler SM, Warr GA, Abid S, Grove RI. Prostacyclin agonists reduce early atherosclerosis in hyperlipidemic hamsters. Octimibate and BMY 42393 suppress monocyte chemotaxis, macrophage cholesteryl ester accumulation, scavenger receptor activity, and tumor necrosis factor production. Arteriosclerosis Thromb 1993; 13:435–444.

166. Morishita H, Yui Y, Hattori R, Aoyama T, Kawai C. Increased hydrolysis of cholesteryl ester with prostacyclin is potentiated by high-density lipoprotein through the prostacyclin stabolization. J Clin Invest 1990; 86:1885–1891.

167. Orekhov AN, Tertov VV, Kudryashov SA, Khashimov KhA, Smirnov VN. Primary culture of human aortic intima cells as a model for testing antiatherosclerotic drugs. Effects of cyclic AMP, prostaglandins, calcium antagonists, antioxidants and lipid-lowering agents. Atherosclerosis 1986; 60:101–110.

168. Akopov SE, Orekhov AN, Tertov VV, Kashimov KA, Gabrieljan ES, Smirnov VN. Stable analogues of prostacyclin and thromboxane $A_2$ display contradictory influences on atherosclerotic properties of cells cultured from human aorta: The effect of calcium antagonists. Atherosclerosis 1988; 72:245–248.

169. Tertov VV, Orekhov AN, Repin VS, Smirnov VN. Dibutyryl cyclic AMP decreases proliferative activity and the cholesteryl ester content in cultured cells of atherosclerotic human aorta. Biochem Biophys Res Commun 1982; 109:1228–1233.

170. Berk BC, Alexander RW. Vasoactive effects of growth factors. Biochem Pharmacol 1989; 38:219–225.

171. Chamley-Campbell JH, Campbell GR, Ross R. Phenotype-dependent response of cultured aortic smooth muscle to serum mitogens. J Cell Biol 1981; 89:379–383.

172. Campbell JH, Campbell GR. Culture techniques and their applications to studies of vascular smooth muscle. Clin Sci 1993; 85:501–513.

173. Holycross BJ, Blank RS, Thompson MM, Peach MJ, Owens GK. Platelet-derived growth factor-BB-induced suppression of smooth muscle cell differentiation. Circ Res 1992; 71:1525–1532.

174. Coughlin SR, Moskowitz MA, Zetter BR, Antoniades HN, Levine L. Platelet-dependent stimulation of prostacyclin synthesis by platelet-derived growth factor. Nature 1980; 288:600–602.

175. Habenicht AJR, Salbach P, Goerig M, Zeh W, Janssen-Timmen U, Blattner C, King WC, Glomset JA. The LDL-receptor pathway delivers arachidonic acid for eicosanoid formation in cells, stimulated by platelet-derived growth factor. Nature 1990; 345:634–636.

176. Libby P, Warner SJC, Friedman GB. Interleukin 1: A mitogen for human vascular smooth muscle cells that induces the release of growth inhibitory prostanoids. J Clin Invest 1988; 81:487–498.
177. Morisaki N, Kanzaki T, Motoyama N, Saito Y, Yoshida S. Cell cycle-dependent inhibition of DNA synthesis by prostaglandin $I_2$ in cultured rabbit aortic smooth muscle cells. Atherosclerosis 1988; 71:165–171.
178. Murase T, Kozawa O, Miwa M, Tokuda H, Kotoyori J, Kondo K, Oiso Y. Regulation of proliferation by vasopressin in aortic smooth muscle cells: function of protein kinase C. J Hypertens 1992; 10:1505–1511.
179. Dorn GW II, Becker MW. Growth factors downregulate vascular smooth muscle thromboxane receptors independent of cell growth. Am J Physiol Cell Physiol 1992; 262:C927–C933.
180. Kanai N, Lu R, Satriano JA, Bao Y, Wolkoff AW, Schuster VL. Identification and characterization of a prostaglandin transporter. Science 1995; 268: 866–869.
181. Hüttner II, Gwebu ET, Panganamala RV, Sharma HM, Geer JC. Fatty acids and their prostaglandin derivatives: inhibitors of proliferation in aortic smooth muscle cells. Science 1977; 197:289–291.
182. Pietilä K, Moilanen T, Nikkari T. Prostaglandins enhance the synthesis of glycosaminoglycans and inhibit the growth of rabbit aortic smooth muscle cells in culture. Artery 1980; 7:509.
183. Owen NE. Prostacyclin can inhibit DNA synthesis in vascular smooth muscle cells. In: Bailey JM, ed. Prostaglandins, Leukotrienes, and Lipoxins. New York: Plenum Press 1985:193–204.
184. Owen NE. Effect of prostaglandin $E_1$ on DNA synthesis in vascular smooth muscle cells. Am J Physiol Cell Physiol 1986; 250:C584–588.
185. Sinzinger H, Zidek Th, Fitscha P, O'Grady J, Wagner O, Kaliman J. Prostaglandin $I_2$ reduces activation of human arterial smooth muscle cells in-vivo. Prostaglandins 1987; 33:915–918.
186. Uehara Y, Ishimitu T, Kimura K, Ishii M, Ikesa T, Sugimoto T. Regulatory effects of eicosanoids on thymidine uptake by vascular smooth muscle cells of rats. Prostaglandins 1988; 36:847–857.
187. Southgate K, Newby AC. Serum induced proliferation of rabbit aortic smooth muscle cells from the contractile state is inhibited by 8-Br-cAMP but not 8-Br-cGMP. Atherosclerosis 1990; 82:113–123.
188. Assender JW, Southgate KM, Hallett MB, Newby AC. Inhibition of proliferation, but not of $Ca^{2+}$ mobilization, by cyclic AMP and GMP in rabbit aortic smooth muscle cells. Biochem J 1992; 288:527–532.
189. Wiley MH, Feingold KR, Grunfeld C, Quesney-Huneuus V, Wu JM. Evidence for cAMP-independent inhibition of S-phase DNA synthesis by prostaglandins. J Biol Chem 1983; 258:491–496.
190. Stout RW. Cyclic AMP: A potent inhibitor of DNA synthesis in cultured arterial endothelial and smooth muscle cells. Diabetologia 1989; 22:51–55.
191. Cook SJ, McCormick FM. Inhibition by cAMP of Ras-dependent activation of Raf. Science 1993; 262:1069–1072.

192. Wu J, Dent P, Jelinek T, Wolfman A, Weber MJ, Sturgill TW. Inhibition of the EGF-activated MAP kinase signaling pathway by adenosine 3',5'-monophosphate. Science 1993; 262:1065–1069.

193. Sevetson BR, Kong X, Lawrence JC. Increasing cAMP attenuates activation of mitogen-activated protein kinase. Proc Natl Acad Sci USA 1993; 90: 10305–10309.

194. Großer T, Bönisch D, Zucker T-Ph, Schrör K. Iloprost induced inhibition of proliferation of coronary artery smooth muscle cells is abolished by homologous desensitization. Agents Actions 1995; 45(suppl):85–91.

195. Boynton AL, Whitfield JF. The role of cyclic AMP in cell proliferation: a critical assessment of the evidence. Adv Cyclic Nucleotide Res 1983; 15: 193–294.

196. Franks DJ, Plamondon J, Hamet P. An increase in adenylate cyclase activity precedes DNA synthesis in cultured vascular smooth muscle cells. J Cell Physiol 1984; 119:41–45.

197. Loesberg C, van-Wijk R, Zandbergen J, van-Aken WG, van-Mourik JA, De Groot PG. Cell cycle–dependent inhibition of human vascular smooth muscle cell proliferation by prostaglandin $E_1$. Exp Cell Res 1985; 160:117–125.

198. Krane A, MacDermot J, Keen M. Desensitization of adenylate cyclase responses following exposure to IP prostanoid receptor agonists. Homologous and heterologous desensitization exhibit the same time course. Biochem Pharmacol 1994; 47:953–959.

199. Hayes LW, Goguen CA, Stevens AL, Magargal SW, Slakey LL. Enzyme activities in endothelial cells and smooth muscle cells from swine aorta. Proc Natl Acad Sci USA 1979; 76:2532–2535.

200. Lee MW, Severson DL. Signal transduction in vascular smooth muscle: diacyclglycerol second messengers and PKC action. Am J Physiol 1994; 267:C659–C678.

201. Daniel TO, Gibbs VC, Milfay DF, Garovoy MR, Williams LT. Thrombin stimulates c-sis gene expression in microvascular endothelial cells. J Biol Chem 1986; 261:9579–9582.

202. Fager G. Thrombin and proliferation of vascular smooth muscle cells. Circ Res 1995; 77:645–650.

203. Stürzebecher S, Nieuweboer B, Matthes S, Schillinger E. Effects of $PGD_2$, $PGE_1$ and $PGI_2$ analogues on PDGF release and aggregation of human gelfiltered platelets. In: Schrör K, Sinzinger H, eds. Prostaglandins in Clinical Research–Cardiovascular System. Progress in Clinical and Biological Research, Vol. 301. New York: Liss, 1989:365–369.

204. Walker LN, Bowen-Pope DF, Ross R, Reidy MA. Production of platelet-derived growth factor-like molecules by cultured arterial smooth muscle cells accompanies proliferation after arterial injury. Proc Natl Acad Sci USA 1986; 83:7311–7315.

205. Haralson MA. Extracellular matrix and growth factors: An integrated interplay controlling tissue repair and progression to disease. Lab Invest 1993; 69:369–371.

206. van Zanten GH, de Graaf S, Slootweg PJ, Heijnen HFG, Connolly TM, de Groot PG, Sixma JJ. Increased platelet deposition on atherosclerotic coronary arteries. J Clin Invest 1994; 93:615–632.

207. Kato S, Sasaguri Y, Morimatsu M. Down regulation in the production of matrix metalloproteinase 1 by human aortic intimal smooth muscle cells. Biochem Mol Biol Int 1993; 31:239–248.

208. Koh E, Morimoto S, Jiang B, Inoue T, Nabata T, Kitano S, Yasuda O, Fukuo K, Ogihara T. Effects of beraprost sodium, a stable analogue of prostacyclin, on hyperplasia, hypertrophy and glycosaminoglycan synthesis of rat aortic smooth muscle cells. Artery 1993; 20:242–252.

209. Sjolund M, Nilsson J, Palmberg L, Thyberg J. Phenotype modulation of primary cultures of arterial smooth muscle cells. Dual effect of prostaglandin $E_1$. Differentiation 1984; 27:158–162.

210. Isogaya M, Yamada N, Koike H, Ueno Y, Kumagai H, Ochi Y, Okazaki S, Nishio S. Inhibition of restenosis by beraprost sodium (a prostaglandin $I_2$ analogue) in the atherosclerotic rabbit artery after angioplasty. J Cardiovasc Pharmacol 1995; 25:947–952.

211. Levitt NA, Dryjski M, Tluczek J, Bjornsson TD. Evaluation of a prostacyclin analog, iloprost, and a thromboxane $A_2$ receptor antagonist, daltroban, in experimental intimal hyperplasia. Prostaglandins 1991; 41:1–6.

212. Zoldhelyi P, McNatt J, Xu X-M, Loose-Mitchell D, Meidell RS, Clubb FJ, Buja M, Willerson JT, Wu KK. Prevention of arterial thrombosis by adenovirus-mediated transfer of cyclooxygenase gene. Circulation 1996; 93: 10–17.

213. Szczeklik A, Nishanowski R, Skawinski S, Szczeklik J, Gluszko P, Gryglewski RJ. Successful therapy of advanced arteriosclerosis obliterans with prostacyclin. Lancet 1979; 1:1111–1114.

214. de Gaetano, Bertelé V, Cerletti C. Mechanism of action and clinical use of prostanoids. In: Dormandy JA, Stock G, eds. Critical Leg Ischemia, Its Pathophysiology and Management. New York: Springer-Verlag 1990:117–137.

215. European Consensus Document on Critical Limb Ischemia. In: Dormandy JA, Stock G, eds. Critical Leg Ischemia, Its Pathophysiology and Management. New York: Springer-Verlag 1990:I–XLVIII.

216. Bugiardini R, Galvani M, Ferrini D, Gridelli C, Tollemeto D, Macri N, Puddu P, Lenzi S. Myocardial ischemia during intravenous prostacyclin administration: Haemodynamic findings and precautionary measures. Am Heart J 1987; 113:234–240.

217. Bugiardini R, Galvani M, Ferrini D, Gridelli C, Mari L, Puddu P, Lenzi S. Effects of iloprost, a stable prostacyclin analog, on exercise capacity and platelet aggregation in stable angina pectoris. Am J Cardiol 1986; 58:453–459.

218. Sakata K, Hoshino T, Yoshida H, Kaburagi T, Takada A. Effects of beraprost sodium, a new prostaglandin $I_2$ analog, on parameters of hemostasis, fibrinolysis, and myocardial ischemia in patients with exertional angina. Cardiovasc Drugs Ther 1995; 9:601–607.

219. Isaka Y, Handa N, Imaizumi M, Kimura K, Kamada T. Effect of TRK 100, a

stable orally active prostacyclin analogue, on platelet function and plaque size in atherothrombotic strokes. Thromb Haemost 1991; 65:344–350.

220. Zeiher AM, Schachinger V. Coronary endothelial vasodilator dysfunction: clinical relevance and therapeutic implications. Z Kardiol 1994; 83(suppl 4): 7–14.
221. Kirschenbaum MA, Roh DD, Kamanna VS. Effect of nifedipine on renal microvascular cholesterol accumulation and prostacyclin biosynthesis in cholesterol fed rabbits. Atherosclerosis 1991; 91:241–246.
222. Löbel P, Schrör K. Stimulation of vascular prostacyclin and inhibition of platelet function by oral defibrotide in cholesterol-fed rabbits. Atherosclerosis 1989; 90:69–79.
223. Schrör K, Ackermann G, Hohlfeld Th, Löbel P, Ney P, Schröder H, Strobach H. Endothelial protection by defibrotide—a new strategy for treatment of myocardial infarction? Z Kardiol 1989; 6:35–41.

# 2

# Prostacyclin and Thromboxane: Role in Ischemic Heart Disease

**Jawahar L. Mehta and Baichun C. Yang**

*University of Florida, Gainesville, Florida*

## I. FORMATION OF PROSTACYCLIN AND THROMBOXANE $A_2$

Prostaglandins (PGs) derived from arachidonic acid (AA) in almost all tissues are natural substances, which possess broad and potent biological activity. Among PGs, $PGI_2$ and thromboxane ($TxA_2$) are the most important modulators in cardiovascular system.

Arachidonic acid, a polyunsaturated fatty acid with a 20-carbon structure and four double bonds (C20:4), is present in the phospholipid pool of almost all cell membranes. It is released on perturbation in the cellular environment by the action of the enzyme phospholipase $A_2$. This acid is converted to cyclic endoperoxides ($PGG_2$ and $PGH_2$) via the catalysis of cyclooxygenase and undergoes metabolic conversion to a variety of eicosanoids with two double bands ($PGE_2$, $PGF_{2a}$, $PGD_2$, $PGI_2$, and $TxA_2$) depending on the enzyme(s) present in the cell.

Hamberg et al. (1) first described the formation of $TxA_2$ in the thrombocytes (hence the name thromboxane) or platelets. $TxA_2$ is generated by the action of enzyme $TxA_2$ synthase on unstable cyclic endoperoxides ($PGG_2$ and $PGH_2$). It has a half-life of 30 sec and is spontaneously hydrolyzed to inactive $TxB_2$, which is further metabolized via $\beta$-oxidation to form 2,3-dinor-$TxB_2$. $TxB_2$ can also be metabolized to 11-dehydro-$TxB_2$, a circulating metabolite which is excreted in the urine (2). Although primarily synthesized in the platelets, small amounts of $TxA_2$ are also synthesized in the macrophages, lungs, kidneys, blood vessel walls, and heart (3,4). $TxA_2$ is a potent platelet aggregant and vasoconstrictor eicosanoid.

Moncada et al. (5) described the synthesis of $PGI_2$ in the blood vessels by the action of enzyme $PGI_2$ synthase as a major product of the cyclooxygenase cascade. $PGI_2$ has a half-life of 2–3 min at 37°C, and it spontaneously hydrolyzes to inactive 6-keto-$PGF_1\alpha$, which is further metabolized via $\beta$-oxidation to 2,3-dinor-6-keto-$PGF_1\alpha$. $PGI_2$ is synthesized primarily in the blood vessels, but other tissues such as leukocytes, lungs, and heart can also generate small amounts of $PGI_2$ (3,4). Since $PGI_2$ inhibits platelet activation and causes vasodilation, effects opposite to those of $TxA_2$, it has been speculated that $PGI_2$ and $TxA_2$ are major regulators of hemostasis and vascular tone.

## II. ALTERATIONS OF $PGI_2$ AND $TxA_2$ DURING MYOCARDIAL ISCHEMIA

Under normal circumstances, $PGI_2$ is produced by the vascular endothelium in quantities which inhibit spontaneous platelet aggregation. However, if $TxA_2$ production is excessive, the balance between $PGI_2$ and $TxA_2$ may be shifted in favor of platelet aggregation, and in vivo thrombosis may be initiated. Enhanced platelet production of $TxA_2$, with or without decreased vascular formation of $PGI_2$, has been suggested to contribute to coronary artery thrombosis and/or vasospasm. Several animal studies have documented the release of $TxA_2$ during myocardial ischemia/reperfusion. Coker et al. (6) and Walinsky et al. (7) showed $TxB_2$ concentrations increased markedly 5–10 min after coronary artery occlusion and returned to baseline at 30 min despite continued occlusion. This indicates a transient release of $TxA_2$ soon after coronary occlusion. Coker et al. (6) also detected a marked increase in 6-keto-$PGF_1\alpha$ concentration in the local coronary venous plasma soon (approximately 5–10 min) after coronary artery occlusion in dogs. Animals with the highest level of $TxB_2$ had the most arrhythmias, whereas there was a negative correlation between occurrence of arrhythmias and increase in 6-keto-$PGF_1\alpha$. In an isolated rabbit heart model, Stahl et al. (8) showed that ischemia induced by infusion of N-formyl-methionyl-leucyl-phenylalanine, a known stimulus for coronary vasospasm, was accompanied by a significant but small increase in coronary effluent $PGI_2$ concentration and a marked increase in $TxB_2$ concentration. $TxA_2$ is also released during the formation of platelet-rich thrombi in the narrowed coronary arteries of dogs. Tada et al. (9) proposed that a relative reduction in $PGI_2$ release, resulting in an "imbalance" between $PGI_2$ and $TxA_2$, may be a cause of cyclical flow reductions in dogs.

TxA$_2$ release has also been documented in a variety of myocardial isch-emic syndromes in humans as well. There is suggestion of marked increase of TxA$_2$ release and only a modest increase of PGI$_2$ synthesis during exercise in patients with stable angina pectoris (10). Myocardial ischemia induced by atrial pacing is also associated with release of TxA$_2$ in the coronary venous blood (11,12). Elevation of TxB$_2$ in the peripheral and coronary venous blood plasma (12,13) has been demonstrated in patients with unstable an-gina pectoris. Enhanced TxA$_2$ release is also evident just prior to acute coronary occlusion in human (14). Walinsky et al. (7) and others (15) have also documented elevated TxB$_2$ values in the peripheral blood plasma of patients soon after acute myocardial infarction.

Balloon angioplasty in man may also be associated with the release of TxA$_2$ at the site of coronary angioplasty (16). In addition, recent studies have shown the release of TxA$_2$ during thrombolysis (17), indicating that platelet activation and TxA$_2$ release may modulate the response to throm-bolytic agents.

During experimental myocardial ischemia/reperfusion as well as in pa-tients with myocardial ischemia, PGI$_2$ release also increases modestly (10,18–20), which is much less in magnitude than the release of TxA$_2$. Therefore, it appears that there is an imbalance between PGI$_2$ and TxA$_2$. The change in this theoretical balance in favor of TxA$_2$ would favor plate-let aggregation, coronary vasoconstriction, and vasospasm. Mingazet-dinova et al. (21) reported that there is a direct relationship between the degree of imbalance between TxA$_2$, PGI$_2$, PGF$_{2\alpha}$, and PGE$_1$ and concur-rent stable angina pectoris in patients with coronary heart disease. In these studies, a significant increase in the levels of TxB$_2$ and PGF$_{2\alpha}$ was found with relative PGI$_2$ and PGE$_1$ deficiency during graded exercise at the moment of transient myocardial ischemia; the imbalance significantly increased as exercise tolerance decreased. Transient myocardial ischemia induced by transesophageal left atrial pacing revealed unidirectional changes in plasma PGs, as did exercise. On the other hand, this imbal-ance may be the mechanism of platelet hyperactivity in acute myocardial infarction in human (22) and decreased platelet sensitivity to the anti-aggregatory effect of PGI$_2$ in patients with angina pectoris and myocardial infarction (22–24).

FitzGerald et al. (20) described the sporadic increases in the urinary excretion of 2,3-dinor-6-keto-PGF$_{1\alpha}$ in patients with unstable angina in rela-tion to episodes of chest pain. Moreover, in patients with acute myocardial infarction, the peak urinary excretion of this metabolite was correlated with and temporally related to peak creatine phosphokinase, suggesting that increased PGI$_2$ biosynthesis may reflect vascular response to platelet activation.

Chahine et al. (4), using AA and left ventricular microsomes from isolated Langendorff rabbit heart, determined myocardial $PGI_2$ and $TxA_2$ synthase activity during ischemia and reperfusion. They found that left ventricular microsomes were able to synthesize $PGI_2$ as well as $TxA_2$ from arachidonic acid. On the other hand, ischemia depressed both $PGI_2$ and $TxA_2$ synthase activities in cardiac tissue. The depression was more pronounced relative to $TxA_2$ synthase than to $PGI_2$ synthase with no significant difference between ischemic and nonischemic regions. The postischemic reperfusion of the heart counteracted the decrease in $PGI_2$ synthase induced by ischemia which returned to the normal level. Reperfusion also slightly reversed the decrease in $TxA_2$ synthase. However, the diminution in $TxA_2$ synthase activity in the nonischemic myocardium was attenuated after reperfusion, but it remained suppressed. Moreover, ischemia and reperfusion decreased the ratio of $PGI_2/TxA_2$, indirectly suggesting that the marked increase in $TxA_2$ release during acute myocardial ischemia is due to platelet aggregation.

In most of these studies, the release of $TxA_2$ was shown to be associated with the presence of myocardial ischemia and ischemia-related arrhythmias. Obviously, it is difficult to ascertain if $TxA_2$ release is the cause of myocardial ischemia or is a consequence of the ischemic process, reminding one of the "chicken and egg" predicament. Even if it were assumed that $TxA_2$ is released following platelet activation in the narrowed coronary artery, $TxA_2$ could potentially exert a vasoconstrictor influence on the coronary vascular bed downstream.

## III. AMELIORATION OF $PGI_2/TxA_2$ IMBALANCE IN EXPERIMENTAL MYOCARDIAL ISCHEMIA

With the preceding evidence of $TxA_2$ release and $PGI_2/TxA_2$ imbalance during myocardial ischemia, a variety of agents with $PGI_2$ mimic or $TxA_2$ inhibitory activity have been developed over the last decade for potential clinical use. There are abundant data on the use of these agents in experimental myocardial ischemia.

### A. $PGI_2$ and Its Analogues

Animal studies have shown $PGI_2$ to have a beneficial effect in several different models of myocardial ischemia. In an isolated perfused cat heart preparation, the administration of $PGI_2$ during the period of ischemia has been shown to inhibit ischemia-induced creatine kinase release independent of any effect on coronary blood flow or platelet activity (25). $PGI_2$ is known to increase coronary artery blood flow and collateral flow, and limit infarct size and the incidence of postinfarction arrhythmias in dogs with ligated left circumflex coronary arteries (26), and prevent $TxA_2$ analogue (U46,619)–induced ischemic electrocardiographic changes in rats (27). Infusion of $PGI_2$ has also been found to prevent coronary artery thrombosis in response to electrically induced intimal injury (28) and ischemia/reperfusion arrhythmias in vitro (29). In addition to a possible cytoprotective effect, $PGI_2$ may inhibit the release of catecholamines from the intraneuronal stores (30). Catecholamines released during the early phases of myocardial ischemia stimulate platelets to aggregate, reduce their cyclic AMP levels, and enhance myocardial metabolism. Therefore the inhibition of catecholamine release by $PGI_2$ during ischemia is beneficial. Lefer et al. (31) documented that the properties of $PGI_2$ of potential value in acute myocardial ischemia include the reduction of systemic blood pressure without a change in the heart rate, the lowering of coronary vascular and total peripheral resistance, the inhibition of platelet aggregation and the concomitant formation of $TxA_2$, and the reduction of the release of lysosomal enzymes. $PGI_2$ has also been shown to decrease myocardial infarct size via inhibition of neutrophil infiltration and accumulation in myocardium and via inhibition of oxygen-derived free radical generation by neutrophils (32,33). Stable $PGI_2$ analogues, 7-oxo-$PGI_2$ and iloprost (ZK36,374), have been shown to exert similar beneficial effects in acute myocardial ischemia (34,35). Defibrotide and nafazatrom, which stimulate the endogenous formation of $PGI_2$, have also been shown to improve contractile recovery from myocardial stunning (36), prevent experimental thrombosis (37), and the in vivo development of occlusive coronary artery thrombi in conscious dog with electrically induced coronary artery endothelial injury (38).

## B.   $TxA_2$ Synthase Inhibitors and $TxA_2$/Endoperoxide Receptor Antagonists

The enzyme $TxA_2$ synthase is inhibited by imidazole and a variety of pyridine derivatives (39,40). Although the synthesis of $TxA_2$ is decreased, platelet aggregation may not be affected until very high concentrations of $TxA_2$ synthase inhibitors are used, presumably because the uninhibited $TxA_2$ and the accumulated cyclic endoperoxides can still induce platelet aggregation. In addition, the formation of $PGE_2$ and $PGI_2$ increases as the accumulated cyclic endoperoxides are utilized by the endothelial cells or leukocytes (41,42). This shunting of cyclic endoperoxides is evident in vitro as well as in vivo after administration of $TxA_2$ synthase inhibitors (42,43). This $TxA_2$ synthase inhibitor–induced increase in $PGI_2$ may be responsible for the reduction in neutrophil superoxide radical generation which is observed when neutrophils are incubated with platelets in the presence of selective $TxA_2$ synthase inhibitor, U63,557A (44). The reduction in the synthesis of superoxide radicals, which have been incriminated in the extension of myocardial injury, may relate to the decrease in infarct size in animals pretreated with selective $TxA_2$ synthase inhibitor (45–49).

Whereas selective $TxA_2$ synthase inhibitors decrease $TxA_2$ synthesis and increase $PGI_2$ formation, inhibitors of cyclooxygenase enzyme such as aspirin and nonsteroidal anti-inflammatory drugs result in a reduction in both $TxA_2$ and $PGI_2$ (50). Although it was initially proposed that low doses of aspirin may selectively inhibit $TxA_2$ and spare $PGI_2$, more recent studies have failed to show such selective inhibition of $TxA_2$ by any dosage of aspirin (51).

In contrast to the minimal effects of $TxA_2$ synthase inhibitors on platelet aggregation, $TxA_2$/endoperoxide receptor antagonists block platelet aggregation in response to a variety of stimuli in very low concentrations. Theoretically, greater efficacy of $TxA_2$/endoperoxide receptor antagonists probably relates to the blockade of proplatelet aggregatory activity of $TxA_2$ as well as of cyclic endoperoxides. $TxA_2$ synthesis is not inhibited and $PGI_2$ generation is not augmented with the use of $TxA_2$/endoperoxide receptor antagonists. It is possible that excessive synthesis of $PGI_2$, as occurs during use of $TxA_2$ synthase inhibitors, may induce myocardial ischemia by shunting blood away from the ischemic zone. This potential hazard is unlikely to occur with $TxA_2$/endoperoxide receptor antagonists.

A variety of $TxA_2$ synthase inhibitors such as dazoxiben and U63,557A have been shown to reduce myocardial infarct size in dogs, cats, and rats. $TxA_2$/endoperoxide receptor antagonists also reduce myocardial infarct size (48,52–55), and the degree of reduction in infarct size with the use of $TxA_2$ synthase inhibitors or receptor antagonists appears to be similar (48). Furthermore, the use of both $TxA_2$ synthase inhibitors or receptor antagonists is associated with a marked reduction in myocardial leukocyte infiltration and peripheral leukocytosis (47–49,55). A reduction in myocardial leukocyte infiltration and activation could be a factor in myocardial infarct size reduction by $TxA_2$ inhibitors, since aspirin, which also inhibits $TxA_2$ formation, does not limit infarct size and does not affect neutrophil infiltration. The importance of the availability of $TxA_2$ is evident from the studies by Mullane and Fornabio (47), who showed that platelet depletion or pretreatment with aspirin prevents $TxA_2$ inhibitor–induced suppression of neutrophil accumulation and reduction in infarct size in dogs subjected to 90 min of coronary occlusion. Osborne and Lefer (54) showed that the $TxA_2$/endoperoxide receptor antagonist BM13,505 reduces atherogenesis in cholesterol-fed rabbits and also diminishes the severity of ischemic damage resulting from total coronary occlusion. It is also apparent from these studies that the beneficial effects of $TxA_2$ inhibitors are not mediated by a reduction in the indices of myocardial oxygen demand.

In animal models of platelet aggregation occurring in the narrowed coronary arteries, $TxA_2$ synthase inhibitors have been found to be effective in decreasing the frequency and magnitude of blood flow reduction (56). The increase in endogenous $PGI_2$ on administration of $TxA_2$ synthase inhibitor may be important in preventing coronary artery thrombosis. The administration of $TxA_2$/endoperoxide receptor antagonist SQ29,548 or ONO-3,708 also decreases intracoronary platelet deposition in experimentally stenosed coronary arteries (57–59). Since $TxA_2$/endoperoxide receptor antagonists do not increase $PGI_2$ concentrations, it is unlikely that a local deficiency of $PGI_2$ plays a significant role in platelet aggregation–related cyclical flow changes.

In a canine model of electrically induced occlusive coronary artery thrombus, the $TxA_2$ synthase inhibitors OKY-1,581 and CGS-13,080 markedly decrease the incidence of thrombotic occlusion and reduce the weight (or mass) of the thrombus (60,61). The $TxA_2$/endoperoxide receptor antagonists L636,499, SQ29,548, and ONO-3,708 also inhibit the formation of occlusive thrombus on delivery of an electric current in the canine thrombus model (59,62). Furthermore, coronary arterial reocclusion after initial thrombolysis can be inhibited with the use of the $TxA_2$ synthase inhibitor CGS-13,080 (63) or the $TxA_2$/endoperoxide receptor antagonists L636,499 and AH-23,848 (64). However, inhibition of platelet aggregation by monoclonal antibody to the platelet GPIIb/IIIa receptors, which does not affect $TxA_2$ biosynthesis, also inhibits reocclusion (64), suggesting that platelet aggregation limits the response to coronary thrombolysis but that the reocclusion is only partly $TxA_2$ dependent (57).

$TxA_2$ synthase inhibitors as well as $TxA_2$/endoperoxide receptor antagonists reduce arrhythmias which occur during the early phase of reperfusion following coronary occlusion (45,65–66). However, Kramer et al. (67) failed to show an important contribution of $TxA_2$ to arrhythmogenesis during evolving myocardial infarction. In carefully conducted studies in the subacute recovery phase of myocardial infarction, the $TxA_2$ synthase inhibitor CGS-12,970, which reduced $TxA_2$ formation to 15% of baseline, did not protect against the induction of ventricular tachycardia by programmed electrical stimulation (68). Contraction of deendothelialized vascular segments in humans, dogs, and rats in response to aggregating platelets can also be significantly attenuated by $TxA_2$ synthase inhibitors (69) and abolished by $TxA_2$/endoperoxide receptor antagonists. These platelet–vessel wall interactions can also be attenuated by serotonin receptor blockers (70), suggesting that multiple mechanisms are responsible for platelet-induced vasoconstriction.

## IV. CLINICAL TRIALS WITH PGI₂ AND ANALOGUES AND TxA₂ INHIBITORS

Because of the aforementioned beneficial effects of $PGI_2$ and its analogues and $TxA_2$ inhibitors, several trials have been conducted in humans with ischemic heart disease.

### A. PGI₂ and Its Analogues

$PGI_2$ has been given intravenously to normal volunteers (71–73) and patients with angina pectoris (74–77). In normal persons, $PGI_2$ has also been found to be a potent coronary vasodilator and inhibitor of platelet aggregation (71–73). The effects of $PGI_2$ administered to patients with ischemic heart disease have been less consistent than expected from initial animal studies. Infusion of $PGI_2$ to patients with pacing-induced angina pectoris and those with spontaneous angina failed to show any improvement in the angina threshold during the pacing-induced episodes, but it did show a sustained improvement in patients with spontaneous angina (74). In contrast, Bergman et al. (75) found that infusion of $PGI_2$ significantly increases the pacing threshold for angina pectoris, decreases platelet aggregation, systemic vascular resistance, pulmonary vascular resistance, and coronary vascular resistance associated with an increase in heart rate and cardiac output. Bugiardini et al. (77) studied 16 patients with severe coronary stenosis and found that $PGI_2$ caused ischemia in 6 patients and iloprost in 3 patients with a low angina threshold during pacing. Angina disappeared soon after $PGI_2$ was discontinued or after administration of aminophylline after iloprost. The investigators concluded that $PGI_2$ and its analogues may induce ischemia in some patients with coronary artery disease, probably by causing dipyridamole-like maldistribution of flow.

Chierchia et al. (76) failed to show a uniform effect of $PGI_2$ in patients with coronary artery spasm. In five patients with spontaneous angina and three with ergonovine-induced angina, $PGI_2$ failed to reduce the incidence and severity of ischemic episodes despite antiplatelet and vasodilator effects. Only in one patient, who had spontaneous angina due to coronary artery spasm, could they show a beneficial effect of $PGI_2$. Theroux et al. (78) also showed a lack of a beneficial effect of $PGI_2$ in patients with unstable angina, a condition with pronounced platelet aggregation. $PGI_2$ appeared to be detrimental despite its very potent platelet aggregation inhibitory effects.

Grose et al. (79) reported that the intracoronary $PGI_2$ infusion of patients with acute myocardial infarction resulted in partial reperfusion in only one of five patients. Kiernan et al. (80) evaluated the effect of $PGI_2$ infusion in patients with acute myocardial infarction. This was a randomized double-blind study of 45 patients with evidence of myocardial infarction of less than a 16-hr duration. The patients were given a 72-hr infusion of $PGI_2$ or placebo. No significant differences were found between the groups in terms of mortality, the development of congestive heart failure, cardiogenic shock, arrhythmias, recurrent chest pain, reinfarction, peak creatine kinase concentration, or the time to peak creatine kinase concentration. No significant difference in baseline ejection fraction was noted between groups, and no significant change in ejection fraction occurred within each group or between groups.

Thrombolytic agents are effective in the treatment of acute myocardial infarction, but the clinical outcome is limited by the failure consistently to induce reperfusion and by the frequency of reocclusion. The latter may be due, in part, to intense platelet activation in the coronary artery at the site of residual thrombus. $PGI_2$ stimulates platelet adenylate cyclase and inhibits platelet activation to all known agonists; as such it would be expected to enhance the response to thrombolytic therapy. However, a clinical trial failed to confirm this hypothesis. In a pilot study, Topol et al. (81) examined the combination of tissue-type plasminogen activator (t-PA) and iloprost, a $PGI_2$ analogue with a similar profile of biological activity, in patients with acute myocardial infarction. They observed no significant effect on patency at 90 min or reocclusion rates. Furthermore, there was no improvement in left ventricular function over the period of observation in contrast to controls. The lack of a beneficial effect of iloprost in this combination has been demonstrated to be due to the enhanced plasma clearance of t-PA in the liver as hepatic blood flow is enhanced by iloprost (82,83).

The apparent conflict between these reports and the failure to duplicate the beneficial effects suggested by animal studies may be due to several factors. The beneficial effects of $PGI_2$ in patients with effort- or pacing-induced angina could depend on the interplay of several factors, including coronary artery anatomy, collateral flow, the presence or absence of "jeopardized collaterals," the severity of the coronary artery obstruction, and the role of transient platelet aggregation in these patients. For example, in patients with 90% stenosis of the left anterior descending coronary artery, transient platelet aggregation could have a role in increasing the functional severity of the coronary artery narrowing. In such patients, $PGI_2$ might have a beneficial effect. In patients with a 90% stenosis of the left anterior descending coronary artery and a "jeopardized" collateral from the right coronary artery with a proximal 70% narrowing, infusion of $PGI_2$ could by its potent arteriolar vasodilatory effect produce coronary "steal" phenomenon. Similarly, considerable differences may exist among patients with coronary artery spasm. In patients with normal coronary arteries and vasospasm, $PGI_2$ may be totally ineffective; in others with coronary spasm associated with a high-grade proximal lesion, $PGI_2$ might be effective either by its direct coronary vasodilator properties or by its effect on platelet aggregation. The situation is obviously less clear in patients with acute myocardial infarction, who may have wide differences in platelet activation, collateral circulation, and the extent of coronary artery disease. Furthermore, as mentioned earlier, there may not be a critical deficiency of $PGI_2$ to account for the genesis of acute myocardial infarction.

## B.   $TxA_2$ Inhibitors

A number of compounds which selectively block the enzyme $TxA_2$ synthase in platelets, or block the $TxA_2$/endoperoxide receptors, or block both $TxA_2$ synthase and $TxA_2$/endoperoxide receptors have been developed and used in animal and clinical studies. Despite much early promise, the trials of $TxA_2$ synthase inhibitors or receptor blockers have been largely negative in all subsets of coronary heart disease (CAD) (84).

Thaulow et al. (85) showed that the $TxA_2$ synthetase inhibitor dazoxiben, but not aspirin, reduced myocardial ischemia in response to atrial pacing, which was quantified by coronary sinus lactate concentrations and ST segment depression. They speculated that preserved or increased $PGI_2$ production may have contributed to these effects of dazoxiben. However, other trials of the $TxA_2$ synthetase inhibitor dazoxiben (86) or the $TxA_2$/endoperoxide receptor antagonist AH-23,848 (87) showed no evidence of benefit in patients with stable ischemic heart disease. These observations raise the possibility that $TxA_2$ does not play a critical pathophysiological role in stable angina.

Since $TxA_2$ formation is clearly increased in unstable angina pectoris and in the early stages of acute myocardial infarction, it is possible that $TxA_2$ inhibitors may be effective in these syndromes. At least in one study (88), $TxA_2$ synthetase inhibitor given within 6 hr of the onset of acute myocardial infarction reduced $TxA_2$ synthesis and caused a modest (approximately 25%) decrease in cumulative creatine kinase release.

There are as yet no published trials on the effects of $TxA_2$ inhibitors when used in conjunction with thrombolytic therapy in humans, although these agents are currently being tested in clinical situations. Clearly, reocclusion after initial restoration of coronary blood flow in acute myocardial infarction continues to be a major problem. In a clinical trial of the $TxA_2$ receptor antagonist sulotroban (BM 13,177), 800 mg four times daily versus aspirin in patients undergoing coronary angioplasty, primary success appeared to be less than with aspirin alone ($P$=NS) (89). Follow-up angioplasty at 6 months showed restenosis in 65% of patients in the sulotroban group and in 61% of patients in the placebo group. However, the same $TxA_2$/endoperoxide receptor antagonist, BM 13,177 was shown to reduce saphenous vein graft occlusion from 11.5% (in the placebo group) to 3.1% in a preliminary report (90). Nonetheless, there is a paucity of published trial of $TxA_2$ inhibitors in patients undergoing coronary bypass surgery, although several trials are currently underway in patients undergoing bypass surgery and angioplasty. Both of these conditions are associated with intense platelet activation at the site of endothelial tear. Hopefully, the results of the ongoing trials will clarify the role of $TxA_2$ in coronary reocclusion after bypass surgery and angioplasty.

## V.  DIETARY ALTERATION OF $PGI_2$/$TxA_2$ AND MYOCARDIAL ISCHEMIA

One of the most exciting attempts to alter the balance between $PGI_2$ and $TxA_2$ production stems from the provocative observations by Dyerberg and colleagues (91). These investigators noted that Eskimos have a low incidence of myocardial infarction and an increased tendency to bleed. They suggested that the low incidence of myocardial infarction in this population was due to their ingestion of a diet rich in fish oil. They found that the ingestion of fish oil by Eskimos was associated with an increase in the n-3 unsaturated fatty acid eicosapentanoic acod and a decrease in the n-6 fatty acid arachidonic acid compared with Caucasians, who ingest a diet relatively rich in red meat. Unlike arachidonic acid, eicosapentanoic acid does not induce platelet aggregation in human platelet-rich plasma. Whereas arachidonic acid leads to the formation of $PGI_2$ and $TxA_2$, eicosapentanoic acid leads to the production of $PGI_3$ and $TxA_3$. $PGI_3$ seems to have the same vasodilator and platelet antiaggregatory effects as $PGI_2$. $TxA_3$, in contrast, does not have platelet-aggregating activity. Thus, the balance between the tendency for platelet aggregation, vasoconstriction, and its consequences is "favorably" altered.

Subsequent studies have shown that ingestion of a diet rich in mackerel for 1 week by healthy white men produced similar changes in plasma and platelet fatty acid composition to that found in the Eskimos (92). In another study of healthy white men fed a diet rich in fish oil for 11 weeks, platelet aggregation inhibition was found to persist for at least 11 weeks after the subjects had resumed their normal diet (93). Aspirin taken during the diet had a synergistic effect and further enhanced the decrease in platelet aggregation. These studies have suggested that a combination of dietary alteration and pharmacological alteration, either by inhibition of the cyclooxygenase pathway or, even more promising, by a specific $TxA_2$ synthetase inhibitor, might have an additive effect in further diminishing the likelihood of $TxA_2$ production, platelet aggregation, and their consequences.

The effect of altering $TxA_2$ production by fish oil has also been studied in dogs and rats with experimentally induced myocardial ischemia/reperfusion (94–96). Animals fed diet rich in fish oil diet had a significant increase in n-3 unsaturated fatty acid in their lipids, plasma, and platelets compared with animals fed a control diet. Dogs given fish oil diet had a significant reduction in infarct size resulting from electrically induced thrombus and the incidence of ventricular ectopic beats after infarction. Although these animals had a significant change in plasma and platelet fatty acid composition, it was of interest to note that there was no direct correlation between the size of the thrombus in the coronary artery and the extent of myocardial damage (94). These results led to a speculation that the increase in n-3 unsaturated fatty acid may have altered the vasoreactivity of the microvasculature and diminished any vasoconstriction that occurs after thrombosis. Dietary fish oil supplementation in rats was also shown to attenuate myocardial dysfunction and injury and arrhythmias caused by global ischemia and reperfusion in isolated perfused hearts (95,96). These cardioprotective effects of fish oil supplementation seem to occur independently of blood and plasma components and are related to an indomethacin-sensitive mechanism (96).

The effect of n-3 unsaturated fatty acids on vascular reactivity was studied in rats maintained for 3 weeks on a diet supplemented with fish oil. The aortic strips from rats fed with fish oil had significantly more eicosapentanoic acid and were less responsive to the vasoconstrictor effects of norepinephrine and arachidonate than those from animals fed a control diet (96). After blockade of the cyclooxygenase pathway with indomethacin, the difference in vasoreactivity to norepinephrine between the two groups was abolished. It was postulated that in the vascular strips from the control rats, arachidonic acid is enzymatically converted to the dienoic prostaglandins which contribute to the vasoconstrictor action of norepinephrine, whereas in the fish oil–treated animals, eicosapentanoic acid is released simultaneously with arachidonic acid and a diminution in the formation of dienoic prostaglandin occurs resulting in a reduction in vasoconstriction after norepinephrine administration (96). Further support for this hypothesis can be found in a study of humans fed a Western diet supplemented with cod liver oil (97). The blood pressure and the blood pressure response to norepinephrine administration can be reduced after the diet without major changes in the resting levels of plasma catecholamines, renin, or urinary aldosterone (98). Studies from our laboratory and other groups also show that fish oil potentiates vasorelaxation in response to endothelium-dependent relaxants (99,100) and preserves postischemic capillary perfusion (101). Although further research in this area is needed, it is intriguing to speculate that dietary alteration of prostaglandin synthesis alone or in combination with other pharmacological regulator(s) may play an important role in altering the natural history of ischemic heart disease and its consequences. However, a recent study by Ascherio et al. (102) in large number of normal subjects followed for several years failed to show any benefit of fish consumption on myocardial ischemic events. This large study obviously raises questions on the validity of previous studies showing the benefit of fish consumption (103). We have recently discussed many of the potential pitfalls in the interpretation of epidemiological studies on fish oil and cardiac mortality elsewhere (104).

## VI.  ASPIRIN IN ISCHEMIC HEART

Aspirin is an irreversible inhibitor of the enzyme cyclooxygenase in platelets, resulting in inhibition of $TxA_2$ and $PGI_2$ formation. It is a potent inhibitor of $TxA_2$-dependent platelet aggregation but does not inhibit platelet adhesion on the denuded vascular surface, nor does it inhibit aggregation in response to stimuli such as thrombin, collagen, or large concentrations of catecholamines.

Over four decades ago, it became evident that patients with degenerative joint disease on large doses of aspirin and salicylates had fewer coronary events than the population not taking these agents (105). Subsequently, with clear identification of platelet activation as the basis of thrombus formation in the narrowed coronary arteries, Folts et al. (106) demonstrated the inhibition of platelet-mediated coronary flow reductions by aspirin in the dog.

There is accumulating evidence that aspirin therapy reduces the progression of coronary atherosclerosis (107) and frequency of clinical events in patients with chronic stable angina (108). There is strong evidence of the benefit of aspirin therapy in unstable angina pectoris, a condition in which platelet activation is very profound. Several studies have demonstrated that the administration of aspirin decreases the evolution of acute myocardial infarction and mortality in patients with unstable angina (109,110). This benefit is independent of the dose of aspirin. A number of clinical studies have also demonstrated the benefit of aspirin when initiated alone or with thrombolytic therapy in patients with acute myocardial infarction. Aspirin decreases the frequency of reinfarction as will as total mortality (111,112). On a long-term basis, aspirin reduces the frequency of vascular events in patients with previous myocardial infarction (113). Taken together, these studies clearly indicate that aspirin is very useful in the secondary prevention of clinical events.

Two major trials, one in the United States and another in the United Kingdom, were designed to examine the effect of aspirin in the primary prevention of myocardial infarction. Whereas the U.S. study (114) clearly showed a salutary effect of aspirin, the British study (115) failed to do so, presumably related to the small number of enrollees. The combined results of the two primary prevention trials, however, continued to show a significant benefit of aspirin in the prevention of cardiac events in apparently healthy males (116). Therapy with aspirin has also clearly been shown to reduce acute as well as long-term occlusion of the coronary artery bypass graft (117). Data on the efficacy of aspirin in decreasing the high rate of restenosis after coronary angioplasty, although suggestive, are not as convincing in patients with acute myocardial ischemia (118).

Almost the entire body of data in various studies on the efficacy of antiplatelet drug therapy have been summarized in the recently published Collaborative Overview of Randomized Trials of Antiplatelet Therapy (119,120). The most widely used antiplatelet agent was aspirin, accounting for over two thirds of the data. Overall, aspirin alone reduced the risk of myocardial infarction, stroke, or vascular death by 26%; aspirin in all doses (from <160 to 1500 mg daily) was equally effective. Most of the benefits from antiplatelet therapy were seen in the first 2 years after initiating aspirin therapy. There was no evidence, however, that the treatment stopped being protective beyond 2 years. Similarly, meta-analysis of data in about 8000 patients undergoing vascular graft placement or angioplasty showed antiplatelet therapy reduced vascular reocclusion rate by 41%, which was highly significant (120). Similar results could be obtained whether the antiplatelet drug was started before the procedure or 24 hr afterward. Again, the most widely used drug was aspirin. Although direct comparisons of different therapeutic regimens were weak because of the small number of patients, there was no evidence for superiority of nonaspirin drug therapy over aspirin alone or when added to aspirin.

Since other cyclooxygenase and $TxA_2$ inhibitors have not shown a similar salutary effect on myocardial infarction as aspirin, the beneficial effect of aspirin on coronary heart disease must relate to mechanism(s) other than the inhibition of cyclooxygenase, such as anti-inflammation. Almost 20 years ago, Moschos et al. (121) showed that aspirin reduces arrhythmias in platelet-depleted animals subjected to nonthrombotic coronary artery occlusion by platelet-independent mechanisms. These animal data clearly suggest that the non–platelet-mediated effects of aspirin may play an important role in cardioprotection. Buchanan et al. (122) showed over a decade ago that aspirin can inhibit platelet function independently of the acetylation of cyclooxygenase. Aspirin attenuates interleukin-6 synthesis in leukocytes (123). It also prevents "leukocyte rolling" (moving along the blood vessel wall at low velocity) (124) and decreases nicotine-induced endothelial activation (125) as well as the activity of endothelial nitric oxide inhibitors (126). Other studies (127) have shown that aspirin reduces hypoxia-induced coronary artery vasoconstriction as well as the procontractile effects of activated neutrophils on the pulmonary artery (128). It is well known that catecholamines induce vasoconstriction and lipolysis, and Strom and Coffman (129) showed that aspirin decreases these effects of catecholamines. Aspirin also prolongs bleeding time by a mechanism distinct from the inhibition of cyclooxygenase (130). A recent study shows that a significant part of the effect of aspirin on platelet activation involves a nitric oxide–cyclic AMP–dependent mechanism (131). Williams et al. (132) have shown that endothelial denudation stimulates the proliferation of vasovasorum, and aspirin can prevent vascular growth after deendothelialization. Aspirin also prevents the macrophage-induced activation of fibroblastic cells (133). Recent studies indicate that high doses of aspirin can inhibit vascular smooth muscle proliferation (134,135), which may be the basis of its effect on chronic reocclusion of the bypass grafts for coronary angioplasty (120). We suggest that the beneficial effects of aspirin are not limited to its platelet-inhibitory effects.

## VII. SUMMARY

$PGI_2$ and $TxA_2$ are formed from AA via catalysis of cyclooxygenase. Animal and clinical studies showed that acute myocardial ischemia results in a marked increase in $TxA_2$ release and only a small increase in $PGI_2$, resulting in altered $PGI_2/TxA_2$ balance. Early animal studies showed that $PGI_2$ and its stable analogues, $TxA_2$ synthase inhibitors, and $TxA_2$ receptor antagonists prevent myocardial injury from experimental ischemia/reperfusion. However, clinical trials thus far have not shown significant benefit of $PGI_2$ and its analogues or $TxA_2$ inhibitors in patients with myocardial ischemic events. Some clinical trials show a marginal benefit of $TxA_2$ receptor antagonists in patients with myocardial ischemic events. $TxA_2$ synthase inhibitor plus $TxA_2$ receptor antagonist do not generally appear to be superior to aspirin. The beneficial role of aspirin in myocardial ischemia may be due to its antiplatelet effect as well as its anti-inflammatory effect. We conclude that $PGI_2$ and $TxA_2$ are important modulators of vascular tone and platelet activity, but augmenting $PGI_2$ and inhibiting $TxA_2$ in altering the course of ischemic heart disease remains unclear.

## REFERENCES

1. Hamberg M, Svensson J, Samuelsson B. Thromboxanes: a new group of biologically active compounds derived from prostaglandin endoperoxides. Proc Natl Acad Sci USA 1975; 72:2994–2998.
2. Catella F, Healy D, Lawson JA, FitzGerald GA. 11-Dehydro-thromboxane $B_2$: a novel index of thromboxane $A_2$ formation in the human circulation. Proc Natl Acad Sci USA 1986; 83:5861–5866.
3. Mehta JL, Roberts A. Human vascular tissues produce thromboxane as well as prostacyclin. Am J Physiol 1983; 244:R839–R844.
4. Chahine R, Chanh AP, Lasserre B, Dossou-Gbete V. Myocardial prostacyclin and thromboxane $A_2$ synthetase activities during ischemia and reperfusion in isolated rabbit heart. Prostaglandins Leukot Essent Fatty Acids 1991; 43:261–266.
5. Moncada S, Gryglewski R, Bunting S, Vane JR. An enzyme isolated from arteries transforms prostaglandin endoperoxides to an unstable substance that inhibits platelet aggregation. Nature 1976; 263:663–665.
6. Coker SJ, Parratt JR, Ledingham IM, Zeitlin IJ. Thromboxane and prostacyclin release from ischemic myocardium in relation to arrhythmias. Nature 1981; 91:323–324.
7. Walinsky P, Smith JB, Lefer AM, Lebenthal M, Urban P, Greenspon A, Golddberg S. Thromboxane $A_2$ in acute myocardial infarction. Am Heart J 1984; 108:868–872.
8. Stahl RF, Deutsch E, Fisher CA, Warsaw DS, Addonizio VP. Cardiac ischemia and endothelial function in the isolated rabbit heart. J Surg Res 1989; 47:97–104.
9. Tada M, Esumi K, Yanagishi M, Kuzuya T, Matsuda H, Abe H, Uchida Y, Murao S. Reduction of prostacyclin synthesis as a possible cause of transient flow reduction an a partially constricted canine coronary artery. J Mol Cell Cardiol 1984; 16:1137–1149.
10. Mehta JL, Mehta P, Horalek C. The significance of platelet-vessel wall prostaglandin equilibrium during exercise-induced stress. Am Heart J 1983; 105: 895–900.
11. Lewy RI, Wiener L, Walinsky P, Lefer AM, Silver MJ, et al: Thromboxane release during pacing-induced angina pectoris: possible vasoconstrictor in influence on the coronary vasculature. Circulation 1980; 61:1165–1171.
12. Mehta JL, Mehta P, Feldman RL, Horalek C. Thromboxane release in coronary artery disease: spontaneous versus pacing-induced angina. Am Heart J 1984; 107:859–900.
13. Tada M, Kuzuya T, Inoue M, Kodama K, Mishima M, Yamada M, Inui M, Abe H. Elevation of thromboxane $B_2$ levels in patients with classical and variant angina pectoris. Circulation 1981; 64:1107–1115.
14. Mehta JL, Menta P, Feldman RL. Severe intracoronary thromboxane release preceding acute coronary occlusion. Prostaglandins Leuko Med 1982; 8:599–605.

15. Szczeklik A, Gryglewski RJ, Musial J, Grodzinska L, Serwonska M, Marcinkiewicz E. Thromboxane generation and platelet aggregation in survivals of myocardial infarction. Thromb Haemostas 1978; 40:66–74.
16. Mehta JL, Feldman RL, MacDonald RG, Letts G. Effect of human coronary occlusion on thromboxane $A_2$ and leukotriene $C_4$ release (abst). J Am Coll Cardiol 1986; 7:106A.
17. Fitzgerald DJ, Wright F, FitzGerald GA: Increased thromboxane biosynthesis during coronary thrombolysis: evidence that platelet activation and thromboxane $A_2$ modulate the response to tissue-type plasminogen activator in vivo. Circ Res 1989; 65:83–94.
18. Fang YX, Chen X, Shen N. Beneficial changes in $PGI_2$ and $TxA_2$ by ginsenosides in experimental myocardial infarction. Acta Pharmacol Sinica 1986; 7:226–230.
19. Mochizuki S, Okumura M, Tanaka F, Sato T, Kagami A, Tada N, Nagano M. Ischemia-reperfusion arrhythmias and lipids: effect of human high- and low-density lipoproteins on reperfusion arrhythmias. Cardiovasc Drugs Ther 1991; 5:269–276.
20. FitzGerald DJ, Roy L, Fitzgerald GA. Enhanced prostacyclin and thromboxane $A_2$ synthesis in vivo in ischemic heart disease: non-invasive evidence of sporadic platelet activation in unstable angina. Circulation 1985; 72:111–113.
21. Mingazetdinova LN, Shaimukhametova LT. Thrombocytic-vascular hemostasis at rest and under physical loading in patients with ischemic heart disease. Kardiologiia 1993; 33:12–14.
22. Mueller HS, Rao PS, Greenberg MA, Buttrick PM, Sussman II, Levite HA, Grose RM, Perez-Davila V, Strain JE, Spaet TH. Platelet hyperactivity in acute myocardial infarction in man—effects of prostacyclin. Herz 1986; 11:116–126.
23. Mehta P, Mehta JL. Platelet function studies in coronary heart disease: VIII. Decreased platelet sensitivity to prostacyclin in patients with myocardial ischemia. Thromb Res 1980; 18:273–277.
24. Sinzinger H, Kaliman J, Widhalm K, Patchinger O, Probst P. Value of platelet sensitivity to antiaggregatory prostaglandins ($PGI_2$, $PGE_1$, $PGE_2$) in 50 patients with myocardial infarction at young age. Prostaglandins Med 1981; 7:125–132.
25. Araki H, Lefer AM. Role of prostacyclin in the preservation of ischemic myocardial tissue in the perfused cat heart. Circ Res 1980; 47:757–763.
26. Jugdutt BI: Effect of $PGE_1$, $PGE_2$ and $PGI_2$ on ventricular arrhythmias during myocardial infarction in consious dogs: relation to infarct size. Prostaglandins Med 1981; 7:431–455.
27. Yamamoto T, Kikuta C, Hosoki K. U-46619–induced ischemic electrocardiographic changes in rats: preventive effects of prostacyclin and nitroglycerin. J Pharmacol 1994; 46:558–562.
28. Romson JL, Haack DW, Abrams GD, Lucchesi BR. Prevention of occlusive coronary artery thrombosis by prostacyclin infusion in the dog. Circulation 1981; 64:906–914.
29. Linz W, Lau HH, Beck G, Schokens BA. Influence of the thromboxane synthe-

tase inhibitor HOE 944, prostacyclin and indomethacin on reperfusion arrhythmias, cardiodynamics and metabolism in isolated ischemic rat hearts. Biomed Biochim Acta 1988; 47:S23–26.

30. Schrör K, Addicks K, Darius H, Ohlendorf R, Rösen P. $PGI_2$ inhibits ischemia-induced platelet activation and prevents myocardial damage by inhibition of catecholamine release from adrenergic nerve terminals: evidence for cAMP as common denominator. Thromb Res 1980; 21:175–180.

31. Lefer AM, Ogletree ML, Smith JB, Silver MJ, Nicolaou KC, Barnette WE, Gasic GP. Prostacyclin: a potentially valuable agent for preserving myocardial tissue in acute myocardial ischemia. Science 1978; 200:52–54.

32. Fanton JC, Kines DA. $PGE_2$ and $PGI_2$ modulation of superoxide production by human neutrophils. Biochem Biophys Res Commun 1983; 11:506.

33. Simpson PJ, Mitsos SE, Ventura A, Gallagher KP, Fantone JC, Abrams GD, Schork MA, Lucchesi BR. Prostacyclin protects ischemic reperfused myocardium in the dog by inhibition of neutrophil activation. Am Heart J 1987; 113:129–137.

34. Szekeres L, Tosaki A. Release of 6-keto-$PGF_1$ alpha and thromboxane $B_2$ in late appearing cardioprotection induced by the stable PGI anologue: 7-oxo-$PGI_2$. Mol Cell Biochem 1993; 119:129–132.

35. Schrör K, Ohlendorf R, Darius H. Beneficial effects of a new carbacyclin derivative ZK36,374 in acute myocardial ischemia. J Pharmacol Exp Ther 1981; 219:243–249.

36. Hohlfeld T, Strobach H, Schrör K. Stimulation of prostacyclin synthesis by defibrotide: improved contractile recovery from myocardial "stunning." J Cardiovasc Pharmacol 1991; 17:108–115.

37. Seuter F, Busse WD, Meng K, Hoffmeister F, Moller E, Horstmann H. The antithrombotic activity of BAYg6575. Arznemittelforsch 1979; 29:54–59.

38. Shea MJ, Driscoll EM, Romson JL, Pitt B, Lucchesi BR. The beneficial effects of nafazatrom (BAYg6575) on experimental coronary thrombosis. Am Heart J 1984; 107:629–637.

39. Needleman P, Raz A, Ferrendelli JA, Minkes M. Application of imidazole as a selective inhibitor of thromboxane synthetase in human platelets. Proc Natl Acad Sci USA 1977; 74:1716–1720.

40. Tai H, Lee N, Tai C. Inhibition of thromboxane synthesis and platelet aggregation by pyridine and its derivatives. In Samuelsson B, Ramwell PW, Paoletti R, eds. Advances in Prostaglandin and Thromboxane Research. New York: Raven Press, 1980:447–452.

41. Marcus AJ, Weksler BB, Jaffe EA, Brockman MJ. Synthesis of prostacyclin from platelet-derived endoperoxides by cultured human endothelial cells. J Clin Invest 1980; 66:979–986.

42. Mehta JL, Mehta P, Lawson DL, Ostrowski N, Brigmon L. Influence of selective thromboxane synthetase blocker CGS-13080 on thromboxane and prostacyclin biosynthesis in whole blood: evidence for synthesis of prostacyclin by leukocytes from platelet-derived endoperoxides. J Lab Clin Med 1985; 106:246–252.

43. FitzGerald GA, Brash AR, Oates JA, Pederson AK. Endogenous prostacyclin biosynthesis and platelet function during selective inhibition of thromboxane synthetase in man. J Clin Invest 1983; 71:1336–1346.

44. Mehta JL, Lawson DL, Mehta P. Modulation of human neutrophil superoxide production by selective thromboxane synthetase inhibitor U63,557A. Life Sci 1988; 43:923–928.

45. Burke SE, Lefer AM, Smith GM, Smith JB. Prevention of extension of ischemic damage following acute myocardial ischemia by dazoxiben, a new thromboxane synthetase inhibitor. Br J Clin Pharmacol 1983; 15:97S–101S.

45. Mehta JL, Nichols WW, Schofield R, Donnelly WH, Chandna VK. TxA$_2$ inhibition and ischemia-induced loss of myocardial function and reactive hyperemia. Am J Physiol 1990; 258: H1402–H1408.

46. Lefer AM, Messenger M, Okamatsu S. Salutary actions of thromboxane synthetase inhibition during global myocardial ischemia. Naunyn Schmiedebergs Arch Pharmacol 1982; 321:130–134.

47. Mullane KM, Fornabio D. Thromboxane synthetase inhibitor reduce infarct size by a platelet-dependent, aspirin-sensitive meshanism. Circ Res 1988; 62: 668–678.

48. Nichols WW, Mehta JL, Wargovich TJ, Franzini D, Ward MB, Lawson D. Similar reduction in myocardial neutrophil accumulation and extension of myocardial infarct size following administration of thromboxane synthetase inhibitor or thromboxane receptor antagonist. Angiology 1989; 40:209–221.

49. Wargovich TJ, Mehta JL, Nichols WW, Ward MB, Urban P, Lawson D, Franzini D, Conti CR. Reduction in myocardial neutrophil accumulation and infarct size following administration of thromboxane inhibitor U63,557A. Am Heart J 1987; 114:1078–1085.

50. Mehta JL, Mehta P, Lopez LM, Ostrowski N, Aguila E. Platelet function and biosynthesis of prostacyclin and thromboxane A$_2$ in whole blood upon aspirin administration in man. J Am Coll Cardiol 1984; 4:806–811.

51. Kyrle PA, Eichler HG, Jager U, Lechner K. Inhibition of prostacyclin and thromboxane A$_2$ generation by low-dose aspirin at the site of plug formation in man in vivo. Circulation 1987; 75:1025–1030.

52. Brezinski ME, Yanagisawa A, Darius H, Lefer AM. Anti-ischemic actions of a new thromboxane receptor antagonist during acute myocardial ischemia in cats. Am Heart J 1985; 110:1161–1168.

53. Grover GJ, Schumacher WA. Effect of thromboxane A$_2$ receptor antagonist SQ30741 on ultimate myocardial infarct size, reperfusion injury and coronary flow reserve. J Pharmacol Exp Ther 1989; 248:484–491.

54. Osborne JA, Lefer AM. Cardioprotective actions of thromboxane receptor antagonism in ischemic atherosclerotic rabbits. Am J Physiol 1988; 255: H318–H324.

55. Thiemermann C, Ney P, Schrör K. The thromboxane receptor antagonist, daltrobin, protects the myocardium from ischemic injury resulting in suppression of leukocytosis. Eur J Pharmacol 1988; 155:57–67.

56. Aiken JW, Shebuski RJ, Miller OV, Gorman RR. Endogenous prostacyclin

contributes to the efficacy of a thromboxane synthase inhibitor for preventing coronary artery thrombosis. J Pharmacol Exp Ther 1981; 219:299–308.

57. Ashton J, Schmidt JM, Campbell WB, Ogletree ML, Raheja S, Taylor AL, Fitzgerald C, Buja LM, Willerson JT. Inhibition of cyclic flow variations in stenosed canine coronary arteries by thromboxane $A_2$/prostaglandin $H_2$ receptor antagonists. Circ Res 1986; 59:569–578.

58. Golino P, Buja LM, Ashton JH, Kulkarni P, Taylor AL, Willerson JT. Effect of thromboxane and serotonin receptor antagonists on intracoronary platelet deposition in dogs with experimentally stenosed coronary arteries. Circ Res 1988; 78:701–711.

59. Kondo L, Seo R, Naka M, Kitagawa T, Wakitani K, Sakata M, Kira H, Okegawa T, Kawasaki A. Effects of ONO-3708, an antagonist of the thromboxane $A_2$/prostaglandin endoperoxide receptor, on platelet aggregation and thrombosis. Eur J Pharmacol 1989; 163:253–261.

60. Shea MJ, Driscoll EM, Romson JL, Pitt B, Lucchesi BR. Effects of OKY-1581, a thromboxane synthetase inhibitor, on coronary thrombosis in the conscious dog. Eur J Pharmacol 1984; 105:285–291.

61. Simpson PJ, Smith CB, Rosenthal G, Lucchesi BR. Reduction in the incidence of thrombosis by the thromboxane synthetase inhibitor CGS-13080 in a canine model of coronary artery injury. J Pharmacol Exp Ther 1986; 238:497–501.

62. Fitzgerald DJ, Doran J, Jackson E, FitzGerald GA. Coronary vascular occlusion mediated via thromboxane $A_2$-prostaglandin endoperoxide receptor activation in vivo. J Clin Invest 1986; 77:496–502.

63. Mickelson JK, Simpson PJ, Gallas MT, Lucchesi BR. Thromboxane synthetase inhibition with CGS 13080 improves coronary blood flow after streptokinase-induced thrombolysis. Am Heart J 1987; 113:1345–1352.

64. Fitzgerald DJ, Wright F, FitzGerald GA. Increased thromboxane biosynthesis during coronary thrombolysis: evidence that platelet activation and thromboxane $A_2$ modulate the response to tissue-type plasminogen activator in vivo. Circ Res 1989; 65:83–94.

65. Coker SJ, Parratt JR. AH-23848, a thromboxane antagonist, suppresses ischemia and reperfusion-induced arrhythmias in anaethetized greyhounds. Br J Pharmacol 1985; 86:259–264.

66. Wainwright C, Parratt J. Antiarrhythmic effects of the thromboxane antagonist BM 13,177. Eur J Pharmacol 1987; 133:257–264.

67. Kramer J, Davis A, Dean R, McCluskey E, Needleman P, Corr PB. Thromboxane $A_2$ does not contribute to arrhythmogenesis during evolving myocardial infarction. J Cardiovasc Pharmacol 1985; 7:1069–1075.

68. Kitzen JM, Lynch JJ, Upricharol ACG, Venkatech N, Lucchesi BR: Failure of thromboxane synthetase inhibition to protect the post-infarcted heart against the induction of ventricular tachycardia and ventricular fibrillation in a conscious canine model of sudden coronary death. Pharmacology 1988; 37:171–186.

69. Houston DS, Shepherd JT, Vanhoutte PM. Aggregating human platelets cause direct contraction and endothelium-dependent relaxation of isolated canine coronary arteries. J Clin Invest 1986; 78:539–544.

70. Yang BC, Mehta JL. Prior episode of anoxia attenuates vasorelaxation in response to subsequent episode of anoxia. J Cardiovasc Pharmacol 1994; 28: 387–394.
71. Szczeklik A, Gryglewski RJ, Nizankowski R, Musial J, Picton R, Mruk J. Circulatory and anti-platelet effects of intravenous prostacyclin in healthy men. Pharmacol Res Commun 1978; 10:545–556.
72. Szczeklik J, Szczeklik A, Nizankowski R. Haemodynamic changes induced by prostacyclin in man. Br Heart J 1980; 44:254–258.
73. Data JL, Molony BA, Meinzinger MM, Gorman RR. Intravenous infusion of prostacyclin sodium in man: clinical effects and influence on platelet adenosine diphosphate sensitivity and adenosine 3':5'-cyclic monophosphate levels. Circulation 1981; 64:4–12.
74. Szczeklik A, Szczeklik J, Ninankowski R, Gluszko P. Prostacyclin for acute coronary insufficiency. Artery 1980; 8:7–11.
75. Bergman G, Daly R, Atkinson L, Rothman M, Richardson PJ, Jackson G. Prostacyclin: hemodynamic and metabolic effects in patients with coronary artery disease. Lancet 1981; 1:569–572.
76. Chierchia S, Patrono C, Crea F, Ciabattoni G, De Caterina R, Cinotti GA, Dostante A, Maseri A. Effects of intravenous prostacyclin in variant angina. Circulation 1982; 65:470–477.
77. Bugiardini R, Galvani M, Ferrini D, Gridelli C, Tollemeto D, Macri N, Puddu P, Lenzi S. Myocardial ischemia during intravenous prostacyclin administration: hemodynamic findings and precautionary measures. Am Heart J 1987; 113:234–240.
78. Theroux P, Latour JG, Diodati J, Leger-Gauthier C, Morissette D, Boxch X, de-Lara J, Waters D. Hemodynanic, platelet and clinical responses to prostacyclin in unstable angina. Am J Cardiol 1990; 65:1084–1089.
79. Grose R, Greenberg M, Strain J, Mueller H. Intracoronary prostacyclin in evolving acute myocardial infarction. Am J Cardiol 1985; 55:1265–1266.
80. Kiernan FJ, Kluger J, Regnier JC, Rutkowski M, Fieldman A. Epoprostenol sodium (prostacyclin) infusion in acute myocardial infarction. Br Heart J 1986; 56:428–432.
81. Topol EJ, Ellis SG, Califf RM, George BS, Stump DC, Bates ER, Nabel EG, Walton JA, Candela RJ, Lee KL, Kline EM, Pitt B, TAMI-4 Study Group. Combined tissue-type plasminogen activator and prostacyclin therapy for acute myocardial infarction. J Am Coll Cardiol 1989; 14:877–884.
82. Nicolini FA, Mehta JL, Nichols WW, Saldeen TGP, Grant M. Prostacyclin analog iloprost decreases thrombolytic potential of t-PA in canine coronary thrombosis. Circulation 1990; 81:1115–1122.
83. Kerin DM, Shuh M, Kunitada S, Fitzgerald GA, Fitzgerald DJ. A prostacyclin analog impairs the response to tissue-type plasminogen activator during coronary thrombolysis: evidence for a pharmacokinetic interaction. J Pharmacol Exp Ther 1991; 357:487–492.
84. Mehta JL, Nichols WW. The potential role of thromboxane inhibitors in preventing myocardial ischemic injury. Drugs 1990; 40:657–665.

85. Thaulow E, Dale J, Myhre E. Effects of a selective thromboxane synthetase inhibitor, dazoxiben, and of acetylsalicylic acid in myocardial ischemia in patients with coronary artery disease. Am J Cardiol 1984; 53:1255–1258.
86. Reuben SR, Kuan P, Cairns J, Gyde OH. Effects of dazoxiben on exercise performance in chronic stable angina. Br J Clin Pharmacol 1983; 15S:835–865.
87. De-bono DP, Lumley P, Been M, Keery R, Ince SE, Wooding DF. Effect of the specific thromboxane receptor blocking drug AH-23848 in patients with angina pectoris. Br Heart J 1986; 56:509–517.
88. Tada M, Hoshida S, Kuzuya Y, Inoue M, Minamino T, Abe H. Augmented thromboxane $A_2$ generation and efficacy of its blockade on acute myocardial infarction. Int J Cardiol 1985; 8:301–312.
89. Finci L, Hoflins B, Ludwig B, Bulitta M, Steffenino G, et al. Sultroban during and after coronary angioplasty: a double-blind placebo controlled study. Z Kardiol 1989; 78(suppl 3):50–54.
90. Hacker RW, Torka MC, Yukseltan I, Pohlman V, Meier P, Zimmerman T, Etti H. Reduction of the vein graft occlusion rate after coronary artery bypass surgery by treatment with a thromboxane receptor antagonist. Proc Eur Soc Cardiol (Vienna), 1989; 325.
91. Dyerberg J, Bank HO, Stoffersen E, Moncada S, Vane JR. Eicosapentanoic acid and prevention of thrombosis and atherosclerosis? Lancet 1978; 2:117–119.
92. Siess W, Scherer B, Bohlig B, Roth P, Kurzmann I, Weber PC: Platelet-membrane fatty acids, platelet aggregation, and thromboxane formation during a mackerel diet. Lancet 1980; 1:441–444.
93. Thorngren M, Gustafson A. Effects of 11-week increase in dietary eicosapentaenoic acid on bleeding time, lipids, and platelet aggregation. Lancet 1981; 2:1190–1193.
94. Culp BR, Lands WEM, Lucchesi BR, Pitt B, Romson J. The effect of dietary supplementation of fish oil on experimental myocardial infarction. Prostaglandins 1980; 20:1021–1031.
95. Yang BC, Saldeen TGP, Nichols WW, Mehta JL. Dietary fish oil supplementation attenuates myocardial dysfunction and injury caused by global ischemia and reperfusion in isolated rat hearts. J Nutr 1993; 123:2067–2074.
96. Yang BC, Saldeen TGP, Bryant JL, Nichols WW, Mehta JL. Long-term dietary fish oil supplementation protects against ischemia-reperfusion–induced myocardial dysfunction in isolated rat hearts. Am Heart J 1993; 126:1287–1292.
97. Lockette WE, Webb RC, Culp BR, Pitt B. Vascular reactivity and high dietary eicosapentanoic acid. Prostaglandins 1982; 24:631–640.
98. Lorenz R, Spengler U, Fischer S, Duhm J, Weber PC. Platelet function, thromboxane formation and blood pressure control during supplementation of the western diet with cod liver oil. Circulation 1983; 67:504–511.
99. Shimokawa H, Lam JYT, Chesebro JH, Bowie EJW, Vanhoutte PM. Effects of dietary supplementation with cod-liver oil on endothelium-dependent response in porcine coronary arteries. Circulation 1987; 76:898–905.

100. Lawson DL, Mehta JL, Saldeen K, Mehta P, Saldeen TGP. Omega-3 polyunsaturated fatty acids augment endothelium-dependent vasorelaxation by enhanced EDRF and vasodilator prostaglandins. Eicosanoids 1991; 4:217–223.
101. Lehr HA, Menge MD, Nolte D, Messmer K. Favorable effects of dietary fish oil on capillary perfusion homogeneity after ischemia and reperfusion. Transplant Proc 1991; 23:2356–2358.
102. Ascherio A, Rimm EB, Stamfer MJ, Giovannucci EL, Willett WC. Dietary intake of marine n-3 fatty acids, fish intake, and risk of coronary disease among men. N Engl J Med 1995; 332:977–982.
103. Kromhout D, Bosschieter EB, de Lezenne Coulander C. The inverse relation between fish consumption and 20-year mortality from coronary heart disease. N Engl J Med 1985; 312:1205–1209.
104. Mehta JL, Nicolini FA, Saldeen TGP. Fish oil: panacea or fish tale? J Myocard Isch 1991; 3:13–14.
105. Craven LL. Experiences with aspirin (acetylsalicylic acid) in the nonspecific prophylaxis of coronary thrombosis. Miss Valley Med J 1953; 75:38.
106. Folts JD, Crowell EB Jr, Rowe GG. Platelet aggregation in partially obstructed vessels and its elimination with aspirin. Circulation 1976; 54:365–370.
107. Chesebro JH, Webster MI, Zoldhelyi P, Roche PC, Badimon L, Badimon JJ. Antithrombotic therapy and progression of coronary artery disease: antiplatelet versus antithrombins. Circulation 1992; 86:III-100-III-111.
108. Ridker PM, Manson JE, Gaziano JM, Buring JE, Hennekens CH. Low dose aspirin therapy for chronic stable angina. A randomized, placebo-controlled clinical trial. Ann Intern Med 1991; 114:835–839.
109. Cairns JA, Gent M, Singer J, et al. Aspirin, sulfinpyrazone, or both in unstable angina: results of a Canadian multicenter trial. N Engl J Med 1985; 313:1369–1375.
110. Lewis HD, David JW, Archibald DG, et al. Protective effects of aspirin against acute myocardial infarction and death in men with unstable angina: results of a Veterans Administration cooperative study. N Engl J Med 1983; 309:396–403.
111. ISIS-2 (Second International Study of Infarct Survival) Collaborative Group. Randomized trial of intravenous streptokinase, oral aspirin, both, or neither among 17,187 cases of suspected acute myocardial infarction. Lancet 1988; 2:349–354.
112. The RISC group. Risk of myocardial infarction and death during treatment with low dose aspirin and intravenous heparin in men with unstable coronary artery disease. Lancet 1990; 336:827–830.
113. Elwood PC, Sweetnam PM: Aspirin and secondary mortality after myocardial infarction. Lancet 1979; 2:1313–1315.
114. Steering Committee of the Physicians' Health Study Research Group. Final report on the aspirin component of the ongoing Physicians' Health Study. N Engl J Med 1989; 321:129–135.
115. Peto R, Gray R, Collins R, et al. Randomized trial of the effects of prophylactic daily aspirin among British male doctors. Br Med J 1988; 296:313–316.

116. Hennekens CH, Peto R, Hutchison GB, Doll A. An overview of the British and American aspirin studies. N Engl J Med 1988; 318:923–924.
117. Goldman S, Copeland J, Moritz T, Henderson W, Zadina K, Ovitt T, Doherty J, Read R, Chesler E, Sako Y, Lancaster L, Emery R, et al. Saphenous vein graft patency 1 year after coronary artery bypass surgery and effects of antiplatelet therapy: results of a Veterans Administration cooperative study. Circulation 1989; 80:1190–1197.
118. Barnathan ES, Schwartz JS, Taylor L, Laskey WK, Kleaveland JP. Kussmaul WG, Hirshfeld JW Jr. Aspirin and dipyridamole in the prevention of acute coronary thrombosis complicating coronary angioplasty. Circulation 1987; 76:125–134.
119. Antiplatelet Trialists' Collaboration. Collaborative review of randomized trials of antiplatelet therapy. I: Prevention of death, myocardial infarction, and stroke by prolonged antiplatelet therapy in various categories of patients. Br Med J 1994; 308:81–106.
120. Antiplatelet Trialists' Collaboration. Collaborative overview of antiplatelet treatment. II: Maintenance of vascular graft or arterial patency by antiplatelet therapy. Br J Med 1994; 308:159–168.
121. Moschos CB, Haider B, De La Cruz C Jr, Lyons MM, Regan TJ. Antiarrhythmic effects of aspirin during nonthrombotic coronary occlusion. Circulation 1973; 57:681–687.
122. Buchanan MR, Rischke JA, Hirsh J. Aspirin inhibits platelet function independent of the acetylation of cyclooxygenase. Thromb Res 1982; 25:363–373.
123. Komatsu H, Yaju H, Chiba K, Okumoto T. Inhibition by cyclooxygenase inhibitors of interleukin-6 production by human peripheral blood mononuclear cells. Int J Immunopharmacol 1991; 16:1136–1146.
124. Oude-Egbrink MG, Tangelder GJ, Slaaf DW, Reneman RS. Influence of platelet-vessel wall interactions on leukocyte rolling in vivo. Circ Res 1992; 70:355–363.
125. Blache D, Bouthillier D, Davignon J. Acute influence of smoking on platelet behavior, endothelium, and plasma lipids and normalization by aspirin. Atherosclerosis 1992; 93:179–188.
126. Rosenblum WI, Nishimura H, Nelson GH. L-NMMA in brain microcirculation of mice is inhibited by blockade of cyclooxygenase and by superoxide dismutase. Am J Physiol 1992; 262:H1343–H1349.
127. Toda N, Matsumoto T, Yoshida K. Comparison of hypoxia-induced contraction in human, monkey and dog coronary arteries. Am J Physiol 1992; 262:H678–H683.
128. Patterson CE, Jin N, Packer CS, Rhoades RA. Activated neutrophils alter contractile properties of the pulmonary artery. Am J Respir Cell Mol Biol 1992; 6:260–269.
129. Strom EA, Coffman JD. Effect of aspirin on circulatory responses to catecholamines. Arthritis Rheum 1963; 6:689–695.
130. Gaspari F, Vigano G, Orisio S, Bonati M, Livo M, Remuzzi G. Aspirin

prolongs bleeding time in uremia by a mechanism distinct from platelet cyclooxygenase inhibition. J Clin Invest 1987; 79:1788–1797.

130a. Valdez JC, Perdigon G. Piroxicam, indomethacin and aspirin action on a murine fibrosarcoma. Effects on tumor-associated and peritoneal macrophages. Clin Exp Immumol 1991; 86:315–321.

131. Lopez-Farre A, Caramelo C, Esteban A, Alberola ML, Millas I, Monton M, Casado S. Effects of aspirin on platelet-neutrophil interactions: Role of nitric oxide and endothelin-1. Circulation 1995; 91:2080–2088.

132. Williams JK, Armstrong ML, Heistad DD: Endothelial denudation stimulates proliferation of vasovasorum. J Vasc Med Biol 1990; 2:12–27.

134. Bernhardt J, Rogalla K, Luscher TF, Buhler FR, Resnik TJ. Acetylsalicylic acid, at high concentrations, inhibits vascular smooth muscle cell proliferation. J Cardiovasc Pharmacol 1993; 21:973–976.

135. Kaltenbach M, Kober G, Scherer D. Recurrence rate after successful coronary angioplasty. Eur Heart J 1985; 6:276–281.

# 3

# Clinical Use of Prostacyclins

## John A. Dormandy

*St. George's Hospital and Medical School, London, England*

## Glyn Belcher

*Schering AG, Berlin, Germany*

## I. INTRODUCTION

The medical community's response to the announcement of a new powerful naturally occurring locally active substance produced by the endothelium was colored by the long history of our experience with systemically active hormones secreted by endocrine glands. There must be a series of disease states characterized by faulty underproduction or overproduction of the prostacyclin. So far, no such "logical" disease state has been identified in relation to prostacyclin. Given that one of its principal sites of production and action is the endothelium, diseases of the circulation were the obvious place to look, but abnormal prostacyclin activity has not yet been demonstrated in any of the commoner degenerative peripheral vascular diseases. Undeterred, the search shifted to diseases where administration of additional prostacyclin may counteract the effects of a pathological process. This chapter describes the results so far obtained pursuing this line of reasoning.

Prostacyclin was first administered by Szczeklik and colleagues in 1979 to six patients with severe atherosclerotic disease affecting the legs. Because of its very short half-life in the circulation, prostacyclin had to be infused directly into the affected arteries. The initial response of these six patients in terms of relief of ischemic rest pain and healing of ulcers seemed promising (1).

A number of analogues of prostacyclin and related compounds were synthesized to try and improve stability. In order to obtain reasonable levels in the diseased arterial circulation, prostacyclin and other prostaglandins continued to be given in most studies intra-arterially. This is undoubtedly less convenient and more dangerous than an intravenous infusion, although the reluctance to use intra-arterial infusion is more marked in some countries than others. The development of stable analogues allowed infusions to be given intravenously over several hours. More recently, the problem of prolonged daily infusion, largely precluding use outside hospital, has been tackled by devising new slow-release formulations which allow single intravenous injections over a few minutes to achieve plasma levels lasting several hours (e.g., lipo-$PGE_1$) and by the development of orally active analogues (e.g., oral iloprost and beraprost).

The main thrust of clinical investigations with prostacyclin analogues has remained in patients with severe leg ischemia, as originally tested by Szczeklik 16 years ago. By far the largest number of patients participating in properly designed clinical trials have been patients with rest pain, ulcers, or gangrene due to severe ischemia. The largest body of evidence for the clinical efficacy of prostacyclin analogues is in this indication, which is considered in the first part of this chapter. But prostacyclin analogues have also been used in a number of other diseases, either affecting the circulation or where platelet activity is considered relevant, and these are considered in the second part of this chapter.

## II.   USE IN SEVERE LEG ISCHEMIA

### A.   Clinical Problem of Severe Leg Ischemia

It has been estimated that 1% of men under 50 years of age and 5% over that age have symptomatic arterial disease affecting the legs. In the early stages, this may only manifest itself as intermittent claudication (i.e., limitation of walking), but a proportion of affected patients will progress until they can hardly move without pain even indoors (2). Finally, the blood supply to the legs may become so restricted that they have pain even at rest or frankly nonviable skin with ulceration or gangrene. The term *critical limb ischemia* (CLI) is applied to these final stages where the imminent prospect facing the patient is a major amputation. Neither the prevalence nor the incidence of critical leg ischemia has ever been directly documented in an adequate epidemiological study. However, from small population studies and national figures for amputations, it has been estimated that the incidence of critical leg ischemia is approximately 1000 per million population per year (3). The fear of reaching this stage is something that is at the forefront of all patients' minds when told they have significant ischemic disease of their legs.

The pathophysiology and management of CLI has been a relatively neglected area of medicine until in 1988 when a Consensus Process on Critical Limb Ischaemia began in Europe (3). This brought together a number of specialists in the basic sciences and clinicians in the various disciplines involved with managing these patients. Because the underlying cause in the majority of CLI is atherosclerotic narrowing of the major arteries, traditionally its treatment has been the province of the vascular surgeon, who could possibly remove or bypass the obstruction. But unfortunately, reconstructive arterial surgery is only technically possible in a proportion of these patients, and such surgical intervention carries considerable risk. In the last decade, the increasing use of percutaneous catheter reopening procedures devised by radiologists has opened up another possibility for correcting the basic arterial narrowing (4). Nevertheless, even in centers where such specialized surgical and interventional radiological techniques are available, the fate of the patient with critical leg ischemia is dire. One survey has shown that even in centers of excellence, 19% of such patients have to undergo primary major amputation, 61% have an attempt at primary surgical or radiological treatment of the arterial occlusion, and the remaining 20% receive some type of temporary nonsurgical management. A year after developing CLI, only 56% will be alive with two legs, 26% will have had a major amputation, and the other 18% will be dead (5). The current prognosis for patients with critical leg ischemia is indeed very bleak.

## B. Possible Role of Pharmacotherapy in the Management of Severe Leg Ischemia

The Consensus Process on CLI brought together vascular surgeons and interventional radiologists, who in most countries provide treatment to the majority of these patients, with internists such as angiologists, cardiologists, and diabetologists, to determine the proper contribution from the respective specialities. Too frequently, angiology is still only practiced as a speciality in a few centers, although the pairing of angiologists and vascular surgeons should be as natural as that of cardiologists and cardiac surgeons. Theoretically, pharmacotherapy may be a primary treatment ideally avoiding the need for any form of mechanical intervention. A different role for pharmacotherapy could be an adjuvant to arterial reconstructions, angioplasty, and thrombolysis or to improve healing in more distal amputations.

Unfortunately, there is little solid evidence that any of the older medications widely used in the management of patients with milder manifestations of leg ischaemia (i.e., intermittent claudication) are really effective in the treatment of CLI. Indeed, even their value in the treatment of claudication is still sometimes questioned (6). The same has to be said for such maneuvers as isovolemic hemodilutation.

The use of drugs as adjuvant therapy during and following mechanical forms of therapy is much better established. But the amazing ingenuity of new percutaneous reboring techniques has not been matched by the necessary corrollary of maintaining patency in the reopened arteries. There have been surprisingly few prospective controlled studies of adjuvant pharmacotherapy following peripheral angioplasty.

The place and usefulness of primary pharmacotherapy as an alternative and preferred treatment to surgery or interventional radiology has recently been enhanced by the advent of prostacyclin and its analogues.

## C.  Pathophysiology of Critical Ischemia and Possible Mode of Action of Prostacyclins

Critical ischemic changes in the distal part of the limb are almost always secondary to long-standing proximal arterial blocks and stenoses. These develop gradually over decades, with the distal blood supply being maintained by the development of collateral channels. In patients with CLI, the development of collateral channels has failed to compensate adequately for the progressive arterial occlusions. In diabetics, the proximal atherosclerosis may be accompanied or even largely replaced by a more localized distal antiopathy. Severe leg ischemia is not invariably the outcome of the progressive deterioration. In some patients, it presents acutely as a result of arterial embolizations or more often as an episode of thrombosis superimposed on preexisting stenosing, but nonocclusive, atherosclerosis. The final changes in the microcirculation are the result of a decreased perfusion pressure. Prostacyclin analogues act largely at this microcirculatory level, reversing the changes resulting from a decreased perfusion pressure.

It has been suggested that the microvascular pathophysiology of severe leg ischemia is essentially made up of two components: a deregulation of the microvascular flow-regulating system and an inappropriate activation of the microvascular defense system. The microvascular flow-regulating system regulates and distributes blood flow in the normal microcirculation. It is characterized by the phenomenon of normal vasomotion, which allows regular periodic perfusion of different capillary networks. Endothelium-derived relaxing factor and one or more endothelium-derived constricting factors also play a role in controlling normal microcirculatory flow. The microvascular defense system is primarily a property of the leukocytes and platelets in the circulating blood and also of the endothelium. In health, activation of platelets and leukocytes occurs and there are interactions between them and the endothelium, which is an entirely appropriate defensive response to injury and infection. It is suggested that in critical ischemia there is a breakdown of both these normal regulatory and defense systems. The components of the inappropriate activation of the microvascular defense system include the local release of leukocyte-derived free radicals, proteolytic enzymes, platelet-activating factor, and an interaction between the responses of the activated white cells and platelets with the damaged endothelium. The trigger for this is a marked decrease in the arterial perfusion pressure following occlusion of the large proximal arteries by atherosclerosis. In addition, rheological changes occur in the distal microcirculation. The low shear stress and raised plasma fibrinogen allow erythrocyte aggregation. Similarly, the platelet and leukocyte aggregates also tend to cause microcirculatory occlusion. Leukocyte plugging is believed to be the principal effect of the low perfusion pressure at the level of individual capillaries.

The clinical benefit of prostacyclin analogues could be due to a reestablishment of the microvascular flow-regulating system and deactivation of the microvascular defense system. They can have no immediate effect on the fixed arterial block, and it is still uncertain whether it can substantially increase collateral blood flow. Clinical studies certainly do not suggest that they substantially improve the arterial perfusion pressure distal to the arterial block. They may, however, improve the distribution of what blood flow there is by reversing many of the local microcirculatory changes which had caused occlusion of the capillaries and by reestablishing normal vasomotion. The crucial, and ultimately the only, important question is whether they work in practice. The evidence is reviewed in the next section.

## D.  Clinical Efficacy of Prostacyclins in Severe Leg Ischemia

The fate of individual patients with severe leg ischemia is extremely variable. Although a number of risk factors have been identified, such as distal as well as proximal large vessel disease and the presence of coexistent venous disease, the outcome of standard therapy in individual patients is very uncertain. Even objective measures of the severity of the atherosclerosis affecting the leg arteries, such as the ankle systolic Doppler pressure, correlate poorly with medium-term outcome. It is therefore important to assess the efficacy of pharmacotherapy in large groups of well characterized patients. This necessitates multicenter studies.

The best evidence for clinical efficacy is obtained from randomized, controlled, prospective, double-blind studies, and it is these which are reviewed. In the majority of studies, placebo was used as a comparator.

Such trials have been performed with prostacyclin itself and its stable analogues: iloprost and tapostrene.

In early studies, the effect on rest pain and the healing of ulcers was used as endpoints. Although these are important outcomes, they are difficult to measure objectively. Furthermore, the more serious risk to these patients is loss of life or limb. One or the other is likely to occur in about half the patients within 6 months of developing rest pain, gangrene, or ulcers. A more valid primary endpoint for such trials is therefore the incidence of major amputation or death within 6 months of starting treatment. By comparison, short-term results in terms of change in ulcer size, for instance, are much less convincing. Double-blind placebo-controlled trials with native prostacyclin generally used only these endpoints after treatment of only a few days' duration (7,8). Most of the larger trials with prospective follow-up for major endpoints have used the prostacyclin analogue iloprost.

In this chapter, only published large, prospective placebo-controlled, double-blind clinical trials are considered where some form of objective endpoint has been used and where patients entered had severe ischemia causing rest pain, ulcers, or gangrene. Trials using less than a week's treatment are omitted.

## 1.  Iloprost

Seven hundred and forty patients were entered into six published multicenter trials fitting the above criteria (9–14). Only patients unsuitable for reconstructive surgery were entered; a quarter of the patients had reconstructive operations previously, which had presumably failed. Treatment consisted of intravenous infusion at maximum tolerated dosage for 6–8 hr each day. It was given for 2–4 weeks in the different studies. Three of the trials had a formal follow-up for a total of 6 months in terms of major amputation or death. The severity of the patient group studied is attested by the fact that in the placebo groups who received standard therapy alone, 57% had either died or required a major amputation within 6 months.

All the studies looked at ulcer healing and relief of rest pain at the end of follow-up. On an intention to treat analysis in five of the six studies, more patients showed evidence of ulcer healing in the iloprost group than in the placebo group, and in three studies, the difference was statistically significant ($P < .05$). Again on an intention to treat analysis, more patients were completely free of rest pain at the end of treatment in the iloprost group than in the placebo group; the difference was statistically significant in one study. The most important analysis, however, must be in terms of major amputation or death during treatment and follow-up. The reduction in the rates of major amputation and death by iloprost in the three trials where this information is available (11–13) are remarkably similar: 19 ($P = .02$),

17, and 14%. In summary, therefore, it would seem that a 2- to 4-week course of intravenous iloprost is beneficial in patients with end-stage severe leg ischemia.

## 2. Tapostrene

Similar published evidence for tapostrene is presently less extensive. In one recent study, 111 patients were given intravenous tapostrene or placebo twice daily for 2 hr each over 4 weeks and followed for 6 months. Results for all endpoints were slightly but statistically insignificantly in favor of tapostrene (15).

## 3. $PGE_1$ (Alprostadil, Prostavasin)

Although not a prostacyclin, $PGE_1$ is a prostaglandin with similar effects and has been used in similar clinical indications. It is therefore briefly reviewed here. Although initially $PGE_1$ was used intra-arterially, because it is rapidly metabolized in the lung, it was subsequently believed that intravenous infusion is equally effective. The best results using intra-arterial $PGE_1$ in a controlled study used ATP as the comparator. Sixty-five patients were treated for 3 weeks with no follow-up. Intra-arterial $PGE_1$ was said to be significantly better in terms of reduction in ulcer size and rest pain. During the 3-week treatment period, amputations were required in nine patients in the control group compared with three in the $PGE_1$ group (16).

Most trials with this compound suffered from serious methodological defects. For instance, two large studies of 302 patients with severe leg ischemia were all treated with an infusion of $PGE_1$. There were no control groups of any kind, and the results are therefore of little scientific value (17,18).

Applying the criteria of randomized, placebo-controlled, prospective trial of at least 1 week's treatment, there has been two studies of $PGE_1$. The first was in 23 patients with rest pain, which showed a statistically insignificant benefit in terms of relief of rest pain after 3 weeks of treatment and 4 weeks of follow-up (19). The same group published the following year a similar series with 46 patients; it is unclear whether these series incorporated the earlier patients. The findings now in terms of control of rest pain were statistically significant. The other placebo-controlled study looked at 4 weeks' intravenous treatment with $PGE_1$, and the patients showed a significant reduction in ulcer size and rest pain during treatment (20). The need for amputation during the 6 months after treatment was 11% in the $PGE_1$ groups compared with 27% in the placebo group. The largest controlled study of intravenous $PGE_1$ used pentoxifylline as control and was carried out in 70 patients with ulcers. 82% of the patients showed some evidence of healing during 4 weeks of treatment compared with 51% in the pentoxyifylline group (21). The need for amputation or other intervention in the subsequent 6 months was lower in the $PGE_1$ groups.

Incorporating the $PGE_1$ into lipid microspheres has the advantage of allowing a bolus injection instead of requiring an infusion, and this is also believed to result in higher concentrations of the substance to be localized in the endothelium. Lipo $PGE_1$ has been on the market in Japan for over 10 years. In a recent study of 166 patients with diabetic rest pain or ulcers given at least 2 weeks of injections, twice as many patients showed global improvement in the lipo $PGE_1$–treated group than in the control group. Unfortunately, there was no follow-up nor breakdown of results in terms of complete relief of pain, complete healing of ulcers, major amputation rate, or death (22).

## E.    Possible Future Clinical Uses in Severe Leg Ischemia

Prostacyclin analogues are undoubtedly the most promising form of pharmacological therapy for severe peripheral ischemia to be introduced in the last decade. This is a clinical area which has been somewhat neglected in the past and has been particularly bereft of any established drug therapy with really significant and widely accepted clinical efficacy. There are several exciting areas for the future clinical application of prostacyclin analogues in this area. Only patients with severe ischemia who were unsuitable for surgical reconstruction and catheter reopening procedures, or where these attempts had failed, were entered in the current trials. Given the promising results in these patients, it may now be appropriate to compare pharmacotherapy with reconstructive arterial surgery as primary treatment of severe ischemia. Limbsalvage surgery carries a definite mortality and is frequently unsuccessful, leading directly to a major amputation. It may well be that for high-risk patients, as many of these patients are, pharmacotherapy will be preferred to a precarious arterial operation. At the same time, the use of prostacyclin analogues as an adjunct to limb-salvage surgery needs to be tested. It may well be that an infusion during and after reconstructive surgery may improve patency and decrease mortality. Similarly, the combination of prostacyclin analogues with percutaneous peripheral catheter procedures is an important study that needs to be carried out in the near future. With the present pharmacotherapy following angioplasty, there is still a high incidence of early reocclusion in distal lesions.

Finally, there is the unexplored area of adjuvant pharmacotherapy for major amputations. Even when a major amputation is inevitable, there is much advantage to be gained in terms of rehabilitation and mobility if the amputation can be carried out below rather than above the knee. For this reason, a below-knee amputation is often attempted even when the chances of proper healing below the knee are uncertain. A review of the literature shows that 15% of below-knee amputations have to be revised above the knee and in a further 15% (23) healing is very delayed. It seems logical to try and improve the success of below-knee amputations by an infusion of prostacyclin analogue immediately after surgery when increased skin blood flow is essential for proper healing. So far, a trial of 700 below-knee amputations, looking at the possible benefit of an iloprost infusion for 3 days after surgery, has shown only short-term benefit during the period of infusion. Pharmacotherapy needs to be explored longer term.

All these areas remain to be fully explored with the present intravenous preparation of prostacyclin. But orally effective prostacyclin analogues have begun to be tested in large clinical trials and will open completely new areas of therapy, as well as possibly increasing the efficacy of the intravenous preparations by continuing with long-term oral medication.

## III. OTHER INDICATIONS

Because of the broad pharmacological profile of prostacyclin and its analogues, the compounds have a wide therapeutic potential in the therapy of other conditions where vascular physiology is disturbed and where cellular components of the blood (particularly platelets) are inappropriately activated. There are reports of benefits after the use of prostacyclins in conditions as diverse as the relatively common Raynaud's phenomenon to the extremely rare condition of heparin-associated thrombocytopoenia. For many of the conditions, there is currently no good understanding of the basic pathological processes involved in the diseases, but abnormal endothelial function is thought often to play a pivotal role.

### A. Secondary Raynaud's Phenomenon

The most intensively studied indication with prostacyclin and its analogues is secondary Raynaud's phenomenon. Raynaud's phenomenon as first described (24) involves episodic digital ischemia provoked by cold or emotion. It is clinically manifest by the tricolor reaction of blanching followed by the blueness of cyanosis and the redness of hyperemia, although it is now recognized that not all features need to be present. The phenomenon is relatively common, with a prevalence of about 10% and with women being affected 10 times as often as men (25), and is usually benign. However, in some patients, it can be so severe as to limit normal daily activities, and it can lead to digital ulceration or gangrene and subsequent amputation. Symptoms of the disorder tend to be particularly severe in patients with underlying connective tissue disease; most commonly systemic sclerosis or mixed connective tissue disease where 90% of patients have Raynaud's phenomenon as part of their disease (26). It is in this group of patients that most studies with prostacyclins have been undertaken. An overview of iloprost studies is given in Table 1.

It is known that patients with systemic sclerosis exhibit a number of abnormalities of the endothelium and the cellular components of the blood. Endothelial damage has been demonstrated by the finding of increased plasma levels of von Willebrand factor (27,28). Levels of this factor also correlate with the severity of Raynaud's attacks (29). Hyperfibrinogenemia secondary to an imbalance in endothelium-produced fibrinolytic factors has been reported (30). Turnover of prostacyclin itself is increased (31). Platelet responsiveness and platelet-release factors are increased in patients with systemic sclerosis (32,33), and it has been postulated that this is due to platelet resistance to prostacyclin (34). Increased white blood cell activity has also been demonstrated (35).

It is difficult to be certain which of these various effects could be a primary event and some are clearly secondary to the intermittent vaso-spasm which occurs in secondary Raynaud's phenomenon. However, it has been suggested that the initial lesion is that of endothelial damage which sets in train the vicious cycle of events of vasospasm and further damage which eventually leads to collagen deposition and fibrosis seen in the dis-ease (36). The presence of a serum factor cytotoxic to endothelium in patients with systemic sclerosis (37) would support this hypothesis.

Whatever the initial pathological lesion of secondary Raynaud's phe-nomenon, the resultant mixture of vascular and cellular abnormalities make prostaglandins theoretically attractive candidates as treatments of the disease. Initial reports of success of treatment used $PGE_1$ (38–40), but the only controlled trial failed to demonstrate a statistically significant differ-ence between active and placebo treatment (41). In 1981 Belch et al. (42) published a report showing benefit using $PGI_2$ given for 5 hours in 4 days weekly and followed this by a well-controlled placebo study confirming the result (43). Since then, most studies have used the stable analogue of prostacyclin, iloprost.

An early clinical pharmacological study in patients with systemic sclerosis demonstrated that after three infusions of iloprost of 8 hours daily at a maximum tolerated dosage up to 2 ng/kg/mins, improvements in digital blood flow (measured using photoplethysmography and strain gauge plethysmography) for up to 10 weeks following treatment could be seen (44). A more recent trial has shown similar long-term improvements in capillary density (45). Placebo-controlled trials using the same regimen in a crossover design confirmed that a reduction in symptoms was maintained for over 6 weeks following short-term treatment (46–48). Two further group comparative studies comparing placebo and iloprost given for 6 hrs each day for 5 days (49,50) showed symptomatic improvements in Raynaud's syndrome for 9 weeks following treatment. Iloprost treatment was also found to improve ulcer healing, and the subgroup of patients with ulcers was found to have the greatest benefit compared with placebo on a quality of life scale. Two trials have compared iloprost with nifedipine. In a double-blind, double-dummy trial, both drugs were found to be effective over 16 weeks, but iloprost produced better ulcer healing and had less side effects (51). In an open trial, iloprost was given for 8 hr on 5 consecutive days and then once every 6 weeks for 6 months compared with continuous treatment with nifedipine (52). Iloprost significantly improved frequency and severity of Raynaud's attacks compared with nifedipine. At 6 months, there were 27% less ulcers in the iloprost group compared with 4% more in the nifedipine group. A retrospective study comparing iloprost treatment with previous treatments for Raynaud's demonstrated that iloprost could improve symptoms in patients resistant to other therapies (53). Several isolated reports recommend iloprost infusions in digit-threatening upper limb ischemia due to a variety of other causes.

Currently, intravenous iloprost has gained acceptance as a second-line therapy for patients with severe disease and for patients with severe digit-threatening ischemia. Studies are now underway with orally active prostacyclin analogues, including iloprost and beraprost. It is possible that one of these agents will prove superior to currently available oral therapy and hold out the possibility that not only can the symptoms of Raynaud's syndrome be better treated but also the underlying connective tissue disease itself.

## B.  Other Vascular Pathologies

There are two other diseases involving vascular pathology where controlled trials have been performed with prostacyclin or its analogues. These are intermittent claudication and thromboangiitis obliterans (Buerger's disease). Although the evidence of the use of prostacyclins in the treatment of severe stages of lower limb ischemia is extensive and consistent, controlled trials in intermittent claudication are few and the results mixed. One trial of 106 patients gave prostacyclin or placebo over 8 hours for 5 days (54). At 2 months follow-up, prostacyclin-treated patients showed increased absolute and relative walking distance compared with those treated with placebo. Some small placebo-controlled trials with either iloprost or tapostrene have also shown increases in walking distance after treatment, but others found little effect, and the clinical significance of the results is questioned. It may be that the full potential of prostanoids in this indication will have to await

**Table 1** Controlled Studies with Iloprost in Raynaud's Phenomenon

| Authors | Treatment | Patients | Design | Follow-up | Main outcome |
|---|---|---|---|---|---|
| Yardumian et al., 1987 (46) | 1–3 ng/kg/min 8 hr × 3 | 10 SSc 1 MCTD 1 UCTD | Single blind Placebo controlled Crossover | 6 weeks | Reduction in attacks |
| McHugh et al., 1988 (47) | 2 ng/kg/min 6 hr × 3 | 26 SSc 3 RD | Double blind Placebo controlled Crossover | 6 weeks | Reduction in attacks |
| Kyle et al., 1992 (48) | 2 ng/kg/min 6 hr × 3 | 8 RD 9 SSc 1 MCTD | Double blind Placebo controlled Crossover | 6 weeks | Reduction in attacks |
| Wigley et al., 1992 (49) | 2 ng/kg/min 6 hr × 5 | 35 SSc | Double blind Placebo controlled Group comparison | 9 weeks | Significantly improved ulcer healing |
| Wigley et al., 1994 (50) | 2 ng/kg/min 6 hr × 5 | 131 SSc | Double blind Placebo controlled Group comparison | 9 weeks | Reduction in attacks Improvement in global Raynaud score Improved ulcer healing |

| Rademaker et al., 1989 (51) | 2 ng/kg/min 8 hr × 3 + 8 hr at 8 weeks vs nifedipine 30–60 mg daily | 23 SSc | Double blind Double dummy Group comparison | 16 weeks | Reduction in attacks with both treatments |
| Mascagni et al., 1994 (52) | 2 ng/kg/min 8 hr × 5 + 8 hr every 6 weeks vs nifedipine 46 mg daily | 35 SSc | Open Group comparison | 6 months | Reduction in attacks greater with iloprost; Reduction in severity of attacks greater with iloprost; Ulcer healing greater with iloprost |

SSc, Systemic sclerosis; McTD, mixed connective tissue disease; UCTD, unclassified connective tissue disease; RD, Raynaud's disease.

the possibility for longer term treatment using orally available compounds. Such trials are currently underway.

Buerger's disease is a rare condition of smokers in whom the distal arteries of both the upper and lower limbs are affected by isolated local vascular changes causing stenosis and thrombosis. The condition is seldom amenable to surgery and no medical therapy had proven efficacy. Patients usually progress to amputation. A double-blind study in 133 patients compared 100 mg aspirin daily with iloprost given for 6 hr a day at up to 2 ng/kg/min for 28 days (55). At the end of treatment, iloprost significantly improved ulcer healing and pain relief, which effects were maintained at the 5-month follow-up after therapy. At this time, 88% of iloprost-treated patients reported improvement compared with 21% of patients who received aspirin. Amputations were required in three iloprost-treated patients and eight aspirin-treated patients. This controlled trial is the largest ever undertaken in Buerger's disease, and iloprost is now considered the treatment of choice for such patients.

Although there are no other controlled studies, the use of prostacyclins, and in particular iloprost, has been reported in case reports or series as being beneficial in a number of other vascular conditions. These include, among others frost bite (56), antiphospholipid syndrome (57), rheumatoid ulcers (58), skin flap healing (59), accidental intra-arterial injection of drugs (60), and embolization after coronary thrombolysis (61).

## C.  Restenosis After Percutaneous Angioplasty

Percutaneous transluminal angioplasty is used to dilate short stenotic lesions in the coronary arteries (PTCA) or peripheral arteries (PTA) to improve blood flow without the need for surgery. Although these procedures are extremely effective, in a small proportion of patients, acute thrombosis occurs in the short term and restenosis at the site of dilatation within 6 months in up to 40% of patients. The latter complication has been the subject of much research, but its pathophysiology remains unclear (62). There have also been many attempts to reduce the incidence of restenosis using various pharmacological approaches, but a complete solution remains elusive (62). Local adhesion and aggregation of platelets to the damaged vessel wall with consequent activation of local haemostatic mechanisms is hypothesized to be a potential mechanism which initiates the process leading to restenosis (63,64). Because of this, prostacyclin appears as an attractive agent to test in the prevention of restenosis. Given immediately after angioplasty, it is also considered that prostacyclin's vasodilator effects could also reduce the early complications of vasospasm and thrombosis.

There are four controlled studies using prostacyclin or prostacyclin analogues during PTCA. Knudston et al. (65) gave prostacyclin or placebo single blind into the coronary artery for 15 min. periprocedure in 286 patients. This was followed by a 48-hr infusion given intravenously. At 6 months, there were more patients with restenosis in the placebo group (32%) than in the iloprost group (27%), but the difference was not statistically significant. However, acute vessel closure occurred significantly less often with prostacyclin (3 vs 10%) as did ventricular fibrillation or tachycardia (0 vs 3%). In a double-blind study, prostacyclin or placebo was given intravenously 36 hr following PTCA (66). The incidence of restenosis at 6 months was 31% for prostacyclin and 34% for placebo.

In the largest trial, 659 patients were randomized to receive the prostacyclin analogue ciprostene or placebo (67). Ciprostene was given into the coronary arteries for 15 min prior to PTCA and followed by intravenous infusion for 48 hr. At 6 months, restenosis was found in 34% of ciprostene-treated patients and 44% of placebo patients. Major clinical events (death, myocardial infarction, repeat PTCA, or coronary artery bypass grafting) was reduced from 30% with placebo to 24% with ciprostene. A retrospective reanalysis of angiograms (68) showed the change in minimal lumen diameter was 0.32 mm in the ciprostene group and 0.57 mm in the placebo group. The difference was statistically significant. A smaller study (69) using intracoronary ciprostene or placebo followed by intravenous infusion for 24 hr demonstrated that in 36 patients the mean residual stenosis following PTCA was similar in both treatment groups. At the 6-month follow-up in 24 patients, the mean arterial stenosis had increased to 51% with ciprostene but 83% with placebo.

These clinical trials demonstrate some evidence that the use of prostacyclin can reduce early clinical events and late restenosis after PTCA. However, the best dosage regimen and necessary concomitant antithrombotic medication, which varied between trials, remain to be determined. The possibility of delivering high levels of prostacyclins locally using special catheters or encapsulating the drug in platelets (70) open intriguing possibilities for the future.

## D. Pulmonary Hypertension

Primary pulmonary hypertension is an uncommon condition occurring in young adults, with women being more often affected than men (71). It is associated with a chronic progressive increase in pulmonary vascular resistance and an inability of the pulmonary circulation to adapt to changes during exercise. Eventually this leads to right heart failure and death (72).

Symptomatic treatment with calcium channel blockers has been shown to be effective in the early stages of the disease, but in later stages heart/lung transplantation is the only possibility.

Studies on the acute effects of prostacyclin showed that, with dose adjustment, pulmonary vascular resistance can be reduced and cardiac output increased (73), and this effect is used by some centers to predict response to long-term oral vasodilator therapy (74,75). Because of the favorable short-term hemodynamic effect in some patients, continuous intravenous therapy with the drug was investigated. It was found that such therapy could improve exercise tolerance over the long term (76). Using a tunneled subclavian infusion line and a portable infusion pump, it has been shown that prostacyclin could be given on an ambulatory basis (77,78). Using nonrandomized controls, it was suggested that such treatment could also improve survival (79), and this has now been confirmed in a prospective randomized trial (80,81). Similar acute effects on hemodynamic and long-term effects on exercise tolerance have been demonstrated using iloprost (82,83). This drug has also been used long term to treat patients with pulmonary hypertension secondary to collagen disease (84,85). The use of continuous ambulatory infusions of prostacyclin has offered new hope to patients with severe pulmonary hypertension.

## E.  Platelet Preservation in Extracorporeal Circuits and Other Systems

Because contact between blood and air or synthetic surfaces stimulates platelet aggregation, platelets are sequestered within extracorporeal circuits during cardiopulmonary bypass, renal dialysis, and hemofiltration. Patients are therefore at an increased risk of bleeding, particularly as they are also receiving concomitant heparin. Platelet aggregate embolization potentially leading to end-organ damage can also occur. Prostacyclins have been used as platelet aggregation inhibiters to try to reduce these problems.

In animal experiments, it was shown that prostacyclin could be substituted for heparin as an antithrombotic agent during hemodialysis (86). Using relatively high doses of prostacyclin, similar results were attained in humans (87,88), but hypotension was noted to be a problem and some questioned its feasibility (89). Given in combination with heparin during dialysis, some "heparin-sparing" effect was noted in some studies (90) but not in others (91). Currently, prostacyclin is not routinely used during dialysis but is reserved for patients who have a high risk of bleeding where its concomitant use allows some reduction in the heparin dosage. Similar results have been found using prostacyclin in hemofiltration and charcoal hemoperfusion (92–94). One added advantage in hemofiltration is that with the use of prostacyclin, the life of the filters can be increased.

Both prostacyclin and iloprost have been extensively tested in combination with heparin during cardiopulmonary bypass. Although general reductions in the consumption and activation of platelets were demonstrated, blood loss and transfusion requirements were either only marginally reduced or were not affected (95–98). Disappointingly, neither of these drugs reduced the neurological complications which are seen following cardiopulmonary bypass (99,100), and prostacyclins are not routinely used during these procedures.

One area where a prostacyclin has found common acceptance is in the management of heparin-associated thrombocytopenia. This is a problem occurring in a very small proportion of patients requiring heparin. In these patients, heparin administration causes a consumption of platelets which is associated with a high incidence of thrombotic and thrombembolic events. There is a high morbidity and mortality associated with the syndrome. The use of high doses of iloprost before and during heparinization for various surgical procedures has been shown to reduce the phenomenon (101–103).

Another area where stable prostacyclins have potentially useful effects is in the preservation of platelet numbers and function in platelet concentrates for infusion. Adding micromolar concentrations of iloprost to blood during platelet preparation considerably enhanced the quality of the stored platelets and might also allow longer storage than is currently possible (104,105).

## IV. CONCLUSIONS

The discovery of the endothelial product prostacyclin has lead to an increasing understanding of endothelial function, but for some years prostacyclin and its stable analogues were a potent therapy in search of a disease. Even now their best results are in relatively rare medical conditions. Prostacyclins have also shown promising results in areas where medical therapy was not previously available; in some cases, even modifying surgical practice. This chapter has mentioned some of these but has not, for example, discussed the use of prostacyclin in the intensive care unit for control of postoperative hypertension. Although in some diseases prostacyclins have already changed dramatically medical practice perhaps because of the need for intravenous administration, their full potential has not yet been fully exploited. The development of orally available formulations of prostacyclins which are now being tested may well expand their use and allow new indications to be fully developed.

*Dormandy and Belcher*

# REFERENCES

1. Szczeklik A, Nizakowski A, Skawinski S, et al. Successful therapy of advanced atherosclerosis obliterans with prostacyclin. Lancet 1979; May 26, 1:1111–1114.
2. Dormandy J, Mahir M, Ascady G, et al. Fate of the patient with chronic leg ischaemia. J Cardiovasc Surg 1989; 30:1;50–58.
3. Dormandy J, ed. European Consensus Document on Critical Leg Ischaemia. New York: Springer-Verlag, 1989; 53–69.
4. Krings W, Peters PE. Percutaneous procedures. In: Ed. Dormandy J, Stock G, eds. Critical Leg Ischaemia: Its Pathophysiology and Management. New York: Springer-Verlag, 1989.
5. Wolfe JHN. Defining the outcome of critical ischaemia: A one year perspective study. Br J Surg 1986; 73:321.
6. Housley E. Treating claudication in five words. Br Med J 1988; 296:1483–84.
7. Belch JJF, McArdle B, Pollock JG, et al. Epoprostenol (prostacylcin) and severe arterial disease. A double-blind trial. Lancet 1983; 1:315–317.
8. Nizankowski R, Krolikowski W, Bielatowicz J, et al. Prostacyclin for ischaemic ulcers in peripheral arterial disease. A random assignment, placebo controlled study. Thromb Res 1985; 37:21–28.
9. Brock FE, Abri O, Baitsch G, et al. Iloprost in der Behandlung ischamischer gewebslasionen bei Diabetikern. Schweiz Med Wschr 1990; 120:1477–1482.
10. Diehm C, Abri O, Baitsch G, et al. Iloprost, ein stabiles Prostacyclinderivat, bei artieller Verschlusskrankheit im Stadium IV. Dtsch Med Wochenschr 1989; 114:783–788.
11. Bliss B, Wilkins D, Campbell WB, et al. Treatment of limb threatening ischaemia with intravenous Iloprost: a randomised double-blind placebo controlled study. Eur J Vasc Surg 1991; 5:511–516.
12. Norgren L, Alwmark A, Angqvist KA, et al. A stable prostacyclin analogue (iloprost) in the treatment of ischaemic ulcers of the lower limb. A Scandinavian-Polish placebo-controlled, randomised multicentre study. Eur J Vasc Surg 1990; 4:463–467.
13. Guilmot JL, Diot E. Treatment of lower limb ischaemia due to atherosclerosis in diabetic and non-diabetic patients with Iloprost, a stable analogue of prostacyclin: results of the French multicentre trial. Drug Invest 1991: 3: 351–359.
14. Balzer K, Bechara G, Bisler H, et al. Reduction of ischaemic rest pain in advanced peripheral arterial occlusive disease—a double blind placebo controlled trial with iloprost. Int Angio 1991; 10:229–232,
15. Belch JFF for Scottish-Finish-Swedish PARTNER STUDY group. Taprostene versus placebo as a treatment of patients with critical limb ischaemia: the Scottish-Finish-Swedish partner study. Proceedings of Eurochap, Lund, Sweden, 1994.
16. Trubestein G, von Ludwig M, Diehm C, et al. Prostaglandin $E_1$ bei arterieller Verschlubkrankheit im Stadium III and IV—Ergebnisse einer multizentrischen Studie. Deutsche Medizinische Wochenschrift 1987; 112:955–959.

17. Grub JD, Bartels D, Ohta T, et al. Conservative treatment of inoperable arterial occlusions of the lower extremities with intra-arterial prostaglandin $E_1$. Br J Surg 1982; 69(suppl):S11–S13.
18. Heidrich H, Ranft J, Peters A, et al. Fruhund Spatergebnisse nach intravenoser Prostavasin-Therapie bei peripher-arteriellen Durchblutungs-Storungen mit Ruheschmerz und Nekrose. Vasa 1987; 20(suppl):202–203.
19. Diehm C, Hubsch-Muller C, Stammler F. Intravenose Prostaglandin $E_1$ Therapie bei Patienten mit peripherer arterieller Verschlubkrankheit (AVK) im Stadium III eine doppelblinde, placebo-kontrollierte Studie In: Heidrich H, Bohme H, Rogatti W, eds. Prostaglandin $E_1$-Wirkungen und therapeutische Wirksamkeit. Berlin: Springer-Verlag, 1988:133–143.
20. Stiegler H, Diehm C, Grom E, et al. Placebokontrollierte, doppleblinde studie zur Wirksamkeit von iv Prostaglandin $E_1$ bei Diabetikern mit AVK im Stadium IV. 21st Annual Congress of the German Society of Angiology. Augsburg, September, 1992.
21. Trubestein G, von Bary S, Breddin K, et al. Intravenous prostaglandin $E_1$ versus pentoxifylline therapy in chronic arterial occlusive disease—a controlled randomised multicenter study. Vasa 1989; 28(suppl):44–49.
22. Mizushima Y, Toyota T, Okita K, et al. Recent clinical studies on lipo $PGE_1$ and lipo $PGE_1$: $PGE_1$ and $PGE_2$ incorporated in lipid microspheres, for targeted delivery. J Control Rel 1994; 28:243–249.
23. Dormandy JA, Thomas PRS. What is the natural history of a critically ischaemic patient with and without his leg? In: Greenhalgh RM, Jamieson CW, Nicolaides AN, eds. Limb Salvage and Amputation for Vascular Disease. Philadelphia, Saunders 1988; 11–25.
24. Raynaud M. De l'asphyxre et de la gengrene symetriques des extremites. Paris 1862. (Translated by Thomas Barlow, London: New Sydenham Society, 1988).
25. Porter JM, Bardona EJ, Baur GM, et al. The clinical significance of Raynaud's syndrome. Surgery 1976; 80:756–764.
26. Gifford RW, Hines EA. Raynaud's disease among young women and girls. Circulation 1957; 16:1012–1013.
27. Kahaleh MB, Osborn I, LeRoy EC. Increased factor VIII von Willebrand factor antigen and von Willebrand factor activity in scleroderma and in Raynaud's phenomenon. Ann Rheum Dis 1981; 94:482–484.
28. Belch JJF, Zoma A, Richards L, et al. Vascular damage and factor VIII related antigen in the rheumatic diseases. Rheumatol Int 1987; 7:107–111.
29. Lau CS, McLaren M, Belch JJF. Factor VIII/von Willebrand factor antigen levels correlate with symptom severity in patients with Raynaud's phenomenon. Br J Rheumatol. 1991; 30:433–436.
30. Belch JJF, Drury J, Flannigan P, et al. Abnormal biochemical and cellular parameters in the blood of patients with Raynaud's phenomenon. Scott Med J 1987; 32:12–14.
31. Belch JJF, McLaren M, Anderson J, et al. Increased prostacyclin metabolites and decreased red cell deformability in patients with systemic sclerosis and Raynaud's syndrome. Prostaglandins Leukot Med 1985; 17:1–9.

32.  Reilly IAG, Roy L, Fitzgerald GA. Biosynthesis of thromboxane in patients with systemic sclerosis and Raynaud's phenomenon. Br Med J 1986; 292:1037–1039.
33.  Kahaleh MB, Osborn I, Leroy EC. Elevated levels of circulating platelet aggregates and beta-thromboglobulin in scleroderma. Ann Intern Med 1982; 96: 610–613.
34.  Belch JFF, O'Dowd A, Forbes CF, et al. Platelet sensitivity to a prostacyclin analogue in systemic sclerosis. Br J Rheumatol 1986; 24:346–350.
35.  Lau CS, O'Dowd A, Belch JJF. White blood cell activation in Raynaud's phenomenon of systemic sclerosis and vibration induced white finger syndrome. Ann Rheum Dis 1992; 51:249–252.
36.  Cooke ED, Ward C. Prostanoids in the treatment of Raynaud's syndrome associated with progressive systemis sclerosis. In: Cooke ED, Nicolaides AN, Porter JM, eds. Raynaud's Syndrome: London: Med-Orion, 1991:167–176.
37.  Kahaleh MB, LeRoy EC. Vascular factors in the pathogenesis of systemic sclerosis. In: Jayson MIV, Black CM, eds. Systemic Sclerosis: Scleroderma. Chichester, UK, Wiley, 1988:107–118.
38.  Clifford PC, Martin MFR, Sheddon EJ, et al. Treatment of vasospastic disease with prostaglandin $E_1$. Br Med J 1980; 281:1031–1034.
39.  Allen JA, O'Reilly MJG. Treatment of severe Raynaud's phenomenon with prostaglandin $E_1$. J Med Sci 1981; 150:190.
40.  Kyle V, Parr G, Salisbury R, et al. Prostaglandin $E_1$ vasospastic disease and thermography. Ann Rheum Dis 1985; 44:73–78.
41.  Mohrland JS, Porter JM, Smith EA, et al. A multiclinic, placebo-controlled, double-blind study of prostaglandin $E_1$ in Raynaud's syndrome. Ann Rheum Dis 1985; 44:754–760.
42.  Belch JFF, Newman P, Drury JK, et al. Successful treatment of Raynaud's syndrome with prostacyclin. Thromb Haemost 1981; 45:255–256.
43.  Belch JFF, Drury JK, Capell H, et al. Intermittent epoprostenol (prostacyclin) infusion in patients with Raynaud's syndrome—a double-blind controlled trial. Lancet 1983; 1:313–315.
44.  Rademaker M, Thomas RHM, Provost G, et al. Prolonged increase in digital blood flow following iloprost infusion in patients with systemic sclerosis. Postgrad Med J 1987; 63:617–620.
45.  Arpaia G, Cimminiello C, Sardina M et al. Microcirculatory effects of iloprost in patients with respected secondary Raynaud's phenomenon. Vasc Surg 1995; 29:37–42.
46.  Yardumian DA, Isenberg DA, Rustin M, et al. Successful treatment of Raynaud's syndrome with iloprost, a chemically stable prostacyclin analogue. Br J Rheumatol 1988; 27:220–226.
47.  McHugh NJ, Csuka M, Watson HR, et al. Infusion of iloprost, a prostacyclin analogue, for treatment of Raynaud's phenomenon in systemic sclerosis. Ann Rheum Dis 1988; 47:43–47.
48.  Kyle MV, Belcher G, Hazleman B. Placebo controlled study showing therapeutic benefit of iloprost in the treatment of Raynaud's phenomenon. J Rheumatol 1992; 19:1403–1406.

49. Wigley F, Seibold J, Wise R et al. Intravenous iloprost treatment of Raynaud's phenomenon and ischaemic ulcers secondary to systemic sclerosis. J Rheumatol 1992; 19:1407–1414.

50. Wigley F, Wise R, Seibold J, et al. Intravenous iloprost infusion in patients with Raynaud's phenomenon secondary to systemic sclerosis. Ann Intern Med 1994; 120:199–206.

51. Rademaker M, Cooke ED, Almond NE, et al. Comparison of intravenous infusions of iloprost and oral nifedipine in treatment of Raynaud's phenomenon in patient with systemic sclerosis: a double blind randomised study. Br Med J 1989; 298:561–564.

52. Mascagni B, Sardina M, Alvino S, et al. Effects of iloprost in comparison to nifedipine in patients with Raynaud's phenomenon secondary to progressive systemic sclerosis. Int Angiol 1994; 13(suppl):81.

53. Watson HR, Belcher G. Retrospective comparison of iloprost with other treatments for secondary Raynaud's phenomenon. Ann Rheum Dis 1991; 50:359–361.

54. Virgolini I, Fitscha P, Linet OI, et al. A double blind placebo controlled trial of intravenous prostacyclin ($PGE_2$) in 108 patients with ischaemic peripheral vascular disease. Prostaglandins 1990; 39:657–664.

55. Fiessinger JN, Schafer M for the TAO Study. Trial of iloprost versus aspirin treatment for the critical limb ischaemia of thromboangitis obliterans. Lancet 1990; 335:555–557.

56. Groechenig E. Treatment of frostbite with iloprost. Lancet 1994; 334:1152–2253.

57. Zahavi J, Charach G, Schafer R, et al. Ischaemic necrotic toes associated with antiphospholipid syndrome and treatment with iloprost. Lancet 1993; 342:862.

58. Veale DJ, Muir AM, Morley KD, et al. Treatment of vasculitic leg ulcers in connective tissue disease with iloprost. Clin Rheum 1995; 14:187–190.

59. Wilson Y, Cawthorn S. Use of iloprost for treatment of skin ischaemia after subcutaneous mastectomy and simultaneous prosthetic reconstruction. Breast 1995; 2:257–258.

60. Tait I, Holdsworth R, Belch JJF, et al. Management of intra-arterial injection injury with iloprost. Lancet 1994; 343:419.

61. Stafford PJ, Strachan CL, Vincent R, et al. Multiple microemboli after disintegration of clot during thrombolysis for acute myocardial infarction. Br Med J 299:1310–1312.

62. Herrman JP, Hermans WRM, Vos S, et al. Pharmacological approaches to the prevention of restenosis following angioplasty. Drugs 1993; 46.

63. Hacker LA. Role of platelets and thrombosis in mechanisms of acute occlusion and restenosis after angioplasty. Am J Cardiol 1987; 60:20b–28b.

64. Chesebro JH, Lam YT, Badimon L, et al. Restenosis after arterial angioplasty in a haemorrheologic response to injury. Am J Cardiol 1987; 60:10b–16b.

65. Knudtson MC, Flintoft VF, Roth D, et al. Effect of short term prostacyclin administration on restenosis after percutaneous transluminal coronary angioplasty. J Am Coll Cardiol 1990; 15:691–697.

66. Gershlick AH, Timmis AD, Rothman MT, et al. Post angioplasty prostacyclin infusion does not reduce the incidence of restenosis. Circulation 1990; 82: 111–497.
67. Demke DM, for the Ciprostene Study Group. Double-blind, placebo-controlled efficacy study of ciprostene (U-61,431F) in percutaneous transluminal coronary angioplasty (PTCA). Br J Haematol 1990; 76:20.
68. The Ciprostene investigators. Ciprostene for restenosis revisited: analysis of angiograms. J Am Coll Cardiol 1993; 21:321a.
69. Darius H, Nixdorff U, Zander J, et al. Effects of Ciprostene on restenosis rate and platelet activation during therapeutic PTCA. Eur Heart J 1991; 12:26.
70. Bunning AP, Penny WJ, Lewis MJ. Reducing platelet adhesions following angioplasty: the effects of platelet encapsulated iloprost delivered locally or intravenously. J Am Coll Cardiol 1995; 25:337a.
71. Rich S, Dantzker DR, Ayres SM, et al. Primary pulmonary hypertension. A national prospective study. Ann Intern Med 1987; 107:216–223.
72. Fuster V, Steele PM, Edwards WD, et al. Primary pulmonary hypertension; natural history and the importance of thrombosis. Circulation 1984; 70:580–587.
73. Guadagni DN, Ikram H, Maslowski AH. Haemodynamic effects of prostacyclin (PGI₂) in pulmonary hypertension. Br Heart J 1981; 45:385–388.
74. Roskovec A, Stardling JR, Shepherd G, et al. Prediction of favourable response to long term vasodilation of pulmonary hypertension by short term administration of epoprostenol (prostacyclin) or nifedipine. Br Heart J 1988; 59:696–705.
75. Reeves JT, Groves BM, Turkevich D. The case for treatment of selected patients with primary pulmonary hypertension. Am Rev Respir Dis 1986; 134:342–346.
76. Higgenbottam TW, Wheeldon D, Wells F, et al. Long term treatment of primary pulmonary hypertension with continuous intravenous epoprostenol (prostacyclin). Lancet 1984; 1:1046–1047.
77. Jones DK, Higgenbottam TW, Wallwork J. Treatment of primary pulmonary hypertension with intravenous epoprostenol (prostacyclin). Br Heart J 1987; 57:270–278.
78. Rubin LJ, Medoza J, Hood M, et al. Treatment of primary pulmonary hypertension with continuous intravenous prostacyclin (epoprostenol). Ann Intern Med 1990; 112:485–491.
79. Higgenbottam TW, Spiegelhalter D, Scott JP, et al. Prostacyclin and heart lung transplantation as a treatment for severe pulmonary hypertension. Br. Heart J 1993; 70:366–370.
80. Butt AY, Cremona G, Sharples L, et al. Continuous prostacyclin infusion of prostacyclin (PGI₂) improve survival in severe pulmonary hypertension. J Am Coll Cardiol 1995:221A.
81. Bardst RJ, Rubin LJ, McGood G et al. Survival in primary pulmonary hypertension with long term continuous intravenous prostacyclin. Ann Intern Med 1994; 121:404–415.
82. Scott JP, Higgenbottam TW, Wallwork J. The acute effect of the synthetic

prostacyclin analogue iloprost in primary pulmonary hypertension. Br J Clin Pharmacol 1990; 6:231–234.

83. Butt AY, Dinh-Xuan AT, Takao M, et al. Long term treatment of severe pulmonary hypertension with prostacyclin analogue iloprost. Eur Resp J 1994: 7(suppl 18):1745.

84. de la Mata J, Gomez MA, Blanco F, et al. Continuous infusion with iloprost for severe pulmonary hypertension in patients with collagen vascular diseases. Arthritis Rheum 1993; 36(suppl):5117

85. Bartram SA, Denton CP, DuBois RM, et al. Use of intravenous prostacyclin to treat pulmonary hypertension associated with systemic sclerosis. Br J Rheumatol 1995; 34(suppl):30.

86. Woods HF, Ash G, Weston MJ, et al. Prostacyclin can replace heparin in haemodialysis in dogs. Lancet 1978; 2:1075–1077.

87. Zusman RM, Robin RH, Cato AE, et al. Haemodialysis using prostacyclin instead of heparin as the sole antithrombotic agent. N Engl J Med 1981; 304:934–939.

88. Smith MC, Danviriyasup K, Crow JW, et al. Prostacyclin substitution for heparin in long-term haemodialysis. Am J Med 1982; 73:669–678.

89. Knudsen F, Nielson AH, Kornerup HJ, et al. Epoprostenol as sole anti-thrombotic treatment during haemodialysis. Lancet 1984; 1:235–236.

90. Turney JH, Williams LC. Fewell MR, et al. Platelet protection and heparin sparing with prostacyclin during regular dialysis therapy. Lancet 1980; 2: 219–222.

91. Dibble JB, Kalra PA, Orchard MA, et al. Prostacyclin and iloprost do not affect action of standard dose heparin on haemostatic function during haemodialysis. Thromb Res 1988; 29:385–392.

92. Gimson AES, Langley PG, Hughes RD, et al. Prostacyclin to prevent platelet activation during charcoal haemoperfusion in fulminant hepatic failure. Lancet 1980; 1:173–175.

93. Legat K, Zimpter M, Steltzer H, et al. Heparin and prostacyclin in haemo-filtration after orthotopic liver transplantation. Transplant Proc 1984; 3:1984.

94. Canaud B, Mion C, Arujo A, et al. Prostacyclin (epoprostanol) as the sole antithrombotic agent in postdilutional haemofiltration. Nephron 1988; 48: 206–212.

95. Walker ID, Davidson JF, Faichney A, et al. A double blind study of prosta-cyclin in cardiopulmonary bypass surgery. Br J Haematol 1981; 49:415–423.

96. Blauth C, Brady A, Arnold J, et al. A double-blind clinical trial of iloprost during cardiopulmonary bypass. Perfusion 1987; 2:271–276.

97. Martin W, Spyt T, Thomas I, et al. Quantification of extracorporeal platelet deposition in cardiopulmonary bypass: Effects of ZK 36374, a prostacyclin analogue. Eur J Nucl Med. 1989; 15:128–132.

98. Spyt T, Wheatley DJ, Walker ID et al. Placebo controlled study of iloprost (ZK 36374) in cardiopulmonary bypass surgery. Perfusion 1988; 3:179–186.

99. Longmore DB, Bennett JG, Hoyle PM, et al. Prostacyclin administration during cardiopulmonary bypass in man. Lancet 1981; 1:800–804.

100. Watson HR, Belcher G, Brierley J, et al. Iloprost in cardiopulmonary bypass procedures. Agents Actions, 1992; 37(suppl):346–353.
101. Kappa J, Horn MK, Fisher CA, et al. Efficacy of iloprost (ZK 36374) versus aspirin in preventing heparin induced platelet activation during cardiac operations. J Thorac Cardiovasc Surg 1987; 94:405–413.
102. Kappa JK, Fischer CA, Berkowitz HD, et al. Heparin-induced platelet activation in sixteen surgical patients: diagnosis and management. J Vasc Surg 1987; 5:101–109.
103. Gruely Y, Lermusiaux P, Lang M, et al. Usefulness of iloprost in the management of heparin associated thrombocytopenia and thrombosis. Thromb Haemost 1989; 62:49.
104. Johnson EJ, Mackie IJ, Machin SJ, et al. Preservation of platelet function in cryopreserved platelet concentrates with prostacyclin. Clin Lab Haematol 1984; 6:141–144.
105. Elias M, Heethuis A, Weggemans M, et al. Stabilization of standard platelet concentrates and minimisation of the platelet storage lesion by a prostacyclin analogue. Ann Haemtol 1992; 64:292–298.

# Nitric Oxide Synthases: Enzymology and Mechanism-Based Inhibitors

**John F. Parkinson and Gary B. Phillips**

*Berlex Biosciences, Inc., Richmond, California*

## I. INTRODUCTION

The discovery of the L-arginine/nitric oxide (NO·) pathway has provided a dramatic increase in our understanding of fundamental physiological processes, including regulation of vascular tone, neurotransmission, and immune function (1–3). Although NO· itself is one of nature's simplest molecules, understanding its role as a signaling molecule and as a destructive tool of the immune/host defense system is extremely complex. This complexity is derived from the exquisite diversity of its chemical reactivity with biological targets (4) and from the mechanisms nature has evolved to control its biosynthesis. As to the latter, it is now apparent that there are at least three major isoforms of nitric oxide synthase (NOS) expressed in mammalian systems which are derived from distinct genes: neuronal NOS (NOS-1), cytokine-inducible NOS (NOS-2), and endothelial NOS (NOS-3). When studying a physiological process subject to regulation by NO·, it is thus essential to appreciate that any given tissue or cell may contain one, two, or all three NOS isoforms which can be regulated independently at several levels via transcriptional, posttranscriptional, and posttranslational mechanisms as well as by direct regulation of enzyme activity.

As with other biological systems, this complexity is very relevant to the vascular biologist, since it has been shown that, depending on physiological or pathophysiological status, several cells of the vascular wall can synthesize NO·, including endothelial cells (5), platelets (6), macrophages (7), and smooth muscle cells (8). Blood vessels are also innervated with NO·-producing neurons which may provide another level for NO·-dependent regulation of vascular function (9). The vessel wall contains all three known NOS isoforms, providing fertile ground for the study of NO· in the regulation of vascular function.

The purpose of this chapter is to focus on the recent advances in our understanding of the enzymology and molecular biology of the nitric oxide synthases and the discovery of mechanism-based isoform-selective NOS inhibitors. These advances have provided more specific tools for research on the expression of the various NOS isoforms at the gene and protein level and for the pharmacological manipulation of NOS activity in vitro and in vivo. Further development of these tools will hopefully lead in the not too distant future to a better understanding of the role of NO· in processes of interest to vascular biologists and to novel NO·-based therapeutics for the treatment of vascular disease.

## II.  NITRIC OXIDE SYNTHASES

### A.  Enzymology and Catalytic Mechanism

Table 1 summarizes the biochemical properties of the three major NOS isoforms as revealed by studies with native or recombinant NOS enzyme preparations (reviewed in refs. 1, 2, and 10). NOS isoforms are homodimeric enzymes requiring FAD, FMN, tetrahydrobiopterin ($BH_4$), and heme as cofactors with NADPH, $O_2$, and L-arginine serving as substrates. Maximal NOS activity also requires the presence of reduced thiols such as dithiothreitol, $\beta$-mercaptoethanol, or glutathione. A further level of complexity is that the neuronal and endothelial enzymes (NOS-1 and NOS-3, respectively) are reversibly activated by $Ca^{2+}$/calmodulin (11, 12), whereas the inducible enzyme (NOS-2) contains calmodulin as a tightly bound subunit and is not activated by $Ca^{2+}$ (13).

All NOS isoforms catalyze the five-electron oxidation of L-arginine to form L-citrulline and NO· in a two-step reaction with N-OH-L-arginine as intermediate. NADPH provides reducing equivalents. The overall stoichiometry of both steps of the reaction is shown in scheme 1 (reviewed in ref. 2). Isotopically labeled arginine and $O_2$ have been used to show that the nitrogen atom in NO· is derived from the guanidino nitrogen of L-arginine and the oxygen atom in citrulline is derived from $O_2$ (14–15). The identity of N-OH-L-arginine as a reaction intermediate was also confirmed by isotopic labeling studies (16).

**Table 1** Enzymology of NOS Isoforms (EC 1.14.13.39)

| | NOS-1 | NOS-2 | NOS-3 |
|---|---|---|---|
| Original name | Neuronal NOS | Inducible NOS | Endothelial NOS |
| Abbreviations | b-NOS, n-NOS, bc-NOS, NOS-I | i-NOS, m-NOS, NOS-II | e-NOS, ec-NOS, NOS-III |
| Subcellular location | Soluble and particulate | Soluble and particulate | Primarily particulate |
| No. of amino acids | 1433[a] | 1153[a] | 1203[a] |
| Subunit size (kD) and structure | 150–160 homodimeric | ~130 homodimeric | 135–140 homodimeric |
| $Ca^{2+}$ dependence | Yes, reversible[b] | No, or partial[b] | Yes, reversible[b] |
| Calmodulin dependence | Yes, reversible[b] | Yes, tightly bound[b] | Yes, reversible[b] |
| Contains heme, FAD, and FMN | Yes | Yes | Yes |
| $BH_4$ affinity | 100–400 nM | 30–100 nM | ~100 nM |
| $K_M$ for L-arginine | ~3 µM | ~3 µM | ~3 µM |
| Requires thiols | Yes | Yes | Yes |
| Specific activity[c] | 100–1000 | 400–1500 | 100–500 |

[a]Amino acid number is species dependent. The number given is for the human isoform as determined by cDNA sequence analysis.
[b]Both NOS-1 and NOS-3 have been shown to be reversibly activated by calcium and calmodulin. NOS-2 contains tightly bound calmodulin and may or may not show a dependence on added calcium depending on species or tissue source.
[c]Nanomoles NO·/min/mg.

Scheme 1: Stoichiometry of the NOS Reaction

L-arginine + $O_2$ + NADPH → N-OH-L-arginine
+ NADP$^+$ + H$_2$O                                                                                          (a)

N-OH-L-arginine + $O_2$ + 0.5 NADPH → L-citrulline + NO·
+ 0.5 NADP$^+$ + H$_2$O                                                                                    (b)

The dependence of NOS activity on flavin nucleotides and BH$_4$ was discovered quite early (17,18), but it was not until the demonstration by three separate groups (19–21) that NOS contained heme that the reaction mechanism could be rationalized in greater detail. It was shown that NOS isoforms contain a heme which can react in the reduced (ferrous) state with carbon monoxide (CO) to form a characteristic thiolate ferrous heme-CO complex with spectral properties essentially identical to the same complex of cytochromes P-450. Subsequent studies showed that both steps in the overall reaction shown in scheme 1 could be inhibited by CO, confirming that the heme was the catalytic center of the enzyme (19,22).

These seminal observations led to the conclusion that NOS isoforms are self-contained electron transfer enzymes in which a flavoprotein reductase mediates sequential electron transfer from NADPH to the heme catalytic center according to scheme 2.

Scheme 2: Electron Transfer in NOS

NADPH → FAD → FMN → Heme ("P-450")

The presence of both a flavoprotein reductase and a P-450–like oxygenase domain in a single enzyme is unprecedented in mammalian systems. Cytochromes P-450 and cytochrome P-450 reductase are separate enzymes. Indeed, the only known precedence for such a structural arrangement is the bacterial fatty acid hydroxylase cytochrome P-450$_{BM-3}$ (23).

The similarity of NOS active site reaction chemistry to cytochrome P-450 monooxygenase chemistry has provided a rationale for NOS catalytic mechanism (reviewed in refs. 10 and 24–26). The conversion of L-arginine to N-OH-L-arginine has been proposed to proceed via standard P-450 chemistry in a manner similar to the formation of N-OH-benzamidine from benzamidine. It is the second step in the NOS reaction, conversion of N-OH-L-arginine to L-citrulline + NO·, which has been most intriguing to enzymologists. This is due to the requirement that N-OH-L-arginine provide an electron for heme reduction in order to account for the observed NADPH stoichiometry for this step (one electron) and the need to generate the NO· radical. Several mechanisms for this step have been proposed (10,24–26).

As with other flavoprotein reductases, NOS isoforms exhibit intrinsic diaphorase activity; that is, the ability to facilitate electron transfer from NADPH to artificial electron acceptors such as ferricyanide, dichlorophenolindophenol, and ferricytochrome c (27). This property of the reductase domain of NOS has proven very useful in the study of three key aspects of NOS enzymology: quaternary structure (dimer ↔ monomer transition), NOS domain structure-function analysis, and regulation of enzyme activity by calmodulin. With NOS-2, it was shown that only dimeric enzyme had NOS activity and that monomers isolated by disruption of dimers with chaotropic agents were inactive for NO· formation but retained intrinsic diaphorase activity (27). Importantly, it was also shown that isolated NOS monomers contained bound FAD and FMN but no bound heme or $BH_4$ and that formation of active dimeric NOS from inactive monomers could be promoted by incubation with arginine, heme, and $BH_4$. Limited proteolysis studies with both NOS-2 and NOS-1 dimers showed that the flavoprotein reductase domain could be separated from the "oxygenase" domain which contained bound heme and $BH_4$ (28,29). With NOS-2, it was shown that the flavoprotein reductase domain was monomeric, whereas the oxygenase domain was dimeric, leading to the proposal that the information required for dimerization was contained within the oxygenase domain and that the NOS dimers are arranged in a head-to-head conformation (Fig. 1).

The role of calmodulin in regulating electron transfer between the flavoprotein and oxygenase domains could be studied directly with NOS-1 owing to the reversibility of calmodulin binding to this isoform (30). In the absence of calmodulin, the addition of NADPH to NOS-1 results in a rapid reduction of the flavins but no reduction of heme or NO· formation; that is, the enzyme could function as a diaphorase but not as NOS. The addition of calmodulin to this "electron-loaded" NOS-1 led to rapid heme reduction and NO·/citrulline formation. This elegant set of experiments showed that calmodulin functions as a switch, permitting electron transfer from the reductase domain to the oxygenase domain. Further experiments along this line, but using enzyme devoid of heme and $BH_4$, have recently shown that binding of calmodulin to NOS-1 also stimulates intradomain electron transfer from NADPH to the flavins (31).

Defining the role of $BH_4$ in the regulation of NOS activity remains enigmatic. In contrast to amino acid hydroxylases which have readily exchangeable $BH_4$, the NOS isoforms contain tightly bound $BH_4$ when isolated (32). Although $BH_4$ has been proposed to play a direct role in NOS catalytic activity, direct evidence for this has been lacking. The amount of bound $BH_4$ appears to correlate with enzyme stability and with coupling NADPH oxidation to NO· formation; that is, $BH_4$-depleted NOS has been

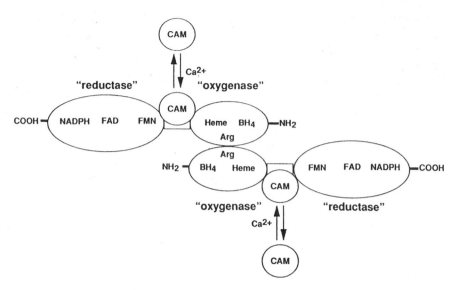

**Figure 1** Head-to-head arrangement of NOS dimers. Schematic representation of NOS dimer assembly. Dimer formation is mediated by the "oxygenase" domain which contains binding sites for heme, $BH_4$, and arginine (Arg). Each oxygenase domain is connected to a "reductase" domain which contains binding sites for NADPH, FAD, and FMN but does not participate in dimerization. The interaction between the oxygenase and reductase domains is further regulated by binding calmodulin (CAM). In the case of NOS-1 and NOS-3, this process is reversible and $Ca^{2+}$ dependent. Calmodulin is associated as a tightly bound subunit in NOS-2 which does not require $Ca^{2+}$ (see Sections II.B and II.C of the text).

shown to generate significant levels of $O_2^{-}/H_2O_2$, presumably through non-specific electron transfer from the heme to $O_2$. Additional hypotheses for a function of $BH_4$ in regulating NOS activity include an allosteric role in promoting arginine binding (33), stabilizing NOS dimers (27), and preventing NOS autoinactivation by NO· (34). Oxidation of bound $BH_4$ to quinonoid $BH_2$ ($qBH_2$) during enzyme catalysis has been proposed (35), raising the possibility that regeneration of $BH_4$ may be a limiting factor for NO· formation.

The dependence of NOS activity on reduced thiols has been largely overlooked. Three recent studies, however, suggest a possible relationship between the $BH_4$ and thiol dependence of NOS. The activity of porcine NOS-1 was shown to be inhibited by numerous thiol-reactive agents and the affinity of the enzyme for $BH_4$ was marginally increased by glutathione (36). The NOS activity, dimer stability, and $BH_4$ binding affinity of recombinant human NOS-3 were all reported to be decreased by a mutation of cysteine 99 to alanine (37). Further evidence supporting a role for thiols in regulating NOS activity was recently provided by the observation that rat NOS-1 could be reversibly inhibited by $Zn^{2+}$ (38). $Zn^{2+}$ blocked NOS activity but did not block diaphorase activity. In addition, evidence for direct blockage of heme reduction by NADPH and perturbation of the heme spectrum were observed in the presence of $Zn^{2+}$, strongly suggesting that $Zn^{2+}$ interacts with the oxygenase domain of NOS-1. It was proposed that the mechanism of $Zn^{2+}$-mediated NOS inhibition was via modification of an active site thiol in proximity to the heme and that cysteine 331 in rat NOS-1 was proposed to be this reactive thiol. This residue corresponds to cysteine 336 in human NOS-1, cysteine 99 in human NOS-3 (see above), and cysteine 115 in human NOS-2. This residue is conserved in all known NOS cDNAs (see below). Whether the thiol-reactive agents described in the study with porcine NOS-1 are reacting with this conserved cysteine residue and thereby decreasing $BH_4$ binding affinity, dimer stability and NOS activity remains to be determined. Taken together, however, these independent observations using three distinct approaches clearly point to an interdependence between an active site thiol, $BH_4$ binding, regulation of the redox, and catalytic status of the heme and enzyme stability.

## B. cDNA Cloning and Structure-Function Analysis of NOS Isoforms

Table 2 summarizes briefly the molecular biology of the human NOS isoforms. For each isoform, full-length or partial cDNAs from other species have been cloned and sequences are available from Genbank. In humans, each NOS isoform is transcribed from a distinct gene with a unique genomic locus. The overall amino acid sequence identity between NOS isoforms is high (50–60%) and, for each isoform, sequence conservation between mammalian species is even higher (>85% for NOS-2 and >95% for NOS-1 and NOS-3). In humans, the intron-exon structure of the NOS genes is remarkably conserved, suggesting that the NOS gene family has evolved from a common ancestor by gene duplication (39). These observations suggest a strong evolutionary pressure for preservation of structure and function. Two recent observations support this hypothesis. Chicken NOS-2 has 67% amino acid identity with NOS-2 and ~50% identity with NOS-1 and NOS-3 (A. Lin and C. McCormick, personal communication). *Drosophila* NOS has 43, 39, and 40% identity with mammalian NOS-1, NOS-2, and NOS-3, respectively, and is $Ca^{2+}$/calmodulin-dependent, suggesting greater similarity to NOS-1 and NOS-3 than NOS-2 (40). The cloning of *Drosophila* NOS demonstrates that the NOS gene family is at

**Table 2** Molecular Biology of NOS Isoforms

|  | Human NOS-1 | Human NOS-2 | Human NOS-3 |
|---|---|---|---|
| Chromosomal localization | 12q24.2 | 17qcen-q12 | 7q35-36 |
| Primary transcript size | ~8.9 kb | ~4.5 kb | ~4.4 kb |
| Alternative transcripts | Yes | ? | ? |
| No. of exons | 29 | 25 | 25 |
| Gene duplications in human genome | No | Yes | No |
| cDNAs for other species | Rat, mouse | Rat, mouse, goat, bovine, chicken | Bovine, mouse, rat |
| Amino acid identity (in mammals) | >95% | >85% | >95% |

least 600 million years old. Further analysis of the evolution of the NOS gene family will require information from a more diverse collection of distantly related NOS sequences.

Analysis of the protein sequences for the mammalian NOS isoforms has revealed a structural organization consistent with the domain structure predicted by enzymology studies. This structure is summarized in Figure 2 using schematic representations of the human NOS isoforms. The N-terminal regions of the NOS isoforms are structurally divergent, showing scant sequence homology. Although divergent in structure, an emerging theme suggests that they serve a common purpose in the regulation of NOS function; that is, targeting to subcellular compartments. This has been clearly shown for NOS-1 in which the N-terminal domain contains a novel "GLGF" motif and is responsible for association of NOS-1 with the dystrophin complex in skeletal muscle (41). Removal of the N-terminal 200 amino acids of NOS-1 does not appear to affect NOS activity. The N-terminus of NOS-3 is myristylated and mutation of the myristylation site (Gly2 → Ala) converts the enzyme from a predominantly membrane-associated enzyme to a soluble enzyme (42). NOS-3 is also palmitoylated at positions Cys15 and/or Cys26, although it remains unclear what contribution this posttranslational modification makes to NOS-3 localization (43). Soluble and particulate associations of NOS-2 have been described, but no detailed study on whether the N-terminus or any other portion of NOS-2 might be involved in regulating these associations has been published.

The remainder of the NOS protein sequence is arranged in the following manner (proceeding from N-terminus to C-terminus): a highly conserved

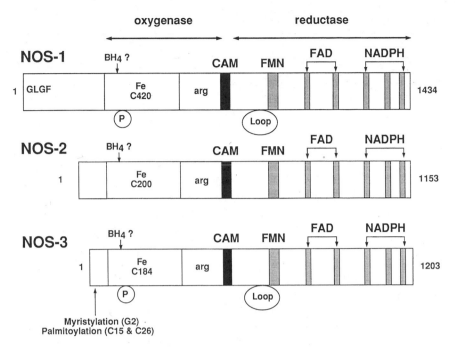

**Figure 2** Domain structure of NOS isoforms deduced from cDNAs. An approximate linear arrangement of the protein sequences for human NOS-1, NOS-2, and NOS-3 as determined by cDNA sequences. Conserved functional elements in the oxygenase and reductase domains of all three NOS isoforms are a putative $BH_4$ binding site ($BH_4$ ?), the heme thiolate cysteine (FeCxxx), an arginine binding site (arg) and nucleotide binding sites for flavin mononucleotide (FMN), flavin adenine dinucleotide (FAD), and reduced nicotinamide adenine dinucleotide phosphate (NADPH). A short sequence of ~44 residues present in the reductase domain of NOS-1 and NOS-3 is absent in NOS-2 (indicated by "Loop"). An amphipathic, helical calmodulin-recognition sequence (CAM) occurs between the oxygenase and reductase domains. NOS-1 and NOS-3 oxygenase domains contain a consensus protein kinase A phosphorylation sequence (P) which is not present in NOS-2. The N-termini of the NOS isoforms are structurally divergent: NOS-1 has a large extension encoding a novel "GLGF" motif involved in binding to accessory proteins such as dystrophin; NOS-3 contains myristylation and palmitoylation sites involved in membrane association.

**Table 3** Domain Organization in Human NOS Isoforms

|                               | NOS-1    | NOS-2    | NOS-3    |
| ----------------------------- | -------- | -------- | -------- |
| NH$_2$-terminal domain        | 1–302    | 1–81     | 1–65     |
| Oxygenase domain              | 303–725  | 82–504   | 66–486   |
| Calmodulin sequence           | 726–759  | 505–538  | 486–519  |
| Flavoprotein reductase domain | 760–1434 | 539–1153 | 520–1203 |

oxygenase domain, a calmodulin-recognition sequence, and a flavoprotein reductase domain (summarized in Table 3). The N-terminal to C-terminal arrangement of oxygenase domain and reductase domain is homologous to the structure of bacterial cytochrome P-450$_{BM-3}$ (23). The unique added feature of NOS is the insertion of a calmodulin-recognition sequence between the oxygenase domain and the reductase domain. All NOS isoforms contain a hydrophobic/basic amphipathic sequence (~33 residues) which is homologous to similar sequences in other calmodulin-dependent enzymes and proteins. The calmodulin-recognition sequence in each NOS isoform is highly conserved from species to species in mammals (100, 73–91, and 94% identity for NOS-1, NOS-2, and NOS-3, respectively) but is less conserved between isoforms (32–60% identity in humans). This divergence may be partly responsible for the differential Ca$^{2+}$/calmodulin dependence of the NOS isoforms.

The flavoprotein reductase domain of NOS contains highly conserved nucleotide binding consensus sequences for the adenine and ribose moieties of the substrate NADPH, the isoalloxazine and pyrophosphate moieties of the cofactor FAD, and also for the cofactor FMN (44). The arrangement of this domain is homologous to other FAD- and FMN-containing flavoprotein reductases such as cytochrome P-450 reductase and sulfite reductase. Derived from ancient genes, these related flavoprotein reductases are expressed throughout biological systems. The reductase domain of NOS-1 has been expressed in *Escherichia coli* and retains cytochrome C reductase activity but does not contain heme (45). Alignment of the NOS-2 sequence with cytochrome P-450 reductase, cytochrome P-450$_{BM-3}$, sulfite reductase, ferredoxin reductase, and flavodoxin indicates that the reductase domain in NOS-2 begins immediately C-terminal to the calmodulin-recognition sequence and extends almost to the C-terminus. In NOS-1 and NOS-3, however, there is an insertion of a hydrophilic, serine-rich loop of 44 residues approximately 70 residues C-terminal to the calmodulin-recognition sequence and immediately N-terminal to the consensus sequence for FMN binding (J. F. Parkinson, unpublished observations). The precise function of this loop remains to be established, but it is likely to be involved in regulating the $Ca^{2+}$/calmodulin dependence of electron flow between the reductase and oxygenase domains of NOS-1 and NOS-3 and may also be responsible for the observed increase in intradomain electron transfer from NADPH to the flavins in the reductase domain of NOS-1 (see above). The insertion of a loop in this region appears to be evolutionarily conserved in NOS isoforms which are reversibly $Ca^{2+}$/calmodulin–dependent, since it is present in *Drosophila* NOS but is absent in chicken NOS-2. The inserted loop in *Drosophila* NOS is somewhat longer (~60 residues) than in mammalian NOS-1 and NOS-3, but it retains the features of being serine rich with high hydrophilicity and surface probability indices (J. F. Parkinson, unpublished observations).

The oxygenase domain (~420 residues) of NOS is highly conserved between isoforms and through evolution: When the sequence of this domain of human NOS-2 is compared with all other published NOS sequences, amino acid identity and similarity are 56–78% and 73–93%, respectively. This domain was initially proposed to be unique to NOS, since comparisons of this region with protein databases did not reveal any striking homology to other proteins. Recent observations suggest, however, that this initial analysis may have been misleading. On the basis of weak homology to the conserved heme binding helix of cytochromes P-450, a cysteine residue which is conserved in all NOS sequences has been proposed to be the axial thiolate heme ligand (21). Subsequent studies with site-directed mutants of this cysteine residue in NOS-1 and NOS-3 have confirmed this proposal (46–47). This cysteine occurs at residue 420, 200, and 184 in human NOS-1, NOS-2 and NOS-3, respectively. The consensus sequence surrounding this cysteine residue, Ala-Trp-Arg-Asn-x-x-Arg-Cys-(Val/Ile)-Gly-Arg-Ile-Gln-Trp, is highly conserved in all NOS isoforms with 11/13 residues being invariant in 10 published NOS sequences. The role of phosphorylation in regulating NOS activity remains controversial, but the oxygenase domain of both NOS-1 and NOS-3 contains a consensus protein kinase A phosphorylation sequence which is conserved in *Drosophila* NOS but is not present in NOS-2 (40). Although ideally placed to modulate oxygenase domain function, no direct evidence that this site is actually phosphorylated under physiological conditions or has any effect on NOS activity have been obtained.

Distant homology of the oxygenase domain of NOS to the pterin and NADPH binding sites of dihydrofolate reductase (DHFR) was recently proposed, suggesting that the $BH_4$ binding site of NOS is contained within the region between the cysteine heme ligand and the calmodulin-recognition sequence (48). This "DHFR module" is 148 residues in length and its potential function was tested by expression in *E. coli* of glutathione–S-transferase (GST) fusion proteins containing rat NOS-1 deletion mutants (49). Surprisingly, a GST fusion protein containing the putative DHFR module of rat NOS-1 (residues 558–721) could not be shown to bind $BH_4$ but did bind [$^3H$]-N-nitro-L-arginine, a potent slow binding inhibitor of NOS-1. A fusion protein containing the DHFR module and the remainder of the putative oxygenase domain (residues 220–721) was shown also to bind [$^3H$-]N-nitro-L-arginine and binding was stimulated by $BH_4$. These data strongly suggest that the C-terminal portion of the oxygenase domain provides the NOS arginine binding site, but they do not locate precisely the $BH_4$ binding site. As mentioned above, however, the NOS oxygenase domain contains a conserved cysteine residue which when mutated to alanine results in decreased $BH_4$ binding affinity and activity of NOS-3 (37). This cysteine (residue 336, 115, and 99 in human NOS-1, NOS-2, and NOS-3, respectively) is N-terminal to the heme thiolate cysteine ligand and is conserved in all known NOS sequences.

## C.  Spectroscopic Probes of NOS Active Site

The heme thiolate catalytic center of NOS provides enzymologists and biophysicists with an extremely useful tool with which to probe the active site of NOS. The properties of the heme in NOS-1 and NOS-2 have been extensively characterized by optical absorption (19–21,50–53) and Raman (54,55) spectroscopy methods. In addition to the CO complex of ferrous heme in NOS, a cyanide complex with ferric heme (50) and complexes of NO· itself with both ferrous and ferric heme (53,55) have been observed. The CO-ferrous heme complex of NOS is flash dissociable, allowing the rate of CO association with the heme in the presence and absence of substrate to be determined by rapid spectroscopic techniques (51). Arginine slows the association rate of CO with the heme by ~12-fold, indicating close proximity of the substrate to the heme. The proximity of the substrate to the heme has also been confirmed by Raman spectroscopy, which showed shifts in both the Fe-NO and Fe-CO stretching frequencies consistent with arginine being positioned directly above the heme (54,55). These results are similar to those observed for cytochromes P-450 in the presence of xenobiotic substrates (56).

A very simple probe of the active site of NOS is optical difference spectroscopy. This simple technique has been used extensively since the 1960s to characterize substrate and inhibitor binding interactions that perturb the heme Soret spectral region of cytochromes P-450 (see ref. 57 for an excellent review). Substrates and substrate analogues typically cause an increase in absorbance at 380–390 nm with a trough at ~420 nm, which is

**Table 4** Difference Spectroscopy with NOS Substrates and Inhibitors

| | NOS-1 | | NOS-2 | |
|---|---|---|---|---|
| Substrate or inhibitor | spectral type | $K_S$ ($\mu M$) | spectral type | $K_S$ ($\mu M$) |
| Arginine | Type I | 2.5 | Type I | ND |
| N-methyl-L-arginine | Type I | 2.5 | ND | ND |
| N-OH-L-arginine | Type I | 0.4–0.8 | ND | ND |
| N-nitro-L-arginine | Type I | ND | ND | ND |
| S-methyl-L-thiocitrulline | Type I | <2.7 | ND | ND |
| L-thiocitrulline | Type II | ND | ND | ND |
| Imidazole | Type II | 160 | Type II | ND |

ND, not determined.
Source: Data compiled from refs. 29, 50, 58, and 59.

termed a type I spectrum. Compounds which bind directly to form a ferric heme ligand complex typically cause an increase at 420–426 nm with a trough at 380–410 nm, which is termed a type II spectrum. These spectral perturbations are dependent on the concentration of compound, showing typical Michaelis-Menton saturation kinetics and permitting determination of $K_S$, a spectral binding constant (not to be confused with $K_M$, which is determined under active enzyme turnover rather than resting conditions). Both NOS-1 and NOS-2 have been shown to give typical type I difference spectra with arginine analogues and type II difference spectra with imidazole and other heme binding compounds (50–52). This provides a simple means for distinguishing the mechanism of action of NOS inhibitors (see also Section III). A summary of data generated using this technique is provided in Table 4. Most of the data have been generated with rat NOS-1 and limited data with mouse NOS-2. One key observation is that L-thiocitrulline forms a type II spectrum with NOS-1, indicating it to be a direct heme ligand, whereas a simple analogue of this compound, S-methyl-L-thiocitrulline, forms a type I spectrum, indicating a simple substrate-type interaction but no direct heme ligation (58).

## D. Future Directions for NOS Enzymology Research

Considerable progress has been made in understanding the structure and function of the family of NOS isoforms. Recent progress in expressing full-length active NOS (60) and NOS domains (50) in high-yield heterologous expression systems, such as *E. coli,* beckons a new ear in NOS enzymology research. These achievements will provide the large amounts of material required for detailed structure-function analyses. The application of rapid mutagenesis techniques combined with direct radioligand binding assays for arginine and $BH_4$ will soon lead to the identification of the arginine and $BH_4$ binding sites of the oxygenase domain and protein residues critical for these interactions. The ultimate goal will be to crystallize one or all of the NOS isoforms in order to obtain high-resolution x-ray coordinates of the active site. Several groups are aggressively pursuing this goal using NOS isoforms expressed in *E. coli*. It is reasonable to expect that this goal will be achieved in the near future.

## III.  MECHANISM-BASED NOS INHIBITORS

A number of approaches to inhibiting NOS activity have been proposed (see ref. 1 for a review). These include limiting arginine uptake by cells, inhibiting the de novo or salvage pathways of $BH_4$ synthesis, isoform-selective calmodulin antagonists, and flavoprotein reductase inhibitors. Each of these approaches has its merits and requires further exploration. One shortcoming of all these approaches, however, is that they lack specificity to NOS and have the potential adversely to affect other biological processes. As reviewed in Section II, the active site of NOS is unique in biological systems, as far as we know. It is reasonable to assume that the safety of a therapeutic will be related to the degree to which it is specific for its target versus other systems. For this reason, drug discovery efforts in the field of NOS inhibitors have focused on mechanism-based enzyme inhibitors directed at the active site of NOS. Recently, significant progress has been made on the discovery of potent NOS inhibitors with reasonable selectivity between isoforms. This section focuses on a review of these developments.

### A.  Arginine Analogues

The standard inhibitors of NOS are structurally related to the substrate arginine. Many compounds that are in this category have been published, but three stand out as useful tools. N-methyl-L-arginine (NMA: compound 1) is a standard nonselective inhibitor with which most other compounds are compared. N-nitro-L-arginine (NNA, compound 2) is the standard for NOS-1 selective inhibition and aminoguanidine (AG; compound 3) is the standard for NOS-2 selective inhibition. Although these inhibitors are cited more than others, they have been previously reviewed and are discussed here except for comparison purposes (10). A recent paper on N-nitro-L-arginine methyl ester, another widely used standard inhibitor, reported that this compound is not the active entity but is a prodrug of NNA (61).

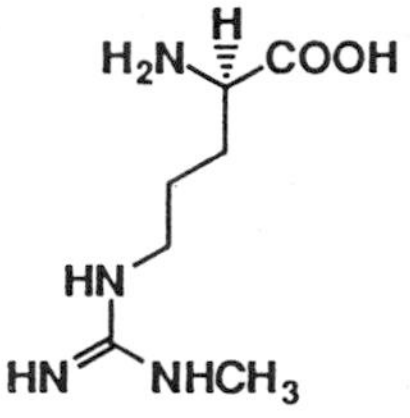

$H_2N$ $H$ COOH
HN
HN NHCH$_3$

**1**

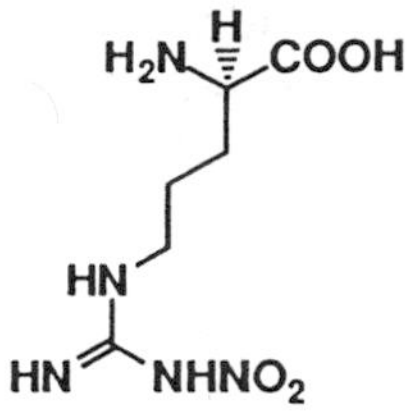

$H_2N$ $H$ COOH
HN
HN NHNO$_2$

**2**

NH
$H_2N$ N NH$_2$
H

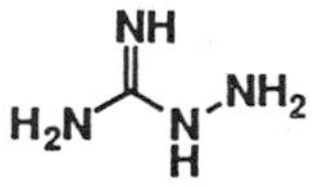

**3**

Two interesting arginine analogues are L-thiocitrulline (52,62; compound 4) and S-methyl-L-thiocitrulline (62,63; compound 5). Thiocitrulline has a type II difference spectrum that is characteristic of a compound coordinating directly to the sixth coordination site of the heme Fe. The thiourea is not basic and cannot form a salt bridge with an acidic residue as can the guanidine of arginine. On the other hand, the thiourea can form hydrogen bonds similar to those a guanidine can form. The inactivity of the isosteric citrulline indicates that the sulfur is critical for binding. The more potent and more basic S-methyl-L-thiocitrulline (compound 5) is also competitive with arginine. S-methyl-L-thiocitrulline is isosteric and less basic than NMA but significantly more potent: $K_i$, human NOS-1/NOS-2/NOS-3: 1.2/40/11 nM (63). An unspecified sulfur binding may be invoked to explain the increased potency of S-methyl-L-thiocitrulline over NMA (see Fig. 4C).

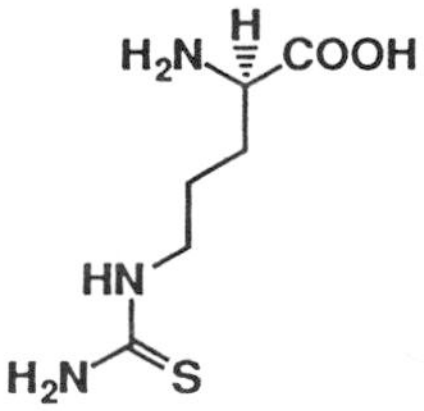

$H_2N$ $H$ COOH
HN
$H_2N$ S

**4**

$H_2N$ $H$ COOH
HN
HN SCH$_3$

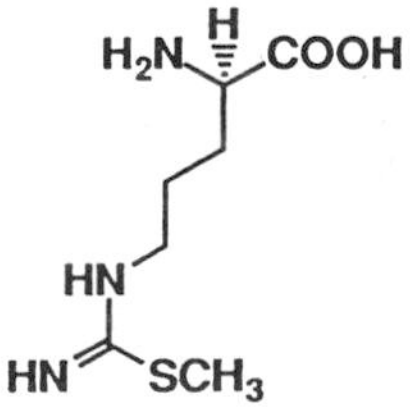

**5**

Two compounds, 1-(iminoethyl)-ornithine (64,65; compound 6) and amino acid 7 (63) illustrate the importance of the guanidine nitrogens. 1-(Iminoethyl)-ornithine is an inhibitor of NOS with similar potency to NMA: IC$_{50}$ rat NOS-1/mouse NOS-2: 3.9/2.2 $\mu$M. Interstingly, lengthening the chain by one carbon (compound 8) gives a NOS-2 selective compound: IC$_{50}$ rat NOS-1/mouse NOS-2: 92 3.3 $\mu$M (65). The results from these two compounds indicate at least minor differences in the active sites of these two enzymes. Replacement of the chain nitrogen with sulfur (63) or methylene (10) results in inactive compounds. This result indicates that the chain nitrogen (NH) is important for binding, presumably through either a hydrogen bond or binding to an acidic residue (see Fig. 4A).

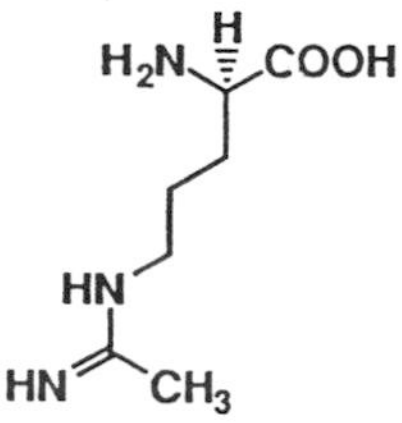

6 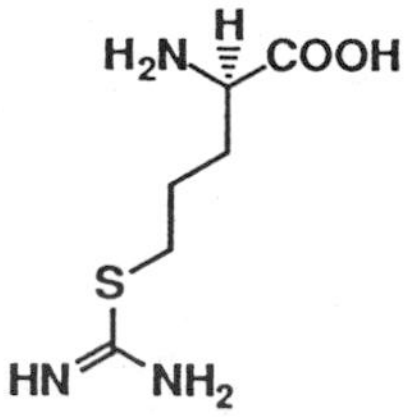                                     7 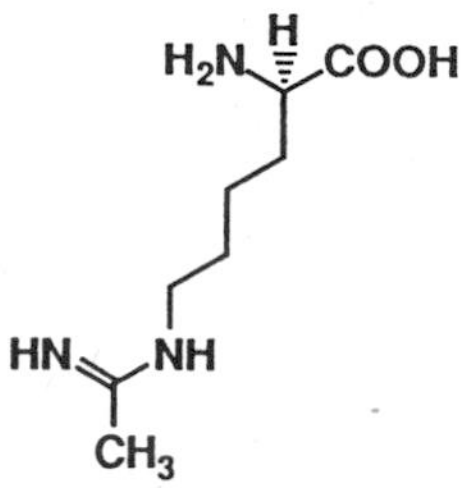                                     8

In order to better understand the arginine binding site, analogues of the mechanism-based inhibitor N-allyl-L-arginine (compound 9) were prepared (66,67). Against bovine NOS-1 it was found that the ester and parent compound have similar potencies, but the acetamide of the amino acid nitrogen is significantly less potent. The conclusion was that the amine moiety is more important for binding than the acid function. Although this conclusion may be true, interpretation of the results of the ester rely on a lack of hydrolysis to the acid, which was not examined.

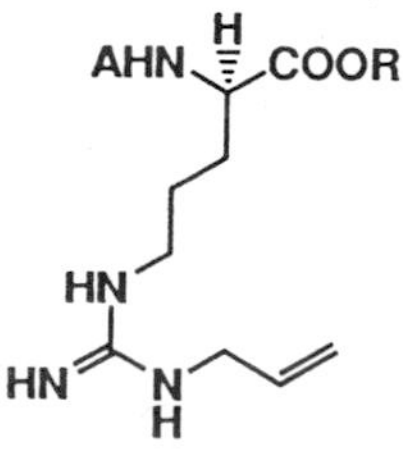

R=H, A=H
R=H, A=COCH$_3$
R=Me, A=H

9

## B.  Amidine-Containing Inhibitors

This series of compounds is being grouped together because they all contain an amidine moiety (C[-=NH]NH$_2$) and the fact that this group is also contained within the guanidine moiety of arginine. There is experimental evidence for some of these compounds to be competitive with arginine, but evidence has not been reported for all of them. No implication is being made that these compounds have the same mechanism or that they bind to the same site as arginine. The grouping is a matter of convenience and to illustrate the structural similarity of the inhibitors.

One group of compounds that have been reported by a number of workers is the isothioureas (ITUs; 68–70). The first and most complete description of these compounds is by the Wellcome group (68). They report very large activity differences for small structural variations. For example, the difference for compound 10, where R = isopropyl and isobutyl against the human enzymes is two orders of magnitude: $K_i$ NOS-1/NOS-2/NOS-3 is 37/10/22 and 6400/1300/8300 nM, respectively. It appears that the site where the alkyl group is situated can only accommodate a small amount of steric bulk, although some is needed, since R = isopropyl is more potent than R = Me ($K_i$ NOS-1/NOS-2/NOS-3: 160/120/200 nM. These compounds show only hints of selectivity for NOS-2 with the human isoforms, but better selectivity in a species mixed group of enzymes: R = Et, rat NOS-1/mouse NOS-2/bovine NOS-3: 250/13/370 nM (69). Binding studies of compound 10 (R = Et) have been performed and the compound was found to bind with a type I spectra against mouse NOS-2. Garvey et al. have proposed that these compounds bind with the SR group pointing toward the heme, the R group in a small hydrophobic pocket, and the nitrogens binding to the same site as the nonreacting guanidine nitrogens present in arginine (68).

The Wellcome group has also reported on bis-ITUs (68). Compound 11 has selectivity for human NOS-2 ($K_i$ NOS-1/NOS-2/NOS-3: 250/47/9000 nM). In the same series, a very potent and partially selective NOS-1 inhibitor was reported (compound 12: $K_i$ NOS-1/NOS-2/NOS-3: 1.3/8.7/90.0 nM). The symmetrical nature of these compounds raises the intriguing possibility that this type of inhibitor may be binding to both active sites of the dimeric enzyme, but no confirmatory evidence of this yet exists. The binding mode of one of the isothioureas has been proposed to be similar to the binding of the ITU of compound 10, but the binding of the rest of the molecule may be more interesting, since it is imparting selectivity to the molecule.

10                    11                              12

Some cyclic ITUs have been reported to inhibit NOS (68,70). 2-Aminothiazole (compound 13, R = H) and 2-aminothiazoline (compound 14) are reported to inhibit NOS ($K_i$ NOS-1/NOS-2/NOS-3: 12/48/10 and 0.41/0.26/0.35 $\mu$M, respectively). Neither compound has significant selectivity, but they are competitive with arginine. The potency of the thiazole is increased significantly by placement of a methyl group in the 5 position (compound 13, R = Me). Related cyclic ITUs have been reported by a group at Abbott (69,70). They have optimized the compounds toward NOS-2 selectivity. The most potent and selective thiazine is shown (compound 15, R = Me, rat NOS-1/mouse NOS-2/bovine NOS-3: 34/3.6/150 nM). They found that the methyl group imparted a 100-fold activity increase against NOS-2, but the increase against both constitutive isoforms was less (compound 15, R = H, NOS-1/NOS-2/NOS-3: 540/30/1200 nM). The corresponding oxygen heterocycles were significantly less active against NOS-2, once again as in thiocitrulline, indicating the importance of sulfur for binding (70).

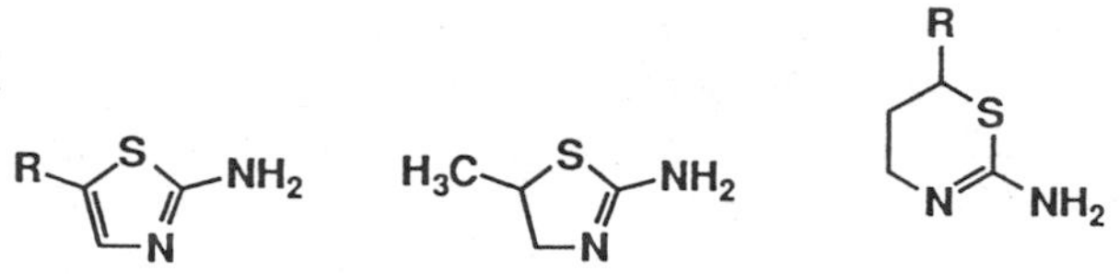

A group from Searle has reported on a series of related cyclic amidines. They seem to have optimized for NOS-2 selectivity (71). The most selective compound reported is the seven-membered ring, compound 16 (rat NOS-1/ mouse NOS-2: 7800/81 nM). A large potency difference was observed with changing the position of the alkyl group, as illustrated in Fig. 3. Listed is a group of six-membered ring cyclic amidines that differ only in the positioning of the methyl group. As with the ITUs, a small steric modification by differential placement of a methyl group on the inhibitor imparts large differences in potency. A series of acyclic amidines has also been reported (72).

2-Aminopyridines (aromatized cyclic amidines) have also been reported to be selective inhibitors of NOS-2 (70; see Fig. 3). The best compound in the series was 2-aminopicoline (compound 17, NOS-1/NOS-2/NOS-3: 250/25/

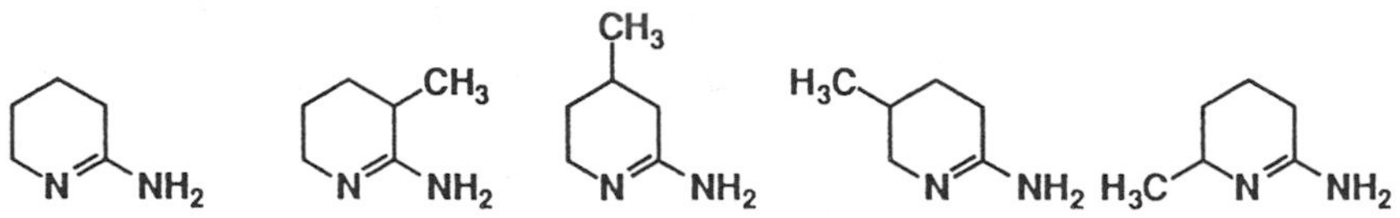

| 600 nM | 1500 nM | 55 nM | 2000 nM | 160 nM |

**Figure 3** Activities of six-membered ring analogues. Structures of six related analogues of a six-membered ring NOS inhibitor. Inhibitor potencies indicated (nM) are against NOS-2. The figure illustrates that small structural changes; that is, incorporation and location of a methyl group, cause large differences in inhibitor potency.

320 nM). Although the methyl group enhanced potency by a factor of 30 over 2-aminopyridine, further substitution at the 4 position caused a decrease in potency.

16        17

While preparing analogues of AG and looking for NOS-2 selective compounds, diaminobenzimidazole (compound 18) was found to be NOS-1 selective: R = Me, rat NOS-1/human NOS-2/human NOS-3: 5.8/>100/>100 $\mu$M (73). Substituting an isopropyl group (compound 18, R = CH[CH$_3$]$_2$) for the methyl "destroyed" activity. The related unsubstituted compound was less active (compound 18, R = H, IC$_{50}$ rat NOS-1/human NOS-2/human NOS-3: 77/25/>100 $\mu$M) and was shown to be competitive with arginine.

2-Iminobiotin, compound 19, was investigated as an arginine analogue and found weakly to inhibit NOS: K$_i$, rat NOS-1/mouse NOS-2: 38/22 $\mu$M (74) and was found to be competitive with arginine. Biotin and thiobiotin, analagous compounds to citrulline and thiocitrulline from arginine, were both inactive. The acid moiety was found not to be important for binding.

A group of bisamidines that are very potent and selective inhibitors of NOS-1 has been reported (75–77). Beginning with a weak, nonselective lead, Macdonald and colleagues have been able to produce very potent and selective compounds (compound 20; K$_i$ NOS-1/NOS-2/NOS-3: 2/14000/370 nM) (74). At present, there have been no claims on the mechanism of action of these compounds.

18             19             20

## C. Heterocyclic Inhibitors

Imidazole (compound 21) and imidazole-containing compounds are well known for binding heme containing enzymes (78) and NOS is no exception (see Section II.C; 79–86). Imidazole is a weak, reversible, arginine competitive inhibitor of bovine NOS-1 that acts as the sixth ligand of the heme (49; see Section II.C). Some imidazole-containing antifungal agents have been described to inhibit NOS-1 with their predominant mode of action arising from a hydrophobic interaction with the calmodulin binding site (80). Not surprisingly, with this mechanism, these compounds do not inhibit mouse NOS-2, which has the calmodulin much more tightly bound (83). 1-Phenylimidazole (compound 22) has been shown to be a selective inhibitor of NOS-2 over the constitutive isoforms: $K_i$, GH$_3$ NOS-1/mouse NOS-2/ bovine NOS-3: 40/0.7/50 $\mu$M (83). 1-Phenylimidazole is presumed to interact with the heme in a manner analogous to imidazole, but no evidence of this interaction has been reported. 1-Phenylimidazole has been found to be competitive with tetrahydrobiopterin (BH$_4$) but not with arginine in NOS-2. Against NOS-3, it was found to be competitive with both BH$_4$ and arginine (81). Unlike the unsubstituted compound, 1-(trifluoromethylphenyl)-imidazole (compound 23) is reported to be selective only against NOS-3: IC$_{50}$, rat NOS-1/mouse NOS-2/bovine NOS-3: 27/28/1000 $\mu$M (86).

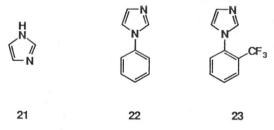

21                        22                        23

Structure activity relationship studies have been done on various indazole agents, and 7-nitroindazole (compound 24, 7-NI) was reported to be a potent and relatively selective inhibitor of NOS-1: $K_i$, GH$_3$ NOS-1/ mouse NOS-2/bovine NOS-3: 0.16/1.6/0.8 $\mu$M (85–89). Interestingly, 7-NI inhibits NOS-1 competitively with respect to arginine and BH$_4$ (88), whereas NOS-2 and NOS-3 were found to be inhibited competitively only with respect to BH$_4$ (81). Wolff and colleagues proposed that the indazole binds to the heme iron based mainly on the structural similarities to benzimidazole and imidazole, but no spectroscopic evidence to support this proposal has yet been reported (81). Regardless of whether the heterocycle is interacting with the heme, a proximal relationship of the arginine and BH$_4$ binding sites is implicated, and a potential difference of location of these two sites in the isoforms may be utilized for subsequent design of isoform-selective compounds. Subsequent studies have found a more potent analogue with less selectivity, 3-bromo-7-nitroindazole (compound 25): IC$_{50}$, rat NOS-1/rat NOS-2/bovine NOS-3: 0.17/0.86/0.62 $\mu$M (89).

24                                25

## D.  Active Site Models

At present, there are no data about the enzyme active site from x-ray analysis or other physical chemical means that can provide clear directions for rational design of NOS inhibitors. What is known from enzymology studies is that the arginine binds very close to the heme (see Section II). The precise three-dimensional relationship between arginine and the heme is not known. In addition, only one compound which combines a heme binding functional group with arginine has been successfully synthesized and shown to bind the heme; that is, thiocitrulline.

The only way to gather information is to build the active site from the inhibitors that are known to interact there. The arginine inhibitors are an excellent place to start, since small differences have been made to the inhibitors that may possibly be extrapolated to small modifications in the developing active site (see Fig. 4). The basicity of the guanidine moiety does not seem to be critical, since NNA and S-methyl-L-thiocitrulline, less basic compounds, both bind. The chain NH does seem to be important for some hydrogen binding interaction. The nonreacting nitrogen does not seem to be important for binding since N-(1-iminoethyl)-L-ornithine is a potent inhibitor. Owing mainly to interpretation of the data from the ITUs, the reactive nitrogen is located in a hydrophobic pocket that can only tolerate small alkyl groups. The binding of thiocitrulline is slightly different in that the sulfur is bonded directly to the heme (see Fig. 4B).

There seems to be a strong unspecified sulfur binding site. Sulfur-containing compounds, such as S-methyl-L-thiocitrulline and the isothio-ureas (compounds 10–12), bind tightly (see Fig. 4C). No speculation to the cause of this tight binding has been made. The acyclic ITUs may also hydrogen bond to the same site mentioned above for the chain NH. A common feature of the amidines is the dramatic activity difference noted with minor modifications in the inhibitor structure. The ITUs (compound 10) show a potency increase from R = methyl to ethyl and then a drop-off going to R = propyl. A similar sensitivity structure has been noted in the aminopyridines and the cyclic amidines. These differences indicate a small binding site, at least in the dimensions explored thus far. Interestingly, in overlapping the

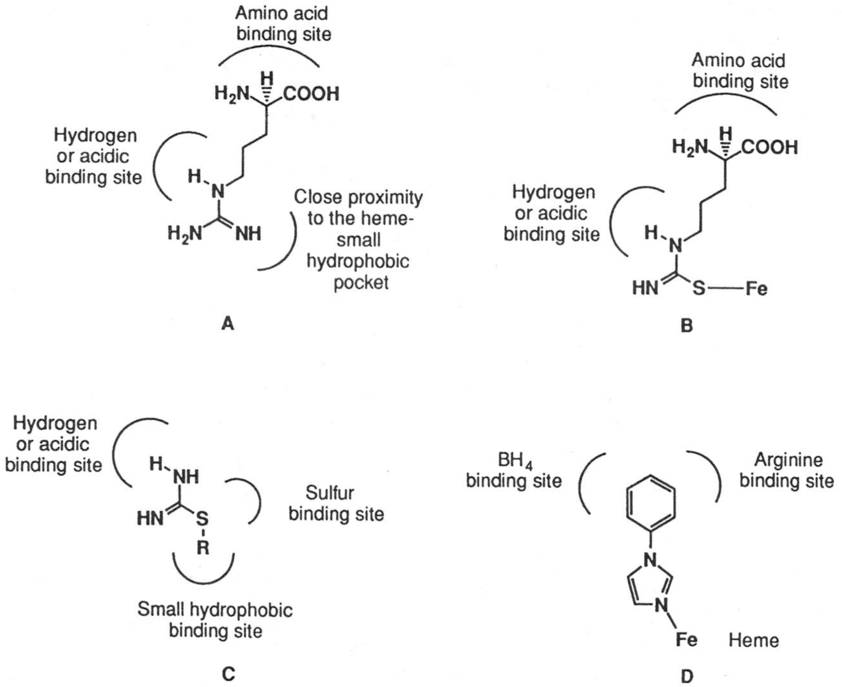

**Figure 4** Models for active site binding interactions of NOS inhibitors. Proposed binding site of some inhibitors. (A) The proposed binding site of arginine and its analogues. The basicity of the guanidine moiety does not seem to be critical for binding, but the chain NH does seem to be important for some hydrogen binding interaction. The nonreacting nitrogen does not seem to be important for binding. (B) The proposed binding site of thiocitrulline. The binding of thiocitrulline is slightly different than arginine in that the sulfur is bonded directly to the heme. (C) Proposed binding of isothioureas (ITUs). The acyclic ITUs, like arginine, may also hydrogen bond to the same site mentioned above for the chain NH. (D) Proposed binding of phenylimidazole. Phenylimidazole has been postulated to interact with the heme. It has also been found to be competitive with $BH_4$ and arginine in some isoforms indicating possible interaction with both of these binding sites.

structures of the aminopyridines and ITUs at the two nitrogens, the four-position of the aminopyridines can overlap with the R group of the ITUs.

1-Phenylimidazole (see Fig. 4D) and 7-NI–containing compounds present different binding schemes owing to their different structures. They also seem to present different binding schemes depending on the isoform being investigated. This is implicated by their apparent competition with $BH_4$.

Whether binding to the $BH_4$ site imparts competitive binding to the arginine site via an allosteric interaction or direct occupation of the arginine site is not known. Both heterocycles are postulated to interact with the heme, but supporting evidence is only available for imidazole.

## E.  Future Directions for Discovery of NOS Inhibitors

Many of the seminal observations on the in vitro and in vivo roles of the L-arginine/nitric oxide pathway in regulating biological systems were made with three very simple L-arginine analogue substrate-based inhibitors: NMA, NNL, and AG (reviewed in ref. 1). These compounds lack, however, the potency and selectivity limits to be considered as viable therapeutics. In addition, their lack of selectivity limits their in vitro and in vivo use in pharmacology experiments aimed at understanding which NOS isoform is involved in a particular biological system. These shortcomings have prompted an aggressive search for more selective tools with the ultimate aim of developing isoform-selective NOS inhibitors as therapeutics.

As can be seen from this chapter, a structurally diverse array of new mechanism-based NOS inhibitors have recently been discovered. In some cases, considerable potency enhancements have been achieved; that is, from low $\mu M$ to low nM inhibitors. In other cases, selectivity has also been improved with compounds achieving 100- to 1000-fold selectivity. These achievements are significant and suggest that development of isoform-selective NOS inhibitors with high potency (low nM) and selectivity (~1000-fold) is achievable. They also confirm that despite a high degree of sequence homology, the active sites of the three NOS isoforms are structurally distinct. The structural basis for these distinctions, however, still remains elusive. To understand and refine inhibitor binding interactions at the active site of NOS, further clarification is needed of the three-dimensional spatial relationships between arginine, heme, and $BH_4$ and the active site amino acids involved in substrate and cofactor binding. This improved understanding, possibly together with a NOS crystal structure, should lead to rational design of isoform-selective NOS inhibitors.

## ACKNOWLEDGMENTS

We would like to thank Drs. Arthur Lin and Charles McCormick (Cornell University, Ithaca, NY) for providing a full-length sequence for chicken NOS-2 in advance of publication. We would also like to thank Drs. Dennis Stuehr (Cleveland Clinic Foundation, Cleveland, OH) and Kirk McMillan (Pharmacopeia Inc., Princeton, NJ) for useful comments and insights on the structure and function of NOS isoforms.

# REFERENCES

1. Nathan C. Nitric oxide as a secretory product of mammalian cells. FASEB J 1992; 6:3051–3064.
2. Feldman PL, Griffith OW, Stuehr DJ. The surprising life of nitric oxide. Chem Eng News 1993; 71:26–38.
3. Bredt DS, Snyder SH. Nitric oxide: a physiologic messenger molecule. Ann Rev Biochem 1994; 63:175–195.
4. Stamler JS, Singel DJ, Loscalzo J. Biochemistry of nitric oxide and its redox-activated forms. Science 1992; 258:1898–1902.
5. Palmer RM, Ferrige AG, Moncada S. Nitric oxide release accounts for the biological activity of endothelium-derived relaxing factor. Nature 1987; 327:524–526.
6. Malinski T, Radomski MW, Taha Z, et al. Direct electrochemical measurement of nitric oxide released from human platelets. Biochem Biophys Res Commun 1993; 194:960–965.
7. Stuehr DJ, Gross SS, Sakuma I, et al. Activated murine macrophages secrete a metabolite of arginine with the bioactivity of endothelium-derived relaxing factor and the chemical reactivity of nitric oxide. J Exp Med 1989; 169:1011–1020.
8. Busse R, Mülsch A. Induction of nitric oxide synthase by cytokines in vascular smooth muscle cells. FEBS Lett 1990; 275: 87–90.
9. Tomimoto H, Nishimura M, Suenaga T, et al. Distribution of nitric oxide synthase in the human cerebral blood vessels and brain tissues. J Cereb Blood Flow Metab 1994; 14:930–938.
10. Kerwin JF, Lancaster JR, Feldman PL. Nitric oxide: a new paradigm for second messengers. J Med Chem 1995; 38:4343–4362.
11. Bredt DS, Snyder SH. Isolation of nitric oxide synthetase, a calmodulin-requiring enzyme. Proc Natl Acad Sci USA 1990; 87:682–685.
12. Pollock JS, Forstermann U, Mitchell JA, et al. Purification and characterization of particulate endothelium-derived relaxing factor synthase from cultured and native bovine aortic endothelial cells. Proc Natl Acad Sci USA 1991; 88:10480–10484.
13. Cho HJ, Xie QW, Calaycay J, et al. Calmodulin is a subunit of nitric oxide synthase from macrophages. J Exp Med 1992: 176:599–604.
14. Iyengar R, Stuehr DJ, Marletta MA. Macrophage synthesis of nitrite, nitrate, and N-nitrosamines: precursors and role of the respiratory burst. Proc Natl Acad Sci USA 1987; 84:6369–6373.
15. Kwon NS, Natahn CF, Gilker C, et al. L-citrulline production from L-arginine by macrophage nitric oxide synthase. The ureido oxygen derives from dioxygen. J Biol Chem 1990; 265:13442–12445.
16. Stuehr DJ, Kwon NS, Nathan CF, et al. N-omega-hydroxy-L-arginine is an intermediate in the biosynthesis of nitric oxide from L-arginine. J Biol Chem 1991; 266:6259–6263.
17. Kwon NS, Nathan CF, Stuehr, DJ. Reduced biopterin as a cofactor in the generation of nitrogen oxides by murine macrophages. J Biol Chem 1989; 264:20496–20501.
18. Stuehr DJ, Cho HJ, Kwon NS, et al. Purification and characterization of the

cytokine-induced macrophage nitric oxide synthase: an FAD- and FMN-containing flavoprotein. Proc Natl Acad Sci USA 1991; 88:7773–7777.

19. White KA, Marletta MA. Nitric oxide synthase is a cytochrome P-450 type hemoprotein. Biochemistry 1992; 31:6627–6631.

20. Stuehr DJ, Ikeda-Saito M. Spectral characterization of brain and macrophage nitric oxide synthases. Cytochrome P-450–like hemeproteins that contain a flavin semiquinone radical. J Biol Chem 1992; 267:20547–20550.

21. McMillan K, Bredt DS, Hirsch DJ, et al. Cloned, expressed rat cerebellar nitric oxide synthase contains stoichiometric amounts of heme, which binds carbon monoxide. Proc Natl Acad Sci USA 1992; 89:11141–11145.

22. Pufahl RA, Marletta MA. Oxidation of NG-hydroxy-L-arginine by nitric oxide synthase: evidence for the involvement of the heme in catalysis. Biochem Biophys Res Commun 1993; 193:963–970.

23. Narhi LO, Fulco AJ. Identification and characterization of two functional domains in cytochrome P-450BM-3, a catalytically self-sufficient monooxygenase induced by barbiturates in Bacillus megaterium. J Biol Chem 1987; 262:6683–6690.

24. Marletta MA. Nitric oxide synthase structure and mechanism. J Biol Chem 1993; 268:12231–12234.

25. Feldman PL, Griffith OW, Hong H, et al. Irreversible inactivation of macrophage and brain nitric oxide synthase by L-N$^G$-methylarginine requires NADPH-dependent hydroxylation. J Med Chem 1993; 36:491–496.

26. Korth HG, Sustmann R, Thater C, et al. On the mechanism of the nitric oxide synthase-catalyzed conversion of N-omega-hydroxyl-L-arginine to citrulline and nitric oxide. J Biol Chem 1994; 269:17776–17779.

27. Baek KJ, Thiel BA, Lucas S, et al. Macrophage nitric oxide synthase subunits. Purification, characterization, and role of prosthetic groups and substrate in regulating their association into a dimeric enzyme. J Biol Chem 1993; 268:21120–21129.

28. Sheta EA, McMillan K, Masters BS. Evidence for a biodomain structure of constitutive cerebellar nitric oxide synthase. J Biol Chem 1994; 269:15147–15153.

29. Ghosh DK, Stuehr DJ. Macrophage NO synthase: characterization of isolated oxygenase and reductase domains reveals a head-to-head subunit interaction. Biochemistry 1995; 34:801–807.

30. Abu-Soud HM, Stuehr DJ. Nitric oxide synthases reveal a role for calmodulin in controlling electron transfer. Proc Natl Acad Sci USA 1993; 90:10769–10772.

31. Abu-Soud HM, Yoho LL, Stuehr DJ. Calmodulin controls neuronal nitric-oxide synthase by a dual mechanism. Activation of intra- and interdomain electron transfer. J Biol Chem 1994; 269:32047–32050.

32. Hevel JM, Marletta MA. Macrophage nitric oxide synthase: relationship between enzyme-bound tetrahydrobiopterin and synthase activity. Biochemistry 1992; 31:7160–7165.

33. Klatt P, Schmid M, Leopold E, et al. The pteridine binding site of brain nitric oxide synthase. Tetrahydrobiopterin binding kinetics, specificity, and allosteric interaction with the substrate domain. J Biol Chem 1994; 269:13861–13866.

34. Griscavage JM, Fukuto JM, Komori Y, et al. Nitric oxide inhibits neuronal nitric oxide synthase by interacting with the heme prosthetic group. Role of tetrahydrobiopterin in modulating the inhibitory action of nitric oxide. J Biol Chem 1994; 269:21644–21649.

35. Stuehr DJ, Kwon NS, Nathan CF. FAD and GSH participate in macrophage synthesis of nitric oxide. Biochem Biophys Res Commun 1990; 168:558–565.

36. Hofmann H, Schmidt, HHHW. Thiol dependence of nitric oxide synthase. Biochemistry 1995; 34:13443–13452.

37. Chen P-F, Tsai A-L, Wu KK. Cysteine 99 of endothelial nitric oxide synthase (NOS-III) is critical for tetrahydrobiopterin-dependent NOS-III stability and activity. Biochem Biophys Res Commun 1995; 215:1119–1129.

38. Persechini A, McMillan K, Masters BSS. Inhibition of nitric oxide synthase by $Zn^{2+}$ ion. Biochemistry 1995; 34:15091–15095.

39. Hall AV, Antoniou H, Wang Y, et al. Structural organization of the human neuronal nitric oxide synthase gene (NOS1). J Biol Chem 1994; 269:33082–33090.

40. Regulski M, Tully T. Molecular and biochemical characterization of dNOS: a Drosophila $Ca^{2+}$/calmodulin-dependent nitric oxide synthase. Biochemistry 1995; 92:9072–9076.

41. Brenman JE, Chao DS, Xia H, et al. Nitric oxide synthase complexed with dystrophin and absent from skeletal muscle sarcolemma in Duchenne muscular dystrophy. Cell 1995; 82:743–752.

42. Busconi L, Michel T. Endothelial nitric oxide synthase. N-terminal myristoylation determines subcellular localization. J Biol Chem 1993; 268:8410–8413.

43. Liu J, Garcia-Cardena G, Sessa WC. Biosynthesis and palmitoylation of endothelial nitric oxide synthase: mutagenesis of palmitoylation sites, cysteines-15 and/or -26, argues against depalmitoylation-induced translocation of the enzyme. Biochemistry 1995; 34:12333–12340.

44. Bredt DS, Hwang PM, Glatt CE, et al. Cloned and expressed nitric oxide synthase structurally resembles cytochrome P-450 reductase. Nature 1991; 351:714–718.

45. McMillan K, Masters BSS. Prokaryotic expression of the heme- and flavin-binding domains of rat neuronal nitric oxide synthase as distinct polypeptides: identification of the heme-binding proximal thiolate ligand as cysteine-415. Biochemistry 1995; 34:3686–3693.

46. Chen P-F, Tsai A-L, Wu KK. Cysteine 184 of endothelial nitric oxide synthase is involved in heme coordination and catalytic activity. J Biol Chem 1994; 269:25062–25066.

47. Richards MK, Marletta MA. Characterization of neuronal nitric oxide synthase and a C415H mutant, purified from a baculovirus overexpression system. Biochemistry 1994; 33:14723–14732.

48. Salerno JC, Morales AJ. Sequence and structural homology in NO synthase: identification of the biopterin binding site. In: Ignarro L, Murad F, eds. Biochemistry and Molecular Biology of Nitric Oxide, First International Conference (abstr). University of California, Los Angeles, 1994:72.

49. Nishimura JS, Martasek P, McMillan K, et al. Modular structure of neuronal nitric oxide synthase: localization of the arginine binding site and modulation by pterin. Biochem Biophys Res Commun 1995; 210:288–294.

50. McMillan K, Masters BS. Optical difference spectrophotometry as a probe of rat brain nitric oxide synthase heme-substrate interaction. Biochemistry 1993; 32:9875–9880.

51. Matsuoka A, Stuehr DJ, Olson JS, et al. L-arginine and calmodulin regulation of the heme iron reactivity in neuronal nitric oxide synthase. J Biol Chem 1994; 269:20335–20339.

52. Frey C, Narayanan K, McMillan K, et al. L-thiocitrulline. A stereospecific, heme-binding inhibitor of nitric-oxide synthases. J Biol Chem 1994; 269: 26083–26091.

53. Hurshman AR, Marletta MA. Nitric oxide complexes of inducible nitric oxide synthase: spectral characterization and effect on catalytic activity. Biochemistry 1995; 34:5627–5634.

54. Wang J, Stuehr DJ, Ikeda-Saito M, et al. Heme coordination and structure of the catalytic site in nitric oxide synthase. J Biol Chem 1993; 268:22255–22258.

55. Wang J, Rousseau DL, Abu-Soud HM, et al. Heme coordination of NO in NO synthase. Proc Natl Acad Sci USA 1994; 91:10512–10516.

56. Ray GB, Li X-Y, Ibers JA, et al. How far can proteins bend the Fe-CO unit? Distal polar steric effects in heme proteins and models. J Am Chem Soc 1994; 116:162–176.

57. Schenkman JB, Sligar SG, Cinti DL. Substrate interaction with cytochrome P-450. Pharmacol Ther 1981; 12:43–71.

58. Narayanan K, Spack L, McMillan K, et al. S-alkyl-L-thiocitrullines. Potent stereoselective inhibitors of nitric oxide synthase with strong pressor activity in vivo. J Biol Chem 1995; 270:11103–11110.

59. Abu-Soud HM, Feldman PL, Clark P, et al. Electron transfer in the nitric-oxide synthases. Characterization of L-arginine analogs that block heme iron reduction. J Biol Chem 1994; 269:32318–32326.

60. Roman LJ, Sheta EA, Martasek P, et al. High-level expression of functional rat neuronal nitric oxide synthase in Escherichia coli. Proc Natl Acad Sci USA 1995; 92:8428–8432.

61. Southan GJ, Gross SS, Vane JR. Esters and amides of $N^G$-nitro-L-arginine act as prodrugs in their inhibition of inducible nitric oxide synthase. In: Moncada S, et al., eds. The Biology of Nitric Oxide, Vol. 4. Enzymology, Biochemistry and Immunology. Portland Press, Chapel Hill, NC, 1995:4–7.

62. Narayanan K, Griffith OW. Synthesis of L-thiocitrulline, L-homothiocitrulline, and S-methyl-L-thiocitrulline: a new class of potent nitric oxide synthase inhibitors. J Med Chem 1994; 37:885–887.

63. Furfine ES, Harmon MF, Paith JE, et al. Potent and selective inhibition of human nitric oxide synthases. Selective inhibition of neuronal nitric oxide synthase by S-methyl-L-thiocitrulline and S-ethyl-L-thiocitrulline. J Biol Chem 1994; 269:26677–26683.

64. McCall TB, Feelisch M, Palmer RM, et al. Identification of N-iminoethyl-L-

ornithine as an irreversible inhibitor of nitric oxide synthase in phagocytic cells. Br J Pharmacol 1991; 102:234–238.

65. Moore WM, Webber RK, Jerome GM, et al. L-N6-(1-iminoethyl)lysine: a selective inhibitor of inducible nitric oxide synthase. J Med Chem 1994; 37: 3886–3888.

66. Olken NM, Marletta MA. $N^G$-allyl- and $N^G$-cyclopropyl-L-arginine: two novel inhibitors of macrophage nitric oxide synthase. J Med Chem 1992; 35: 1137–1144.

67. Robertson JG, Bernatowicz MS, Dhalla AM, et al. Inhibition of bovine brain nitric oxide synthase by a-amino and a-carboxyl derivatives of $N^G$-allyl-L-arginine. Bioorg Chem 1995; 23:144–151.

68. Garvey EP, Oplinger JA, Tanoury GJ, et al. Potent and selective inhibition of human nitric oxide synthases. Inhibition by non-amino acid isothioureas. J Biol Chem 1994; 269:26669–26676.

69. Nakane M, Klinghofer V, Kuk JE, et al. Novel potent and selective inhibitors of inducible nitric oxide synthase. Mol Pharm 1995; 47:831–834.

70. Basha FZ, et al. Presented at the 210th National Meeting of the American Chemical Society, Chicago, August 1995; paper MEDI 244.

71. Hansen DW, Currie MG, Hallinan EA, et al. Amidino derivatives useful as nitric oxide synthase inhibitors. 1995; WO patent 95/11231.

72. Tjoeng FS, Fok KF, Webber RK. Amidino derivatives useful as nitric oxide synthase inhibitors. 1995; WO patent 95/11014.

73. Henley P, Tinker AC. 1,2-Diaminobenzimidazoles: selective inhibitors of nitric oxide synthase derived from aminoguanidine. Bioorg Med Chem Lett 1995; 5:1573–1576.

74. Sup SJ, Green BG, Grant SK. 2-Iminobiotin is an inhibitor of nitric oxide synthases. Biochem Biophys Res Commun 1994; 204:962–968.

75. Macdonald JE. Brain selective antagonists of nitric oxide synthase. Presentation at the 4th Annual International Business Communications Conference on Nitric Oxide; Philadelphia, March, 1995.

76. Macdonald JE, Gentile RJ, Murray RJ. Guanadine derivatives useful in therapy. 1994; WO patent 94/21621.

77. Gentile RJ, Murray RJ, MacDonald JE, et al. Amidine derivatives with nitric oxide synthetase activities. 1995; WO patent 95/05363.

78. Cole PA, Robinson CH. Mechanism and inhibition of cytochrome P-450 aromatase. J Med Chem 1990; 33:2933–2942.

79. Wolff DJ, Datto GA, Samatovicz RA, et al. Calmodulin-dependent nitric-oxide synthase. Mechanism of inhibition by imidazole and phenylimidazoles. J Biol Chem 1993; 268:9425–9429.

80. Wolff DJ, Datto GA, Samatovicz RA. The dual mode of inhibition of calmodulin-dependent nitric-oxide synthase by anti-fungal imidazole agents. J Biol Chem 1993; 268:9430–9436.

81. Wolff DJ, Lubeskie A, Umansky S. The inhibition of the constitutive bovine endothelial nitric oxide synthase by imidazole and indazole agents. Arch Biochem Biophys 1994; 314:360–366.

82. Mayer B, Klatt P, Werner ER, et al. Identification of imidazole as L-arginine-competitive inhibitor of porcine brain nitric oxide synthase. FEBS Lett 1994; 350:199–202.

83. Wolff DJ, Gribin BJ. Interferon-gamma–inducible murine macrophage nitric oxide synthase: studies on the mechanism of inhibition by imidazole agents. Arch Biochem Biophys 1994; 311:293–299.

84. Handy RLC, Wallace P, Gaffen ZA, et al. The antinociceptive effect of 1-(2-trifluoromethylphenyl)-imidazole, a potent inhibitor of neuronal nitric oxide synthase in vitro, in the mouse. Br J Pharmacol 1995; 116:2349–2350.

85. Babbedge RC, Bland-Ward PA, Hart SL, et al. Inhibition of rat cerebellar nitric oxide synthase by 7-nitro indazole and related substituted indazoles. Br J Pharmacol 1993; 108:225–228.

86. Moore PK, Wallace P, Gaffen Z, et al. Characterization of the novel nitric oxide synthase inhibitor 7-nitro indazole and related indazoles: antinociceptive and cardiovascular effects. Br J Pharmacol 1993; 108:219–224.

87. Moore PK, Babbedge RC, Wallace P, et al. 7-Nitro indazole, an inhibitor of nitric oxide synthase, exhibits anti-nociceptive activity in the mouse without increasing blood pressure. Br J Pharmacol 1993; 108:296–297.

88. Wolff DJ, Gribin BJ. The inhibition of the constitutive and inducible nitric oxide synthase isoforms by indazole agents. Arch Biochem Biophys 1994; 311:300–306.

89. Bland-Ward PA, Moore PK. 7-Nitro indazole derivatives are potent inhibitors of brain, endothelium and inducible isoforms of nitric oxide synthase. Life Sci 1995; 57:131–135.

# Endothelin: From Basic to Pathophysiological Research

**Katsutoshi Goto**

*Institute of Basic Medical Sciences, The University of Tsukuba,
Tsukuba, Ibaraki, Japan*

## I. INTRODUCTION

Endothelin, a 21–amino acid peptide, was first isolated from the culture supernatant of porcine aortic endothelial cells and was shown to possess unusually potent vasoconstrictor and pressor activities (1). This peptide, which was originally termed porcine endothelin and is now referred to as endothelin-1, has a molecular weight of 2492, free amino and carboxyl termini, and two intrachain disulfide bonds between residues $Cys^1$-$Cys^{15}$ and $Cys^3$-$Cys^{11}$.

Since the initial isolation, endothelin-1 has been shown to be encoded in the genome of several mammalian species, including humans. Analysis of the human genome revealed that two other endothelin isopeptides are encoded in separate genes, endothelin-2 and endothelin-3 (2). These isoforms of endothelin show a high degree of primary amino acid sequence identity; all are 21–amino acid polypeptides containing two intrachain disulfide bonds, and all contain an identical hydrophobic C-terminal hexapeptide sequence. The three endothelin isopeptides share a remarkable resemblance, both in structure and biological activity, to the sarafotoxins, a family of isopeptides isolated from the venom of the snake *Atractaspis engaddensis*, suggesting a possible common evolutionary origin (3).

The genes encoding the three endothelin isopeptides are expressed with different patterns in a wide variety of tissues, suggesting that the peptides may participate independently in complex cardiovascular regulatory mechanisms (4). In addition to their cardiovascular actions, endothelin isopeptides also act on nonvascular tissues, including respiratory tissues, kidney, endocrine glands, and peripheral and central nervous system, and are considered to be closely related to physiological control as well as having pathophysiological implications in various tissues (5,6). With such a variety of actions, it is not hard to understand why the endothelin isopeptides have stimulated much research activities in both academia and industry. Recent advances in the development of endothelin receptor antagonists have accelerated the pace of investigations of the true pathophysiological roles of endogenous endothelins in mature animals and humans. As a result, the physiological and pathophysiological roles of endothelin-1 have been gradually uncovered. Nevertheless, there is still a paucity of comparative information on endothelin-2 and endothelin-3.

The production of endothelin-deficient (7) and endothelin receptor–deficient (8) mice by means of gene targeting has shown unexpectedly that the endothelins have crucial roles in normal embryonic development. Endothelin-1–deficient mice, for instance, have craniofacial and cardiac abnormalities at birth and die of respiratory failure soon after birth (7). These molecular biological studies open up an entirely new field of research on endothelins, but they are beyond the scope of this chapter.

## II.  BIOSYNTHESIS OF ENDOTHELIN AND ITS REGULATION

Sequence analysis of porcine endothelin-1 cDNA revealed the existence of a single gene copy that encoded for a precursor, preproendothelin. Human preproendothelin-1 is a 212–amino acid protein that is proteolytically cleaved at paired basic amino acids, specifically at an adjacent position of $Lys^{51}$-$Arg^{52}$ and $Arg^{92}$-$Arg^{93}$ by a dibasic pair–specific endopeptidase, furin (9), thereby producing a 38–amino acid residue intermediate peptide, termed "big endothelin-1." Big endothelin-1 is subsequently cleaved at $Trp^{21}$-$Val^{22}$ by a novel endopeptidase, which appears to be specific for endothelin and was putatively termed endothelin-converting enzyme (ECE) (Fig. 1). In vascular endothelial cells, endothelin-1 is secreted via the constitutive pathway, and the rate-limiting step of its biosynthesis is thought to be at the level of transcription (1). Endothelin-1 gene expression in vascular endothelial cells has been shown to be stimulated by a number of chemical stimuli, such as growth factors, thrombin (10), transforming growth factor $\beta$ (TGG-$\beta$) (11), cytokines (e.g., tumor necrosis factor-$\alpha$ [TNF-$\alpha$] [12], interleukin-1 [Il-1] [13]), vasoactive substances

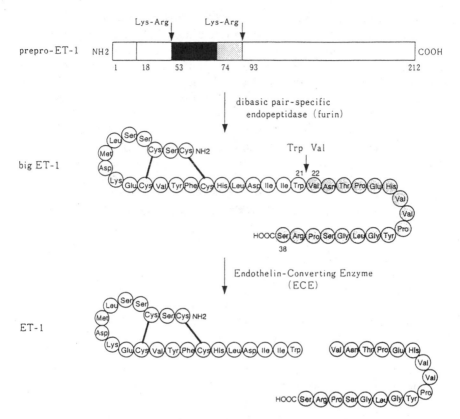

**Figure 1** The biosynthesis and intracellular processing of endothelin-1 (ET-1) from prepro-ET-1. Endothelin-converting enzyme (ECE) specifically catalyzes the conversion of big ET-1 to ET-1.

(e.g., norepinephrine, angiotensin II, vasopressin, bradykinin [14,15]), and physical stimuli (e.g., shear stress) (16).

Whether big endothelin-1 is cleaved intracellularly or extracellularly has been a matter of controversy. Endothelial cells possess a membrane-bound neutral metalloprotease exhibiting ECE activity (17) which is inhibited by a relatively high concentration of phosphoramidon (18). Both in vivo or in vitro, exogenously applied big endothelin-1 is rapidly converted, suggesting that the conversion takes place at the cell surface (19). However, the precise mechanism of conversion still remains to be elucidated.

Recently, by sequencing the ECE fragment purified from the bovine adrenal cortex and using a cDNA product obtained by a reverse transcription-polymerase chain reaction as a probe, the ECE-1 gene was cloned from bovine adrenal cortex cDNA libraries (20). The structure of the ECE-1 gene reflects a 758–amino acid metalloprotease enzyme containing a single membrane-spanning sequence with only a 56-residue N-terminal cytoplasmic tail and an extracellular C-terminal of 681–amino acid residues that contains the catalytic domain. Amino acid residues 593–601 match the highly conserved consensus sequence of a zinc binding motif, HEXXH, which is shared by many known metalloproteases. The ECE-1 protein has 10 predicted sites for N-glycosylation in the extracellular domain, suggesting that ECE-1 behaves as a highly glycosylated protein. Northern blot analysis demonstrated a ubiquitous distribution of a 4.4-kb fragment of mRNA for this enzyme, with the highest expression in endothelium, ovary, testis, and adrenal medulla. This enzyme appears to be associated with the plasma membrane and Golgi complex and to process big endothelin-1 more efficiently than either big endothelin-2 or big endothelin-3, suggesting the possible existence of multiple substrate-specific mammalian isozymes. Furthermore, certain endothelin-producing cell types, most notably neurons, do not exhibit expression of ECE-1 mRNA, again suggesting the possibility that different ECE isozymes may be expressed in neural tissues.

Achieving proper characterization of the pathways involved in endothelin biosynthesis has proved a more difficult goal than we might have predicted. After spending more than six years working toward to goal, cloning and characterization of ECE have been successfully achieved. ECE has been considered to be a potential target for selectively interrupting the biosynthesis of endothelin; although this approach has proven extremely difficult, a N- and C-terminal–truncated analogue of big endothelin-1 (1-38), (Phe[22]) big endothelin-1 (19-37) has recently been shown to be a potent inhibitor of ECE-1 which is at least 30-fold more potent than phosphoramidon in blocking big endothelin-1–induced vasoconstriction in the kidney (21).

## III. ENDOTHELIN RECEPTORS AND SIGNAL TRANSDUCTION

It was originally shown that intravenously administered endothelin-1 produced an initial transient fall and subsequent elevation of systemic blood pressure in anesthetized rats (1). The initial depressor response and the later pressor response were thought to be mediated by different mechanisms; although endothelin-1 is more potent than endothelin-3 in vasoconstrictive activity, both isopeptides are almost equipotent with respect to the initial depressor activity (2). A straightforward interpretation of these findings is that the receptors mediating these opposing responses may be different; one a vascular smooth muscle receptor with a strong preference for endothelin-1 over endothelin-3, and the other an endothelial cell type receptor to which both peptides bind equally. A similar dissociation of the pharmacological potency order of the three endothelin isopeptides has also been observed in a variety of tissues other than the vascular system.

Endothelin-induced responses may be divided into two major groups according to the pharmacological potency order of the three isopeptides (22–34). In the first group of responses, which includes vasoconstriction, bronchoconstriction, uterine smooth muscle contraction, and stimulation of aldosterone secretion, endothelin-1 and endothelin-2 act as far more potent agonists than endothelin-3. In the second group, which includes endothelium-dependent vasorelaxation and inhibition of ex vivo platelet aggregation, the three isopeptides have almost equal potency. These observations suggest that there are at least two distinct ET receptors mediating these two distinct groups of pharmacological responses (Table 1).

Cross-linking experiments between radiolabeled endothelin and the endothelin binding studies in various tissues provided the first biochemical evidence for the existence of multiple endothelin binding sites (35,36). In other experiments on radioligand affinity in membrane fractions prepared from vascular smooth muscle cells (27), chick heart (36), rat lung (37), rat mesangial cells (38), human placenta (39), and bovine cerebellum (40), the existence of at least two distinct subtypes of endothelin receptor was also suggested by the different relative affinities of the endothelin isopeptides.

Two cDNA clones that encode endothelin receptors have been isolated from rat (41) and bovine (42) lungs simultaneously by employing direct expression cloning techniques. Another endothelin receptor cDNA was also cloned from rat A10 cells (43). Subsequently, human homologues of these receptors were isolated by cross hybridization using these cDNAs as probes (44,45). According to the relative binding affinities of the three endothelin isopeptides for the receptors when expressed in transfected mammalian cells, these receptors can be classified into two groups. The order of affinity of endothelins for the first receptor type, designated $ET_A$, is endothelin-1≥endothelin-2>>endothelin-3. The second receptor type, designated $ET_B$, shows equipotent affinity for all three endothelins and for sarafotoxins (5). These results are consistent with the results of previous pharmacological and biochemical experiments and herein provide the molecular basis for the existence of two distinct endothelin receptor subtypes (Fig. 2).

Are there still more subtypes of endothelin receptor? In pharmacological and radioligand binding experiments, the existence of a receptor specific for endothelin-3 has been first demonstrated in cultured bovine endothelial cells (46) and cultured rat anterior pituitary cells (47). Subse-

**Table 1**  Classification of Pharmacological Responses Induced by ET-1 and ET-3 in Various Tisues

| Response | Tissue or organ (species) | Assay | Reference |
|---|---|---|---|
| Type I (ET-1>ET-3) | Vascular smooth muscle cells | E.g., pressor effect in vivo, contraction, PI generation, binding assay | 2 |
| | Bronchial smooth muscle (human) | Contraction | 22 |
| | Smooth muscle of gall bladder (human) | Contraction | 23 |
| | Uterine smooth muscle (rat) | Contraction, PI generation, binding assay | 24 |
| | Cardiac muscle (neonatal rat) | PI generation, binding assay | 25 |
| | Adrenocortical cells (zona glomerulosa, bovine) | Stimulation of aldosterone secretion, binding assay | 26 |
| | C6 glioma cells (rat) | PI generation, binding assay | 27 |
| | Fibroblast cells (human, mouse) | $Ca^{2+}$ transient, binding assay | 28 |
| | Osteoblast cells (rat) | E.g., DNA synthesis, PI generation, binding assay | 29 |
| Type II (ET-1=ET-3) | Whole animal (rat) | Initial depressor response in vivo | 2 |
| | Mesenteric artery (rat) | Transient relaxation, EDRF release | 30 |
| | Smooth muscle of renal pelvis (human) | Contraction | 23 |
| | Stomach (rat) | Ulcerogenicity | 31 |
| | Whole animal (rabbit) | Inhibition of ex vivo platelet aggregation | 32 |
| | Cerebral cortex, cerebellum (rat) | PI generation | 33 |
| | Astrocytes (rat) | PI generation, $Ca^{2+}$ transient | 34 |
| | Mesangium cells (rat) | PI generation, binding assay | 27 |

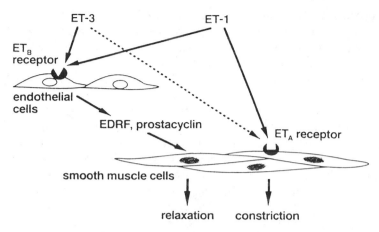

**Figure 2** Schematic presentation of vasodilation and vasoconstriction induced by ET-1 or ET-3. The $ET_A$ receptor on smooth muscle has high affinity for ET-1 but low affinity for ET-3, inducing vasoconstriction. The $ET_B$ receptor on the endothelium has equal affinity for both peptides, releasing EDRF or prostacyclin. Responses induced by ETs depend on balance of activities at $ET_A$ and $ET_B$ receptors.

quently, much pharmacological evidence has accumulated to suggest that there may exist further subtypes or sub-subtypes of endothelin receptor (48). However, there has been no report so far on isolation of the cDNA clones encoding the receptor specific for endothelin-3 from mammalian tissues. Furthermore, Southern blot analysis of human genomic DNAs with cloned cDNA probes suggests that each endothelin receptor cDNA probe can cross hybridize with only two different genomic DNA fragments even under the condition of reduced stringency (45). Thus, it appears that mammalian genomes contain only two closely related genes that encode endothelin receptors, which may correspond to $ET_A$ and $ET_B$, and it is likely that the third receptor gene, if it exists in mammalian genomes, has little similarity to the two cloned receptors.

From the dermal melanophore of *Xenopus laevis,* a receptor has been cloned that shows functional selectivity for endothelin-3 over endothelin-1, and this was termed $ET_C$. This receptor has 47 and 53% primary amino acid homology to mammalian $ET_A$ and $ET_B$ receptors, respectively (49). However, the difference in affinity to the expressed receptor between endothelin-3 and endothelin-1 was not as great as expected. Further, the expressed receptor showed only low affinity for both endothelin-3 and endothelin-1, with $K_d$ values several orders of magnitude lower than those of most published receptors for both endothelin isopeptides. Another endothelin receptor has been cloned from *Xenopus laevis* heart (50). The isolated cDNA encoded a protein of 415 amino acids which showed 74, 60, and 50% primary amino acid sequence identity with human $ET_A$, $ET_B$, and *Xenopus laevis* $ET_C$ receptors, respectively. The characteristics of this receptor are similar to those of the mammalian $ET_A$ receptor in that endothelin-3 showed weaker affinity than endothelin-1, and sarafotoxin 6c showed hardly any affinity. Since BQ-123, the $ET_A$-selective antagonist, was found to be ineffective in inhibiting [125]I–endothelin-1 binding, this *Xenopus laevis* receptor might be an amphibian variant of the mammalian $ET_A$ receptor.

Exposure of cultured smooth muscle cells (51), Swiss 3T3 cells (52), and glomerular mesangial cells (53) to endothelin-1 for a long time causes a marked decrease in [125]I–endothelin-1 binding sites, indicating an autologous downregulation of endothelin receptors. As observed with other vasoconstrictor substances, internalization of the endothelin receptor complex has been proposed as the mechanism for downregulation (54). After internalization, the ligand-receptor complex is thought to be sequestered into lysosomal compartments where the acidic environment promotes ligand dissociation (51). In rat osteosarcoma ROS 17/2 cells, rapid downregulation (within several hours) of the $ET_B$ receptor has been demonstrated (55). A decrease in $ET_B$ receptor mRNA was also induced by addition of either phorbol esters or ionomycin to the culture medium; this effect possibly results from a decrease in the stability of $ET_B$ receptor mRNA rather than from inactivation of mRNA transcription.

Functionally, both $ET_A$ and $ET_B$ receptors may be coupled to phospholipase C (PLC) via GTP binding proteins (56,57). Activation of PLC causes phosphatidyl inositol hydrolysis and rapid formation of 1,4,5-inositol triphosphate ($IP_3$) and sustained accumulation of 1,2-diacylglycerol (DG). $IP_3$ is an important intracellular signaling molecule that stimulates the release of $Ca^{2+}$ from intracellular stores in the sites' sarcoplasmic reticulum. Numerous in vitro studies demonstrated that upon application of endothelin-1, arterial smooth muscle cells show a rapid transient increase in intracellular $Ca^{2+}$ concentration $[Ca^{2+}]i$ and a subsequent sustained increase in $[Ca^{2+}]i$ (58). The initial transient phase of $[Ca^{2+}]i$ response is not dependent on the presence of external $Ca^{2+}$ and is the result of $IP_3$-induced mobilization of $Ca^{2+}$ from intracellular stores. In contrast, the sustained increase of $[Ca^{2+}]i$ appears to be due to an influx of extracellular $Ca^{2+}$ through either dihydropyridine-sensitive voltage-dependent L-type $Ca^{2+}$ channels (59,60) or receptor-operated (nonselective) cation channels that are insensitive to dihydropyridine (61). Following stimulation of endothelin receptors, the cation channels might be opened either by direct coupling with the GTP binding protein subunit or via certain intracellular signal transduction, but the precise mechanism remains to be elucidated.

As the short-term changes in cell function produced by endothelin receptor activation, other than the increase in $[Ca^{2+}]i$, activation of phospholipase $A_2$ (62) and D (63) and arachidonic acid metabolism have been demonstrated. The activation of phospholipase D appears to contribute to the sustained DG accumulation, which may lead to prolonged activation of protein kinase C (PKC) (64). In vascular smooth muscle and cardiac muscle cells, a change in intracellular pH (alkalinization) is also induced via stimulation of $Na^+$-$H^+$ exchange, which seems to be a consequence of PKC activation (65).

In addition to being a potent vasoconstrictor, endothelin-1 is a potent mitogen in, for example, cultured vascular smooth muscle cells (66), cardiac myocytes (67), and glomerular mesangial cells (68). Endothelin-1 also induces the expression of several proto-oncogenes (c-*fos,* c-*myc,* c-*jun*) (69). The proliferative and hypertrophic potential of endothelin-1 raises the possibility that endothelin-1 may contribute to the cardiovascular remodeling associated with various pathophysiological states. Since endothelin-1, but not sarafotoxin S6c, a selective $ET_B$ agonist, produces cellular proliferation which is inhibited by BQ-123, the $ET_A$ receptor is thought to be coupled to the mitogenic effects of endothelin isopeptides (70). However, it has been found that cultured rat aortic vascular smooth muscle cells possess predominantly $ET_A$ receptors between passage 10–15, and $ET_B$ receptors between passage 30–35 (71). In this case, the later-passaged cells appeared to be linked to the mitogenic response. Such phenotypic changes in endothelin receptors might occur in certain pathophysiological conditions, such as atherosclerosis and neointima formation. Thus, which endothelin receptor subtype is responsible for the mitogenic effect is still a matter of controversy.

In these long-term effects of endothelin, elevation of $[Ca^{2+}]i$, activation of PKC, and tyrosine and threonine phosphorylation of mitogen-activated protein kinase (MAPK) have been proposed to play crucial roles (72). Irrespective of the exact mechanisms of action, endothelin isopeptides may participate in long-term adaptive changes in various tissues via these signaling pathways; for example, vascular remodeling, including neointima formation, cardiac hypertrophy, chronic heart failure, glomerulonephritis, and bone remodeling. In cultured vascular smooth muscle cells, even though endothelin-1 alone did not show mitogenic effects, it strongly potentiated, for example, the mitogenic activities of PDGF (73) and calf serum (74). These findings suggest that endothelin-1 may be a potent competence and/or progression factor, stimulating transition from $G_0$ to $G_1$ in the cell cycle, leading to increased DNA synthesis in certain conditions and to mitogenesis in combination with other growth factors, particularly in in vivo situations.

## IV.  ENDOTHELIN RECEPTOR ANTAGONISTS

In order to develop new agonists and antagonists, as in the case of many bioactive peptides, modification of the endothelin and sarafotoxin amino acid sequences has been attempted and resulted in not only production of a series of agonists with varying potency but also gave rise to a number of antagonists that are either selective or nonselective for endothelin receptor subtypes. An important milestone in the development of useful tools for the study of endothelin was the isolation of a cyclic pentapeptide BE-18257B from the fermentation products of *Streptomyces misakiensis* (75). Further modification of BE-18257B has led to the identification of the cyclic pentapeptide BQ-123 (Banyu) with higher affinity for $ET_A$ receptor (76). Because of its competitive and selective nature, high potency, and aqueous solubility (77), BQ-123 has been widely used not only for in vitro pharmacological as well as biochemical studies but also for the investigation of potential physiological and/or pathophysiological roles of endogenous endothelin. A cyclic hexapeptide, TAK-044 (Takeda), is a synthetic compound that exhibits antagonistic activity on both $ET_A$ and $ET_B$ receptors (78) (Fig. 3).

Subsequent structure-activity studies using BQ-123 have led to the development of a series of potent $ET_A$ receptor–selective linear tripeptides, FR139317 (Fujisawa) (79), BQ-610 (Banyu) (80), PD151242 (Parke-Davis) (81), and the hexapeptide, TTA-386 (Takeda) (82). Further modifications along these lines resulted in the production of an $ET_B$ receptor–selective agonist, BQ-3020 (Banyu), and an $ET_B$ receptor–selective antagonist, BQ-788 (Banyu) (83). IRL 1620 (84) and IRL 2500 (Ciba-Geigy) (85) are other linear peptides exhibiting $ET_B$ receptor–selective agonistic and antagonistic actions, respectively. A linear hexapeptide, PD145065 (Parke-Davis) (86) exhibits antagonistic activities against both $ET_A$ and $ET_B$ receptors. These peptide agonists and antagonists have also been used in a wide variety of pharmacological and biochemical research on endothelin isopeptides (Fig. 4). Although small, relatively potent, and selective peptide antagonists of endothelin receptors have proven to be extremely valuable tools for the characterization of the endothelin receptors and for the determination of their tissue distribution, there are well-known limitations of the use of peptides in vivo for the chronic treatment of animal disease models and for clinical application in human patients. Thus, much effort has been directed toward the discovery of nonpeptide endothelin receptor antagonists.

The first nonpeptide endothelin receptor antagonist for practical use was Ro 46-2005 (Hoffmann-La Roche), which was shown to inhibit the binding of [125]I–endothelin-1 to human vascular smooth muscle cells ($ET_A$ receptors) and rat aortic endothelial cells ($ET_B$ receptors) with $IC_{50}$ values of 220 and

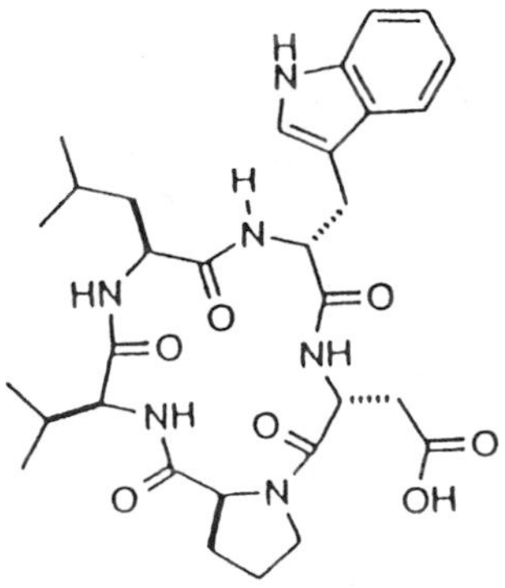

BQ– 123

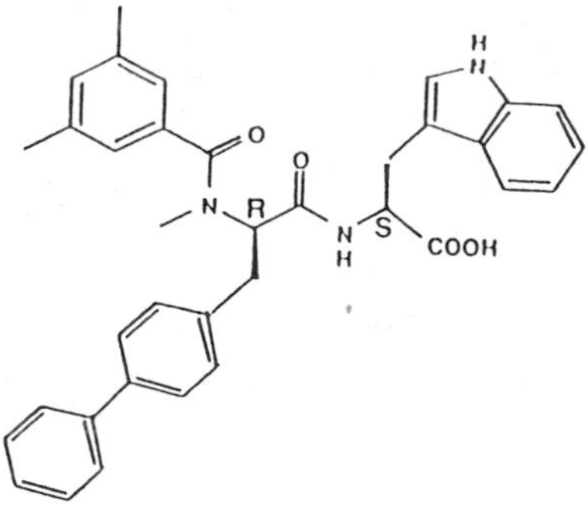

IRL 2500

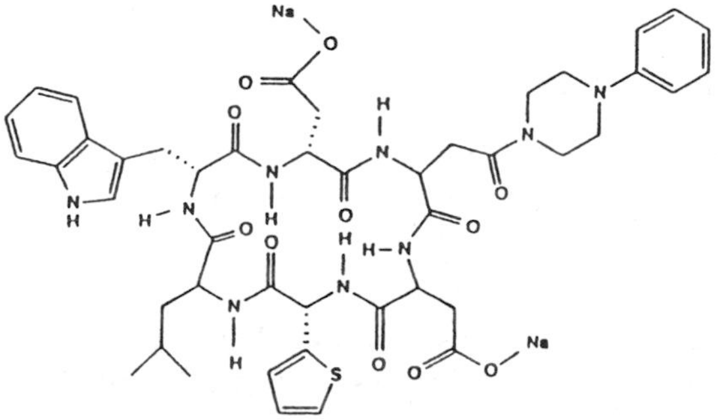

TAK– 044

**Figure 3** Molecular structures of endothelin receptor antagonists of cyclic tripeptide (BQ-123), cyclic hexapeptide (TAK-044), and linear tripeptide (IRL 2500).

1000 nM, respectively (87). Ro 46-2005 was produced by structural modification of a sulfonamide lead compound first synthesized as part of an antidiabetic effort and was identified as a nonselective antagonist of endothelin receptors. Although Ro 46-2005 had no effect on blood pressure in normotensive rats, it did show a long-lasting blood pressure–

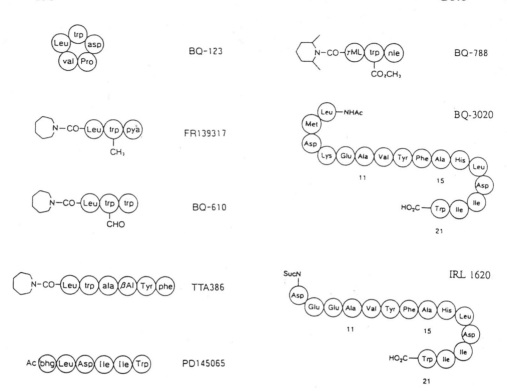

**Figure 4**  Amino acid sequences of various peptide agonists and antagonists for endothelin receptor. Capital letter; L-amino acid; Lowercase; D-amino acid.

lowering effects when orally administered as a bolus to sodium-depleted squirrel monkeys (10–100 mg/kg). This was the first demonstration that the oral administration of an endothelin receptor antagonist is actually efficacious to lower systemic blood pressure. Subsequent structure-activity relationships in this series led to the discovery of Ro 47-0203, bosentan (Hoffmann-LaRoche), a far more potent and more $ET_A$ receptor selective antagonist, with $K_i$ values (affinity) of 6.5 and 343 nM for $ET_A$ and $ET_B$ receptors, respectively (88). When administered either orally or intravenously, Ro 47-0203 did inhibit both the initial transient depressor ($ET_B$) and the following prolonged pressor ($ET_A$) responses induced by intravenously injected endothelin-1.

Using $^1H$ NMR-derived conformational models of ET-1, a rational approach was made in search of new nonpeptide antagonists of endothelin receptors. Screening of a chemical bank led to the identification of SK&F 66861 (SmithKline Beecham), another important lead structure of diphenylindane compounds (89). Comparison of the three-dimensional structure of this compound to low-energy $^1$H NMR-based conformations of endothelin-1 suggested that the 1- and 3-phenyl groups of SK&F 66861 are mimics of a combination of two of the aromatic side chains of Try$^{13}$, Phe$^{14}$ and Trp$^{21}$ in endothelin-1. Three-dimensional peptidomimetic simulation has been further continued. As a result, an extremely potent and highly specific nonpeptide endothelin receptor antagonist, SB 209670 (SmithKline Beecham), has been synthesized and characterized (90). The $K_i$ values of SB 209670 in inhibiting $^{125}$I-endothelin binding to cloned human endothelin receptor subtypes $ET_A$ and $ET_B$ are 0.2 and 18 nM, respectively. Intraduodenal administration of SB 209670 produced a dose-dependent reduction of blood pressure in spontaneously hypertensive rats, which continued for 24–48 hr. SB 209670 also protected against ischemia-induced neuronal degeneration in a gerbil stroke model (intracerebroventricular administration) and attenuated neointima formation following rat carotid artery balloon angioplasty (intraperitoneal administration).

At the 4th International Conference on Endothelin held in London in April 1995, further orally active nonpeptide antagonists of endothelin receptors were presented, including PD155080 and PD156707 (Parke-Davis) (91,92), L-751,281 and L-754,142 (Merke), BMS-182874 (Bristol-Myers Squibb). These new nonpeptide antagonists of endothelin receptors are under extensive investigation and are expected to be marketed in the near future (Fig. 5).

## V. PATHOPHYSIOLOGICAL ROLES OF ENDOGENOUS ENDOTHELINS

Endothelin-1 causes potent vasoconstriction and long-lasting elevation of blood pressure (1). Thus, endogenous endothelin-1 is assumed to modulate the vascular tone and regional blood flow as a circulating hormone or to exert its actions locally within the vascular wall and on the endothelium in an autocrine or paracrine fashion. This assumption may be naturally extended to the possible implication of endothelin-1 in the development of systemic hypertension. If endothelin-1 is actually involved in the pathophysiology of the hypertension, it could result from, for example, excessive production, reduced degradation, enhanced sensitivity or augmented responsiveness of vascular smooth muscle cells to the peptide (93), enhanced secretion of neurohumoral mediators of blood pressure regulation (e.g., norepinephrine, renin, angiotensin II), or diminished production of counterbalancing vasodilating mediators (94). Endothelin-1 is also thought to cause vascular wall thickening owing to its potent prolif-

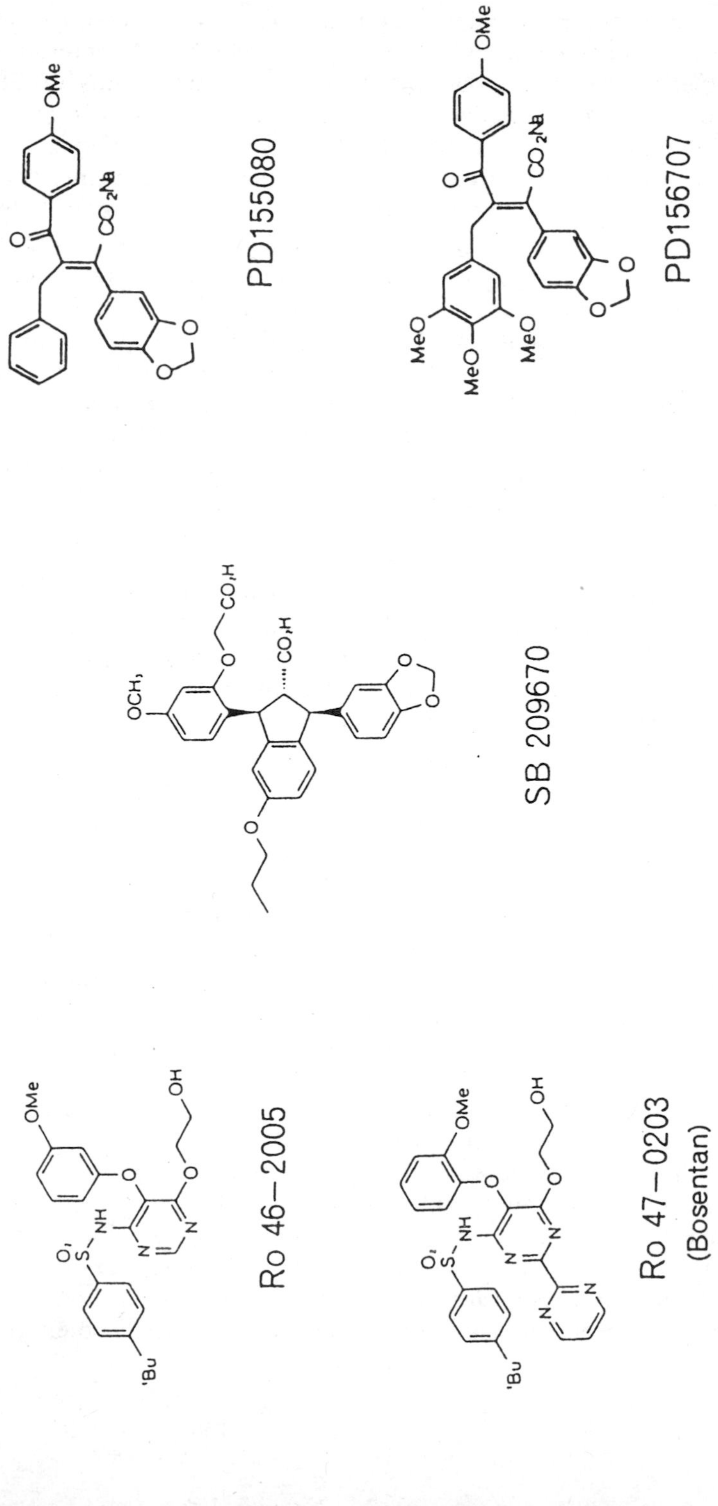

**Figure 5**  Molecular structures of nonpeptide endothelin receptor antagonists.

erative effects (95). Either one of these activities of endothelin-1 or a combination of these mechanisms may occur throughout the evolution of hypertension.

There are currently many reports regarding plasma levels of immunoreactive endothelin-1, and the results are fairly divergent (96). These observations have gradually given rise to the such negative supposition that endothelin-1 may not play any significant pathophysiological roles in the development of hypertension. Nevertheless, even if no appreciable change in plasma levels was detected, a significant correlation between the concentration of immunoreactive endothelin-1 in vascular tissue and the level of systemic blood pressure has been demonstrated in deoxycorticosterone acetate (DOCA)–salt–induced hypertensive rats (97). Furthermore, in this DOCA-salt–induced hypertension model, the elevated blood pressure was markedly reduced by $ET_A$ receptor antagonists, for example, BQ-123 (98), FR-139317 (99), and also by an endothelin-converting enzyme inhibitor, phosphoramidon (100).

Although the effects of peptide antagonists for endothelin receptors in spontaneously hypertensive rats (SHR) are currently controversial (101–103), the nonpeptide antagonist, SB 209670 has recently been shown to exert significant and long-lasting hypotensive actions following intraduodenal administration in this particular model of hypertension (90). The nonpeptide antagonists have been demonstrated to be effective in lowering the blood pressure in various animal models of hypertension; for example, sodium depletion–induced hypertension in squirrel monkeys (87), and renal hypertension in dogs (104). From these results, it can be speculated that endogenous endothelin-1 may be implicated in the pathogenesis of some types of hypertension in humans. However, we have to await the results of further studies in humans to confirm these observations.

The enhanced production of endothelin-1 and the effectiveness of endothelin receptor antagonists have been demonstrated in a number of other diseases, such as acute myocardial infarction (105,106), pulmonary hypertension (107–109), neurogenic pulmonary edema (110), cerebral vasospasm following subarachnoid hemorrhage (111,112), acute renal failure (113), and peptic ulcer (114,115). In addition to these acute effects, endothelin-1 is considered to exert chronic effects and to be deeply implicated in the proliferative responses associated with vascular diseases (116,117). Endothelin-1 has been reported to stimulate c-*fos* and c-*myc* expression (118), increase the incorporation of [³H]-thymidine into DNA, and cause proliferation of vascular smooth muscle cells (119), capillary endothelial cells (120), and fibroblasts. In vascular smooth muscle cells as well as in cardiac myocytes, endothelin-1 induces the expression of mRNA encoding PDGF and TGF-$\beta$ (122). Recent evidence suggests that the primary role of endothelin-1 in the pathophysiology of vascular disease is in the promotion of the synthesis and secretion of the glycoproteins, thrombospondin, fibronection, and tenascin, thereby leading to the modification of extracellular constituents in cardiovascular tissues (123). Of particular interest in this connection, SB 209670 has been shown to attenuate strongly neointima formation following rat carotid artery balloon angioplasty (90).

In patients with chronic heart failure, a condition frequently associated with high plasma endothelin-1 concentration (124,125), intravenous infusion of bosentan, a nonpeptide endothelin receptor antagonist, was shown to produce marked improvement of hemodynamic parameters; reductions in mean arterial, pulmonary arterial, right atrial and pulmonary artery wedge pressures, decreases in systemic and pulmonary vascular resistance, and resultant increases in cardiac output and stroke volume (126). These observations provide clear evidence that endothelin-1 contributes to the maintenance of vascular tone in such patients. Interestingly, in patients with acute myocardial infarction which often leads to chronic heart failure, the plasma level of endothelin-1 appears to be an indicator of long-term prognosis; the higher the plasma level of endothelin-1, the higher the long-term mortality (127). In the left coronary artery–ligated rat model of chronic heart failure, it has also been shown that endothelin-1 contributes to both maintenance and aggravation of chronic heart failure, most probably owing to an enhanced production of endothelin-1 in cardiac tissues (128). These findings suggest that interference with the endothelin-1 system by either specific receptor antagonists or endothelin-1–converting enzyme inhibitors may prove to be useful not only for the further delineation of the role of endogenous endothelin-1 in circulatory pathophysiology but also in new therapeutic approaches associated with high plasma or tissue levels of endothelin-1.

## REFERENCES

1. Yanagisawa M, Kurihara H, Kimura S, et al. A novel potent vasoconstrictor peptide produced by vascular endothelial cells. Nature 1988; 332:411–415.
2. Inoue A, Yanagisawa M, Kimura S, et al. The human endothelin family: three structurally and pharmacologically distinct isopeptides predicted by three separate genes. Proc Natl Sci USA 1989; 86:2863–2867.
3. Takasaki C, Tamiya N, Bdolah A, et al. Sarafotoxins S6: several isotoxins from *Atractaspis engaddensis* (burrowing asp) venom that affect the heart. Toxicon 1988; 26:543–548.
4. Sakurai T, Yanagisawa M, Inoue A, et al. cDNA cloning, sequence analysis and tissue distribution of rat preproendothelin-1 mRNA. Biochem Biophys Res Commun 1991; 75:44–47.

5. Sakurai T, Yanagisawa M, Masaki T. Molecular characterization of endothelin receptors. Trends Pharmacol Sci 1992; 13:103–108.

6. Rubabnyi GM, Polokoff MA. Endothelins: molecular biology, biochemistry, pharmacology, physiology, and pathophysiology. Pharmacol Rev 1994; 46: 325–415.

7. Kurihara Y, Kurihara H, Suzuki H, et al. Elevated blood pressure and craniofacial abnormalities in mice deficient in endothelin-1. Nature 1994; 368:703–710.

8. Hosoda K, Hammer RE, Giad A, et al. Targeted and natural (piebald-lethal) mutations of endothelin-B receptor gene produce megacolon associated with spotted coat color in mice. Cell 1994; 79:P1267–1276.

9. Denault J-B, Claing A, D'Orleans-Juste P, et al. Processing of proendothelin-1 by human furin convertase. FEBS Lett 1995; 362:276–280.

10. Emori T, Hirata Y, Imai T, et al. Cellular mechanisms of thrombin on endothelin-1 biosynthesis and release in bovine endothelial cell. Biochem Pharmacol 1992; 44:2409–2411.

11. Kurihara H, Yoshizumi M, Sugiyama T, et al. Transforming growth factor beta stimulates the expression of endothelin mRNA from vascular endothelial cells. Biochem Biophys Res Commun 1989; 159:1435–1440.

12. Marsden PA, Brenner BM. Transcriptional regulation of the endothelin gene by TNF alpha. Am J Physiol 1992; 262:C854–C861.

13. Maemura K, Kurihara H, Morita T, et al. Production of endothelin-1 in vascular endothelial cells is regulated by factors associated with vascular injury. Gerontology 1992; 38(suppl 1):29–35.

14. Marsden PA, Dorfman DM, Collins T, et al. Regulated expression of endothelin-1 in glomerular capillary endothelial cells. Am J Physiol 1991; 261: F117–F125.

15. Imai T, Hirata Y, Emori T, et al. Induction of endothelin-1 gene by angiotensin and vasopressin in endothelial cells. Hypertension 1992; 19:753–757.

16. Malek A, Izumo S. Physiological fluid shear stress causes downregulation of endothelin-1 mRNA in bovine aortic endothelium. Am J Physiol 1992; 263:C389–C396.

17. Ohnaka K, Takayanagi R, Yamauchi T, et al. Identification and characterization of endothelin converting activity in cultured bovine endothelial cells. Biochem Biophys Res Commun 1990; 168:1128–1136.

18. Ikegawa R, Matsumura Y, Tsukahara Y, et al. Phosphoramidon, a metalloproteinase inhibitor, suppresses the secretion of endothelin from cultured endothelial cells by inhibiting a big endothelin-1 converting enzyme. Biochem Biophys Res Commun 1990; 171:669–675.

19. Fukuroda T, Noguchi K, Tsuchida S, et al. Inhibition of biological actions of big endothelin-1 by phosphoroamidon. Biochem Biophys Res Commun 1990; 172:390–395.

20. Xu D, Emoto N, Giaid A, et al. ECE-1: a membrane-bound metalloprotease that catalyzes the proteolytic activation of big endothelin-1. Cell 1994; 78: 473–485.

21. Claing A, Neugebauer W, Yana M, et al. [Phe$^{22}$]-big endothelin-1[19-17]: a new and potent inhibitor of the endothelin-converting enzyme. J Cardiovasc Pharmacol 1995; 26(suppl 3):S72–S74.
22. Adenier C, Sarria B, Naline E, et al. Contractile activity of three endothelins (ET 1, ET 2 and ET 3) on the human isolated bronchus. Br J Pharmacol 1990; 100:168–172.
23. Maggi C, Giuliani S, Patacchini R, et al. Contractile responses of the human urinary bladder, renal pelvis and renal artery to endothelins and sarafotoxin S6b. Gen Pharmacol 1990; 21:247–249.
24. Bousso-Mittler D, Galton R and Sokolovsky M. Endothelin/sarafotoxin receptor heterogeneity: evidence for different glycosylation in receptors from different tissues. Biochem Biophys Res Commun 1991; 178:921–956.
25. Galron R, Kloog Y, Bdolah A, et al. Different pathways of endothelin/sarafotoxin stimulated phosphoinositide hydrolysis in myosites. Eur J Pharmacol 1990; 188:85–88.
26. Gomez-Sanchez CE, Cozza EN, Foeching MF, et al. Endothelin receptor subtypes and stimulation of aldosterone secretion. Hypertension 1990; 15:744–747.
27. Martin ER, Brenner BM and Ballermann BJ, et al. Heterogeneity of cell surface endothelin receptors. J Biol Chem 1990;265:14044–14049.
28. Ohnishi-Suzuki A, Yamaguchi K, Kasuhara M, et al. Comparison of biological activities of endothelin-1, -2 and -3 in murine and human fibroblast cell lines. Biochem Biophys Res Commun 1990; 166:608–614.
29. Takuwa Y, Masaki T, Yamashita K. The effects of the endothelin family on cultured osteoblastic cells from rat calvariae. Biochem Biophys Res Commun 1990; 170:998–1005.
30. Warner TD, Mitchell JA, De Nucci G, et al. Endothelin 1 and endothelin 3 release EDRF from isolated perfused arterial vessels of the rat and rabbit. J Cardiovasc Pharmacol 1989; 13(suppl 5):S85–S88.
31. Wallace JL, Keena CM, McNaughton WK, et al. Comparison of the effects of endothelin 1 and endothelin 3 on the rat stomach. Eur J Pharmacol 1989; 167:41–47.
32. Lidbury PS, Thiemermann C, Thomas GR, et al. Endothelin-3: selectivity as an anti-aggregatory peptide in vivo. Eur J Pharmacol 1989; 166:335–338.
33. Crawford ML, Hiley CR, Young JM. Characteristics of endothelin 1 and endothelin 3 stimulation of phosphoinositide breakdown differ between regions of guinea pig and rat brain. Naunyn Schmiedebergs Arch Pharmacol 1990; 341:268–271.
34. Marsault R, Vigne P, Breittmayer JP, et al. Astrocytes are target cells for endothelin and sarafotoxin. J Neurochem 1990; 54:2142–2144.
35. Calron R, Bdolah A, Kochva E, et al. Kinetic and cross linking studies indicate different receptors for endothelins and sarafotoxins in the ileum and cerebellum. FEBS Lett 1991; 283:11–14.
36. Watanabe H, Miyazaki H, Kondoh M, et al. Two distinct types of endothelin receptors are present on chick cardiac membranes. Biochem Biophys Res Commun 1989; 161:1252–1259.

37. Masuda Y. Two different forms of endothelin receptors in rat lung. FEBS Lett 1989; 257:208–210.
38. Sugiura M, Snajdar RM, Schwartzberg M, et al. Identification of two types of specific endothelin receptors in rat mesangial cell. Biochem Biophys Res Commun 1989; 162:1396–1401.
39. Nakajo S, Sugiura M, Inagami T, et al. Native forms of endothelin receptor in human placental membrane. Biochem Biophys Res Commun 1990; 167: 280–286.
40. Schvartz I, Ittoop O, Hazum E. Bovine cerebellum : solubilization and identification. Endocrinology 1990; 126:3218–3222.
41. Arai H, Hori S, Aramori I, et al. Cloning and expression of a cDNA encoding an endothelin receptor. Nature 1990; 348:730–732.
42. Sakurai T, Yanagisawa M, Takuwa Y, et al. Cloning of a cDNA encoding a non isopeptide selective subtype of the endothelin receptor. Nature 1990; 348:372–375.
43. Lin HY, Kaji EH, Winkel GK, et al. Cloning and functional expression of a vascular smooth muscle endothelin receptor. Proc Natl Acad Sci USA 1991; 88:3185–3189.
44. Hosoda K, Nakao K, Tamura N, et al. Organization, structure, chromosomal assignment, and expression of the gene encoding the human endothelin A receptor. J Biol Chem 1992; 267:18797–18804.
45. Sakamoto A, Yanagisawa M, Sakurai T, et al. Cloning and functional expression of human cDNA for $ET_B$ endothelin receptor. Biochem Biophys Res Commun 1991; 178:656–663.
46. Emori T, Hirata Y, Marumo F. Specific receptors for endothelin 3 in cultured bovine endothelial cells and its cellular mechanism of action. FEBS Lett 1990; 263:261–264.
47. Samson WK, Skala K, Huang FL, et al. Central nervous system action of endothelin 3 to inhibit water drinking in the rat. Brain Res 1991; 539:347–351.
48. Sudjarwo SA, Hori H, Tanaka T, et al. Subtypes of endothelin $ET_A$ and $ET_B$ receptors mediating venous smooth muscle contraction. Biochem Biophys Res Commun 1994; 200:627–633.
49. Karne S, Jayawickreme CK, Lerner MR. Cloning and characterization of an endothelin-3 specific receptor ($ET_C$ receptor) from *Xenopus laevis* dermal melanophores. J Biol Chem 1993; 268:19126–19133.
50. Kumar C, Mwangi V, Nuthulaganti P, et al. Cloning and characterization of a novel endothelin receptor from *Xenopus* heart. J Biol Chem 1994; 269: 13414–13420.
51. Hirata Y, Yoshimi H, Takaichi S, et al. Binding and receptor down regulation of a novel vasoconstrictor endothelin in cultured rat vascular smooth muscle cells. FEBS Lett 1988; 239:13–17.
52. Devesly P, Phillips PE, Johns A, et al. Receptor kinetics differ for endothelin 1 and endothelin 2 binding to Swiss 3T3 fibroblasts. Biochem Biophys Res Commun 1990; 172:126–134.
53. Thomas CP, Baldi E, Simonson MS, et al. Endothelin receptors and coupled

GTP binding proteins in glomerular mesangial cells. J Cardiovasc Pharmacol 1991; 17(suppl 7):S79–S84.

54. Resink TJ, Scott-Burden T, Buhler FR. Activation of multiple signal transduction pathways by endothelin in cultured human vascular smooth muscle cells. Eur J Biochem 1990; 189:415–421.
55. Sakurai T, Morimoto Y, Kasuya Y, et al. Level of ET$_B$ receptor mRNA is down-regulated by endothelin through decreasing the intracellular stability of mRNA molecules. Biochem Biophys Res Commun 1992; 186:342–347.
56. Badr KF, Murray JJ, Breyer MD, et al. Mesangial cell, glomerular and renal vascular responses to endothelin in the rat kidney. Elucidation of signal transduction pathways. J Clin Invest 1989; 83:336–342.
57. Takuwa Y, Kasuya Y, Takuwa N, et al. Endothelin receptor is coupled to phospholipase C via a pertussis toxin insensitive guanine nucleotide binding regulatory protein in vascular smooth muscle cells. J Clin Invest 1990; 85:653–658.
58. Simonson MS, Dunn MJ. Cellular signaling by peptides of the endothelin gene family. FASEB J 1990; 4:2989–3000.
59. Silberberg SD, Poder TC, Lacerda A. Endothelin increases single channel calcium currents in coronary arterial smooth muscle cells. FEBS Lett 1989; 247:68–72.
60. Goto K, Yanagisawa M, Kimura S, et al. Endothelin activates the dihydropyridine sensitive, voltage dependent Ca$^{2+}$ channel in vascular smooth muscle. Proc Natl Acad Sci USA 1989; 86:3915–3918.
61. Inoue Y, Oike M, Nakao K, et al. Endothelin augments unitary calcium channel currents on the smooth muscle cell membrane of guinea pig portal vein. J Physiol (Lon) 1990; 423:171–191.
62. Resink TJ, Scott-Burden T, Buhler FR. Activation of multiple signal transduction pathways by endothelin in cultured human vascular smooth muscle cells. Eur J Biochem 1990; 189:415–421.
63. Liu Y, Geisburhler B, Jones AW. Activation of multiple mechanisms including phospholipase D by endothelin-1 in rat aorta. Am J Physiol 1992; 262:C941–C946.
64. Griendling KK, Tsuda T, Alexander RW. Endothelin stimulates diacyglycerol accumulation and activates protein kinase C in cultured vascular smooth muscle cells. J Biol Chem 1989; 8237–8240.
65. Lonchampt MO, Pinelis S, Goulin J, et al. Proliferation and Na$^+$/H$^+$ exchange activation by endothelin in vascular smooth muscle cells. Am J Hypertens 1991; 4:776–779.
66. Chua BH, Krebs CJ, Chu CC, et al. Endothelin stimulates protein synthesis in smooth muscle cells. Am J Physiol 1992; 262:E412–E416.
67. Bogoyevitch MA, Glennon PE, Sugden PH. Endothelin 1, phorbol esters and phenylephirine stimulate MAP kinase activities in ventricular cardiomyocytes. FEBS Lett 1993; 317:271–275.
68. Simonson MS, John JM, Dunn MJ. Differential regulation of *fos* and *jun* gene expression and AP 1 *cis* element activity by endothelin isopeptides. Possible

implication for mitogenic signaling by endothelin. J Biol Chem 1992; 267: 8643–8649.

69. Simonson MS. Endothelins: multifunctional renal peptides. Physiol Rev 1993; 73:375–411.

70. Ohlstein EH, Arleth A, Bryan H, et al. The selective endothelin $ET_A$ receptor antagonist BQ123 antagonizes endothelin 1 mediated mitogensis. Eur J Pharmacol 1992; 225:347–350.

71. Eguchi S, Hirata Y, Imai T, et al. Phenotypic change of endothelin receptor subtype in cultured rat vascular smooth muscle cells. Endocrinology 1994; 134:222–226.

72. Simonson MS, Wang Y, Jones J, et al. Protein kinase C regulates activation of mitogen-activated protein kinase and induction of proto oncogene c-*fos* by endothelin-1. J Cardiovasc Pharmacol 1992; 20(suppl 12):S29–S31.

73. Koide M, Kawahara Y, Tsuda T, et al. Endothelin 1 stimulates tyrosine phospholylation and the activities of two mitogen activated protein kinases in cultured vascular smooth muscle cells. J Hypertens 1992; 10:1173–1182.

74. Janakidevi K, Fisher MA, Del Vecchio PJ, et al. Endothelin 1 stimulates DNA synthesis and proliferation of pulmonary artery smooth muscle cells. Am J Physiol 1992; 263:C1295–1301.

75. Ihara M, Fukuroda T, Saeki T, et al. An endothelin receptor ($ET_A$) antagonist isolated from *Streptomyces misakiensis*. Biochem Biophys Res Commun 1991; 178:132–137.

76. Ihara M, Noguchi K, Saeki T, et al. Biological profiles of highly potent novel endothelin antagonists selective for the $ET_A$ receptor. Life Sci 1992; 50:247–255.

77. Ishikawa K, Fukami T, Nagase T, et al. Cyclic pentapeptide endothelin antagonist with high $ET_A$ selectivity. J Med Chem 1992; 35:2139–2145.

78. Ikeda S, Awane Y, Kusumoto K, et al. A new endothelin receptor antagonist, TAK-044, shows long-lasting inhibition of both $ET_A$ and $ET_B$-mediated blood pressure responses in rats. J Pharmacol Exp Ther 1994; 270:728–733.

79. Aramori I, Nrei T, Shoubo M, et al. Subtype selectivity of a novel endothelin antagonist, FR 139317, for the two endothelin receptors in transfected Chinese hamster ovary cells. Mol Pharmacol 1993; 43:127–131.

80. Ishikawa K, Fukami T, Hayama T, et al. Endothelin antagonistic cyclic pentapeptides with high selectivity for $ET_A$ receptor. In: Smith JA, Rivier JE, eds. Peptides: Chemistry and Biology. 12th Am Peptide Symposium Escom Science Publishers, The Netherlands, 1992:812–819.

81. Davenport AP, Kuc RE, Fitzgerald F, et al. [$^{125}$I]-PD151241: a selective radioligand for human $ET_A$ receptors. Br J Pharmacol 1994; 111:4–6.

82. Kitada C, Ohtaki T, Masuda Y, et al. Design and synthesis of $ET_A$ receptor antagonists and study of $ET_A$ receptor distribution. J Cardiovasc Pharamacol 1993; 22(suppl 8):S128–S130.

83. Ishikawa K, Ihara M, Noguchi K, et al. Biochemical and pharmacological profile of a potent and selective endothelin B-receptor antagonists, BQ-788. Proc Natl Acad Sci USA 1994; 91:4892–4896.

84. James AF, Urade Y, Webb RL, et al. IRL 1620, succinyl-[Glu$^9$, Ala$^{11, 15}$]-endothelin-1(8-21), a highly specific agonist of the ET$_B$ receptor. Cardiovasc Drug Rev 1993; 11:257–270.

85. Webb RL, Navarrete AD, Ksander GM, et al. Effects of the ET$_B$-selective antagonist IRL 2500 in conscious spontaneously hypertensive and Wistar-Kyoto rats. J Cardiovasc Pharmacol 1995; 26(suppl 3):S389–S392.

86. Doherty AM, Cody WL, He JX, et al. Design of C-terminal peptide antagonists of endothelin: structure-activity relationships of ET-1[16-21, D-His16]. Bioorg Med Chem Lett 1993; 3:497–502.

87. Clozel M, Breu V, Burri K, et al. Pathophysiological role of endothelin revealed by the first orally active endothelin receptor antagonist. Nature 1993; 365:759–761.

88. Clozel M, Breu V, Gray GA, et al. Pharmacological characterization of bosentan, a new potent orally active nonpeptide endothelin antagonist. J Pharamacol Exp Ther 1994; 270:228–235.

89. Elliott JD, Lago MA, Cousins RD, et al. 1,3-Diarylindan-2-carboxylic acids, potent and selective non-peptide endothelin receptor antagonists. J Med Chem 1994; 37:1553–1557.

90. Ohlstein EL, Nambi P, Douglas SA, et al. SB 209670, a rationally designed potent nonpeptide endothelin receptor antagonist. Proc Natl Acad Sci USA 1994; 91:8052–8056.

91. Doherty AM, Patt WC, Repine J, et al. Structure-activity relationships of a novel series of orally active nonpeptide ET$_A$ and ET$_{A/B}$ endothelin receptor-selective antagonists. J Cardiovasc Pharamacol 1995; 26(suppl 3):S358–S361.

92. Maguire JJ, Kuc RE, Doherty AM, et al. Potency of PD155080, an orally active ET$_A$ receptor antagonist, determined for human endothelin receptors. J Cardiovasc Pharmacol 1995; 26(suppl 3): S362–S364.

93. Vanhoutte PM. Is endothelin involved in the pathogenesis of hypertension? Hypertension 1993; 21:747–758.

94. Otsuka A, Mikami H, Katahira K, et al. Changes in plasma renin activity and aldosterone concentration in response to endothelin injection in dogs. Acta Endrocrinol 1989; 121:361–364.

95. Hirata Y, Takagi N, Fukuda Y, et al. Endothelin is a potent mitogen for rat vascular smooth muscle cells. Atherosclerosis 1989; 78:225–228.

96. Battistini B, D'Orleans-Juste P, Sirois P. Biology of diseases, Endothelin: circulating plasma levels and presence in other biological fluids. Laboratory Invest 1993; 6:600–628.

97. Fujita K, Matsumura Y, Kita S, et al. Role of endothelin-1 and the ET$_A$ receptor in the maintenance of deoxycorticosterone acetate-salt-induced hypertension. Br J Pharmacol 1995; 114:925–930.

98. Warner TD, Allcock GH, Vane JR. Reversal of established responses to endothelin-1 in vivo and in vitro by the endothelin receptor antagonists, BQ123 and PD145065. Br J Pharmacol 1994; 112:207–213.

99. Matsumura Y, Fujita K, Miyazaki Y, et al. Involvement of endothelin-1 in

deoxycorticosterone acetate-salt-induced hypertension and cardiovascular hypertrophy. J Cardiovasc Pharmacol 1995; 26(suppl 3):S456–S458.

100. Vemulapalli S, Watkins RW, Brown A, et al. Disparate effects of phosphoramidon on blood pressure in SHR and DOCA-salt hypertensive rats. Life Sci 1993; 53:783–793.

101. Nishikibe M, Tsuchida S, Okada M, et al. Antihypertensive effects of a newly synthesized endothelin antagonist, BQ-123, in a genetic hypertensive model. Life Sci 1993; 52:717–724.

102. Sogabe K. Nirei H, Shoubo M, et al. Pharmacological profile of FR139317, a novel endothelin ET$_A$ receptor antagonist. J Pharmacol Exp Ther 1993; 264:1040–1046.

103. Ohlstein EH, Douglas SA, Ezekiel M, et al. Antihypertensive effects of the endothelin antagonist BQ-123 in conscious spontaneously hypertensive rats. J Cardiovasc Pharmacol 1993; 22(suppl 8):S321–S323.

104. Donckier J, Stoleru L, Hayashida W, et al. Role of endogenous endothelin-1 in experimental renal hypertension in dogs. Circulation 1995; 92:106–113.

105. Miyauchi T, Yanagisawa M, Tomizawa T, et al. Increased plasma concentrations of endothelin-1 and big endothelin-1 in acute myocardial infarction. Lancet 1989; 2:53–54.

106. Watanabe T, Awane Y, Ikeda S, et al. Pharmacology of a non-selective ET$_A$ and ET$_B$ receptor antagonist, TAK-044 and the inhibition of myocardial infarct size in rats. Br J Pharmacol 1995; 114:949–954.

107. Giaid A, Michel R, Stewwart DJ, et al. Expression of endothelin-1 in lungs of patients with crytogenic fibrosing alveolitis. Lancet 1993; 341:1550–1554.

108. Giaid A, Yanagisawa M, Langleben D, et al. Expression of endothelin-1 in lungs with pulmonary hypertension. N Engl J Med 1993; 328:1732–1739.

109. Miyauchi T, Yorikane R, Sakai S, et al. Contribution of endogenous endothelin-1 to the progression of cariopulmonary alterations in rats with monocrotaline-induced pulmonary hypertension. Circ Res 1993; 73:887–897.

110. Herbst C, Tippler B, Shams H, et al. A role for endothelin in bicuculline-induced neurogenic pulmonary oedema in rats. Br J Pharmacol 1995; 115:753–760.

111. Shigeno T, Clozel M, Sakai S, et al. The effect of bosentan, a new potent endothelin receptor antagonist, on the pathogenesis of cerebral vasospasm. Neursurgery 1995; 37:87–91.

112. Hirose H, Ide K, Sakaki T, et al. The role of endothelin and nitric oxide in modulation of normal and spastic cerebral vascular tone in the dog. Eur J Pharmacol 1995; 277:77–87.

113. Gellai M, Jugus M, Fletcher T, et al. Reversal of post ischemic acute renal failure with a selective endothelin$_A$ receptor antagonist in the rat. J Clin Invest 1994; 93:900–906.

114. Masuda E, Kawano S, Nagano K, et al. Role of endogenous endothelin in pathogenesis of ethanol induced gastric mucosal injury in rats. Am J Physiol 1993; 265:G474–G481.

115. Whittle BJR. Neuronal and endothelium-derived mediators in the modula-

tion of the gastric microcirculation: integrity in the balance. Br J Pharmacol 1993; 110:3–17.

116. Dashwood MR, Allen SP, Lunn TN, et al. The effect of the ET$_A$ receptor antagonist, FR139317, on [$^{125}$I]-ET-1 binding to the atherosclerotic human coronary artery. Br J Pharmacol 1994; 112:386–390.

117. Douglas SA, Vickery-Clark LM, Storer BL, et al. A role for endogenous endothelin-1 in neointimal formation following rat carotid artery balloon angioplasty: protective effects of the non-peptide endothelin receptor antagonist SB 269670. Circ Res 1994; 75:190–196.

118. Pribnow D, Muldoon LL, Fajado M, et al. Endothelin induces transcription of *fos/jun* family genes: a prominent role for calcium ion. Mol Endocrinol 1992; 6:1003–1012.

119. Janakidevi K, Fisher MA, Del Vecchio PJ, et al. Endothelin 1 stimulates DNA synthesis and proliferation of pulmonary artery smooth muscle. Am J Physiol 1992; 263:C1295–C1301.

120. Shichiri M, Hirata Y, Nakajima M, et al. Endothelin-1 is an autocrine-paracrine growth factor for human cancer cell lines. J Clin Invest 1991; 87: 1867–1871.

121. Takuwa N, Takuwa Y, Yanagisawa M, et al. A novel vasoactive peptide endothelin stimulates mitogenesis through inositol lipid turnover in Swiss 3T3 fibroblasts. J Biol Chem 1989; 264:7856–7861.

122. Hahn AWA, Resink TJ, Bernhardt J, et al. Stimulation of autocrine platelet derived growth factor-AA homodimer and transforming growth factor in vascular smooth muscle cells by vasoconstrictive peptides. Biochem Biophys Res Commun 1991; 178:1451–1456.

123. Hahn AWA, Resink TJ, Kern F, et al. Peptide vasoconstrictors, vessel structure, and vascular smooth proliferation. J Cardiovasc Pharmacol 1993; 22(suppl 8):S37–S40.

124. Cody RJ, Haas GJ, Binkley PF, et al. Plasma endothelin correlates with the extent of pulmonary hypertension in patients with chronic congestive heart failure. Circulation 1992; 85:504–509.

125. Cacoub P, Dornet R, Nataf A, et al. Plasma endothelin and pulmonary pressures in patients with congestive heart failure. Am Heart J 1993; 126: 1484–1488.

126. Kiowski W, Sutsch G, Hunziker P, et al. Evidence for endothelin-1-mediated vasoconstriction in severe chronic heart failure. Lancet 1995; 346:732–736.

127. Omland T, Lie RT, Aakvaag A, et al. Plasma endothelin determination as a prognostic indicator of 1-year mortality after acute myocardial infarction. Circulation 1994; 89:1573–1579.

128. Sakai S, Miyauchi T, Sakurai T, et al. Endogenous endothelin-1 participates in the maintenance of cardiac function in rats with congestive heart failure – marked increase in endothelin-1 production in the failing heart. Circulation 1996; 93:1214–1222.

# 6

# Transmigration of Leukocytes

**B. Stein, Y. Khew-Goodall, J. Gamble, and M. A. Vadas**

*Hanson Centre for Cancer Research, Institute of Medical and Veterinary Science, Adelaide, South Australia, Australia*

## I.  INTRODUCTION

Migration of cells through a vascular endothelial monolayer is essential in two of the central pathological processes, inflammation and metastasis. Migration of inflammatory cells, particularly of neutrophils, is the most studied form, and forms a basis for understanding the migration of other cell types.

This chapter concentrates on neutrophil transmigration, limiting its focus to the process of moving across the endothelial monolayer, and steps immediately surrounding that process. We will refine the current models of transmigration by proposing a more detailed model for passage across the endothelial monolayer and, where possible, discuss specific molecular mechanisms.

### A.  Transmigration

1.  Normal Endothelium

Normally, the endothelium exists in a resting state, without adherent or transmigrating cells (1). This is consistently reproduced in vitro, where neutrophil migration across resting endothelium is insignificant (2–4).

Specialized endothelia characterized by their morphology (high endothelium) as part of recirculation, an aspect of immune surveillance, allow lymphocyte transmigration without additional perturbation. These specialized aspects of transmigration (5,6) do not form part of the main thrust of this chapter, and will not be considered further.

## 2. Two Types of Transmigration

Neutrophils in vitro can migrate across resting or unactivated endothelium if an exogenous chemokinetic or chemotactic stimulus is present (3,7,8). For example, the addition of a gradient of interleukin-8 (IL-8) or N-formyl-methioninyl-leucinyl-phenylalanine (fMLP) results dose-dependent transmigration, which at optimal concentrations of the chemoattractant results in 50–90% of the neutrophils transmigrating (8–10). Huang and Silverstein (7) have termed this "leucocyte driven" transmigration, but as the leukocytes are responding to exogenous chemoattractants, we feel chemotactic transmigration is a more accurate description.

The pathophysiological hallmark of established inflammatory transmigration is endothelial activation—an event requiring transcription and protein synthesis. This results in upregulation of adhesion molecules, production of inflammatory mediators, and endothelial secretion of chemoattractants and transmigration. Endothelial chemoattractants (summarized in Table 1) are critical for transmigration. They are secreted in significant amounts; for example, the IL-8 secreted from IL-1–activated endothelial cells reaches concentrations of about 1 nM in vitro (11), close to the peak of the chemotactic dose-response curve. The stimulus for endothelial activation in vivo is probably local production of cytokines and other inflammatory mediators released on tissue injury.

To differentiate clearly these two types of transmigration, we will refer to them as type I (exogenous or nonendothelial chemoattractant) and type II (cytokine activated, endothelial chemoattractant). These differences are summarized in Table 2 and Figure 1. Type I and Type II transmigration are both important pathophysiological events. Type I transmigration is probably the mechanism by which early responses to tissue injury are generated, and type II transmigration enables the generation of later, more prolonged

**Table 1**  Classes of Chemoattractants Produced by the Endothelium

| Class | Example | Example target cell |
|---|---|---|
| Arachidonic acid metabolites | $LTB_4$ | Neutrophils, eosinophils |
| Ether lipids | PAF | Neutrophils, eosinophils |
| CXC chemokines | IL-8 | Neutrophils, lymphocytes |
| CC chemokines | MCP-1 | Monocytes, T-cells, eosinophils |

**Table 2** Difference in Type I and Type II Transmigration

|  | Type I | Type II |
|---|---|---|
| Synonyms | Chemoattractant transmigration, leukocyte-dependent transmigration | Cytokine-activated transmigration, endothelium-dependent transmigration |
| Time for activation | Minutes | Hours |
| Duration of action | Hours | Days |
| Stimulus | Exogenous chemoattractants | Activation of the endothelium; e.g., by cytokines |
| Chemoattractants | Exogenous | Local (endothelial production) |
| Requires protein synthesis | No | Yes |
| Upregulation of endothelial adhesion molecules | ? | Yes |
| PECAM-1 dependent | Probably not | Yes |
| IAP dependent | Yes | Yes |
| CD18 dependent | Yes | Yes |
| ICAM-1 dependent | Yes | Yes |
| Dependent on second messengers, especially [Ca$^{2+}$]i | Yes | Yes |
| In vivo correlate | Early response to infection and tissue injury | Established inflammatory focus |

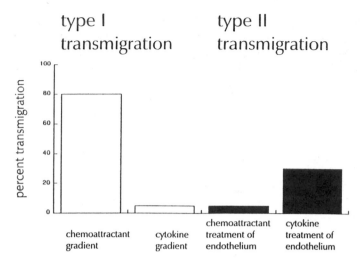

**Figure 1**    An illustration of the differences between type I and type II transmigration.

responses. Type I transmigration has been studied less than type II transmigration, and as summarized in Table 2, the mechanisms may not be the same.

### 3.   Transmigration in Vivo: Three Steps

Transmigration has been conceptualized as involving three steps: rolling, activation or triggering resulting in firm adhesion, which is followed by migration across the endothelium and into the tissues (12,13).

A view of transmigration can be obtained in vivo by intravital microscopy of several tissues: for example, the exteriorized mesentery. On exposing the mesentery, the postcapillary venules are seen to contain a number of leukocytes that are peripheral to the central stream of blood flow and moving more slowly. They are in contact with the vessel wall, along which they roll. The preparation itself provides sufficient stimulation to the endothelium to induce rolling (14). Rolling consists of adhesive interactions that are sufficient to slow the leukocyte but not sufficient to overcome blood flow and stop the leukocyte. If an additional stimulus is provided, for example, by induction of an inflammatory response with cytokines such as IL-1 or tumor necrosis factor-$\alpha$ (TNF-$\alpha$) or application of a chemoattractant such as fMLP, large numbers of leukocytes will become firmly adherent to the side of the vessel, forming a layer like pebbles in a stream. In contrast to the adhesion involved in rolling, firm adhesion is associated with sufficient strength of adhesion to overcome blood flow. In contrast to rolling, firm adhesion is associated with flattening and spreading of the leukocyte. With progression of an inflammatory response, the vessel may become occluded by adherent leukocytes, and blood flow may essentially stop. Firm adhesion is usually rapidly followed by migration across the endothelial monolayer. After transmigration, there is often a "hold-up" of cells at the basement membrane (1,15). Leukocytes remain adherent to the basal aspect of the endothelium and may form a temporary sheath around the vessel before moving out into the tissues (1).

## 4. Molecular Mediators of the Three Steps of Transmigration

Rolling slows the leukocyte, allowing it to come into greater contact with the endothelium. Rolling is critical, as the molecules responsible for firm adhesion cannot interact with their ligands if the leukocyte is moving rapidly (16). It involves repetitive, transient molecular interactions. These predominantly involve members of the selectin class of adhesion molecules (17), but certain integrin adhesion molecules, if located on the tips of leukocyte microvilli, may perform the same task (18). Some of the critical molecules in transmigration and their endothelial distribution are outlined in Table 3 and Figure 2.

With increased endothelial contact, it is hypothesized that receptors on the leukocyte bind chemoattractants produced by the endothelium, which

**Table 3** Some Important Molecules in Transmigration

| Molecule | Synonyms | Location |
|---|---|---|
| PECAM-1 | CD31 | Neutrophils, monocytes, some T-cell subtypes, eosinophils, endothelium |
| $\beta_2$-integrin | CD18 | All leukocytes |
| $\alpha_L$-chain of $\beta_2$-integrin | CD11a, LFA-1 | All leukocytes |
| $\alpha_m$-chain of $\beta_2$-integrin | CD11b, Mac-1 | NK cells, neutrophils, monocytes, eosinophils |
| $\alpha_4\beta_1$-integrin | CD49d/CD29, VLA-4 | Lymphocytes, monocytes, eosinophils |
| ICAM-1 | CD54 | Endothelium, monocytes, some T cells |
| IAP | CD47 | All leukocytes, endothelium |
| VCAM-1 | CD106 | Cytokine-activated endothelium |

are outlined in Table 1. Chemoattractant stimulation together with signaling generated by binding to adhesion molecules results in activation of members of the integrin class of adhesion molecules on the leukocyte, particularly the $\beta_2$-integrins. Integrin activation is thought to be generated by alterations in affinity rather than upregulation of integrin numbers. Integrins on the activated leukocyte are able to interact with their ligands on the endothelium–members of the immunoglobulin superfamily of adhesion molecules–and form a strong adhesive bond, bringing the cell to a halt. This third step is then followed by migration across the endothelial cell monolayer (12,13).

## 5. Static and Dynamic Transmigration: Effects of Blood Flow

In vivo, adhesion and transmigration takes place under shear stress from blood flow. This was estimated to be about 5 dynes/cm (219), the force used in many in vitro models, but more recent work has suggested stresses in the range of 17–29 dynes/cm (220). This stress may be lower once inflammation is established, and the capillary is almost occluded by adherent leukocytes (14,21), but it cannot be ignored early in the inflammatory response. Thus, there must be a set of mechanisms to deal with flow stresses in transmigration.

The role of some molecules may differ in flow situations. For example, antibodies to intracellular adhesion molecule-1 (ICAM-1) and CD18 significantly decrease neutrophil transmigration in both static and flow models. In contrast, ICAM-1 and CD18 are important in firm adhesion in static models but not in flow models (16).

## 6. Transmigration Is a Final Result of Many Factors

A number of interactions occur between the leukocyte and the endothelium during transit from the bloodstream to the tissues. Abolition of interactions that precede transit across the endothelium may reduce the number of cells that transmigrate, without affecting the mechanism by which cells move across the endothelium. For example, inhibition of selectin binding significantly reduces transmigration. This does not imply that selectins are involved in the passage across the monolayer. It reflects the requirement for selectin-mediated slowing of leukocyte flow velocity which in turn is required for firm adhesion (16). This can make it difficult to localize the role of a particular molecule in the transmigration process.

This chapter concentrates on mechanisms that specifically operate after firm binding has occurred, and alterations in steps leading up to firm adhesion that result in decreased transmigration are not generally discussed here.

## II.   THE PROCESS OF TRANSMIGRATION

### A.   Firm Adhesion: Necessary, but Not Sufficient, for Transmigration

**1.   Only Firmly Adherent Cells Transmigrate**

As discussed in Section I.A.3, the initial adhesive interactions between leukocyte and endothelium result in rolling, which is necessary to allow slowing of the leukocyte. On activation of leukocyte integrins, the leukocyte is able to adhere to the vessel wall against the force of blood flow. This firm adhesion is a prerequisite for transmigration. Both in vivo (reviewed in ref. 1) and in vitro experiments (2,14) clearly show that only firmly adherent cells will transmigrate.

**2.   Firm Adhesion Is Separate from Transmigration**

*Leukocyte Adhesion Alone Does Not Trigger Transmigration.*   Firm adhesion per se is not enough to promote transmigration–treating neutrophils with TNF-$\alpha$, for example, induces firm adhesion to resting human umbilical vein endothelial cells (HUVECs), but does not promote transmigration. Similarly, binding induced by other mechanisms, for example, via immunoglobulin Fc receptors does not induce transmigration (4). Thus, there is not an inherent leukocyte-dependent mechanism that is triggered on binding and results in transmigration, which suggests a leukocyte alteration separate from firm adhesion is required for transmigration.

Other strategies also suggest that binding and transmigration can be separated, and that binding is necessary but not sufficient for transmigration. These data imply that a further endothelial event is also required subsequent to firm adhesion. We postulate this involves a signal altering the endothelium to allow transmigration.

*Inhibiting Chemoattractants May Reduce Type II Transmigration Without Decreasing Firm Adhesion.*   Endothelial and exogenous chemoattractants are critical in transmigration. As chemoattractant inhibitors may decrease transmigration without altering firm adhesion, this provides another argument that adhesion and transmigration are separate events. For example, Kuijpers et al. found that IL-1 pretreatment of HUVECs induced both neutrophil adherence and transmigration. Transmigration was decreased in a dose-dependent manner by the platelet-activating factor (PAF) antagonist WEB 2086, but adhesion was unaffected (22). Hill et al. reported similar findings to those of Kuijpers using WEB 2086 and the newer more potent PAF antagonist YM 264 (23). In vivo, the firm adhesion resulting from IL-1 activation of rat mesenteric vessels was not affected, but transmigration was reduced by 60% by pretreatment with either of two PAF antagonists (24). In contrast, Smart et al. (25) found that WEB 2086 had little effect on neutrophil transmigration across TNF-$\alpha$–activated HUVECs. Our results and those of Brevario et al. (26) are similar to Smart et al. (11). Hill et al. have suggested that the discrepant effects of PAF antagonists is due to the antagonists used–higher doses of less potent antagonists used by, for example, Brevario et al. (26), might have caused nonspecific effects on firm adhesion, reducing both firm adhesion and transmigration.

Kuijpers et al. also reported that IL-8 antisera reduced transmigration without altering firm adhesion (22). We found no inhibition of adhesion, but we did find significantly reduced inflammatory transmigration when IL-8 effects were inhibited by desensitization of neutrophils (27). This is in contrast to Huber et al. (28), who reported an inhibition of adhesion and transmigration, but this may reflect differences in the in vitro model the various groups used.

Although there are disagreements, there are a number of results showing dissociation of adhesion and transmigration using chemoattractant inhibition.

*Antibodies to CD47 Reduce Type I and II Transmigration Without Altering Firm Adhesion.*   We have recently shown that blocking the function of neutrophil CD47 (integrin-associated protein) also reduces chemotactic and inflammatory transmigration (29) (see Section II.C.4). In recent experiments, we have found that neutrophil adhesion is normal (B. Stein, Y. Khew-Goodall, E. Brown, F. Lindberg, J. Gamble, M. Vadas, in preparation). This is both a novel mediator of transmigration and another mechanism demonstrating that adhesion and transmigration are separate.

*Perturbation of Intracellular Signaling Can Inhibit Types I and II Transmigration Without Altering Firm Adhesion.*   Probably the strongest argument in favor of adhesion and transmigration being separate events comes from direct alteration of second messengers in intracellular signaling pathways. Adhesion of neutrophils and monocytic U937 cells induces a rise in endothelial cell [$Ca^{2+}$]i (30,31). By buffering intracellular calcium, transmigration to either an fMLP gradient or across IL-1–activated HUVECs was decreased by over 85%, but neutrophil adhesion was unaltered (30). This argues strongly for an extra endothelial step after binding, which requires signaling.

Another system in which alteration of transmigration is separate from adhesion, probably mediated via alterations in intracellular signaling, was reported by Oppenheimer-Marks. Treatment of endothelial cells with prostaglandin $E_2$ (PGE$_2$) decreased T-lymphocyte transmigration in a dose-dependent fashion across stimulated and resting endothelium, without altering adhesion, or expression of E-selectin and vascular cell adhesion molecule-1 (VCAM-1) (32). This effect may be mediated by cAMP, as it was increased by adding dibutryl cAMP or by inhibition of phospho-diesterase activity with 3-isobutyl-1-methylxanthine (IBMX).

*Conclusion.* The requirement for intact second-messenger pathways in endothelial cells for neutrophils to traverse both resting and activated endothelium strongly suggests that a further endothelial event is needed after firm binding for both type I and type II transmigration. This event is signal dependent. The dissociation of adhesion and transmigration seen with inhibition of CD47 function supports this notion. Firm adhesion by leukocytes is a necessary signal for the endothelium, although it is probably not sufficient.

The inability of firm adhesion per se to cause transmigration suggests that as well as signals generated by firm adhesion, another signal is required for leukocyte transmigration. Although the data from chemo-attractant inhibition are not as convincing, they are generally in keeping with this thesis. In contrast to the hypothesis of the three-step model, the dissection of binding and transmigration suggests that endothelial chemoattractant signaling plays a critical role after firm binding, promoting type II transmigration, and not just as a primary cause of firm binding (13,33).

## 3. Do All Stimulated Cells Transmigrate?

In type I transmigration (chemoattractant and resting HUVECs) in vitro, the majority of neutrophils will migrate (9,27). Those that do not may reflect cells inactivated during the preparatory process, contaminants from other leukocyte types, or possibly reflect differences in inherent migratory capacity.

Using 1 nM IL-8, almost all neutrophils can be induced to transmigrate (9,27). This suggests there is not a large population of inherently nonmigratory neutrophils. Chemoattractants vary in potency (34), which might explain some differences between chemotactic transmigration systems. In contrast to IL-8, fMLP generally induces ~40% of neutrophils to transmigrate (34). Given the similarities in receptors, signaling, and other functional activation (35), the greater potency of IL-8 is interesting.

In contrast to type I transmigration, only 25–50% of neutrophils transmigrate across cytokine-activated endothelium (type II transmigration) (2–4) despite the ability of the activated endothelium to generate large amounts of chemoattractants. Of the nontransmigrating cells, the majority fail to adhere; the others become dissociated from the endothelium within 10–60 min (2). The origin of the limitation on transmigration in some systems is not clear. Adding an external gradient of fMLP, C5a, or leukotriene B$_4$ (LTB$_4$) to IL-1–stimulated endothelium increased the proportion of cells that transmigrated (3,4,36), but this increase was on the order of 10%, and in no situation did the majority of neutrophils transmigrate. Similar findings have been noted with TNF-$\alpha$ stimulation of HUVECs (3). It is unlikely this represents inadequate endothelial activation. Adding both IL-1 and TNF-$\alpha$ does not increase transmigration, and IL-1 and TNF$\alpha$ both have steep dose-response curves with a plateau at relatively low doses (3). The limitation may be a leukocyte-based phenomenon, as the proportion of neutrophils transmigrating is independent of the number added (2,3); however, the findings in type I transmigration suggest an endothelial origin. It is possible that type II transmigration reveals some subtle endothelial characteristic that may or may not be an in vitro artifact.

## B. Adhesion to the Monolayer and Movement to the Interendothelial Cleft

Furie (2) observed that initial adherence to the endothelium was random and not predisposed to the interendothelial junctions. As the leukocyte transmigrates through the interendothelial junction, there must be some means to locate it. A mechanism for this is suggested by in vivo observations (1,37) that adherent leukocytes crawl over the endothelial surface, seeming to probe for an opening, before transmigrating. This suggests two components operate—motility, for which adhesion is required, and guidance.

### 1. Moving to the Interendothelial Cleft

Crawling involves a series of attachments and detachments from the substrate, development of tension through the cytoskeleton (38), and active remodeling of the cytoskeleton (39,40). Without adhesion, crawling and all the subsequent movement-dependent steps in transmigration will be inhibited. Agents which affect the cytoskeleton, like taxol (32), inhibit transmigration, presumably by preventing crawling. Less obviously, interference with detachment from the substrate, as is seen with upregulation of $\beta_1$-integrin function, may prevent crawling, with the leukocyte being "glued" in one spot (38,41).

### 2. Specific Molecules Involved in Transmigration

Adhesion molecules probably provide the adherence mechanism for most leukocyte movement (Table 1 outlines some of the critical molecules). In contrast to platelet endothelial cell adhesion molecule-1 (PECAM-1), which seems particularly important to migration through the interendothelial junction, there are several adhesion molecules whose role is not unequivocally localized to one step of the process. These molecules may act in adhesive interactions required for crawling to the interendothelial junction, or they may function in passage through the interendothelial junction.

*ICAM-1 (CD54).* ICAM-1 is a member of the immunoglobulin superfamily of adhesion molecules containing five immunoglobulin-like domains. It is one of the principal ligands for the leukocyte $\beta_2$-integrin CD11a/CD18 (LFA-1) which binds to the $NH_2$ terminal Ig domain (42). CD11b/CD18 (Mac-1), another leukocyte $\beta_2$- integrin, binds to the third Ig domain (43): its binding affinity is inversely proportional to the glycosylation state of the region (43). It is constitutively expressed on endothelial cells, and is significantly upregulated by cytokine stimulation (44). The time course of cytokine-induced upregulation is prolonged. Expression gradually increases, peaking at 12 hr, but remaining significantly elevated until 72 hr (45). The cytoplasmic tail is capable of binding to the cytoskeleton via $\alpha$-actinin (46) allowing immobilization in the membrane.

In vivo, ICAM-1 knockout mice show significant impairment in neutrophil migration into an inflamed peritoneum (47,48), and ICAM-1 antibodies reduce acute and chronic inflammation in a number of animal models (45). ICAM-1 antibodies reduce type II transmigration of neutrophils in vitro by over 85% (49,50). ICAM-1 is also important in type I transmigration. Antibodies inhibit neutrophil chemotactic transmigration by $\sim$55% (8). ICAM-1 seems more important in transmigration of neutrophils in flow situations where antibodies do not inhibit adhesion but do reduce transmigration by >85% (16).

ICAM-1 is involved in transmigration of many leukocyte subtypes. As well as reducing neutrophil transmigration, antibodies reduce transmigration of resting and activated T-cells across resting HUVECs by 50% and across cytokine-activated HUVECs by about 40% (51). Although their efficacy alone was not reported, a combination of ICAM-1 and CD18 antibodies reduced migration of monocytes in a combination chemotactic and inflammatory transmigration model by 50–75% (52,53). This combination did not alter basal transmigration (52).

In T-cell transmigration ICAM-1 is localized to the interendothelial cleft and in the regions of T-cell–endothelium contact (51). The localization of ICAM-1 in T-cell transmigration (51) suggests that ICAM-1 is involved in the passage through the interendothelial cleft. As blocking ICAM-1 function is not associated with accumulation of leukocytes at the interendothelial junction, as seen with PECAM-1, it suggests that its role is not limited to passage through the interendothelial cleft. ICAM-1 may be required for crawling across the endothelium to the interendothelial junction, as it is predominantly located on the apical surface of resting endothelial cells (54,55), and during cytokine activation it is upregulated on the apical surface (55). Activation with $H_2O_2$ is associated with redistribution of ICAM-1 to basal surfaces (54), although the physiological relevance of this is unclear. The expression of ICAM-1 on such cells as fibroblasts and epithelium (56) may provide an adhesive ligand for leukocytes migrating through tissues.

### $\beta_2$-Integrins.

CD-18.   Three different $\alpha$ chains, $\alpha_L$ (CD11a), $\alpha_M$ (CD11b), and $\alpha_X$ (CD11c) share the common $\beta_2$-integrin chain, which is expressed on all leukocytes. The CD11/CD18 complex is one of the critical determinants of neutrophil transmigration, and it plays an important role in transmigration of other leukocyte subsets.

The functional importance of CD18 is exemplified by a congenital deficiency syndrome, leukocyte adhesion deficiency syndrome type I (LAD I), reviewed by Anderson et al. (57). Afflicted individuals have profoundly abnormal responses to infectious challenges developing nonresolving infections. Histologically there is no neutrophil influx, although monocyte, eosinophil, and lymphocyte responses are relatively preserved. In vitro, LAD I patients' neutrophils adhere and transmigrate poorly. There are some situations in vivo in which some transmigration does occur. Inflammation in the lung can generate some neutrophil influx, suggesting that a CD18-independent mechanism of neutrophil transmigration exists (57) (see below).

The use of $\beta_2$-integrin antibodies in animal models generally confirms a phenotype similar to that of patients with LAD I syndrome. As in LAD deficiency, in some circumstances neutrophil transmigration can still occur (58). CD18 antibodies are also effective inhibitors of transmigration in vitro (Table 4); however, the degree of inhibition seen in neutrophils is consistently greater than other leukocyte populations. This appears related to the ability of monocytes, eosinophils, and lymphocytes to use alternative adhesive systems, primarily mediated through VLA-4 (see below).

Where their effects have been examined, combinations of CD11a and CD11b antibodies are very similar to CD18 antibodies (8,59–61). Antibodies to the CD11a and CD11b subunits alone are not as potent as antibodies to CD18.

CD11a (LFA-1).   $\alpha_L \beta_2$-integrin (LFA-1, CD11a/CD18) is expressed on all leukocytes. Its ligands are ICAM-1 and ICAM-2 on the endothelium, with binding sites on their distal Ig homology regions. It is involved in a broad array of adhesive functions; for example, T helper cell interactions, as well as leukocyte-endothelium interactions (62). Circulating leukocytes constitutively express LFA-1 in an inactive conformation. Activation is required for ligand binding (63). This activation can be generated by intracellular signals from, for example, chemoattractants–"inside-out" signaling. In addition, cross linking of LFA-1 can induce signals–"outside-in" signaling (64,65).

Blocking antibodies to CD11a do inhibit transmigration (see Table 4) but to a lesser degree and with greater variability than antibodies to CD18. Monoclonal antibodies can reduce inflammation in vivo, but their efficacy depends on the model. For example, monoclonal antibodies reduce IgG immune complex lung injury but not IgG immune complex glomerulonephritis in the rat (66).

CD11b (Mac I). $\alpha_M \beta_2$-integrin (Mac-1, CD11b/CD 18, complement receptor-3) is expressed on neutrophils, monocytes, and natural killer (NK) cells. It is expressed on the cell surface and is stored in secondary and tertiary granules (67,68). Inflammatory mediators cause increases in cell surface expression, although functional upregulation does not require quantitative upregulation. It binds to fibrinogen, C3bi, a number of microbial determinants, for example, the filamentous hemaglutinin of *Bordetella pertussis,* factor X, and ICAM-1 (69). As well as contributing to phagocytosis, binding to surfaces through CD11b leads to massive activation of the respiratory burst in primed neutrophils. Monoclonal antibody studies have shown several different functional epitopes, with some antibodies inhibiting adhesion more than aggregation and vice versa (70).

Despite the significant inhibition of such functions as chemotaxis in vitro, antibodies to CD11b are not particularly effective in inhibiting transmigration in vitro (see Table 4), although van Epps (71) did record significant inhibition of resting T-cell migration across activated endothelium. CD11b monoclonal antibodies can inhibit inflammation in vivo, but in contrast to CD11a antibodies, CD11b antibodies reduce IgG immune complex glomerulonephritis but not IgG immune complex lung injury (66).

CD11a and CD11b: Conclusion.   CD11a is thus critical in neutrophil transmigration and important in transmigration of other leukocyte subtypes. CD11b antibodies alone are not as potent inhibitors of neutrophil transmigration in vitro, but they add significantly to the effect of CD11a antibodies in vitro. In vivo, both CD11a and CD11b monoclonal antibodies can reduce inflammation, suggesting a dependence on the inflammatory stimulus and organ involved.

CD11c (p150,95).   $\alpha\chi\beta_2$-integrin (p150,95, CD11c/CD18) is expressed on neutrophils, monocytes, and macrophages. It does not appear to be necessary for transmigration, as blocking antibodies do not reduce neutrophil or NK cell transmigration (50,72), nor do antibodies reduce monocyte adhesion to endothelial cells (73).

VLA-4 ($\alpha_4\beta_1$-integrin, CD49d/CD29).   VLA-4 is expressed by most leukocytes, but it is observed on neutrophils only under special conditions (see Section II.B.2). It binds to fibronectin in the HepII/IIICS region (74).

**Table 4** Type I and Type II Transmigration: Inhibition by Blocking Antibodies

| Type | Molecule | High | Moderate | Low | Not significant |
|---|---|---|---|---|---|
| I | CD18 | Neutrophils (8) | Monocytes (52,53) | | |
| I | ICAM-1 | Neutrophils (8) | | | |
| I | CD11a | | | | |
| I | CD11b | | Neutrophils (8) | | |
| I | VLA-4 | | Eosinophils (in vivo) (209) | Neutrophils (8) Monocytes (in vivo) (78) | Monocytes (in vivo) (78) |
| II | CD18 | Neutrophils (49,60,210) T cells (71) Eosinophils (82) | Monocytes (73) NK cells (72) | Monocytes (100,101) | |
| II | ICAM-1 | Neutrophils (49,50) | Resting T cells Activated T cells (51) | Eosinophils (82) | |
| II | CD11a | Resting T cells (71) Neutrophils (59,61,211) | Resting T cells (51,71) Activated T cells (51) | Eosinophils (82) Monocytes (in vivo) (78) | Monocytes (in vivo) (78) |
| II | CD11b | Resting T cells (71) | Eosinophils (82) | Neutrophils (8,49,50) | Eosinophils (81,82) Neutrophils (73) |
| II | VLA-4 | | Resting T cells (51) NK cells (72) Monocytes (53,76) Primed Eosinophils (83) | Monocytes (73) | Activated T cells (51) |

HepII is the major proteoglycan binding domain, whereas HepIIICS is a region subject to alternative splicing. There are three distinct $\alpha_4\beta_1$ binding domains in the HepII/IIICS region, two in the HepIIICS region (peptides CS-1 and CS-5) and one in the HepII region. The affinity of CS-1 binding is about 20 times stronger than CS-5, which is of the same order of magnitude as binding to the HepII area. Alternatively spliced fibronectin variants are produced by endothelial cells in culture (41), which may be upregulated by cytokine activation (75). The other ligand of VLA-4 is the immunoglobulin superfamily member VCAM-1, of which domains I and IV are important in binding. VCAM-1 is alternatively spliced into a molecule containing six or seven Ig domains by removal of domain IV. VCAM-1 binding occurs with approximately four times greater affinity than binding to fibronectin.

The involvement of VLA-4 in transmigration in vitro is variable. It appears not to be involved in neutrophil transmigration (73) nor in transmigration of activated T cells (51). VLA-4 antibodies do not reduce transmigration of resting T cells across resting endothelium, not do they reduce transmigration of monocytes across resting endothelium (51,53,76,77). Type II transmigration of resting T cells and NK cells are reduced by 40 and 30%, respectively (51,72). As firm adhesion is reduced to a similar extent, it is unclear whether this is a specific effect on passage across the endothelium. With monocyte type II transmigration investigators report variable results. In vitro, Meerschaert reported antibodies to CD18 and VLA-4 in concert inhibited transmigration across IL-1–activated HUVECs by up to 98%, but individually they did not significantly inhibit either process (76). This seems to involve inhibition of firm adhesion rather than movement across the monolayer, as adhesion was inhibited to a similar extent. Hakkert et al. (73) also reported that VLA-4 antibodies had no effects on binding or transmigration of monocytes, but when added to a CD18 antibody, VLA-4 antibodies increased inhibition of adhesion by about 20% and transmigration by about 10%. Chuluyan (53) also reported no significant effect of CD18 antibodies alone but noted 90% inhibition of monocyte adhesion and transmigration across cytokine-activated endothelium when $\alpha_4$-integrin antibodies and CD18 antibodies were used in concert. VLA-4 may play a role in type I transmigration of monocytes, as monoclonal antibodies are able to inhibit migration to dermal chemoattractants by 20–30% (78). Eosinophil adhesion to cytokine-activated endothelial cells involves VLA-4 adhesion to VCAM-1 (79,80). Type II migration in vitro was not significantly inhibited by VLA-4 antibodies alone (81,82), but after IL-4 priming, VLA-4 antibodies significantly reduced transmigration (83).

Of the two VLA-4 ligands, antibodies to VCAM-1 alone do not inhibit transmigration of T cells (51) nor of monocytes (52), but adding VCAM-1 antibodies and CS-1 peptide to CD18 antibodies does increase the blockade of adhesion to levels similar to that of VLA-4 and CD18 antibodies in combination (72,76), suggesting both $\alpha_4\beta_1$ ligands are used by NK cells and monocytes.

*Other Molecules.* There are other adhesion molecules of potential importance in transmigration. CD44 and CD43 seem likely candidates, although further data are needed.

CD44. CD44 is expressed on neutrophils, monocytes, NK cells, and T cells. It binds to hyaluronan, a component of many extracellular matrices, as well as other ligands. It has been implicated in many migratory processes, including metastasis (84), with some isoforms conferring greater metastatic potential (85).

CD44 has been implicated in migration of activated but not resting T cells across cytokine-activated HUVECs (86), and blocking antibodies have been reported to reduce lymphocytic infiltration in a murine arthritis model (87), but its role in transmigration of other leukocyte types is not clear. It is likely that CD44 also has a role beyond the endothelium, as discussed in Section II.E.3.

CD43. Sialophorin (CD43) is a large, heavily sialylated, cell surface glycoprotein present only on hematopoietic cells. It has been reported to be a counterreceptor for ICAM-1 (88), and it may function as a signaling molecule, as ligation can induce cell activation (89). Neutrophil aggregation is triggered by CD43 antibodies via a $\beta_2$-integrin–dependent pathway (90). CD43 knockout mice show increased adhesion of T cells to fibronectin and ICAM-1 and increased proliferative responses in vitro (91). These observations suggest a potential role for this molecule in transmigration as an inhibitor of adhesion, and that it needs to be lost or downregulated to allow maximal adhesion to develop.

*$\beta_2$-integrin–Independent Transmigration of Neutrophils.*

In Vivo Models. Rabbits pretreated with CD18 antibodies challenged with intrabronchial *Streptococcus pneumoniae* or hydrochloric acid were able to develop a neutrophil influx into the lung, whereas the same stimuli instilled into the peritoneal cavity did not induce local inflammation (58). The importance of the type of stimulus as well as the location of inflammation was shown by experiments using *Escherichia coli*—neither live organisms nor endotoxin induced neutrophil influx when given intrabronchially in CD18 antibody pretreated animals (58). There are other models of this process, for example, delayed-type hypersensitivity induced inflammation in rat joints but not in skin (92).

Determination of a mechanism is complicated by the dependence of the phenomenon on the stimulus, the vascular bed involved, and the species of experimental animal used. CD18-dependent and CD18-independent stimuli induce different changes in adhesion molecules on both endothelium and neutrophils (93,94), but their role is unclear. Complement appears important in some models, although this adds little to a possible mechanism (95). IL-8 may mediate neutrophil influx in acid-induced lung damage, but it is not clear if it mediates only $\beta_2$-integrin–independent transmigration (96).

In Vitro Models. Recently, Issekutz et al. demonstrated CD18-independent transmigration of neutrophils in vitro (97). The phenomenon was seen only when CD18 antibody-treated neutrophils were induced to transmigrate across cytokine-activated HUVECs which also had a chemotactic gradient of C5a or $LTB_4$ but not IL-8 or fMLP. Kubes et al. (98) reported that CD18 antibody–treated neutrophils stimulated with cytochalasin B and fMLP expressed $\beta_1$-integrin, as did untreated neutrophils that had undergone transmigration. This suggests a $\beta_1$-integrin–dependent contribution; however, in contrast to monocyte CD18-independent transmigration, $\alpha_4$- and $\beta_1$-integrin antibodies did not reduce neutrophil CD18-independent transmigration in the Issekutz model. $\beta_3$-integrins may play a role in some kinds of type I transmigration, as CD18 antibodies do not inhibit adhesion or chemotaxis of neutrophils toward the extracellular matrix protein entactin, but antibodies to the $\beta_3$-integrin do (99); however, such antibodies were not inhibitory in the Issekutz model (97).

The mechanism of transmigration in the Issekutz model remains unclear. Antibodies to $\beta_1$-integrin, IL-8, and PAF antagonists had no inhibitory effect. A combination of all these inhibitors with antibodies to $\beta_3$-integrin was also ineffective. Antibodies to PECAM-1, ICAM-1, P-selectin, and VCAM-1 did not inhibit transmigration, but some inhibition was seen with E-selectin antibodies.

Conclusion. $\beta_2$-integrin–independent transmigration of neutrophils appears clinically important. The mechanism is not yet understood, but a cryptic $\beta_1$-integrin–mediated event is possible. The models of $\beta_2$-integrin–independent transmigration may also be useful in examining PECAM-1–independent neutrophil transmigration.

## 3. Finding the Interendothelial Cleft

Adherent leukocytes move toward the interendothelial cleft with speed and apparent purpose (100). This argues against a chemoattractant-stimulated random walk as a mechanism for finding the junction and argues for the existence of directional information.

*Contact Guidance.* There are several different directional cues potentially available to the leukocyte. For the transmigrating leukocyte, the topography of the endothelial cell itself may contain directional information. Endothelial cells exposed to shear align themselves in the direction of the force (101). Using atomic force microscopy, Barbee et al. showed that, under shear stress, endothelial cells are ridged (102), with the ridges aligned in the direction of flow. The ridges are about 50 nm in height and 200–1000 nm in width and are more prominent at the cell periphery. Many cells, including neutrophils (103), can use topographical information as a guide to migration (104). Guidance cues from structures of this order of magnitude have been revealed by advances in microfabrication techniques (105). This ridging may then provide directional information. Contact guidance may also be provided by other shapes. Although neutrophils do not readily align themselves along cylinders, they do so along grooves (106) such as may occur at the intercellular junction.

*Tensile Guidance.* In a matrix of fibrin that is under tension, neutrophils move parallel to the fiber axes in preference (106). In this system, there are clearly geometrical cues, but there may well be cues from differences in rigidity, as fibers subject to a tensile strain will be more rigid, and this may provide contact guidance (107). Experimentally, this effect is difficult to separate from that of alignment along a surface. However in a three-dimensional matrix of aligned fibrils, a protrusion in the direction of fiber alignment will meet less resistance than one perpendicular to fiber alignment (103). This effect could occur in the cleft itself, although the direction of tension in the matrix may not be directed away from the lumen. Thus, this mechanism must be considered speculative, as must guidance clues from differences in cellular rigidity (107).

*Haptotaxis.* In addition to contact guidance, guidance can come from gradients of varying kinds. Haptotaxis requires gradients of adhesiveness (108) and has been shown to induce cell migration in vitro (107). E-selectin is haptotactic to neutrophils (109), thrombospondin is haptotactic to monocytes and neutrophils (110,111), and fibronectin, vitronectin, and collage IV are haptotactic for activated T cells (112). Evidence for in vivo relevance of haptotaxis has been provided in embryological systems but has not conclusively been demonstrated for transmigration. In vitro, HL-60 cell adhesion to IL-1–stimulated HUVECs was assessed with atomic force microscopy. The strength of adhesion was greater in the junctional than in the cytoplasmic region. Adhesion was significantly inhibited by E-selectin antibodies, suggesting there may be a gradient of adhesion in vivo (113). The greater concentration of extracellular matrix proteins in the cleft (see Sections II.C.1 and II.C.6) may also provide a haptotactic gradient. Similarly, the distribution of PECAM-1, maximal in the interendothelial junctional region, suggests a potential for haptotactic guidance, although this has not been directly examined.

*Blood Flow and Establishment of Chemotactic Gradients: "Chemohaptotaxis."* Zigmond (114) has shown that a stable gradient in required for chemotaxis. A problem potentially arises early in inflammation when there is blood flow. Blood flow might remove chemoattractants, making a gradient of soluble material unstable. In contrast, as endothelial cells secrete some chemoattractants in both directions, blood flow might disperse the component secreted into the lumen, maintaining a gradient of chemoattractant. It has been debated whether chemoattractants can act in the bloodstream or are diluted by blood flow and are relatively ineffective.

Binding to a surface would ensure a concentration gradient immune to the effects of flow. Many chemoattractants have anionic or hydrophobic sites that are potential sites for surface binding (115). PAF, for example, is predominantly inserted in the endothelial cell membrane (22), and IL-8 can bind to the extracellular matrix or basement membrane and to endothelial cells (116), probably via its heparin binding-domain (28), although the proportions of free and bound material are not clear (116).

Surface-bound chemokines may also have other modes of action. IL-8 and C5a, but not fMLP, are haptotactic in vitro (117). Although chemotactic gradients exist across the endothelium, the extent to which they provide guidance to the cleft is uncertain. We are unaware of any demonstration of gradients of surface-bound chemokines leading to the cleft nor of a gradient extending through the cleft.

Should blood flow stop, there will be accumulation of chemoattractant in the lumen where it may act as a chemokinetic rather than a chemotactic agent. In this latter state, desensitization may occur (27), downregulating leukocyte responses to the agent—this may be an in vivo limitation on transmigration.

Chemoattractants are important in transmigration, but it may well be that their guidance role is in or past the cleft, and their ability to activate leukocytes is critical before and in the cleft.

## C. Leukocytes Migrate Through the Interendothelial Cleft

Ultrastructural studies in vivo (1) and in vitro (2,14) show that adherent neutrophils extrude pseudopodia that indent the surface of the endothelium and extrude between neighboring cells. Despite the potentially formidable barrier formed by the multiple adhesion systems in the interendothelial cleft, movement through the monolayer is rapid—occurring within 30 sec (118). Monocytes in transit are tightly apposed to the endothelial monolayer (119). Similar findings have been noted with neutrophils and lymphocytes. Once monocytes have extended pseudopods into the interendothelial cleft, they are resistant to removal with cation chelators (100). This suggests non–integrin-mediated mechanisms may be involved.

1.   Structure of the Interendothelial Cleft

Endothelial cells are polygonal and extended in the direction of blood flow along the long axis of the vessel (120). The interendothelial cell cleft is little longer than a straight line joining the surface to the basement membrane (120), between 0.12 and 0.64 $\mu$m in length (120,121), although it is often tortuous (122). Endothelial cells are strongly adherent to the basement membrane and adhere to each other via adherens, tight, and gap junctions (122, 123). The intercellular junctions, especially adherens junctions, form a continuous belt around the cell (122). Intracellularly actin and myosin are close to the cleft in vivo and in vitro and may regulate junction opening via endothelial contraction (124). The principal extracellular molecules involved in interendothelial adhesion appear to be $\alpha_2\beta_2$-integrins and $\alpha_5\beta_1$-integrins, PECAM-1, and VE-cadherin (also known as cadherin-5) (125–129).

*Integrins.*   Immunofluorescence studies (125) have revealed two integrins, $\alpha_2\beta_1$ and $\alpha_5\beta_1$ in the cleft. Their principal ligands are fibronectin, collagen, and laminin. The organization of these two integrins and their ligands in the interendothelial cleft is unclear. Collagen, laminin, thrombospondin, and fibronectin are all produced by endothelial cells and found in the cell-cell interaction rims (127,130–132) and might serve as integrin ligands.

Antibodies to $\alpha_2\beta_1$- or $\alpha_5\beta_1$-integrin increase endothelial permeability (125) as do RGD peptides (133), but antibodies to the various matrix components do not. There is some evidence that these integrins bind to endothelial cells, as endothelial cell aggregation in suspension can be inhibited by anti–$\alpha_5\beta_1$-integrin antibodies and peptides containing an RGD motif (125).

*Cadherins.*   Cadherins are a family of adhesion molecules (reviewed in ref. 134) that bind homophilically and heterophilically in a cation-dependent and protease-sensitive manner. Endothelial cells express three cadherins: N-, P-, and VE-cadherin. The first is diffusely spread across the cell (135), the second is present in trace amounts (136), and the last is specifically localized to the interendothelial cell junction (126). VE-cadherin seems important in maintaining endothelial permeability, as monolayers of transfected cells show calcium-dependent reductions in permeability (16).

*Immunoglobulin Superfamily of Adhesion Molecules.*   PECAM-1 is a member of the immunoglobulin superfamily of adhesion molecules (reviewed in refs. 137 and 138). It is concentrated at the interendothelial junction in monolayers (125). PECAM-1 expression is widespread, with highest levels being seen on endothelial cells and platelets, but significant expression is also seen on myeloid and lymphoid lineages (56).

The PECAM-1 molecule is a single-chain membrane spanning glycoprotein of 130 kD molecular weight with six extracellular Ig-like domains of the C2 subclass (139). Homophilic interactions appear to require all six Ig domains, as loss of 1 domain disables binding (140). Active binding sites are proposed to reside in domains 2–3 and 5–6 (141). Heterophilic binding is cation dependent and is impaired by sulfated glycosaminoglycans. The second Ig domain contains a heparin binding consensus sequence and appears necessary for heterophilic interactions. A ligand for this interaction on lymphokine-activated killer cells has recently been shown to be the $\alpha_V\beta_3$-integrin (140).

Unlike many other endothelial cell adhesion molecules, expression is not significantly upregulated by activation with TNF-$\alpha$ or interferon-$\gamma$ (INF-$\gamma$) (142). Romer et al. reported that high doses of cytokines (TNF-$\alpha$ 2000 U/ml, IFN-$\gamma$ 1000 U/ml) resulted in reduced intensity of expression at HUVECs intercellular contact rims, which they interpreted as a redistribution of PECAM-1 (142). $H_2O_2$-treated HUVECs show redistribution of PECAM-1 away from the cleft and toward the basal surface of the HUVECs (54); however, this is associated with endothelial retraction, and it is difficult to extrapolate this data to more physiological situations. In contrast to Romer et al.'s data (142), Davidson et al. presented an abstract showing PECAM-1 was not redistributed during cytokine or chemotactic transmigration (143). Clarification of these findings are clearly important to our understanding of PECAM-1 changes in transmigration.

As well as changes in distribution, PECAM-1 association with the cytoskeleton might be altered by activation. Romer et al. (142) also noted the reduction in PECAM-1 intensity to be associated with a reduction in the cytoskeletal associated fraction in contradiction to the findings of Lampugnani et al. (127). This may be related to different extraction buffers used by the two groups, and it requires further elucidation.

The PECAM-1 cytoplasmic tail has five potential phosphorylation sites (137), suggesting another mechanism for regulation. Phosphorylation of PECAM-1 has been reported after platelet activation and is associated with reduced mobility on the membrane. Phosphorylation is also seen after endothelial activation, and this suggests this is a likely mechanism for regulating PECAM-1 function (137).

*Organization of Molecular Systems.* Ultrastructural and confocal microscopic studies (129) show PECAM-1 to be located more basally in the junction than VE-cadherin. PECAM-1 is not associated with electron microscopic adherens junctions in contrast to VE-cadherin. PECAM-1 appears in the junction some hours after VE-cadherin, but unlike the cadherin, cation chelation does not lead to its redistribution.

## 2.   PECAM-1 Is Critical in Passage Through the Cleft

PECAM-1 is clearly important in the passage through the cleft. Anti–PECAM-1 antibodies reduce monocyte transmigration through resting endothelium, and both monocyte and neutrophil transmigration through cytokine-activated endothelium by 70–90% (137,144). Binding to endothelium is not affected. The effects are seen if endothelial cells or leukocytes or both are treated with antibodies. In vivo, small doses of monoclonal antibodies to murine PECAM-1 are as effective as CD11b antibodies in preventing neutrophil influx in thioglycollate-induced peritonitis, and similarly have an effect lasting at least 48 hr (137,145). The efficacy of PECAM-1 antibodies in vivo has been confirmed in other inflammatory models (137,146).

The neutrophils and monocytes that are blocked in transmigration accumulate at the cleft (144), where they remain firmly adherent. Electron microscopy of the monocytes showed that most had at least a small pseudopod inserted into the cleft (144). In vivo, the mesenteric vessels of treated animals contain an excess of adherent neutrophils (145). This strongly suggests a role for PECAM-1 in passage through the interendothelial junction.

Monoclonal antibodies mapped to domains 1–2 inhibit transmigration, but other monoclonal antibodies are not inhibitory (147) (C. Bernard, L. Noack, J. Gamble, M. Vadas, in preparation). In view of the role of $\alpha_V\beta_3$-integrin as a lymphokine-activated killer cell ligand for PECAM-1 (140), we have examined the role of $\alpha_V\beta_3$-integrin in neutrophil transmigration. Using cyclic peptides which inhibit $\alpha_V\beta_3$-integrin–mediated melanoma adhesion, we have seen no effect on neutrophil transmigration across cytokine-activated HUVECs. It would be of interest to examine the role of $\alpha_V\beta_3$-integrin in lymphocyte transmigration and to examine alternative $\alpha_V\beta_3$-integrin inhibitors in neutrophil transmigration.

Lymphocyte transmigration has not been examined using the standard HUVEC system. Using changes in the proportion of PECAM-1-expressing cells after transmigration as a surrogate measure of PECAM-1 dependence, Bird et al. (148) were not able to show a role for PECAM-1 in lymphocyte transmigration. This finding is of importance but needs confirmation in a standard assay.

## 3.   PECAM-1–Independent Transmigration

The residual transmigration of 10–30% after PECAM-1 inhibition suggests that other mechanisms operate in passage through the cleft in type II transmigration. There are no candidate molecules whose role in transmigration is solely in passage through the interendothelial junction. Other molecules, for example, ICAM-1, might account for some of the PECAM-1– independent transmigration, but there is insufficient direct evidence to comment further.

In contrast to type II (inflammatory) transmigration, in type I (chemotactic) transmigration induced by IL-8 and $LTB_4$, PECAM-1 antibodies are not effective in decreasing transmigration (C. Bernard, L. Noack, J. Gamble, M. Vadas, in preparation). This suggests that different mechanisms operate in the two processes, and examination of PECAM-1–independent inflammatory transmigration may yield clues as to the mechanism operating in type I transmigration.

4.  Role of CD47 (Integrin-Associated Protein) in Transmigration

Integrin-associated protein (IAP, CD47) is a single-chain protein that, on the basis of its primary structure, has five potential membrane-spanning regions, a number of potential glycosylation sites, and a large extra-cytoplasmic amino-terminus with homology to the IgV domain of the immunoglobulin superfamily (149,150). It was originally isolated by coimmunoprecipitation with a $\beta_3$-integrin–related molecule, the leukocyte-response integrin (151). It is expressed widely, and its expression is not limited to cells expressing integrins (152).

Blocking antibodies have shown a variety of functions. It is required for the rise in $[Ca^{2+}]i$ seen when endothelial cells bind to extracellular matrix components, but it is not required for endothelial cell adhesion, integrin-mediated increases in $pH_i$, or tyrosine phosphorylation, nor is it required for the influx of $Ca^{2+}$ triggered by histamine stimulation (153). Neutrophil chemotaxis and adhesion to entactin are IAP and $\beta_3$-integrin dependent (99). Generation of the respiratory burst triggered by $\beta_3$-integrin binding is also IAP dependent (154). In monocytes, the enhanced binding seen on activation of CD11b/CD18 by binding to an RGD site of bacterial origin also requires IAP function (155). Not all $\beta_3$-integrins are functionally associated with IAP: Platelet GpIIa/IIIb–dependent functions are not IAP dependent (156). Recently, Blystone et al. (157,158) described $\alpha_V\beta_3$-integrin–mediated modulation of $\alpha_5\beta_1$-integrin–dependent phagocytosis with no alteration of $\alpha_5\beta_1$-integrin–dependent adhesion. The modulation of phagocytosis could be mimicked by antibodies to IAP. These observations have led to the suggestions that IAP functions as a calcium channel (153) or as a signal transduction unit, modulating the effect of integrin function (154), possibly via interaction with the cytoplasmic tail of the $\beta_3$-integrin (157).

Cooper et al. have shown the critical dependence of transmigration on

IAP function (29). Treatment of either HUVECs or neutrophils inhibited cytokine-activated transmigration by >80% and inhibited neutrophil chemotaxis. Although there are no data specifically to link it to passage through the cleft, the lack of inhibition of adhesion and its effects on [Ca$^{2+}$]i provide some suggestion that it is critical in this phase of migration. The mechanism of action is not clear; however, in further work we have not found any inhibition of chemoattractant stimulated adhesion or superoxide generation, suggesting these effects are not mediated via $\beta_2$-integrins (B. Stein, E. Brown, F. Lindberg, J. Gamble, M.A. Vadas, in preparation). We have not tested antibodies to $\beta_3$-integrin, but peptides that inhibit $\beta_3$-integrin–mediated endothelial cell functions do not inhibit transmigration (B. Stein M.A. Vadas, unpublished observations). Elucidating the mechanism of action of this molecule in transmigration will be of considerable interest.

## 5.  Negotiating the Interendothelial Cell Cleft

Although neutrophils can be induced to release many factors, it is clear some of them play no role in transmigration. Products of the respiratory burst do not appear necessary, as the neutrophils of patients with chronic granulomatous disease are able to accumulate in the tissues despite their incompetence in generating an oxidative burst.

Proteolysis of the barrier does not appear to be important. Direct evidence shows inhibition of elastase does not prevent transmigration (2,159). Similarly, inhibition of urokinase or depletion of plasmin or plasminogen does not inhibit transmigration (7), although the urokinase receptor appears to have a role in signaling functions as inhibition of receptor function with monoclonal antibodies inhibits monocyte chemotaxis to fMLP and adhesion to activated HUVECs. This appears to be through an interaction with CD11b/CD18, with which the urokinase receptor associates (reviewed in ref. 160). Indirect evidence that proteolysis is not required is provided by Huber et al. (15). These investigators were examining neutrophil transmigration and penetration of the basement membrane of an in vitro blood vessel model. They noted that inhibitors of many enzyme systems (see Section II.E.2) did not affect neutrophil penetration through their construct, implying there was little effect on transmigration (15).

Although it seems unlikely, other enzymes may be important. Release of granule enzymes, such as cathepsin G (7), are associated with endothelial cell injury or increases in permeability, which are not seen in vitro. This suggests if granule enzymes are involved, they are regulated in some way and not released indiscriminately.

In conclusion, given the density of adhesive bonds between endothelial cells, the cleft is a significant barrier. The precise mechanism involved in passage is unclear. In type II transmigration, as opposed to type I transmigration, some, if not all, leukocyte subtypes require PECAM-1.

### 6. Extracellular Matrix in the Interendothelial Cleft

Apart from a role as a ligand for leukocyte integrins (see Section II.B.2), the extracellular matrix in the cleft may have role as a source of traction for the transmigrating cell. In addition to functioning as a ligand for leukocyte integrins, cells crawling in a three-dimensional matrix can use the geometrical characteristics of a mesh for traction—protruding a pseudopod through a narrow region and allowing it to expand distally provides a source of adhesion that does not require specific adhesion molecules (107). Although T cells are able to penetrate a three-dimensional matrix despite inhibition of adhesion to a two-dimensional surface of the same material (161), suggesting that such a mechanism may be involved, proof that meshwork effects are important is difficult.

As outlined above, the matrix may also function as a guidance source, directly through haptotaxis, and contact guidance, and may provide a chemotactic gradient through chemoattractants bound to it.

## D. Transmigration Does Not Necessarily Increase Endothelial Permeability

Although many inflammatory mediators can increase endothelial permeability (123), transmigration can occur without increasing permeability. In vitro electrical resistance and microscopic integrity is maintained during transmigration (7), as is impermeability to albumin (4). Transmigration in vivo also preserves macromolecular impermeability (1).

### 1. Relationship Between Impermeability and Transmigration

There is a correlation between macromolecular permeability changes and cytoskeletal changes. For example, bradykinin and thrombin increase permeability and cause retraction of the actin-dense peripheral band (162). Disruption of the band with cytochalasin B causes similar increases in permeability (162). Second-messenger systems also play a role; increases in intracellular calcium with calcium ionophore treatment or activation of protein kinase C via phorbol myristate acetate (PMA) increases permeability, with corresponding retraction in actin fibers (162). In contrast, $\beta$-adrenergic agonists and purinergic agonists cause decreases in permeability and cause protrusion of the dense peripheral band. Stabilization of the cytoskeleton with phalloidin has similar effects on both the impermeability and the actin band. Modulators of second-messenger systems also have similar effects, with dibutryl cAMP and forskolin decreasing permeability (162–164).

Cytoskeletal function also appears important in transmigration. Agents known to increase impermeability and increase the peripheral actin band are associated with decreases in transmigration. Doukas et al. (165) have shown that abolition of cytoskeletal rearrangement with phalloidin decreases transmigration and cytochalasin treatment increases transmigration. This suggests modulation of the cytoskeleton is the important event. Other indirect modulators of cytoskeletal function like norepinephrine and serotonin both significantly decrease migration across bovine aortic endothelial cells induced by fMLP, as well as basal neutrophil migration, without altering firm adhesion (165). Similarly, increases in cAMP and decreases in $[Ca^{2+}]i$ levels in endothelial cells which increase impermeability and increase peripheral actin density have been shown to reduce chemotactic transmigration (30). It is possible that the effects of norepinephrine and serotonin are regulated by reduction of the baseline production of chemokinetic eicosanoid metabolites like Thromboxane $B_2$ ($TxB_2$) (164); however, this would not explain the inhibitory effects of phalloidin. Changes in permeability might alter the gradient of chemoattractant and decrease transmigration. It is difficult to assess whether the effect should inhibit or enhance transmigration because of a dose-dependent effect, as at higher doses the barrier function provided by endothelial cells maintains a better chemoattractant gradient and increases transmigration. Furthermore, cytokines like TNF-$\alpha$ can also affect the actin band (166) without changing permeability, suggesting that the cytoskeletal changes are the important phenomenon.

This suggests that endothelial cells can regulate the interendothelial junction, either increasing or decreasing its macromolecular and cellular permeability. It also suggests that this is regulated via cytoskeletal rearrangements. These alterations have mainly been noted in the context of type I transmigration using agents which produce rapid, relatively transient responses. Agents with more prolonged effects, for example, TNF-$\alpha$, can also affect the actin band (166), suggesting that active modulation of the interendothelial junction occurs in type II transmigration as well.

## E. Events Immediately After Transit

### 1. Consequences of Migration Across the Endothelial Monolayer

Leukocytes exhibit a number of functional changes in response to transmigration. Some of these are identical to those induced by exposure to chemoattractants. For example, PAF induces neutrophil degranulation, shedding of L-selectin, and upregulation of CD11b (67). In contrast, Walker et al. reported that transmigration of eosinophils upregulated CD11b and CD35, slightly decreased CD11a, CD29, and CD32 and primed the eosinophil respiratory burst (167), findings that could not be entirely reproduced by supernatants produced by IL-1–stimulated HUVECs and chemoattractants. Kubes et al. reported that transmigration of neutrophils induces expression of cell surface $\beta_1$-integrin and $\alpha_4\beta_1$-integrin (98). As neutrophils do not usually express $\beta_1$-integrin, this finding is of great interest and may reflect novel mechanisms for interaction between the neutrophil and the endothelium.

The stimulus for these changes may involve outside-in signaling from adhesion to HUVECs. In the eosinophil, Walker et al. noted upregulation of CD11b on exposure to membrane fragments of IL-1–activated HUVECs and similar changes on adhesion to HUVECs that were not inhibited by antibodies to E-selectin, VCAM-1 or ICAM-1 nor by PAF antagonists (167). In a similar manner, the stimulus may involve integrin-mediated signaling on exposure of the transmigrated leukocyte to basement membrane or extracellular matrix components in the interendothelial cleft or beyond. These molecules have been reported to induce a variety of functional changes (reviewed in ref. 168); for example, upregulation of cytokine synthesis by neutrophils and monocytes, priming of the neutrophil respiratory burst, and stimulation of phagocytosis. As previously discussed, exposure of neutrophils to entactin induced expression of $\beta_3$-integrin (99) on the cell surface and induced CD18–independent migration. Although transmigration in vivo will expose leukocytes to basement membrane and extracellular matrix molecules, in vitro, Huber et al. noted it took approximately 3 weeks for the basement membrane secreted by endothelial cells to resemble the basement membrane in vivo (15). Whether the matrix secreted by endothelial cells used in most transmigration systems is sufficient to trigger such changes is not clear. It is possible that some conflicting results reflect differences in extracellular matrix between HUVECs growing on amniotic membrane and those growing on fibronectin-coated surfaces.

## 2. Migration Across the Basement Membrane

After transmigration, leukocytes pause at the basement membrane and further migration is delayed until the basement membrane is penetrated (1,15). Neutrophils remain adherent to the basal aspect of the endothelium and may form a temporary sheath around the vessel before moving out into the tissues (1). In contrast to adhesion and earlier steps in transmigration, relatively little is known about penetration of the basement membrane.

Neutrophils in vitro can adhere to basement membrane components such as enactin (99). Huber et al. used prolonged HUVEC culture to generate an in vitro model of basement membrane passage (15) to test these observations. They noted that transmigration of large numbers of neutrophils did not result in morphological alterations of the basement membrane but did increase its permeability. The permeability defect was repaired within 4 hr in a process dependent on transcription and protein synthesis by endothelial cells. Penetration was not dependent on protein synthesis. The investigators were not able to inhibit membrane penetration with inhibitors of plasminogen activator, plasmin, neutral metalloendo-protease, cysteine proteases, aspartate proteases, nor serine proteases. They added an excess of heparin or recombinant tissue inhibitors of metalloproteases (TIMP) to neutralize neutrophil heparanase and met-alloproteinases and saw no reduction in penetration of the basement mem-brane. In contrast, Leppert et al. (169) used specific inhibitors of metal-loproteinases and showed that migration of resting and IL-2–activated T cells across a Matrigel barrier required gelatinase B (92-kD type IV colla-genase, matrix metalloproteinase-9), which is constitutively expressed by T cells. Activated T cells also produce the structurally related gelatinase A (72-kD type IV collagenase, matrix metalloproteinase-2), which may also be involved in basement membrane degradation (169,170). Although they are interesting, these results may not be relevant in vivo, as inhibition of enzymes used by neutrophils to degrade isolated basement membrane com-ponents were not important in the vessel construct of Huber et al. (15).

Leppert et al. did note that migration of T cells through their basement membrane construct was not random, but that cells tended to migrate through an area through which a previous cell had passed (169). Whether this represents a focal loss of resistance to migration, generation of a chemohaptotactic gradient from release of matrix-bound factors, or a com-bination of these remains to be seen, but it may be an important model of directional clues in tissues.

## 3.   Migration into the Tissues

Although the specific molecular details are not yet well understood, PECAM-1 is important in monocyte migration into the extracellular matrix after transmigration. Unlike passage through the junction, which is inhibited by antibodies to domains 1–2 but not by antibodies to domain 6, heparin and antibodies to domain 6 inhibit migration through the extracellular matrix (147). Migration through three-dimensional matrices is increased by the presence of hyaluron, a CD44 ligand. Activating monoclonal antibodies (161) have a similar effect, and it is likely that CD44 has a role in migration through the extracellular matrix. Although not specifically examined, it is likely that $\beta_2$-integrins and VLA-4 will be important in this process.

## III. MODEL FOR PASSAGE THROUGH THE INTERENDOTHELIAL CLEFT

### A. Movement Through the Cleft: The "Zipper"

As discussed in Section II.C.1 and II.C.5, the interendothelial junction forms a significant barrier to transmigration, but transmigration does not result in detectable changes in endothelial permeability (7) nor morphological sequelae. A mechanism which maintains impermeability and does not cause persisting morphological change must exist to allow transmigration.

As transmigration is associated with intimate contact between endothelial cells and leukocytes, a possible mechanism involves the transmigrating cell interacting with the interendothelial junction like a zipper. As the pseudopod of the migrating cell intrudes into the cleft, it disrupts endothelial-endothelial adhesion and replaces it with endothelial-leukocyte-endothelial adhesion (Fig. 2). So, for example, the PECAM-PECAM–based adhesion between two endothelial cells could temporarily become an endothelial PECAM-neutrophil PECAM interaction as the neutrophil moves through the cleft. If the interaction is strong enough, its permeability would be maintained. The large number and high density of adhesion molecules in the cleft seems ideal to provide strong adhesion and maintain a permeability barrier. These interactions would also provide the migrating cell with a firm anchor for traction. A "zipper" would provide a mechanism for overcoming the barrier of the interendothelial junction. A prediction of this model would be that regulation of the endothelial barrier could both increase and decrease transmigration.

### 1. The "Zipper"

We hypothesize that formation of a zipper interaction requires some change in the interendothelial junction. This probably involves regulation of adhesive forces between endothelial cells in association with active cytoskeletal rearrangement, which allows formation of the zipper interaction between the transmigrating cell and the endothelium.

*Potential Zipper Mechanisms.* There is insufficient information to allow for a good understanding of the process, but there are several candidate mechanisms.

Alteration of adhesion molecules would allow rapid changes in barrier functions of the endothelium and would be a good candidate mechanism. The altered phosphorylation of PECAM-1 seen with endothelium activation and the changes in PECAM-1 association with the cytoskeleton seen with high-dose cytokine activation (142) might facilitate passage by reducing the intercellular adhesive forces in the junction. This is in keeping with

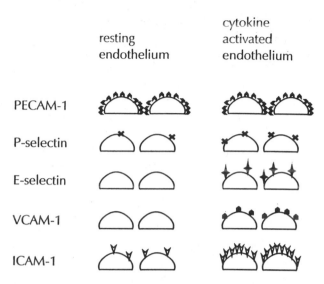

**Figure 2** A schematic representation of the distribution of adhesion molecules of endothelium.

a recent abstract which reported that VE-cadherin on activated en-dothelium is redistributed during neutrophil transmigration, and these changes were preceded by loss of β-catenin from the junction, suggesting loss of attachment to the cytoskeleton (143).

The inhibition of transmigration by phalloidin (165) suggests that cy-toskeletal function is important in a situation where there is no de-tectable retraction. A combination of cytoskeletal contraction together with a reduction in interendothelial adhesion through downregulation of PECAM-1 and dissociation of cadherins and PECAM-1 from the cyto-skeleton would ease the passage of a migrating cell through the endo-thelial monolayer.

*Utility of the Model.* This model could account for a number of features of transmigration. Increases in adhesion between endothelial cells would pre-vent zipper interactions by increasing the endothelial barrier, and this might decrease transmigration. As the barrier to permeability is mediated by intercellular adhesion molecules, as discussed in Section II.C, an in-crease in interendothelial adhesion could also decrease permeability. This would explain the findings discussed in Section II.D; namely, agents which decrease permeability decrease transmigration. For example, $PGE_2$ and vasoactive amines like serotonin and norepinephrine that decrease perme-

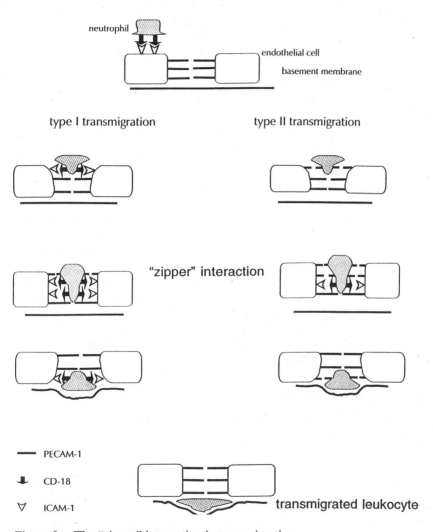

**Figure 3** The "zipper" interaction in transmigration.

ability also reduce chemotactic transmigration. Alterations in second messengers also regulate permeability—calcium ionophore increases it and cAMP decreases it (165,171)—and these effects are matched by the inhibition in inflammatory and chemotactic transmigration induced by preventing a rise in $[Ca^{2+}]i$ and by increasing intracellular cAMP (30,163). Finally, prevention of actin remodeling by phalloidin decreases transmigration and permeability (165). We propose this is a manifestation of interference with zipper function.

This model also emphasizes the importance of the endothelial cytoskeleton in the maintenance of an endothelial barrier, as discussed in Section II.D. Disruption of the cytoskeleton with cytochalasin D results in endothelial retraction with disruption of the interendothelial junction and loss of the barrier function. This is associated with increases in permeability and increases in transmigration. The decreases in transmigration seen with phalloidin treatment of endothelial cells (165) is in keeping with inhibition of zipper function from impaired cytoskeletal rearrangement.

*Endothelium Is Active in Types I and II Transmigration.*   The endothelium is clearly active in type II transmigration in vitro, producing chemoattractants and altering expression of adhesion molecules. In contrast, the endothelium has been hypothesized to have no active role in type I transmigration in vitro (7), because unstimulated neutrophils do not migrate across resting endothelium. As inhibition of endothelial cytoskeletal rearrangement and intracellular signaling in endothelial cells are required for type I transmigration (reviewed in Sections II.A.2 and II.D.1), there is clearly an endothelial component in vitro. We hypothesize that the endothelial activity in type I transmigration is the formation of a zipper interaction allowing transmigration to occur. We would predict that similar events are required in transmigration of unstimulated T cells and monocytes across resting endothelium.

## 2.   Potential Mechanisms for Generating a Zipper Interaction

The model we propose requires an interaction between leukocyte and endothelium resulting in formation of a zipper interaction as part of a process of moving across the endothelial monolayer. As discussed in Section II.A.2, signaling is required for transmigration, and it seems likely that one of the results of signaling is formation of a zipper interaction. The nature of the signaling mechanism is not known, but there are several candidate mechanisms.

*Paracrine or Juxtracrine Molecules.*   Signaling from soluble mediators might accomplish two roles. First, endothelial stimulation might open the interendothelial junction and reduce the endothelial barrier. This is seen with agents like histamine that induce endothelial retraction, which they appear to do by altering regulatory molecules of cytoskeletal contractile elements, for example, altering the phosphorylation state of myosin light chain kinase (172). This may increase transmigration, as cytochalasin B, which induces endothelial retraction, increases neutrophil transmigration (165). Second, it is possible that signaling from soluble factors is responsible for activating the endothelium so that a zipper interaction can occur. This would not necessarily be accompanied by an increase in permeability, and to our knowledge has not been directly demonstrated.

*Adhesion Molecules.* Signaling as a result of adhesion molecules binding to their ligands (reviewed in ref. 64) clearly occurs in the context of transmigration in both leukocytes and in the endothelium.

Endothelial cells respond in a number of ways to leukocyte binding. Rises in endothelial cell $[Ca^{2+}]i$ (30) are induced by binding of neutrophils but not red cells nor inert microspheres (31). This was abolished by pretreating neutrophils with CD18 antibodies (31). T-cell binding to endothelial cells induces an increase in p60$^{src}$ tyrosine kinase activity, with phosphorylation of several proteins, particularly cortactin, an actin binding protein (173). This appeared to be mediated through ICAM-1, as identical changes were noted when activating monoclonal antibodies were used. Calcium fluxes are not the only response to leukocyte binding. For example, monocyte binding to resting endothelial cells induces the secretion of large amounts of MIP-1$\alpha$, which can be inhibited by antibodies to ICAM-1 but not VCAM-1 (174). Leukocytes also respond to binding to endothelium. For example, binding to endothelium induces an increase in neutrophil $[Ca^{2+}]i$. If this increase is prevented by calcium chelators, CD11b upregulation is impaired (175).

There appears to be an adhesion molecule–mediated cross talk between the leukocyte and the endothelium. For example, on firm adhesion of NK cells to endothelium, there was an initial change in NK cell $[Ca^{2+}]i$ and an oscillatory change in endothelial $[Ca^{2+}]i$ which occurred after strong adhesion. If the NK cell $[Ca^{2+}]i$ changes were prevented, the endothelial $[Ca^{2+}]i$ changes did not occur. Antibodies to ICAM-1 or LFA-1 could prevent the changes in endothelial $[Ca^{2+}]i$, suggesting these adhesion molecules are the active participants (176).

These data are all consistent with binding providing signals to the endothelium. As discussed in Section II.A.2, perturbation of endothelial intracellular signaling, particularly that involving $[Ca^{2+}]i$, profoundly inhibits transmigration, although the mechanism has not been established. We suggest that such signaling is necessary for formation of the zipper.

*Gap Junctions.* Another possible mechanism of communication is via gap junctions, as these aqueous channels linking cells allow direct communication between adjacent cells. The channels are made up of six protein subunits, the connexins. There is significant heterogeneity in the tissue distribution of gap junctions and in the connexins comprising them (reviewed in ref. 177). During firm adhesion, extensive contact occurs between leukocyte and endothelium, with areas of close apposition. Gap junctions could form in such areas and would allow rapid communication between the cells, providing a good mechanism for modulation of the endothelial barrier.

Indirect evidence for gap junction formation has been found. Endothelial cells in small arteries express connexin 37 and 40 and HUVECs express connexin 43 and 40 (178). Lymphocytes and neutrophils and monocytes have been reported not to express connexin 37 (179). Jara et al. (180) also showed no expression of connexin 43 in unstimulated leukocytes but noted upregulation by immunofluorescence and Western blotting after lipopolysacharide (LPS) activation of monocytes and neutrophils but not of lymphocytes. In a Hamster cheek pouch ischemia reperfusion model, these investigators showed immunostaining for connexin 43 on adherent leukocytes in ischemic areas but not on adherent leukocytes in control areas. More direct evidence was provided by electron microscopy, where there were areas of close contact consistent with gap junctions, but they did not use dye transfer to examine function. Previous electron microscopic studies have shown gap junctions on venous and capillary endothelium (181), and Guinan et al. (182) have shown dye transfer between lymphocytes and endothelial cells. However, other workers have reported that monocytes do not express connexin 43 mRNA, nor do they transfer dye to endothelial cells (183).

It is thus not entirely clear that gap junctions are important in transmigration, although they would provide a mechanism for the rapid communication needed for coordinated interactions between the transmigrating cell and the endothelium involved in zipper interactions.

## B.  Problem of Endothelial Heterogeneity

It is clear that the high endothelial venules in lymph nodes are specialized for lymphocyte transmigration (184), and specific mechanisms may exist in such "habitual" regions of transmigration. There are significant variations in endothelial morphology (181), responses to growth factors (185), expression of adhesion molecules and gap junctions (185,186), and transmigration (1) between different parts of the circulation. These differences between vascular beds are not extensively addressed by our theoretical or current in vitro experimental models. The effect of endothelial heterogeneity is an important area where our understanding, particularly of migration across the endothelium, needs to be extended.

## IV. THERAPEUTIC IMPLICATIONS OF ALTERATION OF LEUKOCYTE TRANSMIGRATION

Transmigration is a complex process. Specific "antitransmigratory" treatments may not be possible, although it is possible to interfere with transmigration by specific inhibition of adhesion.

### A. Clinical Considerations for Transmigration Inhibition

1. Potential Problems with Inhibition of Transmigration

Inhibition of transmigration for prolonged periods, as would be necessary in chronic diseases, may well be attended with significant increases in infection, and possibly neoplasia, as transmigration is a critical part of host defense and immune surveillance. Furthermore, many of the reagents of established value in animal models are monoclonal antibodies of mouse origin. Recurrent use of such reagents is frequently associated with an immune response to the antibody, which may decrease their efficacy. This suggests that the ideal situation for altering transmigration is an acute, single event, preferably one in which there are no effective treatment approaches. Animal experience suggests that such an approach, for example, with ICAM-1 antibodies, is not associated with increases in the risk of infection (187).

2. Acute Inflammatory Disorders

Several leukocyte subtypes are involved in inflammatory disorders; for example, eosinophils in allergic responses and monocytes in chronic inflammation and atherogenesis. As neutrophils play a critical role in most acute inflammatory states, we will concentrate on inhibitors of neutrophil transmigration.

There has been an increasing appreciation of the role of neutrophil and endothelial activation in multiple clinical situations; for example, hemorrhagic shock, thrombosis, and embolism. Although these situations of ischemia-reperfusion do not only involve problems with adhesion and transmigration, they do involve a component of disregulation of these mechanisms (reviewed in refs. 188 and 189). The advantages of applying antitransmigration treatment in these disorders is that they are common and cause significant mortality; and in some, like stroke and multiple trauma, there are no established alternatives.

There are many animal models of ischemia-reperfusion (reviewed in ref. 190). Benefit has been shown in stroke, myocardial infarction, remote lung injury following gut ischemia, soft tissue ischemia, and multiple trauma or hemorrhagic shock. Most interventions have used monoclonal antibodies to ICAM-1 and $\beta_2$-integrins, approaches that alter transmigration but may also have other effects, such as downregulation of neutrophil superoxide production. The inhibition of P-selectin in animal models has also shown benefit in ischemia-reperfusion (191), suggesting the beneficial effects are not solely from the inhibition of other aspects of leukocyte physiology. Although the mechanism may not be entirely specific, this would seem an ideal situation to consider for human trial. Another advantage of these disorders is the presence of models showing the benefit of antitransmigration treatment applied after injury, thus mimicking the typical clinical situation. In myocardial infarction, ischemia-reperfusion can be predicted to occur after thrombolytic therapy, and in this situation pretreatment prior to ischemia-reperfusion is also possible.

### 3. Chronic Inflammatory Disorders

The potential side effects from inhibiting transmigration suggest that although chronic inflammatory disorders could be treated in this manner, they are more difficult targets. This suggests that inhibition of transmigration might be more valuable in exacerbations of this disease and could still be of genuine value even if they are not able to prevent disease progression. For example, in solid organ transplantation, acute rejection is a serious problem with significant rates of graft failure. Modulation of this event alone would be a useful advance.

## B. Agents of Potential Interest

### 1. Inhibitors of Chemoattractants

Chemoattractants are critical to both types I and II transmigration. Prevention of all chemoattractant generation would essentially abolish type I transmigration, although the large number of chemoattractants generated in injured tissue may limit this approach. Type II transmigration of neutrophils is heavily dependent on endothelial IL-8 production. IL-8 antibodies have been used in animal models to reduce inflammatory lung and glomerular injury (192,193), and IL-8 mutants have been constructed that are competitive inhibitors (194). This may provide a method of generating relatively cell-specific inhibition of transmigration.

### 2. Inhibitors of Adhesion Molecule Function

*Monoclonal Antibodies to Adhesion Molecules.* Monoclonal antibodies are established therapeutic agents (195). The animal models showing the efficacy of $\beta_2$-integrin, PECAM-1, and ICAM-1 antibodies suggest these to be logical starting points for phase I trials. The ability of CD18 and ICAM-1 antibodies to inhibit both type I and type II transmigration suggests broad therapeutic roles. In contrast, the apparent limitation of PECAM-1 to type

II transmigration may limit its value as a therapeutic target, although this has not been evident in animal models.

It is possible that adhesion proteins that are not absolutely required for transmigration, for example, P-selectin, might be better targets as inhibition may produce less risk of side effects like infection that are related to abolition of physiological function (196).

*Other Inhibitors of Adhesion Molecule Function.*

Neutrophil-Inhibitory Factor.   The hookworm protein neutrophil-inhibitory factor (NIF) binds to the I domain of CD11b and acts in similar fashion to anti-CD11b monoclonal antibodies (197). It has shown efficacy in animal models of ischemia-reperfusion (198) (M. Moyle Corvas International, personal communication), but as a foreign protein, its use may be limited by immunological neutralization.

Small Molecules as Inhibitors of Adhesion Molecules.   Several groups are trying to avoid the problems of monoclonal antibodies by finding small peptides or other molecules that are equivalent inhibitors of adhesion molecule function.

Peptide inhibitors of integrin function containing the RGD motif are troubled by lack of specificity, but a specific inhibitor of VLA-4 has been described (199) and used in animal models of asthma (200), and it may be a prototype for other integrin inhibitors. Small molecular weight selectin inhibitors have also been effective in vivo. They reduced both chemoattractant-induced inflammation and thioglycollate peritonitis (201).

### 3.   Inhibitors of Endothelial Activation

All the above approaches to inhibition have concentrated on inhibiting the function of adhesion molecules that have been upregulated in response to inflammation or other stimuli. The prevention of endothelial responses to inflammatory activators may also be of value. In addition to antibodies to cytokines like TNF-$\alpha$, there are other agents which appear to inhibit this process.

*Flavonoids.*   Flavonoids are potent anti inflammatory substances found in high concentrations in citrus fruits and vegetables (202). They have been recently been shown to inhibit cytokine upregulation of ICAM-1, VCAM-1, and E-selectin in vitro (203). One of the more potent flavonoids, apigenin, also inhibited synthesis of prostaglandin, IL-8, and IL-6. In a rat inflammation model and a murine delayed-type hypersensitivity model, apigenin was efficacious. This is a potentially interesting class of agents.

*Proteosome Pathway.*   Several peptide aldehydes are capable of inhibiting the catalytic activity of proteosomes, as well as lysosomal proteases. Read et al. (204) reported that the proteosome inhibitor MG132 (carbenzoxylleucinyl-leucinyl-H) reversibly inhibits TNF-$\alpha$–induced upregulation of E-selectin, VCAM-1, and ICAM-1 expression on HUVECs, but did not downregulate IL-8 mRNA synthesis. Pretreatment with micromolar concentrations reduced neutrophil adhesion to TNF-$\alpha$–activated HUVECs by ~55% and inhibited transmigration by over 85%. These figures are similar to the effects of ICAM-1 antibodies, and it is possible that the effects on neutrophil transmigration reflect the downregulation of ICAM-1. Lymphocyte adhesion was decreased by ~90%. As baseline lymphocyte transmigration was very low, an accurate assessment of its effects on transmigration was not possible.

Unfortunately, inhibition of transmigration requires addition of MG132 before or with cytokine (204). This limits its potential as a therapeutic agent, but this class of compounds is an example of an agents that interfere with endothelial activation and may yield innovative inhibitors of transmigration.

### 4.   Other Potential Inhibitors of Transmigration

Therapeutic approaches may also aim at processes after migrating across the endothelium. For example, to enter the tissues, leukocytes must transit the basement membrane; thus inhibitors of basement membrane transit might be useful in inhibiting transmigration. At present, there is insufficient understanding of the process to suggest potential therapeutic agents.

### C.   Clinical Trials of Antitransmigratory Approaches

In contrast to the large number of animal models of ischemia-reperfusion using many different reagents (45), there are few human trials.

The most extensive experience has been with a mouse anti–ICAM-1 antibody (reviewed in ref. 205). In a phase I-II trial, it was used in addition to immunosuppression with azathioprine, steroids, and cyclosporin A in high-risk recipients of cadaveric renal transplants to prevent graft rejection (206). The original study treated 18 patients, who had comparable results to historical controls. Given the study design, it is difficult to assess efficacy; however, it is interesting that patients achieving target levels had a less delayed graft failure and less acute rejection. Sixteen of the 18 patients developed human antimouse antibodies. With the establishment of an optimal dosing regimen, this agent is now in a randomized double-blind placebo controlled study in 200 renal transplant recipients. A phase I-II trial has now been completed, but not yet reported, in liver transplantation (205). This antibody has also been used in a phase I-II study in longstanding, severe rheumatoid arthritis, which has been reported in abstract form (207). Twenty-three patients have been treated with a 4-day dosing regimen which was well tolerated. Thirteen patients showed a reduction in inflammatory markers and clinical indices of disease activity. Responses did not appear to be durable, with most progressing after 60–90 days.

The other reported human trial used anti-CD11a antibodies in the conditioning regimen for HLA-mismatched allogenic bone marrow transplantation (208) for metabolic and immunodeficiency diseases. They reported no significant problems and comparable engraftment and survival rates to a historical control group.

## D. Future Directions

### 1. Clinical Trials

Human trials show the potential for therapeutic approaches based on alteration of transmigration. Two important directions need exploration. First, other phase I clinical trials are imperative. The positive animal models and established use of some reagents in other disorders suggests there should not be large theoretical barriers to initiation of these trials. Ischemia-reperfusion disorders where there are no established alternatives, such as stroke and multiple trauma, would seem to be likely targets. Second, the large-scale trial in renal transplantation will allow more precise estimates of toxicity and efficacy. There is, however, a need for further clinical data detailing the expression and distribution of adhesion molecules in different disease states. These data will enable a more precisely targeted approach to therapy and will be essential if multiple antimigratory or antiadhesive agents are to be employed in combination.

### 2. New Directions

Transmigration is a multistep process involving many different leukocyte subtypes. This suggests that the use of multiple inhibitors may be needed to achieve therapeutic goals.

Specific inhibition of transmigration without altering other leukocyte functions is an important goal. This might be achieved through the discovery of inhibitors of specific transmigration molecules, such as PECAM-1 and its isoforms. It might be achieved through the use of multiple reagents, targeting different aspects of the process.

Generation of cellular specificity is an important goal. It is likely to be an important part of controlling undesired effects of transmigration, without inhibiting the necessary host defense functions of transmigration. This might be possible through targeting multiple aspects of the process, although a deeper understanding of the generation of cellular specificity is needed to have the best chance of achieving this.

## V. CRITICAL QUESTIONS IN FUTURE TRANSMIGRATION RESEARCH

Although much is understood about early events in transmigration, particularly rolling and firm adhesion, several major questions are raised by observations of transmigration.

The first group of questions relates to the process of transmigration. First, how does a firmly adherent cell become a migratory cell capable of moving across the endothelium. Second, migratory cells must move through the interendothelial junction. As discussed in Section II.C.1, the density and variety of intercellular adhesions make this a formidable barrier. How it is rapidly crossed without altering its functional characteristics is unclear. Finally, having migrated through the endothelium, the mechanism of ongoing migration through the basement membrane and tissue is not well understood.

The second group of questions relates to the cellular specificity of transmigration. Different inflammatory stimuli result in migration of different populations of leukocytes, and with evolution of an inflammatory response, the population of transmigrating cells changes (21). The mechanism by which cellular specificity is generated and the mechanism by which the evolution of cellular migration into an inflammatory reaction takes place are also not deeply understood.

## REFERENCES

1. Grant L. The sticking and emigration of white blood cells in inflammation. In: Zweifach B, Grant L, McCluskey L, eds. The Inflammatory Process. 2nd ed. New York: Academic Press, 1973:205–249.
2. Furie MB, Naprstek BL, Silverstein SC. Migration of neutrophils across monolayers of cultured microvascular endothelial cells. J Cell Sci 1987; 88: 161–175.
3. Furie MB, McHugh DD. Migration of neutrophils across endothelial monolayers is stimulated by treatment of the monolayers with interleukin-1 or tumor necrosis factor-$\alpha$. J Immunol 1989; 143:3309–3317.
4. Moser R, Schleiffenbaum B, Groscurth P, Fehr J. Interleukin 1 and tumor necrosis factor stimulate human vascular endothelial cells to promote transendothelial neutrophil passage. J Clin Invest 1989; 83:444–455.
5. Imhoff BA, Dunon D. Leukocyte migration and adhesion. Adv Immunol 1995; 58:345–416.
6. De Bruyn PPH, Cho Y. Structure and function of high endothelial postcapillary venules in lymphocyte circulation. Curr Topics Pathol 1990; 84:85–101.
7. Huang AJ, Silverstein SC. Mechanisms of neutrophil migration across the

endothelium. In: Simionescu N, Simionescu M, eds. Endothelial Cell Dysfunctions. New York: Plenum Press, 1992:201–232.

8. Furie MB, Tancinco MC, Smith CW. Monoclonal antibodies to leukocyte integrins CD11a/CD18 and CD11b/CD18 or intercellular adhesion molecule-1 inhibit chemoattractant-stimulated neutrophil transendothelial migration in vitro. Blood 1991; 78:2089–2097.

9. Smith WB, Gamble JR, Clark Lewis I, Vadas MA. Interleukin-8 induces neutrophil transendothelial migration. Immunology 1991; 72:65–72.

10. Smith WB, Gamble JR, Vadas MA. The role of granulocyte-macrophage and granulocyte colony-stimulating factors in neutrophil transendothelial migration: comparison with interleukin-8. Exp Hematol 1994; 22:329–334.

11. Smith WB. The mechanisms and regulation of neutrophil transendothelial migration. Ph.D. dissertation, University of Adelaide, Australia, 1994.

12. Springer TA. Traffic signals for lymphocyte recirculation and leukocyte emigration: the multistep paradigm. Cell 1994; 76:301–314.

13. Butcher EC. Leukocyte-endothelial cell recognition: three (or more) steps to specificity and diversity. Cell 1991; 67:1033–1036.

14. Smith CW. Transendothelial migration. In: Harlan JM, Liu DY, eds. Adhesion: Its Role in Inflammatory Disease. New York: Freeman, 1992:83–116.

15. Huber AR, Weiss SJ. Disruption of the subendothelial basement membrane during neutrophil diapedesis in an in vitro construct of a blood vessel wall. J Clin Invest 1989; 83:1122–1136.

16. Lawrence MB, Smith CW, Eskin SG, McIntire LV. Effect of venous shear stress on CD18-mediated neutrophil adhesion to cultured endothelium. Blood 1990; 75:227–237.

17. Bevilacqua MP, Nelson RM. Selectins. J Clin Invest 1993; 91:379–387.

18. Berlin C, Bargatze RF, Campbell JJ, et al. Alpha 4 integrins mediate lymphocyte attachment and rolling under physiologic flow. Cell 1995; 80:413–422.

19. Atherton A, Born GVR. Relationship between the velocity of rolling granulocytes and that of the blood flow in venules. J Physiol (Lond.) 1973; 233:157.

20. Tangelder GJ, Arfors KE. Inhibition of leukocyte rolling in venules by protamine and sulfated polysaccharides. Blood 1991; 77:1565.

21. Movat HZ. The Inflammatory Reaction. Amsterdam: Elsevier, 1985.

22. Kuijpers TW, Hakkert BC, Hart MH, Roos D. Neutrophil migration across monolayers of cytokine-prestimulated endothelial cells: a role for platelet-activating factor and IL-8. J Cell Biol 1992; 117:565–572.

23. Hill ME, Bird IN, Daniels RH, Elmore MA, Finnen MJ. Endothelial cell–associated platelet-activating factor primes neutrophils for enhanced superoxide production and arachidonic acid release during adhesion to but not transmigration across IL-1 beta-treated endothelial monolayers. J Immunol 1994; 153:3673–3683.

24. Nourshargh S, Larkin SW, Das A, Williams TJ. Interleukin-1-induced leukocyte extravasation across rat mesenteric microvessels is mediated by platelet-activating factor. Blood 1995; 85:2553–2558.

25. Smart SJ, Casale TB. TNF-alpha-induced transendothelial neutrophil migration is IL-8 dependent. Am J Physiol 1994; 266:L238–L245.
26. Brevario F, Bertocchi F, Dejana E, Bussolino F. IL-1 induced adhesion of polymorphonuclear leukocytes to cultured endothelial cells: role for platelet-activating factor. J Immunol 1988; 141:3391.
27. Smith WB, Gamble JR, Clark Lewis I, Vadas MA. Chemotactic desensitization of neutrophils demonstrates interleukin-8 (IL-8)–dependent and IL-8–independent mechanisms of transmigration through cytokine-activated endothelium. Immunology 1993; 78:491–497.
28. Huber AR, Kunkel SL, Todd RF, Weiss SJ. Regulation of transendothelial neutrophil migration by endogenous interleukin-8. Science 1991; 254:99–102.
29. Cooper D, Lindberg FP, Gamble JR, Brown EJ, Vadas MA. Transendothelial migration of neutrophils involves integrin-associated protein (CD47). Proc Natl Acad Sci USA 1995; 92:3978–3982.
30. Huang AJ, Manning JE, Bandak TM, Ratau MC, Hanser KR, Silverstein SC. Endothelial cell cytosolic free calcium regulates neutrophil migration across monolayers of endothelial cells. J Cell Biol 1993; 120:1371–1380.
31. Ziegelstein RC, Corda S, Pili R, et al. Initial contact and subsequent adhesion of human neutrophils or monocytes to human aortic endothelial cells releases an endothelial intracellular calcium store. Circulation 1994; 90:1899–1907.
32. Oppenheimer-Marks N, Kavanaugh AF, Lipsky PE. Inhibition of the trans-endothelial migration of human T lymphocytes by prostaglandin E2. J Immunol 1994; 152:5703–5713.
33. Shimizu Y, Newman W, Tanaka Y, Shaw S. Lymphocyte interactions with endothelial cells. Immunol Today 1992; 13:106–112.
34. Casale TB, Abbas MK, Carolan EJ. Degree of neutrophil chemotaxis is dependent on the chemoattractant and barrier. Am J Respir Cell Mol Biol 1992; 7:112–117.
35. Baggiolini M, Boulay F, Badwey JA, Curnutte JT. Activation of neutrophil leukocytes: chemoattractant receptors and respiratory burst. FASEB J 1993; 7:1004–1010.
36. Furie MB, Burns MJ, Tancinco MC, Benjamin CD, Lobb RR. E-selectin (endothelial-leukocyte adhesion molecule-1) is not required for the migration of neutrophils across IL-1–stimulated endothelium in vitro. J Immunol 1992; 148:2395–2404.
37. Harlan JM, Winn RK, Vedder NB, Doerschuk CM, Rice CL. *In vivo* models of leukocyte adherence to endothelium. In: Harlan JM, Liu DY, eds. Adhesion: Its Role in Inflammatory Disease. New York: Freeman, 1992:117–150.
38. Harris AK. Locomotion of tissue culture cells considered in relation to ameboid locomotion. Int Rev Cytol 1994; 150:35–68.
39. Stossel TP. On the crawling of animal cells. Science 1993; 260:1086–1094.
40. Devreotes PN. Chemotaxis in eukaryotic cells: a focus on leukocytes and *Dictyostelium*. Annu Rev Cell Biol 1988; 4:649–686.
41. Kuijpers TW, Mul EP, Blom M, et al. Freezing adhesion molecules in a state of high-avidity binding blocks eosinophil migration. J Exp Med 1993; 178:279–284.

42. Staunton DE, Dustin ML, Erickson HP, Springer TA. The arrangement of the immunoglobulin-like domains of ICAM-1 and the binding sites for LFA-1 and rhinovirus. Cell 1990; 61:243.

43. Diamond MS, Staunton DE, Marlin SD, Springer TA. Binding of the integrin Mac-1 (CD-11b/CD-18) to the third immunoglobulin like domain of ICAM-1 (CD 54) and its regulation by glycosylation. Cell 1991; 65:961.

44. Dustin ML, Rothlein R, Bhan AK, Dinarello CA, Springer TA. Induction by IL-1 and interferon-gamma: tissue distribution, biochemistry, and function of a natural adherence molecule (ICAM-1). J Immunol 1986; 137:245–254.

45. Carlos TM, Harlan JM. Leukocyte-endothelial adhesion molecules. Blood 1994; 84:2068–2101.

46. Carpen O, Pallai P, Staunton DE, Springer TA. Association of intercellular adhesion molecule-1 (ICAM-1) with actin-containing cytoskeleton and alpha-actinin. J Cell Biol 1992; 118:1223–1234.

47. Bullard DC, Qin L, Lorenzo I, et al. P-selectin/ICAM-1 double mutant mice: acute emigration of neutrophils into the peritoneum is completely absent but is normal into pulmonary alveoli. J Clin Invest 1995; 95:1782–1788.

48. Sligh JE, Ballantyne CM, Rich SS, et al. Inflammatory and immune responses are impaired in ICAM-1 deficient mice. Proc Natl Acad Sci USA 1993; 90: 8529–8533.

49. Smith CW, Rothlein R, Hughes BJ, et al. Recognition of an endothelial determinent for CD-18 dependent human neutrophil adherence and transendothelial migration. J Clin Invest 1988; 82:1746–1756.

50. Luscinskas FW, Cybulsky MI, Kiely JM, Peckins CS, Davis VM, Gimbrone MAJ. Cytokine-activated human endothelial monolayers support enhanced neutrophil transmigration via a mechanism involving both endothelial-leukocyte adhesion molecule-1 and intercellular adhesion molecule-1. J Immunol 1991; 146:1617–1625.

51. Oppenheimer-Marks N, Davis LS, Bogue DT, Ramberg J, Lipsky PE. Differential utilization of ICAM-1 and VCAM-1 during the adhesion and transendothelial migration of human T lymphocytes. J Immunol 1991; 147:2913–2921.

52. Chuluyan HE, Issekutz AC. VLA-4 integrin can mediate CD11/CD18–independent transendothelial migration of human monocytes. J Clin Invest 1993; 92:2768–2777.

53. Chuluyan HE, Osborn L, Lobb R, Issekutz AC. Domains 1 and 4 of vascular cell adhesion molecule-1 (CD-106) both support very late activation antigen-4 (CD-49d/CD-29)-dependent monocyte transendothelial migration. J Immunol 1995; 155:3135–3144.

54. Bradley JR, Thiru S, Pober JS. Hydrogen peroxide-induced endothelial retraction is accompanied by a loss of the normal spatial organization of endothelial cell adhesion molecules. Am J Pathol 1995; 147:627–641.

55. Almenar-Queralt A, Duperray A, Miles L, Felez J, Altieri DC. Apical topography and modulation of ICAM-1 expression on activated endothelium. Am J Pathol 1995; 147:1278–1288.

56. Shaw S. Leukocyte differentiation antigen database (database). (International

workshop on leukocyte differentiation antigens). Bethesda: Available from S. Shaw National Institutes of Health on disk; NIH ftp site (balrog.nci.nih.gov), 1994.

57. Anderson DC, Springer TA. Leucocyte adhesion deficiency: An inherited defect in the Mac-1, LFA-1, and p150,95 glycoproteins. Ann Rev Med 1987; 38:175–194.

58. Doerschuk CM, Winn RK, Coxson HO, Harlan JM. CD-18 dependent and independent mechanisms of neutrophil emigration in the pulmonary and systemic microcirculation of rabbits. J Immunol 1990; 144:2327–2333.

59. Issekutz AC, Issekutz TB. The contribution of LFA-1 (CD11a/CD18) and Mac-1 (CD11b/CD18) to the in vivo migration of polymorphonuclear leucocytes to inflammatory reactions in the rat. Immunology 1992; 76:655–661.

60. Anderson DC, Rothlein R, Marlin SD, Krater SS, Smith CW. Impaired transendothelial migration by neonatal neutrophils: abnormalities of Mac-1 (CD11b/CD18)-dependent adherence reactions. Blood 1990; 76:2613–2621.

61. Smith CW, Marlin SD, Rothlein R, Toman C, Anderson DC. Cooperative interactions of LFA-1 and Mac-1 with intercellular adhesion molecule-1 in facilitating adherence and transendothelial migration of human neutrophils in vitro. J Clin Invest 1989; 83:2008–2017.

62. Kishimoto TK, Anderson DC. The role of integrins in inflammation. In: Gallin JI, Goldstein IM, Snyderman R, eds. Inflammation. Basic Principles and Clinical Correlates. 2nd ed. New York: Raven Press, 1992:353–406.

63. Dustin ML, Springer TA. T-cell receptor cross-linking transiently stimulates adhesiveness through LFA-1. Nature 1989; 341:619–624.

64. Hynes RO. Integrins: versatility, modulation, and signaling in cell adhesion. Cell 1992; 69:11–25.

65. Arroyo AG, Campanero MR, Sanchez-Mateos P, Zapata JM, Ursa MA, del Pozo MA. Induction of tyrosine phosphorylation during ICAM-3 and LFA-1 mediated intercellular adhesion and its regulation by the CD-45 tyrosine phosphatase. J Cell Biol 1994; 126:1277–1286.

66. Albelda SM, Smith CW, Ward PA. Adhesion molecules and inflammatory injury. FASEB J 1994; 8:504–512.

67. Edwards SW. Biochemistry and Physiology of the Neutrophil. Cambridge, UK: Cambridge University, 1994.

68. Jones DH, Schmalstieg FC, Dempsty K, et al. Subcellular distribution and mobilization of Mac-1 (CD11b/CD18) in neonatal neutrophils. Blood 1990; 75:488–498.

69. Diamond MS, Staunton DE, de Fougerolles AR, et al. ICAM-1 (CD54): a counterreceptor for Mac-1 (CD11b/CD18). J Cell Biol 1990; 111:3129–3139.

70. Diamond MS, Johnson SC, Dustin ML, McCaffery P, Springer TA. Differential effects on leukocyte functions of CD-11a, CD-11b, and CD-18 monoclonal antibodies. In: Knapp W, Dorken B, Gilks WR, et al., eds. Leukocyte Typing IV. London: Oxford University, 1989:570–574.

71. Van Epps DE, Potter J, Vachula M, Smith CW, Anderson DC. Suppression of

human lymphocyte chemotaxis and transendothelial migration by anti-LFA-1 antibody. J Immunol 1989; 143:3207–3210.

72. Bianchi G, Sironi M, Ghibaudi E, et al. Migration of natural killer cells across endothelial cell monolayers. J Immunol 1993; 151:5135–5144.

73. Hakkert BC, Kuijpers TW, Leeuwenberg JF, van Mourik JA, Roos D. Neutrophil and monocyte adherence to and migration across monolayers of cytokine-activated endothelial cells: the contribution of CD18, ELAM-1, and VLA-4. Blood 1991; 78:2721–2726.

74. Humphries MJ, Sheridan J, Mould AP, Newham P. Mechanisms of VCAM-1 and fibronectin binding to integrin $\alpha_4\beta_1$: implications for rational drug design. In: Marsh J, Goode JA, eds. Ciba Foundation Symposium 189: Cell Adhesion and Human Disease. Chichester, UK: Wiley, 1995:177–194.

75. Elices MJ, Tsai V, Strahl D, et al. Expression and functional significance of alternatively spliced CS1 fibronectin in rheumatoid arthritis vasculature. J Clin Invest 1994; 93:405–416.

76. Meerschaert J, Furie MB. Monocytes use either CD11/CD18 or VLA-4 to migrate across human endothelium in vitro. J Immunol 1994; 152:1915–1926.

77. Meerschaert J, Furie MB. The adhesion molecules used by monocytes for migration across endothelium include CD11a/CD18, CD11b/CD18, and VLA-4 on monocytes and ICAM-1, VCAM-1, and other ligands on endothelium. J Immunol 1995; 154:4099–4112.

78. Issekutz TB. In vivo monocyte migration to acute inflammatory reactions. IL-1$\alpha$, TNF-$\alpha$, IFN-$\gamma$, and C5a utilizes LFA-1, Mac-1, and VLA-4. J Immunol 1995; 154:6533–6540.

79. Bochner BS, Luscinskas FW, Gimbrone MA, Jr, et al. Adhesion of human basophils, eosinophils, and neutrophils to interleukin 1-activated human vascular endothelial cells: contributions of endothelial cell adhesion molecules. J Exp Med 1991; 173:1553–1557.

80. Schleimer RP, Sterbinsky SA, Kaiser J, et al. IL-4 induces adherence of human eosinophils and basophils but not neutrophils to endothelium. Association with expression of VCAM-1. J Immunol 1992; 148:1086–1092.

81. Moser R, Fehr J, Olgiati L, Bruijnzeel PL. Migration of primed human eosinophils across cytokine-activated endothelial cell monolayers. Blood 1992; 79:2937–2945.

82. Ebisawa M, Bochner BS, Georas SN, Schleimer RP. Eosinophil transendothelial migration induced by cytokines. I. Role of endothelial and eosinophil adhesion molecules in IL-1 beta–induced transendothelial migration. J Immunol 1992; 149:4021–4028.

83. Moser R, Fehr J, Bruijnzeel PL. IL-4 controls the selective endothelium-driven transmigration of eosinophils from allergic individuals. J Immunol 1992; 149:1432–1438.

84. Knudson CB, Knudson W. Hyaluronan-binding proteins in development, tissue homeostasis, and disease. FASEB J 1993; 7:1233–1241.

85. Sleeman J, Moll J, Sherman L, Dall P, Pals ST, Ponta H. The role of CD-44 splice variants in human metastatic cancer. In: Marsh J, Goode JA, eds. Ciba

Foundation Symposium 189: Cell Adhesion and Human Disease. Chichester, UK: Wiley, 1995:142–151.

86. Oppenheimer-Marks N, Davis LS, Lipsky PE. Human T lymphocyte adhesion to endothelial cells and transendothelial migration. Alteration of receptor use relates to the activation status of both the T cell and the endothelial cell. J Immunol 1990; 145:140–148.

87. Mikecz K, Brennon FR, Kim JH, Glant TT. Anti-CD44 treatment abrogates tissue oedema and leukocyte infiltration in murine arthritis. Nature Med 1995; 1:558–563.

88. Rosenstein Y, Park JK, Hahn WC, Rosen FS, Bierer BE, Burakoff SJ. CD43, a molecule defective in Wiskott-Aldrich syndrome, binds ICAM-1. Nature 1991; 354:233.

89. Mentzer SJ, Remopld-O'Donnell E, Crimmins MAV, Bierer BE, Rosen FS, Burakoff SJ. Sialophorin, a surface glycoprotein defective in Wiskott-Aldrich syndrome, is involved in human T-lymphocyte proliferation. J Exp Med 1987; 165:1383.

90. Rosenkrantz AR, Majdic O, Stöckl J, Pickl W, Stockinger H, Knapp W. Induction of neutrophil homotypic adhesin via sialophorin (CD-43), a surface sialoglycoprotein restricted to haematopoietic cells. Immunology 1993; 80: 431–438.

91. Manjunath N, Correa M, Ardman M, Ardman B. Negative regulation of T-cell adhesion and activation by CD43. Nature 1995; 377:535–538.

92. Gao JX, Issekutz AC, Issekutz TB. Neutrophils migrate to delayed-type hypersensitivity reactions in joints, but not in skin. Mechanism is leukocyte function-associated antigen-1-/Mac-1-independent. J Immunol 1994; 153:5689–5697.

93. Burns AR, Takei F, Doerschuk CM. Quantification of ICAM-1 expression in mouse lung during pneumonia. J Immunol 1994; 153:3189–3198.

94. Burns AR, Doerschuk CM. Quantitation of L-selectin and CD18 expression on rabbit neutrophils during CD18-independent and CD18-dependent emigration in the lung. J Immunol 1994; 153:3177–3188.

95. Tipping PG, Cornthwaite LJ, Holdsworth SR. Beta 2 integrin independent neutrophil recruitment and injury in anti-GBM glomerulonephritis in rabbits. Immunol Cell Biol 1994; 72:471–479.

96. Folkesson HG, Matthay MA, Hébert CA, Broaddus VC. Acid aspiration-induced lung injury in rabbits is mediated by interleukin-8-dependent mechanisms. J Clin Invest 96; 107:116.

97. Issekutz AC, Chuluyan HE, Lopes N. CD11/CD18-independent transendothelial migration of human polymorphonulcear leukocytes and moncytes: involvement of distinct and unique mechanisms. J Leukoc Biol 1995; 57: 553–561.

98. Kubes P, Niu X, Smith CW, Kehrli ME, Reinhardt PH, Woodman RC. A novel $\beta$1-dependent adhesion pathway on neutrophils: a mechanism invoked by dihydrocytochalasin B or endothelial transmigration. FASEB J 1995; 9: 1103–1111.

99. Senior RM, Gresham HD, Griffin GL, Brown EJ, Chung AE. Entactin stimu-

lates neutrophil adhesion and chemotaxis through interactions between its arg-gly-asp (RGD) domain and the leukocyte response integrin. J Clin Invest 1992; 90:2251–2257.

100. Muller WA, Weigl SA. Monocyte-selective transendothelial migration: dissection of the binding and transmigration phases by an in vitro assay. J Exp Med 1992; 176:819–828.

101. Davies PF. Flow-mediated endothelial mechanotransduction. Physiol Rev 1995; 75:519–560.

102. Barbee KA, Davies PF, Lal R. Shear stress-induced reorganisation of surface topography of living endothelial cells imaged by atomic microscopy. Circ Res 1994; 74:163–171.

103. Wilkinson PC, Lackie JM. The influence of contact guidance on chemotaxis of human neutrophil leukocytes. Exp Cell Res 1983; 145:255–264.

104. Clark P, Connolly P, Curtis ASG, Dow JAT, Wilkinson CDW. Topographic control of cell behaviour: II. multiple grooved substrata. Development 1990; 108:635–644.

105. Clark P, Connolly P, Moores GR. Cell guidance by micropatterned adhesiveness in vitro. J Cell Sci 1992; 103:287–292.

106. Wilkinson PC, Shields JM, Haston WS. Contact guidance of human neutrophil leucocytes. Exp Cell Res 1982; 140:55.

107. Lackie JM. Cell Movement and Cell Behaviour. London: Unwin & Allen, 1986.

108. Carter SB. Principles of cell motility: the direction of cell movement and cancer invasion. Nature 1965; 208:1183–1187.

109. Lo SK, Lee S, Ramos RA, et al. Endothelial-leukocyte adhesion molecule 1 stimulates the adhesive activity of leukocyte integrin CR3 (CD11b/CD18, Mac-1, alpha m beta 2) on human neutrophils. J Exp Med 1991; 173:1493–1500.

110. Mansfield PJ, Suchard SJ. Thrombospondin promotes both chemotaxis and haptotaxis in neutrophil-like HL-60 cells. J Immunol 1993; 150:1959–1970.

111. Mansfield PJ, Suchard SJ. Thrombospondin promotes chemotaxis and haptotaxis of human peripheral blood monocytes. J Immunol 1994; 153:4219–4229.

112. Hauzenberger D, Klominek J, Sundqvist KG. Functional specialization of fibronectin-binding beta 1-integrins in T lymphocyte migration. J Immunol 1994; 153:960–971.

113. Sung KL, Saldivar E, Phillips L. Interleukin-1 beta induces differential adhesiveness on human endothelial cell surfaces. Biochem Biophys Res Commun 1994; 202:866–872.

114. Zigmond S. Chemotaxis by polymorphonuclear leukocytes. J Cell Biol 1978; 77:269–287.

115. Miller MD, Krangel MS. Biology and biochemistry of the chemokines: a family of chemotactic and inflammatory cytokines. Crit Rev Immunol 1992; 12:17–46.

116. Schöenbeck U, Brandt E, Petersen F, Flad H-D, Loppnow H. IL-8 specifi-

cally binds to endothelial but not to smooth muscle cells. J Immunol 1995; 154:2375–2383.

117. Rot A. Endothelial cell binding of NAP-1/IL-8: role in neutrophil emigration. Immunol Today 1992; 13:291–294.

118. Beesley JE, Pearson JD, Hutchings A, Carleton JS, Gordon JL. Interaction of leukocytes with vascular cells in culture. J Cell Sci 1978; 33:85–101.

119. Pawlowsky NA, Kaplan G, Abraham E, Cohn ZA. The selective binding and transmigration of monocytes through the junctional complexes of human endothelium. J Exp Med 1988; 168:1865.

120. Adamson RH. Microvascular endothelial cell shape and size in situ. Microvasc Res 1993; 46:77–88.

121. Adamson RH. Permeability of frog mesenteric capillaries after partial pronase digestion of the endothelial glycocalyx. J Physiol (Lond) 1990; 428:1–13.

122. Franke WW, Cowin P, Grund C, Kuhn C, Kapprell H-P. The endothelial junction: the plaque and its components. In: Simionescu N, Simionescu M, eds. Endothelial Cell Biology in Health and Disease. New York: Plenum, 1988:147–166.

123. Caveda L, Corada M, Padura IM, et al. Structural characteristics and functional role of endothelial cell to cell junctions. Endothelium 1994; 2:1–10.

124. Goeckeler ZM, Wysolmerski RB. Myosin light chain kinase-regulated endothelial cell contraction: the relationship between isometric tension, actin polymerization, and myosin phosphorylation. J Cell Biol 1995; 130:613–627.

125. Lampugnani MG, Resnati M, Dejana E, Marchisio PC. The role of integrins in the maintenance of endothelial monolayer integrity. J Cell Biol 1991; 112:479–490.

126. Lampugnani MG, Resnati M, Raiteri M, et al. A novel endothelial-specific membrane protein is a marker of cell-cell contacts. J Cell Biol 1992; 118: 1511–1522.

127. Lampugnani MG, Corada M, Caveda L, et al. The molecular organization of endothelial cell to cell junctions: differential association of plakoglobin, beta-catenin, and alpha-catenin with vascular endothelial cadherin (VE-cadherin). J Cell Biol 1995; 129:203–217.

128. Albelda SM, Muller WA, Buck CA, Newman PJ. Molecular and cellular properties of PECAM-1 (endoCAM/CD31): a novel vascular cell-cell adhesion molecule. J Cell Biol 1991; 114:1059–1068.

129. Ayalon O, Sabanai H, Lampugnani MG, Dejana E, Geiger B. Spatial and temporal relationships between cadherins and PECAM-1 in cell-cell junctions of human endothelial cells. J Cell Biol 1994; 126:247–258.

130. Volker W, Schon P, Vischer P. Binding and endocytosis of thrombospondin and thrombospondin fragments in endothelial cell cultures analysed by cuprolinic blue staining, colloidal gold labeling, and silver enhancement techniques. J Histochem Cytochem 1991; 39:1385–1394.

131. Kowalczyk AP, McKeown-Longo PJ. Basolateral distribution of fibronectin matrix assembly sites on vascular endothelial monolayers is regulated by substratum fibronectin. J Cell Physiol 1992; 152:126–134.

132. Kowalczyk AP, Tulloh RH, McKeown-Longo PJ. Polarized fibronectin secretion and localised matrix assembly sites correlate with subendothelial matrix formation. Blood 1990; 75:2335–2342.
133. Qiao R, Yan W, Lum H, Malik AB. Arg-gly-asp peptide increase endothelial hydraulic conductivity: comparison with thrombin response. Am J Physiol 1995; 269:C110–C117.
134. Takeichi M. Cadherins: a molecular family important in selective cell-cell adhesion. Annu Rev Biochem 1990; 59:237–252.
135. Salomon D, Ayalon O, Patel King R, Hynes RO, Geiger B. Extrajunctional distribution of N-cadherin in cultured human endothelial cells. J Cell Sci 1992; 102:7–17.
136. Liaw CW, Cannon C, Power MD, Kiboneta PK, Rubin LL. Identification and cloning of two species of cadherins in bovine endothelial cells. EMBO J 1990; 9:2701–2708.
137. Muller WA. The role of PECAM-1 (CD31) in leukocyte migration: studies in vitro and in vivo. J Leukoc Biol 1995; 57:523–528.
138. DeLisser HM, Newman PJ, Albelda SM. Platelet endothelial cell adhesion molecule (CD31). Curr Top Microbiol Immunol 1993; 184:37–45.
139. Newman PJ, Berndt MC, Gorski J, et al. PECAM-1 (CD31) cloning and relation to adhesion molecules of the immunoglobulin gene superfamily. Science 1990; 247:1219–1222.
140. Piali L, Hammel P, Uherek C, et al. CD-31/PECAM-1 is a ligand for $\alpha_V\beta_3$ integrin involved in adhesion of leucocytes to endothelium. J Cell Biol 1995; 130:451–460.
141. Fawcett J, Buckley C, Holness CL, et al. Mapping the homotypic binding sites in CD31 and the role of CD31 adhesion in the formation of interendothelial cell contacts. J Cell Biol 1995; 128:1229–1241.
142. Romer LH, McLean MV, Yan HC, Daise M, Sun J, DeLisser HM. IFN-gamma and TNF-alpha induce redistribution of PECAM-1 (CD-31) on human endothelial cells. J Immunol 1995; 154:6582–6592.
143. Davidson MK, Harrison J, Furie MB. Endothelial junctional events during neutrophil transmigration (abstr). FASEB J 1995; 9:A269.
144. Muller WA, Weigl SA, Deng X, Phillips DM. PECAM-1 is required for transendothelial migration of leukocytes. J Exp Med 1993; 178:449–460.
145. Bogen S, Pak J, Garifallou M, Deng X, Muller WA. Monoclonal antibody to murine PECAM-1 (CD-31) blocks acute inflammation in vivo. J Exp Med 1994; 1059:1064.
146. Vaporciyan AA, DeLisser HM, Yan HC, et al. Involvement of platelet-endothelial cell adhesion molecule-1 in neutrophil recruitment in vivo. Science 1993; 262:1580–1582.
147. Liao F, Huynh HK, Eiroa A, Greene T, Polizzi E, Muller WA. Migration of monocytes across endothelium and passage through extra-cellular matrix involve separate molecular domains of PECAM-1. J Exp Med 1995; 182:1337–1343.
148. Bird IN, Spragg JH, Ager A, Matthews N. Studies of lymphocyte trans-

endothelial migration: analysis of migrated cell phenotypes with regard to CD31 (PECAM-1), CD45RA and CD45RO. Immunology 1993; 80:553–560.

149. Lindberg FP, Gresham HD, Schwarz E, Brown EJ. Molecular cloning of integrin-association protein: an immunoglobulin superfamily member with multiple membrane spanning domains implicated in $\alpha_V\beta_3$-dependent ligand binding. J Cell Biol 1993; 123:485–496.

150. Lindberg FP, Lublin DM, Telen MJ, et al. Rh-related antigen CD-47 is the signal-transducer integrin-associated protein. J Biol Chem 1994; 269:1567–1570.

151. Brown F, Hooper L, Ho T, Gresham H. Integrin-associated protein: a 50-kD plasma membrane antigen physically and functionally associated with integrins. J Cell Biol 1990; 111:2785–2794.

152. Rosales C, Gresham HD, Brown EJ. Expression of the 50-kDa integrin-associated protein on myeloid cells and erythrocytes. J Immunol 1992; 149:2759–2764.

153. Schwartz MA, Brown EJ, Fazeli B. A 50-kD integrin-associated protein is required for integrin-regulated calcium entry in endothelial cells. J Biol Chem 1993; 268:19931–19934.

154. Zhou M, Brown EJ. Leukocyte response integrin and Integrin-associated protein act as a signal transduction unit in generation of a phagocyte respiratory burst. J Exp Med 1993; 178:1165–1174.

155. Ishibashi Y, Claus S, Relman DA. *Bordetella pertussis* filamentous hemagglutinin interacts with a leukocyte signal transduction complex and stimulates bacterial adherence to monocyte CR3 (CD-11b/CD-18). J Exp Med 1994; 180:1225–1233.

156. Fujimoto T, Fujimura K, Noda K, Takafuta T, Shimomura T, Kuramoto A. 50-kD Integrin-Associated Protein does not detectably influence several functions of glycoprotein IIb-IIIa complex in human platelets. Blood 1995; 86:2174–2182.

157. Blystone SD, Lindberg FP, LaFlamme SE, Brown EJ. Integrin $\beta_3$ cytoplasmic tail is necessary and sufficient for regulation of $\alpha_5\beta_1$ phagocytosis by $\alpha_V\beta_3$ and integrin-associated protein. J Cell Biol 1995; 130:745–754.

158. Blystone SD, Graham IL, Lindberg FP, Brown EJ. Integrin $\alpha_V\beta_3$ differentially regulates adhesive and phagocytic functions of the fibronectin receptor $\alpha_5\beta_1$. J Cell Biol 1994; 127:1129–1137.

159. Furie MB, Cramer EB, Naprstek BL, Silverstein SC. Cultured endothelial cell monolayers that restrict the transendothelial passage of macromolecules and electrical current. J Cell Biol 1984; 98:1033–1042.

160. Altieri DC. Proteases and protease receptors in modulation of leukocyte effector functions. J Leukoc Biol 1995; 58:120–127.

161. Friedl P, Noble PB, Zanker KS. T lymphocyte locomotion in a three-dimensional collagen matrix. Expression and function of cell adhesion molecules. J Immunol 1995; 154:4973–4985.

162. Haselton FR, Alexander JS, Mueller SN, Fishman AP. Modulation of endothelial paracellular permeability: a mechanistic approach. In: Simionescu

N, Simionescu M, Eds. Endothelial Cell Dysfunctions. New York: Plenum Press, 1992:103–128.

163. Langeler EG, Van Hinsberg VWM. Norepinephrine and iloprost improve barrier function of human endothelial cell monolayers: role of cAMP. Am J Physiol 1991; 260:C1052–C1059.

164. Doukas J, Hechtman HB, Shepro D. Vasoactive amines and eicosanoids interactively regulate both polymorphonuclear leukocyte diapedesis and albumin permeability in vitro. Microvasc Res 1989; 37:125–137.

165. Doukas J, Shepro D, Hechtman H. Vasoactive amines directly modify endothelial cells to affect polymorphonuclear leukocyte diapedesis in vitro. Blood 1987; 69:1563–1569.

166. Moloney L, Armstrong L. Cytoskeletal reorganizations in human umbilical vein endothelial cells as a result of cytokine exposure. Exp Cell Res 1991; 196:40–48.

167. Walker C, Rihs S, Braun RK, Betz S, Bruijnzeel PL. Increased expression of CD11b and functional changes in eosinophils after migration across endothelial cell monolayers. J Immunol 1993; 150:4061–4071.

168. Pakianathan DR. Extracellular matrix proteins and leukocyte function. J Leukoc Biol 1995; 57:699–702.

169. Leppert D, Waubant E, Galardy R, Bunnett NW, Hauser SL. T cell gelatinases mediate basement membrane transmigration in vitro. J Immunol 1995; 154:4379–4389.

170. Simon MM, Kramer MD, Prester M, Gay S. Mouse T-cell associated serine proteinase 1 degrades collagen type IV: a structural basis for the migration of lymphocytes through vascular basement membranes. Immunology 1991; 73:117–119.

171. Doukas J, Hechtman H, Shepro D. Endothelial-secreted arachidonic acid metabolites modulate polymorphonuclear leukocyte chemotaxis and diapedesis in vitro. Blood 1988; 71:771–779.

172. Garcia JGN, Davis HW, Patterson CE. Regulation of endothelial gap formation and barrier dysfunction: role of myosin light chain phosphorylation. J Cell Physiol 1995; 163:510–522.

173. Durieu-Trautmann O, Chaverot N, Cazaubon S, Strossberg AD, Courad PO. Intercellular adhesion molecule 1 activation induces tyrosine phosphorylation of the cytoskeleton-associated protein cortactin in brain microvessel endothelial cells. J Biol Chem 1994; 269:12536–12540.

174. Lukacs NW, Strieter RM, Elner VM, Evanoff HL, Burdick M, Kunkel SL. Intercellular adhesion molecule-1 mediates the expression of monocyte-derived MIP-1 alpha during monocyte-endothelial cell interactions. Blood 1994; 83:1174–1178.

175. Kuijpers TW, Hoogerwerf M, Roos D. Neutrophil migration across monolayers of resting or cytokine-activated endothelial cells. Role of intracellular calcium changes and fusion of specific granules with the plasma membrane. J Immunol 1992; 148:72–77.

176. Pfau S, Leitenberg D, Rinder H, Smith BR, Pardi R, Bender JR. Lympho-

cyte adhesion-dependent calcium signaling in human endothelial cells. J Cell Biol 1995; 128:969–978.

177. Beyer EC. Gap junctions. Int Rev Cytol 1993; 137:1–38.
178. Reed KE, Westphale EM, Larson DM, Want HZ, Veenstra RD, Beyer EC. Molecular cloning and functional expression of connexin37, an endothelial cell gap junction protein. J Clin Invest 1993; 91:997–1004.
179. Bruzzone R, Haefliger JA, Gimlich RL, Paul DL. Connexin40, a component of gap junctions in vascular endothelium, is retricted in its ability to interact with other connexins. Mol Biol Cell 1993; 4:7–20.
180. Jara PI, Boric MP, Saez JC. Leukocytes express connexin 43 after activation with lipopolysaccharide and appear to form gap junctions with endothelial cells after ischemia-reperfusion. Proc Natl Acad Sci USA 1995; 92:7011–7015.
181. Palade GE. The microvascular endothelium revisited. In: Simionescu N, Simionescu M, eds. Endothelial Cell Biology in Health and Disease. New York: Plenum Press, 1988:3–22.
182. Guinan EC, Smith B, Davies PF, Pober JS. Cytoplasmic transfer between endothelium and lymphocytes. Am J Pathol 1988; 132:406–409.
183. Polacek D, Lal R, Volin MV, Davies PF. Gap junctional communication between vascular cells. Induction of connexin 43 messenger RNA in macrophage foam cells of atherosclerotic lesions. Am J Pathol 1993; 142:593–606.
184. Mebius RE, Watson S, Kraal G. High endothelial venules: regulation of activity and specificity. Behring Inst Mitt 1993; 92:8–14.
185. Brindle NPJ. Growth factors in endothelial regeneration. Cardiac Res 1993; 27:1162–1172.
186. Pepper MS, Montesano R, el Aoumari A, Gros D, Orci L, Meda P. Coupling and connexin 43 expression in microvascular and large vessel endothelial cells. Am J Physiol 1992; 262:C1246–C1257.
187. Mileski WJ, Winn RK, Vedder NB, Pohlmann TH, Harlan JM, Rice CL. Inhibition of CD-18-dependent neutrophil adherence reduces organ injury after hemorrhagic shock in non-human primates. Surgery 1990; 108:205–212.
188. Grace PA. Ischaemia-reperfusion injury. Br J Surg 1994; 81:637–647.
189. Granger DN, Kubes P. The microcirculation and inflammation: modulation of leukocyte-endothelial cell adhesion. J Leukoc Biol 1994; 55:662–675.
190. Winn RK, Sharar SR, Vedder NB, Harlan JM. Leukocyte and endothelial molecules in ischaemia/reperfusion injuries. In: Marsh J, Goode JA, eds. Ciba Foundation Symposium 189: Cell Adhesion Molecules and Human Disease. Chichester, UK, Wiley, 1995:63–76.
191. Weyrich AS, Ma X-L, Albertine KH, Lefer AM. In vivo neutralization of P-selectin protects feline heart and endothelium in myocardial ischaemia and reperfusion injury. J Clin Invest 1993; 91:2620–2929.
192. Wu XB, Wittwer AJ, Carr LS, Crippes BA, Delarco JE, Lefkowith JB. Cytokine-induced neutrophil chemoattractant mediates neutrophil influx in immune complex glomerulonephritis in rat. J Clin Invest 1994; 94:337–344.
193. Mulligan MS, Jones ML, Bolanowski MA, et al. Inhibition of lung inflamma-

tory reactions in rats by an anti-human IL-8 antibody. J Immunol 1993; 150:5585–5595.

194. Clarke-Lewis I, Kim KS, Rajarathnam K, et al. Structure-activity relationships of chemokines. J Leukoc Biol 1995; 57:703–711.

195. EPIC. Use of a monoclonal antibody directed against the platelet glycoprotein IIb/IIIa in high-risk coronary angioplasty. N Engl J Med 1994; 330:956–961.

196. Sharar SR, Sasaki SS, Flaherty LC, Paulson JC, Harlan JM, Winn RK. P-selectin blockade does not impair host defence against bacterial peritonitis and soft tissue infection in rabbits. J Immunol 1993; 151:4982–4988.

197. Moyle M, Foster DL, McGrath DE, et al. A hookworm glycoprotein that inhibits neutrophil function is a ligand of the integrin CD-11b/CD-18. J Biol Chem 1994; 269:10008–10015.

198. Barnard JW, Biro MG, Lo SK, et al. Neutrophil inhibitory factor prevents neutrophil-dependent lung injury. J Immunol 1995; 155:4876–4881.

199. Nowlin DM, Gorcsan F, Moscinski M, Chiang SL, Lobl TJ, Cardarelli PM. A novel cyclic pentapeptide inhibits alpha 4 beta 1 and alpha 5 beta 1 integrin-mediated cell adhesion. J Biol Chem 1993; 268:20352–20359.

200. Elices MJ. The integrin $\alpha_4\beta_1$ (VLA-4) as a therapeutic target. In: Marsh J, Goode JA, eds. Ciba Foundation Symposium 189: Cell Adhesion and Human Disease. Chichester, UK: Wiley, 1995:79–90.

201. Cecconi O, Nelson RM, Roberts WG, et al. Inositol polyanions—non-carbohydrate inhibitors of L- and P-selectin that block inflammation. J Biol Chem 1994; 269:15060–15066.

202. Read MA. Flavonoids—naturally occurring anti-inflammatory agents. Am J Pathol 1995; 147:235–237.

203. Gerritsen ME, Carley WW, Rangers G, et al. Flavonoids inhibit cytokine induced endothelial cell adhesion protein gene expression. Am J Pathol 1995; 147:278–292.

204. Read MA, Neish AS, Luscinskas FW, Palombella VJ, Maniatis T, Collins T. The proteasome pathway is required for cytokine-induced endothelial-leukocyte adhesion molecule expression. Immunity 1995; 2:493–506.

205. Rothlein R, Jaeger JR. Treatment of inflammatory diseases with a monoclonal antibody to intercellular adhesion molecule 1. In: Marsh J, Goode JA, eds. Ciba Foundation Symposium 189: Cell Adhesion and Human Disease. Chichester, UK: Wiley, 1995:200–211.

206. Haug CE, Colvin RB, Delmonico FL, et al. A phase I trial of immunosuppression with anti-ICAM-1 (CD-54) mAb in renal allograft recipients. Transplantation 1993; 55:766–773.

207. Kavanaugh A, Nichols LA, Lipsky PE, et al. Treatment of refractory rheumatoid arthritis with an anti CD-54 (intercellular adhesion molecule 1 ICAM-1) monoclonal antibody (abstr). Arthritis Rheum 1992; 35:S43.

208. Fisher A, Lisowska-Grospierre B, Anderson DC, Springer TA. Leukocyte adhesion deficiency: molecular basis and functional consequences. In: Rosen FS, Seligman M, eds. Immunodeficiency Reviews. London Harwood, 1988: 39–54.

209. Faccioli LH, Nourshargh S, Moqbel R, et al. The accumulation of 111In-eosinophils induced by inflammatory mediators, in vivo. Immunology 1991; 73:222–227.
210. Tanaka Y, Adams DH, Shaw S. Proteoglycans on endothelial cells present adhesion-inducing cytokines to leukocytes. Immunol Today 1993; 14:111–115.
211. Hakkert BC, Rentenaar JM, Van Aken WG, Roos D, van Mourik JA. A three-dimensional model system to study the interactions between human leukocytes and endothelial cells. Eur J Immunol 1990; 20:2775–2781.

# 7

# Transforming Growth Factor-β and Cardiovascular Protection

**David J. Grainger and James C. Metcalfe**

*University of Cambridge, Cambridge, England*

## I. INTRODUCTION

The development of clinically significant atherosclerosis is correlated with a wide variety of genetic and lifestyle risk factors. Set against this undoubted complexity of the atherogenic process, we have proposed that the cytokine transforming growth factor-β (TGF-β) has a dominant protective action on the coronary arteries ("the protective cytokine hypothesis") (1,2). The evidence relating to this hypothesis, which provides a potential key to the prevention and treatment of atherosclerosis, is described in this chapter.

The protective cytokine hypothesis postulates the TGF-β actively maintains the normal physiological phenotype of the endothelial cells and smooth muscle cells in the arterial vessel wall and inhibits the activation of the cells by atherogenic agents. The hypothesis has provided a framework to rationalize the atherogenic actions of an apparently disparate group of risk factors correlated with the development of atherosclerosis through their ability to reduce the level of active TGF-β available to protect the vessel wall. In broad outline, the hypothesis therefore implies that a variety of different combinations of risk factors can act in concert to suppress TGF-β below the protective level, leaving the arteries susceptible to atherogenic agents which cause the development of lipid-filled lesions susceptible to thrombotic rupture. A corollary of the hypothesis is that although loss of the protective effect of TGF-β may generally be necessary

for the development of clinically significant atherosclerosis, it is not sufficient to cause atherogenesis. Risk factors capable of driving the development of lipid-filled lesions when the TGF-$\beta$ activity is below a critical
threshold are also required. Some at least of these risk factors may be
regulated independently of the TGF-$\beta$ activity.

Examples to illustrate how active TGF-$\beta$ and risk factors may vary with
age for high- and low-risk individuals are shown in Figure 1a and 1b. We do
not know whether individuals convert from low to high risk by progressive
loss of active TGF-$\beta$ levels with increasing age (Fig. 1c), although preliminary evidence suggests that men below the age of 30 may have higher levels
of active TGF-$\beta$ than older men. However, there is evidence that levels of
other risk factors associated with atherosclerosis are increased with age.
The hypothesis also offers an explanation of how individuals with high
levels of known risk factors may nevertheless be free of clinically significant
disease if they have protective levels of TGF-$\beta$.

In this chapter, we describe how the hypothesis from in vitro data for the
effects of TGF-$\beta$ on vascular cells and how the biochemical pathway proposed to link conventional risk factors for atherosclerosis to TGF-$\beta$ activity
and to vascular cell phenotype was tested in vivo in animal models and in
the human population. We also consider the potential diagnostic and prognostic value of TGF-$\beta$ levels in the human population and the identification
of dietary factors and drugs which modulate TGF-$\beta$ activity in mouse models of atherosclerosis and in humans and their potential effects on the
development of the disease.

## II.  TGF-$\beta$

### A.  Isoforms

TGF-$\beta$ is the prototype of a superfamily of growth factors and cytokines that
is subdivided on the basis of their structural similarities. The functions of
these proteins are beginning to be unraveled by the use of gene knockout and
transgenic mice, and many members of the superfamily have roles in pattern
formation and tissue specification in embryonic development (3). The three
mammalian isoforms of the TGF-$\beta$ family ($\beta$1, $\beta$2, and $\beta$3) are strongly
related in primary sequence and structure and are highly conserved through
evolution. The three isoforms have very similar biological activities in vitro
and in vivo (4,5), but their expression patterns and post-translational regulation differ significantly, suggesting that their functions in vivo may differ.
The active form of the proteins consists of a 25-kD homodimer with a single
interchain disulfide bond and is released proteolytically from latent, inactive
forms of the protein.

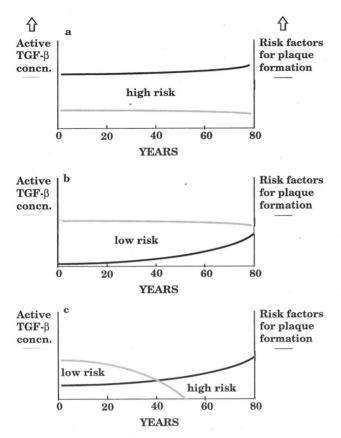

**Figure 1** Models of the relationship between the risk of developing atherosclerosis and TGF-β activity. Factors which regulate TGF-β activity (e.g., genes, lipoprotein [a], PAI-1) are discussed in the text. Risk factors involved in the formation of atherosclerotic plaques when TGF-β activity is suppressed probably include LDL and fibrinogen. Some of these risk factors, for example, fibrinogen, may themselves be regulated by TGF-β activity. (a) Very high levels of risk factors for plaque formation (e.g., lipid levels in familial hypercholesterolemia) relative to TGF-β activity are associated with a high-risk profile from a very early age. (b) High levels of TGF-β activity are assumed to provide long-term protection against normal levels of risk factors which cause plaque formation. (c) If TGF-β activity can decline with age as indicated, an individual may shift from a low-risk profile to a high-risk profile. Note that the risk of developing disease after TGF-β activity is suppressed will depend on the levels of risk factors which cause plaque formation (see text).

## B.   Synthesis and Activation

TGF-$\beta$ is synthesized by cells as latent, precursor forms (6,7), and the availability of active TGF-$\beta$ to protect the arterial vessel wall depends on several factors. These include the synthesis of the latent forms of the cytokine, the efficiency of the activation process, the lifetime of active TGF-$\beta$, and the delivery of the TGF-$\beta$ at the arterial sites required to exert a protective effect.

The synthesis and activation of TGF-$\beta$ protein is complex, involving several processing events that are likely to be similar for the three isoforms but have been most studied for TGF-$\beta$1 (8). The first event is probably removal of a hydrophobic signal sequence to give pro–TGF-$\beta$1. The pro–TGF-$\beta$1 is cleaved within the cell between the C-terminal 112 amino acids and the larger N-terminal peptide. After cleavage, the N-terminal peptides, termed the latency associated peptides (LAPs), remain noncovalently associated with the C-terminal peptides (6). TGF-$\beta$1 is secreted from cells in this latent, inactive form of ~ 110 kD or as a larger complex in which a latent TGF-$\beta$ binding protein (LTBP) is covalently attached through a disulfide bond to a LAP (9). The LTBP is not necessary for latency, but it may facilitate secretion from cells and may also be required for cell-mediated activation of the TGF-$\beta$1 and for correct extracellular delivery. Large and small latent complexes of all three human isoforms of TGF-$\beta$ are secreted by cells in vitro, and variants of the major complexes have also been described. There is accumulating evidence that TGF-$\beta$1 is activated proteolytically in vivo by plasmin (10,11) and possibly by other protease(s) to release the mature 25-kD dimer, but the activation mechanism may also involve the concerted action of mannose-6-phosphate/IGF-II receptor (12), transglutaminase, and the urokinase-type plasminogen-activator receptor.

Studies of monozygous and dizygous twins have shown that the total concentration of the active and latent forms of TGF-$\beta$ identified in plasma is under strong genetic control with heritablility estimated at ~ 70% (13). The concentration of active TGF-$\beta$ is also genetically determined (heritability estimated at ~ 40%), implying that the major factors regulating activation of TGF-$\beta$ in the human population are also likely to be under genetic control, as discussed later.

## C.   Assays

The forms of TGF-$\beta$ present in platelet-poor plasma are assumed to be the extracellular forms present in the circulation. For many individuals two main plasma forms are detectable which can be separated by cation exchange FPLC (14). One peak corresponded by size analysis to the 25-kD active

active form, confirmed as biologically active by the mink lung cell bioassay, and the other peak was a latent form shown by immunoprecipitation to contain the 25 kD homodimer and LAP but not LTBP (Fig. 2). However, the latent complex behaved anomalously on a sizing column, eluting with an apparent size of <5 kD instead of ~110 kD implied by its peptide composition. This complex was fully activatable by acid activation (pH 2 for 10 min).

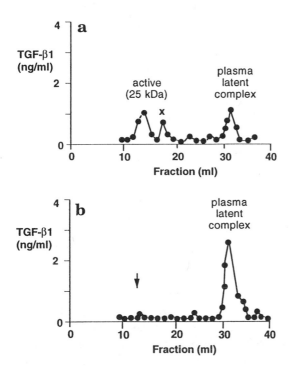

**Figure 2**   Separation of active and latent forms of TGF-β in platelet-poor plasma by cation-exchange FPLC. (a) Plasma from an individual who had approximately equal amounts of active and (a+1)TGF-β by the active and (a+1)TGF-β ELISAs (see text) also had similar amounts of active TGF-β (~25 kD) and plasma latent TGF-β assayed by the R&D Systems Quantikine ELISA after acid/urea activation of all the FPLC fractions (see text). There was no detectable activity where the latent forms(s) of TGF-β in serum made from the same blood sample normally elute. The amounts of peak (X) were too small to determine its composition. (b) Plasma from an individual with no TGF-β eluting at the position for the active form but a substantial amount of the plasma latent complex, consistent with the data for the same sample by the active TGF-β and the (a+1)TGF-β ELISAs. The consistency between the two independent methods of analyzing active and latent forms of TGF-β in plasma provides strong validation of the assays.

Two enzyme-linked immunosorbent assays (ELISAs) were developed which determine the amounts of these two forms of TGF-$\beta$ in platelet-poor plasma (15). The active form of TGF-$\beta$ is assayed using a recombinant, truncated form of the TGF-$\beta$ type II receptor (purified as a soluble GST fusion protein) as the capture reagent (RZX) and a polyclonal anti–TGF-$\beta$ antibody to detect the captured active TGF-$\beta$ with a sensitivity of ~1 ng/ml (40 pM). Typical values for human platelet-poor plasma lie in the range from <1 to 10 ng/ml. The active form of TGF-$\beta$ together with the acid-activatable form of latent TGF-$\beta$, denoted as (a+1) TGF-$\beta$, are assayed using as the capture agent a polyclonal antibody which binds both forms with equal affinity, and the same antibody for detection as in the active TGF-$\beta$ assay. Values for (a+1) TGF-$\beta$ in human platelet-poor plasma are typically <1–30 ng/ml (15).

## D.  Origin and Lifetime

Although it has been assumed that the TGF-$\beta$ pools found in platelet-poor plasma are likely to be derived from platelets, since they contain the main pool of TGF-$\beta$ in blood, two observations have suggested that platelets may not be the main or sole source of TGF-$\beta$ in circulation. Only the TGF-$\beta$1 isoform has been detected in human platelets (16). However, using an ELISA modified to be specific for TGF-$\beta$3, we have detected significant amounts of this isoform in approximately 10–20% of human plasma samples. The origin of the TGF-$\beta$3, and by implication of the TGF-$\beta$1, in the circulation is uncertain.

The only form of TGF-$\beta$1 previously reported in platelets was a large latent complex containing the 25-kD dimer, LAP, and LTBP. However, we have shown that platelets also contain a small latent TGF-$\beta$ complex, which is present in approximately equal proportions to the large latent complex (17). The reason that this platelet form of TGF-$\beta$ was not previously detected is that when TGF-$\beta$ is released by activation of isolated platelets (e.g., by thrombin), the small latent complex is retained by an RGD binding site on the LAP, probably by binding to the platelet gpIIb/IIIa protein, and only the large latent complex is released. The small latent complex is released if the platelets are activated in the presence of RGD peptide and contains the 25-kD dimer and LAP, but not LTBP, by immunoprecipitation analysis. The complex is ~110 kD by size analysis (17), which is consistent with its peptide composition, and therefore differs from the complex with the same peptide components in platelet-poor plasma which eluted with an apparent size of <5 kD (14). If the latent complex is derived from either of the latent complexes in platelets, it has either been substantially modified after release, or it is strongly associated with another intrinsic component or with a plasma component.

When serum is prepared, the small latent complex in the platelets is retained entirely in the clot by the RGD binding site and only the large latent complex is released into the serum. The small latent complex can be released from the clot by RGD peptide or by treatment with plasmin, which activates and releases the TGF-β, and it may provide a slow release mechanism for active TGF-β in wound healing (17). The large latent complex is separated from the plasma forms of TGF-β by cation-exchange FPLC and has an apparent size of 240 kD, corresponding to its peptide composition by immunoprecipitation of a 25-kD dimer, LAPs, and LTBP (14). In contrast to the small latent complex, the large latent complex in serum is not recognized by the capture antibody in the ELISA for (a+1)TGF-β, and hence the (a+1)TGF-β values obtained from platelet-poor plasma and serum prepared from the same blood sample are very similar (15). This very fortunate selectivity of the (a+1)TGF-β ELISA capture antibody enabled us to use serum samples to measure only the forms of TGF-β present in plasma, although the serum samples typically contain ~50 ng/ml of the large latent TGF-β complex. Furthermore, the large latent complex in serum is not activated by the acid treatment (pH 2 for 10 min) which activates the small latent complex. The active TGF-β ELISA values obtained after acid activation of both serum and plasma obtained from the same blood sample are therefore very similar and correspond closely to the (a+1)TGF-β value for the same samples before acid activation. This acid-activation procedure therefore provides a powerful experimental test of the internal consistency of the ELISA TGF-β values for plasma and serum samples (15).

The question of where TGF-β in circulation and in the arterial vessel wall is synthesized is of major importance in understanding the physiological regulation of TGF-β in vivo. In particular, we do not know whether most of the TGF-β in circulation is derived from platelets or from other sources. Similarly, we do not know whether TGF-β in circulation is able to permeate the endothelium to act on the underlying smooth muscle cells. However, there is indirect evidence to suggest that the smooth muscle cells synthesize TGF-β and secrete it into the vessel wall, and it is therefore possible that at least some of the TGF-β in circulation is also derived from the vessel wall if significant permeation occurs.

Little is known about the lifetime of endogenous latent or active forms of TGF-β in circulation. High concentrations of active TGF-β injected into the circulation in rats is cleared with a half-time of <3 mins (18), but it is unlikely that this represents the clearance of endogenous TGF-β which can associate with various plasma proteins (e.g., α2-macroglobulin) which will affect the lifetime and distribution of the bound protein (19). Exogenous injected protein may not become associated with the plasma proteins and may also bind rapidly to the low-affinity endoglin TGF-$\beta$ receptors on the endothelial cells throughout the vasculature, effectively removing it from the pool in circulation. This effect, or the presence of another large, low-affinity TGF-$\beta$ binding pool, may account for the much faster clearance rate of high concentrations of injected radiolabeled TGF-$\beta$ compared with lower concentrations of the cytokine (18).

## III.  IN VITRO EFFECTS OF TGF-$\beta$ ON VASCULAR CELL PHENOTYPE AND FUNCTION

### A.  Endothelial Cells

The earliest stage of atherogenesis is thought to be activation of the endothelial cells by atherogenic agents (e.g., oxidized low-density lipo-protein [LDL]) in the current formulation of the "response to injury" hypothesis (20). Several atherogenic agents activate an inflammatory re-sponse in endothelial cells by stimulating expression of adhesion mole-cules for circulating leukocytes such as adhesion molecules ICAM-1, VCAM-1, and E-selectin and by stimulating the production of interleukin-6 (IL-6), IL-8, and nitrous oxide (NO). TGF-$\beta$ has been shown to inhibit leukocyte adhesion to a variety of endothelial cell types both in the presence and absence of inflammatory cytokines, at least in part by inhibiting the expression of adhesion molecules (21). There is conflicting evidence for the effect of TGF-$\beta$ on VCAM-1 expression on endothelial cells, but E-selectin expression is consistently inhibited. TGF-$\beta$ also inhibited the expression of IL-6 and IL-8 by human umbilical vein endothelial cells in response to TNF-$\alpha$ and IL-1$\beta$ (22). The latter cytokines also induce the secretion of latent TGF-$\beta$ by rat pulmonary artery endothelial cells (23), suggesting that autoregulation of the in-flammatory response may be exerted by endothelial cells. In our experi-ments, rat aortic endothelial cells were treated for 24 hr with the pro-inflammatory cytokines tumor necrosis factor-$\alpha$ (TNF-$\alpha$) or IL-1$\beta$ in the presence or absence of TGF-$\beta$. The cells were washed free of the cytokines and exposed to platelets for 1 hr before assaying activation of the platelets by the release of platelet factor 4 (PF-4). PF-4 release was stimulated by prior exposure of the endothelial cells to the inflammatory cytokines, but this effect was completely inhibited by coexposure to TGF-$\beta$. The anti–inflammatory action of TGF-$\beta$ on the interaction of endothelial cells in vitro with other leukocytes and with the atherogenic lipoproteins requires systematic evaluation.

## B.  Vascular Smooth Muscle Cells

In the early stages of lesion development following activation of the endothelial cells and exposure of the underlying smooth muscle cells to potentially atherogenic growth factors and cytokines, it is believed that the underlying smooth muscle cells migrate, undergo a phenotypic change in which they lose the smooth muscle–specific isoforms of myosin heavy chain (SM-MHC) and α-actin which are essential for the contractile function of the cells, and proliferate to form a neointima (20). The details of this process are unresolved. In particular, it is not clear whether all of the medial smooth muscle cells are able to initiate the process or whether a subset of less differentiated ("pup-like") cells (24) undergo selective expansion in the earliest stages of neointima development. Similarly, the relative importance of migration compared with proliferation (and apoptosis) in forming the neointima is unresolved. It is clear that the earliest stages of plaque formation cannot occur without direct involvement of smooth muscle cells but also obvious that net proliferation rates of intimal smooth muscle cells in the subsequent development of atherosclerotic plaques must be very slow given the long time scale over which clinically significant plaques generally develop.

The effects of TGF-β on the migration, dedifferentiation, and proliferation of vascular smooth muscle cells (VSMCs) in vitro have been extensively studied, and the reported responses are generally consistent with an antiatherogenic effect of TGF-β on VSMCs. When VSMCs are isolated by enzyme dispersal from the aorta of several mammalian species and are plated in primary cultures, under most conditions, they rapidly undergo a process of dedifferentiation as defined by the phenotypic changes described above for VSMCs in atherosclerotic plaques. It is of note that dedifferentiation of primary cultures occurs as effectively in serum-free medium under conditions when the cells do not proliferate as in growth-promoting medium (25,26). In vitro dedifferentiation is therefore a response to dispersal of the cells and removing them from an environment which normally maintains their phenotype rather than a response of the cells to entering the cell cycle or proliferating. These observations suggest that the phenotype of the cells is actively maintained in vivo and that dedifferentiation is a response of the cells to loss of the local interactions or factor(s) which maintain the differentiated phenotype. When TGF-β is added to primary VSMC cultures in the presence or absence of serum, it prevents the dedifferentiation process marked by the loss of smooth muscle–specific contractile proteins and maintains the differentiated phenotype of the freshly isolated cells (27). It is therefore plausible that TGF-β exerts the same effect in the arterial vessel wall where we have shown that there is significant TGF-β activity. Further effects of TGF-β on the differentiation of VSMCs in vitro was revealed by VSMC cloning experiments (see below).

TGF-β inhibits the in vitro proliferation of VSMCs stimulated by growth factors in serum-free medium or by serum. In serum-free medium, TGF-β inhibits proliferation by inhibiting activation of essential early gene responses, including c-*myc* (28). Entry into S phase is inhibited and the cells fall out of the cell cycle. However, when cells are stimulated to proliferate by serum in the presence of TGF-β, the cells do not leave the cell cycle, but he G2 phase of the cell cycle is extended with little effect on the duration of the G1 and S phases, and the overall response is that the rate of proliferation is substantially reduced (27). For rat aortic VSMCs, entry into M phase is preceded by a transient rise in cAMP at the end of G2, and in the presence of TGF-β, the cAMP transient is delayed to the same extent as entry into M phase. This effect of TGF-β on the duration of G2 can be fully reversed by addition of forskolin immediately after S phase at concentrations which mimic the twofold increase in cAMP which normally occurs before M phase. The mechanisms of the two distinct effects of TGF-β on the cell cycle of rat aortic VSMCs are not known, but the inhibition of S phase may reflect the interaction of TGF-β with relatively low-affinity receptors at high free concentrations of TGF-β in serum-free medium. Consistent data for the effects of TGF-β on the proliferation of VSMCs in previous studies have been reported, showing inhibition of entry into S phase in serum-free medium (28) and elongation of the cell cycle for serum-stimulated cells (29,30). Although TGF-β inhibits the proliferation of proliferating VSMCs, it causes a small increase in [³H]thymidine incorporation into DNA of neonatal human VSMCs in the absence of serum or other growth factors, but it has no effect at higher concentrations (31). We have observed a similar effect of TGF-β on rat VSMCs in the absence of mitogens, although it has not been shown whether the small increase in [³H]thymidine incorporation results in a subsequent increase in cell number. As for many of the actions of TGF-β, the response appears to depend on the status of the cells, and it is important to bear this in mind when interpreting the in vivo effects of TGF-β.

TGF-β also inhibits the migration of both VSMCs and endothelial cells (32,33). Cocultures of bovine aortic smooth muscle cells and endothelial cells secreted latent TGF-β which was activated by plasmin in the medium and the active TGF-β blocked the migration of both types of cells.

## C. Smooth Muscle Cell Heterogeneity and Phenotype

It has been suggested that atherosclerotic plaques might be formed from a small subset of less differentiated pup-like cells (24,34,35) and that this might explain why the cells in most plaques are monoclonal (36). This explanation implies heterogeneity of the VSMCs in the vessel wall which has also been inferred from a variety of in vitro properties of VSMCs. We found that freshly dispersed rat aortic VSMCs could be resolved into three distinct size populations by flow cytometry (Fig. 3a) (37). Small cells were the dominant phenotype obtained from neonatal (12-day) rats, but there was a progressive shift in distribution to medium-sized cells from the aorta of young adults and to a population consisting predominantly of large cells from older rats. Cells of different phenotypes were cloned from the freshly dispersed rat VSMCs by dilute plating, and colonies derived from single

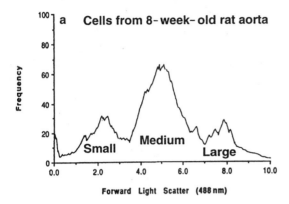

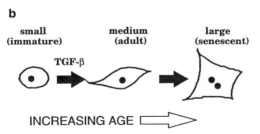

**Figure 3** (a) Resolution of freshly dispersed aortic smooth muscle cells from an 8-week-old rat into three size distributions by flow cytometry. (b) The maturation lineage hypothesis. Small cells, which are the predominant form obtained from 12-day-old rats, are converted irreversibly to the adult, medium-sized cells by TGF-β in vitro and to the large, polyploid cells which do not proliferate by plating the cells at low densities. If cells corresponding to the clonal phenotypes interconvert in vivo as proposed, it is unclear whether proliferation and apoptosis is an obligatory part of the conversion mechanism (see text).

cells were expanded and characterized. A set of clones consisting of cells of the same size as the small cells in the cytometric analysis was obtained which had a cobblestone morphology and properties similar to the pup cell cultures obtained from very young rats. Clones were also obtained consisting of cells of medium size with the spindle-shaped morphology and properties characteristic of the predominant cell type obtained from young adult rats. Clones of cells corresponding in size to the large cells in the freshly dispersed cell population were also established which proliferated very slowly. Cells of similar size but distinct morphology were obtained which did not proliferate but remained as single cells. Further experiments demonstrated that for rats of increasing age, the proportions of the different types of clones obtained corresponded very closely with the distribution of the cells between the three sizes separated by cytometry.

Interconversions of the clonal phenotypes were demonstrated. Clones of cells of the small phenotype were converted to clones of medium-sized cells by a single exposure to TGF-$\beta$ for >12 hr. Conversion was not reversible by removing TGF-$\beta$ and conversion only occurred if the small cell clone was proliferating. The cells proliferated stably in the converted phenotype for many passages, and their phenotype was indistinguishable from that of the medium sized clones. A major proportion of the medium-sized cells were converted irreversibly to large, nonproliferating cells by plating at low density. The biochemical mechanisms triggering this conversion have not been identified.

Based on these observations, we proposed a maturation lineage hypothesis (see Fig. 3b), in which the small cells ("immature" phenotype) are converted to medium-sized cells ("adult" phenotype) and subsequently to large cells ("senescent" phenotype) as the aorta ages (37). However, although interconversions between the phenotypes consistent with the maturation hypothesis can be demonstrated in vitro, it is equally plausible that the changes in proportions of cell types with age occurs in vivo by a process of replacement when the cells proliferate and apoptose.

A striking property of the immature clones which is lost on conversion by TGF-$\beta$ to the adult phenotype is the ability to proliferate by an autocrine mechanism. After conversion, the cells stop making a factor secreted into serum-free medium which enables the immature clonal phenotype to proliferate and also stop proliferating in response to the factor. The factor, which does not correspond in its biochemical and signaling properties to any known VSMC mitogen, is at least as potent in partially purified form as platelet-derived growth factor (PDGF) (37).

We note that if a small subpopulation of cells with the small cell phenotype is retained in the adult vessel wall and is capable of being activated to produce an autocrine growth factor which cannot stimulate the surrounding adult cells, this would be an effective mechanism for the monoclonal expansion of the small cells to form atherosclerotic plaques. However, an alternative explanation for the monoclonality of the cells in plaques is that the VSMCs within the media of the vessel consist of mosaic patches of VSMC clones formed during development, and the plaque cells are generally derived from cells within a single patch of the mosaic and therefore also appear monoclonal (38).

Preliminary experiments revealed another potentially proatherogenic property of the clones with the immature phenotype in that they take up large amounts of labeled LDL. However, this uptake is inhibited by >90% after conversion by TGF-β to the adult phenotype (39). This observation provides in vitro evidence for a potential protective effect of TGF-β on VSMCs, since excessive uptake of LDL into VSMCs occurs in lipid-rich plaques.

The resolution of the various hypotheses described above which were prompted by the in vitro properties of the VSMC clones depends on unambiguous identification of the parental VSMC types within the intact vessel wall which are presumed to generate the different clonal types in vitro. On the basis of the in vitro data, expression of the autocrine growth factor in the vessel wall may enable the parental cells of the clones with the immature phenotype to be identified in vivo.

## D. Mechanisms Controlling Vascular Cell Phenotype

Control of the endothelial cell and VSMC phenotype and function is exerted through the patterns of gene expression in the cells. One mechanism by which VSMCs appear to autoregulate their phenotype is by TGF-β–induced expression of TGF-β mRNA (40), and we suggest that this response may provide a positive-feedback loop by which the cells actively maintain their phenotype. The signaling pathways by which TGF-β regulates gene expression are only beginning to be unraveled, but it is very likely that TGF-β antagonizes the gene activation mechanisms of inflammatory cytokines (e.g., IL-1, TNF-α) exerted through the NFκB pathway. Regulation of this pathway may well mediate the protective effect of TGF-β against atherogenic agents which activate inflammatory responses in the cells of the vessel wall.

## E. Drugs That Stimulate TGF-β Production by Smooth Muscle Cells

The effects of TGF-β on VSMCs prompted a survey of potential therapeutic agents which might stimulate the cells to produce TGF-β using human or rat aortic VSMCs for screening. The production of TGF-β was assayed by ELISA, and the activity of the TGF-$\beta$ was determined by demonstrating reversal of its inhibitory effect on proliferation using a neutralising antibody.

Heparin was found to reduce the rate of proliferation of VSMCs by releasing TGF-$\beta$ activity from fetal calf serum in the medium (41), which is consistent with previous data (42,43). Further screening revealed two drugs, aspirin and the antiestrogen tamoxifen as potential agents to raise TGF-$\beta$ activity in vivo. Aspirin inhibited the proliferation of explant human aortic VSMCs with half-maximal inhibition ($ED_{50}$) at $12 \pm 3$ $\mu$M and maximally inhibited proliferation at 50 $\mu$M (44). The amount of (a+1) TGF-$\beta$ in the medium conditioned on VSMCs for 96 hr was increased from $1.5 \pm 0.4$ ng/ml in the absence of aspirin to $4.9 \pm 1.2$ ng/ml (n = 3; $p < .05$) in the presence of 10 $\mu$M aspirin. Tamoxifen inhibited the proliferation of rat aortic VSMCs with an $ED_{50}$ of 2–5$\mu$M and maximally at a concentration of 10$\mu$M, which increased the active TGF-$\beta$ concentration in the medium from <0.1 to $4.8 \pm 0.9$ ng/ml and the amount of (a+1)TGF-$\beta$ from $2.1 \pm 1.8$ to $13.7 \pm 2.2$ ng/ml (45). Tamoxifen had a similar effect on explant human aortic VSMCs but was more potent than for the rat VSMCs with an $ED_{50}$ of 50 nM (46). The observation that tamoxifen stimulated the production of TGF-$\beta$ by smooth muscle cells was consistent with previous evidence that it caused human breast tumor cells to produce TGF-$\beta$ (47).

## IV.   THE HYPOTHESIS BASED ON IN VITRO EVIDENCE

Taken together, the data for the effects of TGF-$\beta$ on vascular cells in vitro are consistent with a set of antiatherogenic properties: TGF-$\beta$ inhibits the activation of endothelial cells to express adhesion molecules for leukocytes and platelets, and it inhibits the dedifferentiation, migration, and proliferation of VSMCs. Thus on the basis of this in vitro evidence, TGF-$\beta$ might be expected to suppress these responses of vascular cells to inflammatory cytokines, growth factors, and other agents implicated in the atherogenic process. However, if TGF-$\beta$ has a broader protective effect on vascular cells than purely as an anti–inflammatory agent, it might be expected to act directly to downregulate the expression of at least some risk factors. It would also be very likely that some risk factors would act by depressing TGF-$\beta$ activity and that some protective factors would increase TGF-$\beta$ activity. The strength of the hypothesis will depend in part on how many apparently disparate risk factors and protective factors can be accommodated within a framework of being modulated by TGF-$\beta$ or being modulators of TGF-$\beta$ activity.

A key early step in expanding the basis of the in vitro hypothesis came from examining the effects of a known blood risk factor, lipoprotein(a),

[Lp(a)] on VSMC proliferation (48). We found that human aortic VSMCs prepared by enzyme dispersal secreted large amounts of latent TGF-β in culture (49). The cells also produced tissue plasminogen activator (tPA), mainly associated with the cell surface, which activated serum plasminogen in the culture medium to plasmin. The plasmin proteolytically activated the latent TGF-β, which acted back on the cells in an autocrine loop to inhibit their proliferation. Lp(a) consists of an LDL particle covalently linked to the distinguishing protein, apolipoprotein(a) [apo(a)]. An important feature of apo(a) is that it has 80% sequence homology to plasminogen in the corresponding protein domains, and consequently it acts as an indirect inhibitor of tPA by occupying the fibrin binding sites for plasminogen. Addition of either Lp(a) or apo(a) to the human aortic VSMC cultures blocked the conversion of plasminogen to plasmin and therefore the activation of TGF-β, which relieved the autocrine inhibition of proliferation (48). Lp(a) had also previously been shown to relieve the effect of TGF-β on the migration of smooth muscle cells by a similar mechanism (33).

The biochemical pathway linking Lp(a) to the inhibition of TGF-β activation and the consequent proatherogenic effects it might exert on vascular cells are shown in Figure 4. Another blood risk factor, plasminogen-activator inhibitor-1 (PAI-1), is an independent inhibitor of tPA, implying that PAI-1 would be an independent in vitro inhibitor of TGF-β activation. The key issue was whether the in vitro pathway could be shown to operate

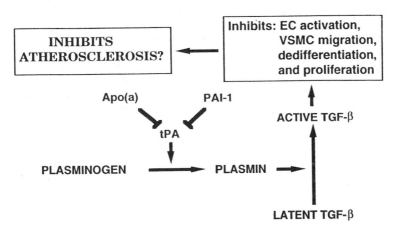

**Figure 4**  The biochemical pathway linking Lp(a) and PAI-1 to inhibition of TGF-β activation and the consequent proatherogenic effects on endothelial cells and smooth muscle cells based initially on in vitro evidence [48] and subsequently tested in vivo (11,56).

in vivo. If elevated Lp(a) or PAI-1 resulted in reduced activation of TGF-$\beta$ in vivo, it would link known risk factors to the modulation of TGF-$\beta$ activity. The underlying assumption that TGF-$\beta$ exerts phenotypic control of vascular cells in vivo also required testing.

## V.  IN VIVO EFFECTS OF TGF-$\beta$ ON VASCULAR CELL PHENOTYPE

### A.  Endothelium

It is technically more difficult to determine the effects of TGF-$\beta$ on the phenotype of vascular cells in the intact vessel wall, but there is evidence to suggest that TGF-$\beta$ has a potent protective effect on the endothelium against inflammatory stimuli. The absence of TGF-$\beta$ in knockout mice results in abnormal embryonic differentiation of the endothelium (50), and in the mice that survive to birth, there is rampant inflammation (51,52). Loss of TGF-$\beta$ activity on the endothelium also results in increased leukocyte binding and extravasation in models of ischemic reperfusion (53,54).

### B.  Vascular Smooth Muscle

The main approaches taken to examine the relationship between VSMC differentiation and TGF-$\beta$ in the vessel wall have depended on the development of quantitative immunofluorescence methods to assay active and latent forms of TGF-$\beta$ and protein markers of VSMC differentiation and activation in sections. Active TGF-$\beta$ is assayed using the R2X receptor domain used for the active TGF-$\beta$ ELISA and (a+ 1)TGF-$\beta$ is assayed using the polyclonal detection antibody used for the (a+ 1)TGF-$\beta$ ELISA (15). Part of the evidence obtained is correlative and is based on studies of rat and human vessels (55). We have found that there is a strong association between active TGF-$\beta$ levels and the amount of SM-MHC and SM-$\alpha$-actin in rat aorta and carotid artery. In particular, the amount of active TGF-$\beta$ and of SM-$\alpha$-actin decreased at vessel branch points, whereas the total amount of active and latent TGF-$\beta$ remained constant, indicating that production of TGF-$\beta$ was not affected. Whether the reduced activation of TGF-$\beta$ is mediated by sheer induced stress at the branch points is unclear. However, it is significant that branch points are preferentially susceptible sites for lesion formation.

Sections of normal human aorta free of macroscopic lesions contained no detectable intracellular or extracellular lipid by microscopic examination. The amounts of latent TGF-$\beta$ in the media and the intima were very similar, but the activation of the TGF-$\beta$ in the intima was suppressed by approximately 50% compared with the media, and there were similar, strongly correlated reductions in the expression of SM-MHC and SM–α-actin (Fig. 5). The cell density was slightly higher (~30%) in the intima than the media (Fig. 5a), and therefore the correlations could not be attributed to a reduced cell density in the intima compared with the media, resulting in reduced accumulation of the proteins. Similar patterns of relative amounts of protein expression for active and latent TGF-β and for SM-MHC and SM–α-actin were observed for the media and intima of aortic plaques, although the amounts of all of the proteins were reduced by ~25% compared with the corresponding amounts in normal media and intima (Fig. 5b–d). In advanced plaques (type VI), there is preliminary evidence that the level of latent TGF-β is further reduced throughout the intima except around the rim of VSMCs underlying the fibrous cap. It is possible that the ability of these cells to produce collagen and matrix proteins to form the fibrous cap may be regulated by the local TGF-β activity produced by the cells.

These observations showed that the activation, but not the production, of latent TGF-β is suppressed in normal and lesion intima compared with normal and plaque media, and that suppression of TGF-β activation and reduced expression of the protein differentiation markers in the intima precedes detectable lipid accumulation. This is a critical point in support of the hypothesis: Reduction in TGF-β activity and dedifferentiation of the VSMCs precede the lipid accumulation which occurs in fatty streak development.

The data for rat and human vessels established clear correlations between TGF-β activity and the expression of protein markers of VSMC differentiation. To examine causal relationships, ways of modulating TGF-β activity were required to determine whether this activity controlled the expression of the VSMC differentiation markers. The ability to modulate TGF-β in vivo also allowed the relationship between TGF-β activity and the formation of vascular lipid lesions to be determined.

## VI. MODULATION OF TGF-β ACTIVITY IN MOUSE MODELS OF ATHEROSCLEROSIS: EFFECT ON PHENOTYPE AND VASCULAR LESIONS

### A.  Effect of Tamoxifen on C57B16 and ApoE Knockout Mice

1.  C57B16 Mice

The in vitro evidence that tamoxifen stimulated the production of TGF-β by VSMCs (45,46) provided a potential method to increase TGF-β activity in the circulation and/or in the vessel wall. The first animal model in which the effects of tamoxifen were examined was the C57B16 mouse (56), which

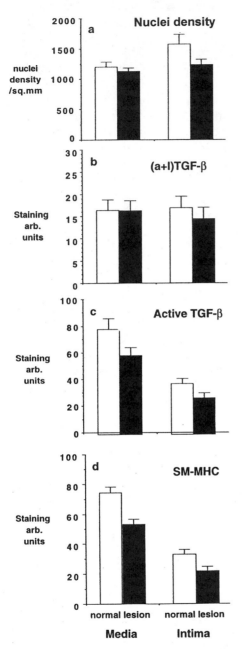

**Figure 5**  The correlation between TGF-β activity and SM-MHC in the media and intima of normal human aorta and atherosclerotic plaques. (a) Nuclei densities. (b) (a+1)TGF-β; (c) active TGF-β and (d) SM-MHC assayed by quantitative immuno-fluorescence (arbitrary units) using agents for the TGF-β assays described in the text. Similar data for the expression of SM−α-actin were obtained to the data for SM-MHC (not shown).

is susceptible to the formation of aortic lipid lesions on a high-fat diet. After 7 days on a high-fat diet containing tamoxifen, which gave a dose equivalent to $1.1 \pm 0.3$ mg/kg body weight per day, adult male mice showed a maximal increase in (a+1)TGF-β of 2.8-fold in serum and 10-fold in the vessel wall. After 7 days (a+1)TGF-β in both the vessel wall and serum declined slowly, so that by 28 days, it was elevated by 2.4-fold in serum and by 5.8-fold in the vessel wall. Active TGF-β also increased in response to tamoxifen, and the kinetics of the initial increases in active TGF-β were very similar to those for (a+1)TGF-β, reaching a maximum at 7 days, with more than 90% of the (a+1)TGF-β in serum and in the aortic wall being in the active form. However, between 7 and 28 days, the active TGF-β in both serum and in the aortic wall declined more rapidly than the (a+1)TGF-β, so that after 28 days, active TGF-β was only elevated by 1.5-fold in serum and 2.2-fold in the aortic wall. These changes in (a+1)TGF-β and in active TGF-β in response to tamoxifen were very similar for mice on normal or high-fat diets. The decrease in the proportion of TGF-β in the active form after 7 days appears to be due to the induction of PAI-1, which may act as a feedback capping mechanism, protecting against excessive increases in the concentration of active TGF-β.

Aortic sections adjacent to the lipid lesions in C57B16 mice on a high-fat diet showed regions of high osteopontin protein accumulation, whereas there was very little osteopontin accumulation (85% reduction) in aortic sections from mice on the high-fat diet with tamoxifen. Osteopontin is expressed by dedifferentiated, proliferating VSMCs in culture (57,60), and tamoxifen therefore suppresses expression of this marker of smooth muscle cell activation. Similar experiments in which the accumulation of SM–α-actin was assayed showed an inverse pattern to that for osteopontin. There were regions of low SM–α-actin expression in adjacent sections to lipid lesions, whereas the amount of SM–α-actin was increased (~35%) in the sections from mice on the high-fat diet with tamoxifen. Thus TGF-β activity is directly correlated with expression of the SM–α-actin differentiation marker for VSMCs.

When adult mice were fed a high-fat diet without tamoxifen for 3 months, there was a five-fold increase in the number of lipid lesions in the aortic wall compared with mice on a normal diet for the same period, but for mice on the high-fat diet containing tamoxifen, there was an 86% reduction in the number of diet-induced lesions and an 88% reduction in the area of the lipid lesions (Fig. 6).

Tamoxifen has a wide range of pharmacological activities (61). In cell culture, it is a potent calmodulin antagonist and a weak inhibitor of protein kinase C. In mice, tamoxifen has full estrogen agonist activity in contrast to its predominantly antiestrogen activity in women. However, in post-

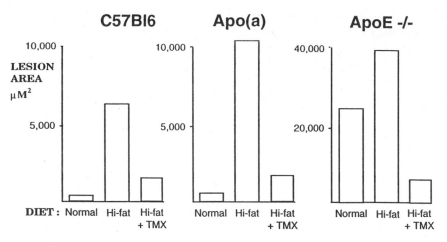

**Figure 6**  The suppression of lipid lesion formation in mouse models of atherosclerosis. C57B16 mice and apo(a) mice were fed a high-fat diet for 3 months with or without tamoxifen (dose ~ 1 mg/kg body weight per day). The diet-induced formation of lipid lesions was substantially reduced (>85%). For apoE knockout mice, the extent of lesion formation was much greater on a normal diet than for C57B16 or apo(a) mice on a high-fat diet (compare scales). Tamoxifen treatment reduced lipid lesion formation substantially for mice on a high-fat diet or a normal diet.

menopausal women, it has an estrogen-like activity in lowering total cholesterol, LDL cholesterol, and Lp(a) concentrations and increasing high-density lipoprotein (HDL) cholesterol [62–64]. Tamoxifen did not significantly affect the levels of 17$\beta$-estradiol or of testosterone in the male C57B16 mice, and indirect evidence suggested that the effects of tamoxifen on the lipid profiles of the mice and on weight gain were unlikely to be the major mechanism by which lipid lesions were prevented. However, methods of elevating TGF-$\beta$ in the artery wall that are more specific than the use of tamoxifen, for example, by transgenic technology, are required to test the protective effect of TGF-$\beta$ rigorously (56).

## 2.  ApoE Knockout Mice

ApoE knockout mice provide a more severe model of atherosclerosis than C57B16 mice (65,66) in that they develop extensive lesions resembling human atherosclerotic plaques irrespective of the fat content of their diet (66,67). Tamoxifen (equivalent to 1.9 mg/kg body weight per day) fed in a normal or high-fat diet reduced the lipid lesion area substantially below the level for mice on a normal diet (see Fig. 6) (68). There were very large changes induced in the lipid profiles of the mice, with total cholesterol reduced by 85%. The proportion of the remaining cholesterol present in very low density lipoprotein (VLDL) remained unchanged, whereas the proportion in LDL decreased by 37% and in HDL increased by 64%. Consistent with this shift from LDL cholesterol to HDL cholesterol distribution, there was a 62% decrease in total triglycerides. The concentrations of active and $(a+1)$TGF-β in aortic sections were increased by tamoxifen by 87 and 24%, respectively. For this model, the increase in TGF-β activity and the changes induced by tamoxifen in lipid profile are both anti-atherogenic, and both may contribute to the reduced formation of lipid lesions.

## B. Effect of Apo(a) on TGF-β Activity and VSMC Differentiation in Transgenic Apo(a) Mice

The biochemical pathway linking apo(a) to the activation of TGF-β suggested that the apo(a) transgenic mouse was an obvious starting point to test both the pathway and, if apo(a) reduced TGF-β activity, whether the VSMCs were less differentiated as a consequence. In the apo(a) mouse, the cDNA for the human apo(a) gene is expressed under the control of the mouse transferrin promoter (67) to direct synthesis of the apo(a) protein to the liver where it is synthesized in humans. Levels of apo(a) similar to those in the normal range for the human population of ~6 mg/dl are present in the circulation, although nearly all of the protein (>95%) is not associated with LDL, because mouse apolipoprotein B100 lacks the appropriate cysteine for disulfide linkage to human apo(a). The apo(a) mouse provides a very clean test tube to analyze the effects of apo(a), since there is no corresponding murine gene (apo[a] is only expressed in the higher primates and in hedgehogs). When the apo(a) transgenic mice are fed a high-fat diet, they develop fatty streaks similar to those observed in the earliest stages of human atherosclerosis, but more complex lesions sufficient to cause luminal stenoses are not formed. The dependence of lesion formation on a high-fat diet provides an important experimental maneuver to distinguish the effects of apo(a) on the vessel wall, including any affect on TGF-β activity, from those which depend on subsequent lipid accumulation.

The apo(a) is not only present in the circulation but is also localized throughout the vessel (70). It is likely that the apo(a) in the vessel wall is taken up from the circulation, since it was not possible to detect expression of the apo(a) gene by in situ hybridization in the vessel wall. However, we cannot eliminate the possibility that at least some of the apo(a) is made by the smooth muscle cells but that the apo(a) mRNA in the cells was below the detection limit. Within a uniform background of apo(a) there are focal sites of high apo(a) accumulation at 10- to 100-fold higher concentrations than the background levels. These focal sites are mainly close to the luminal surface of the vessel, and are significant because they are sites at which lipid accumulates if the mice are subsequently fed a high-fat diet.

Quantitative immunofluorescence assays were developed to measure plasminogen and plasmin activity in the vessel wall to test the proposed biochemical pathway linking apo(a) to TGF-$\beta$ activation and lesion development (see Fig. 4) (10). The presence of apo(a) in the vessel wall had no effect on the levels of plasminogen or of (a+1)TGF-$\beta$, but there was ~70% less plasmin activity and ~60% less TGF-$\beta$ activity compared with normal littermate controls lacking the apo(a) transgene. This was a consistent observation for aortic sections from all of the apo(a) mice and normal littermates examined, providing very strong correlative evidence for the proposed biochemical pathway. Furthermore, the focal sites of high accumulations of apo(a) showed severely inhibited TGF-$\beta$ activity compared with the surrounding areas of vessel, and the smooth muscle cells at the same sites were relatively dedifferentiated with reduced levels of SM–$\alpha$-actin. The activation of the smooth muscle cells at the focal sites was also indicated by the expression of substantial amounts of the protein osteopontin, which was barely detectable in the vessels of normal littermate controls. Osteopontin is expressed in human atherosclerotic plaques (59,60), mainly at sites of calcification where much of the protein appears to be expressed by macrophages. However, macrophages cannot be detected in the lesions of the apo(a) mouse aorta, and it is the smooth muscle cells which express the osteopontin. When the apo(a) mice are fed a high-fat diet, it is also the smooth muscle cells which become engorged with lipid. It should be emphasized, however, that all of the changes in the vessel wall, including focal apo(a) accumulation, severe inhibition of TGF-$\beta$ activation, and expression of osteopontin by the smooth muscle cells, occur when the mice are fed a normal diet. The changes are therefore a response to the presence of apo(a) and do not depend in any way on lipid accumulation.

Further studies of the progression with age of the changes in the vessel wall of mice on a normal diet have led to a proposed mechanism for the focal changes by a positive-feedback loop between apo(a) accumulation and inhibition of TGF-$\beta$ activity (70). An initial accumulation of apo(a) at sites of endothelial cell activation results in a limited inhibition of TGF-$\beta$ activity. The reduced TGF-$\beta$ activity allows further activation of the endothelial cells and hence more accumulation of apo(a) and greater inhibition of TGF-$\beta$ activity. The smooth muscle cells become dedifferentiated and activated. The focal sites therefore increase progressively in size, and if the mice are fed a high-fat diet, then the activated smooth muscle cells take up lipid from the excess present in the circulation. Such a feedback loop may account for the progressive growth of lesions at the sites of focal apo(a) accumulation with increasing age.

## C. Effects of Blocking the Formation of Vascular Lipid Lesions in Transgenic Apo(a) Mice

The mechanistic sequence proposed in the feedback loop is of cycles of focal apo(a) accumulation, TGF-β inactivation, and smooth muscle cell dedifferentiation and activation, leading to lipid accumulation by the smooth muscle cells. This sequence has been tested by blocking the endpoint of lipid accumulation and determining which of the preceding steps in the putative pathway are blocked.

Tamoxifen was shown to prevent lipid lesion formation in C57B16 and apoE knockout mice and was found to have the same effect in apo(a) mice (see Fig. 6) (71). The drug also blocked all of the steps in the pathway from focal apo(a) accumulation to lipid accumulation. The inhibition of focal accumulation of apo(a) by tamoxifen occurs in mice on a normal diet without lipid involvement and is therefore very unlikely to be due to the changes in the lipoprotein profile induced by tamoxifen. It is also unlikely that the inhibition of lipid lesion formation in apo(a) mice on a high-fat diet is due to the changes in the lipoprotein profile, since the changes would not be expected to be proatherogenic. Stabilization of the endothelium and of the differentiated smooth muscle cell phenotype by the increased level of TGF-β in the circulation and/or in the vessel wall is a more plausible explanation. However, as for the C57B16 mice, it will be necessary to test this conclusion by using more specific methods of increasing TGF-β activity in the vessel wall.

Another independent method of preventing vascular lesion formation in the apo(a) mice is by crossing them with transgenic mice overexpressing apolipoprotein A1[71]. The double transgenic mice have the same levels of circulating apo(a) as the apo(a) mice but do not develop vascular lipid lesions on a high-fat diet, which was attributed to the protective effect of the elevated concentration of protective high-density lipoprotein. In these mice, the inhibition of lipid lesion formation is also correlated with inhibition of focal apo(a) accumulation and all of the consequent local changes of TGF-β inactivation and smooth muscle cell dedifferentiation and activation in the vessel wall (70).

The results from these two independent methods of inhibiting lipid lesion formation in the apo(a) mice are therefore consistent with the pathway proposed for the feedback loop which drives progressive lesion development.

## VII. CONTROL OF TGF-β ACTIVITY IN THE HUMAN POPULATION

### A. Genes

As mentioned earlier, studies of 139 pairs of female monozygous and dizygous twins have shown that the concentration of (a+1)TGF-β in circulation is under strong genetic control with an estimated heritability of ~70% and for active TGF-β of ~40% (13). Analysis of the *TGFb1* gene promoter in the twins has so far identified two polymorphisms which are correlated with TGF-β concentration in circulation. One polymorphism is a single base substitution at position −800 from the transcriptional start site (Fig. 7), where an A was substituted for a G in about 11% of alleles. Although this polymorphism was relatively infrequent (only one pair of twins was homozygous for the rarer A allele), there was a significant association ($p < .05$) between the presence of an A allele and lower levels of

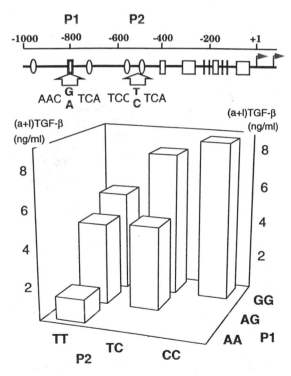

**Figure 7** Correlation of polymorphisms in the *TGFb1 gene* promoter with (a+1)TGF-β concentration in circulation (see text).

(a+1)TGF-β in the circulation (AG genotype: 4.12 ± 1.13 ng/ml; n=52 and GG genotype: 6.68 ± 1.33 ng/ml; n=222). However, this polymorphism was not strongly correlated with active TGF-β in the circulation. A second polymorphism at −509 from the start site with a T substituted for a C has an approximate allele frequency of 30%. The T allele may be associated with high concentrations of (a+1)TGF-β (*p* = .05) and high levels of active TGF-β (*p* = .03). The data indicate that other genetic determinants of (a+1)TGF-β remain to be identified, but it is likely that a significant predisposition to atherosclerosis is linked to particular alleles of the human *TGFb1* gene.

## B. Lp(a) and PAI-1

Studies of TGF-β activation in volunteer groups have shown that the proportion of TGF-β in the active form shows very strong inverse correlations with both Lp(a) and PAI-1 concentration and together they account for a major part of the control of TGF-β activation (Fig. 8) (71). There was, however, a striking difference between men and women in the activation of TGF-β: women consistently showed higher proportions of active TGF-β and activation was not significantly affected by the concentration of Lp(a) or PAI-1. Although this difference is presumably hormonally regulated, the mechanisms by which the effects of Lp(a) and PAI-1 on TGF-β activation are bypassed in women have not been determined. The data suggest that for women there is an alternative, dominant pathway for activation of TGF-β that does not depend on activation of plasminogen by the known plasminogen activators, tPA and uPA. The existence of such pathways, at least in mice, is implied by the viability of plasminogen knockout mice (72) and of the tPA/uPA double-knockout mice (73) compared with the lethal effects of deleting of the TGF-β1 gene in knockout mice. The embryonic TGF-β1 knockout mice show impaired vascular development with abnormal differentiation of the endothelium (50), and those mice which survive beyond birth may be dependent on maternal transfer of TGF-β. If the pathway shown in Figure 4 was the only mechanism by which TGF-β could be activated, then the plasminogen knockout mice and the double tPA/uPA knockout mice would show the same phenotype as the TGF-β1 knockout mice and would not be viable. Clearly latent TGF-β can be activated by protease(s) other than plasmin, and these protease(s), or plasminogen, can be activated by enzymes other than tPA and uPA. It is possible that such pathways predominate in the activation of TGF-β in women.

It is well established that Lp(a) levels are genetically determined in the human population, and since active TGF-β levels show significant heritability, it is likely that the levels of other major determinants of TGF-β activation, including PAI-1, will also be under strong genetic control.

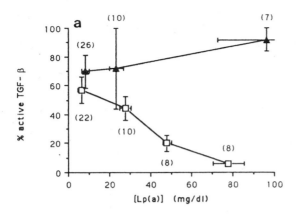

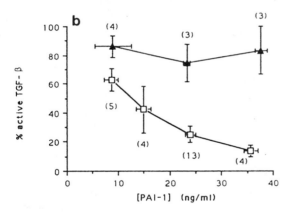

**Figure 8** The relationship between (a) Lp(a) concentration, (b) PAI-1 concentration, and the activation of TGF-$\beta$ in the serum of a volunteer group of donors for (□) men and (▲) women.

## C. TGF-$\beta$ Association with Lipoproteins

An elevated concentration of LDL, which is thought to be the main lipoprotein responsible for depositing cholesterol in the atherosclerotic plaques, has been correlated with the development of atherosclerosis (74). Studies of TGF-$\beta$ in volunteer groups and in patient groups (see below) showed weak independent correlations between TGF-$\beta$ activation and LDL concentration ($p = .10$ and $p = .13$, respectively). These and other observations raised the question of whether lipoproteins other than Lp(a) have a direct effect on TGF-$\beta$ activity in circulation. Lipoproteins were separated from plasma proteins in platelet-poor plasma from 10 healthy volunteers and TGF-β was assayed by the R&D Systems Quantikine ELISA after treatment of the fractions with 5 M urea/1.3 M acetic acid which releases TGF-β from interactions with LAP, LTBP, and lipoproteins (75). For 7 of 10 volunteers, TGF-β was also detected in the lipoprotein fraction, varying from <1 to 39% with a mean of 16%. TGF-β associated with the lipoprotein fraction was not able to bind the TGF-β receptor and was inactive biologically as an inhibitor of mink lung epithelial cell proliferation. Further experiments to determine which of the lipoprotein classes sequestered TGF-β activity showed that for a typical healthy volunteer, the major part of the plasma TGF-β associated with the lipoprotein fraction eluted with a tightly defined subfraction of HDL with the smallest size of all of the cholesterol-containing lipoproteins. Much smaller amounts of TGF-β were associated with the VLDL and LDL fractions. This pattern was typical of all the healthy donors tested (>80% of the lipoprotein TGF-β associated with a subfraction of HDL).

Diabetic patients, particularly those with poor glucose control, often exhibit elevated plasma concentrations of the triglyceride-rich lipoproteins. The proportion of TGF-β in the lipoprotein fraction for 10 diabetic patients with poor glucose control (Hb a1C > 8) was measured (75). These patients had increased total plasma triglyceride levels (by 63%), and the proportion of TGF-β which was associated with lipoprotein, and therefore inactive, was markedly increased (68 ± 21% compared with 16 ± 11% for the health donors). The distribution of the TGF-β between the lipoproteins was also affected, so that major proportions TGF-β were associated with the largest triglyceride-rich particles and smaller, variable amounts with LDL.

These data suggest that if plasma TGF-β activity is important in protecting the vessel wall, then the association of much higher proportions of plasma TGF-β with the most triglyceride rich lipoproteins (particularly VLDL and chylomicrons) and with LDL is an additional mechanism by which diabetics with poor glucose control have an increased risk of cardiovascular disease.

## D.  Effect of Fish Oil on Circulating TGF-β Activity

Dietary supplementation with fish oil has been used clinically to lower the circulating triglyceride concentration in diabetic patients (76) and fish oil is also known to alter the composition of lipoproteins in nondiabetic individuals (77). Fish oil and its putative active components, the ω3 fatty acids, have also been proposed to mediate significant cardiovascular protection. Platelet-poor plasma was prepared from 33 donors prior to and immediately following 4 weeks of dietary supplementation with 2.4 g/day of fish oil. A further plasma sample was prepared 9 weeks after ceasing the supplementation. At the end of 4 weeks, supplementation total triglycerides were reduced (28%) with no effect on total cholesterol. The proportion of TGF-$\beta$ associated with the lipoproteins was reduced from 19 ± 10% to 7 ± 4% ($p <$ .01). After a further 9 weeks without fish oil supplementation, triglycerides had returned to baseline and the proportion of TGF-$\beta$ associated with the lipoprotein pool had increased to 13 ± 9% but had not returned to baseline. Consistent with the changes in lipoprotein associated TGF-$\beta$, the concentration of active TGF-$\beta$ in the plasma increased by 21% ($p<.01$) after 4 weeks of supplementation, which was partially reversed 9 weeks after supplementation ended. These data indicate that increased dietary intake of fish oil reduces the fraction of plasma TGF-$\beta$ sequestered into the lipoprotein pool and increase the concentration of active TGF-$\beta$ in plasma. If this effect is beneficial in protecting the vessel wall, supplementation of the diet with fish oil would be most effective for individuals with high proportions of their TGF-$\beta$ associated with lipoprotein; for example, diabetics with poor glucose control.

## E.  Effect of a Fat Tolerance Test on Circulating TGF-$\beta$ Activity

Since TGF-$\beta$ can associate with lipoprotein particles, we hypothesized that postprandial hyperlipidemia would cause a reduction in bioavailable TGF-$\beta$ and a decrease in active TGF-$\beta$ concentrations. To test this hypothesis, the responses of lipoproteins, TGF-$\beta$ and PAI-1 in 57 healthy white men (57–70 years old) to a fat tolerance test were followed for 8 hr (78). After 8 hr the total amount of TGF-$\beta$1 in plasma, including the lipoprotein-associated pool (assayed by the R&D Systems Quantikine ELISA), increased from 4.9 ± 1.0 ng/ml to 6.1 ± 0.9 ng/ml ($p<.001$), and the lipid-associated TGF-$\beta$1 increased proportionally from 0.8 ± 0.2 ng/ml to 1.0 ± 0.3 ng/ml ($p<.001$). However, the plasma concentration of available active TGF-$\beta$ decreased from 5.4 ± 0.4 ng/ml to 4.9 ± 0.1 ng/ml ($p<.0001$) and PAI-1 levels increased from 6.8 ± 0.8 ng/ml to 10.6 ± 0.7 ng/ml ($p<.0001$). The increase in PAI-1 levels over 8 hr was correlated with the decrease in active TGF-$\beta$ concentrations during the test ($r = -0.55$, $p<.0001$). Postprandial lipidemia is therefore associated with a potentially prothrombotic increase in PAI-1 concentration and a proatherogenic decrease in plasma-active TGF-$\beta$ concentration. Furthermore, the decrease in active TGF-$\beta$ concentrations is likely to be mediated, at least in part, by the postprandial increase in PAI-1 concentrations. The effects of other lifestyle factors on TGF-$\beta$ activity remain to be determined, but it is known that exercise produces a rapid, small decrease in PAI-1 activity, which would be expected to increase the proportion of TGF-β in the active form.

## VIII.   TGF-β AND HUMAN ATHEROSCLEROSIS

### A.   Comparison of Patient Groups

In an initial study, we compared active TGF-β and (a+1)TGF-β in patients with advanced atherosclerosis and with normal coronary arteries by angiography (71). The concentrations of (a+1)TGF-β for the two patient groups showed wide variation with substantial overlap between the two groups (Fig. 9). However, there was a significant number of patients with advanced atherosclerosis who had no detectable (a+1)TGF-β, which is mainly genetically determined. Of the 32 patients with >50% stenoses of all three coronary arteries, 2 had detectable levels of active TGF-β by ELISA (1 ng/ml) and 30 were below the detectable level with <1 ng/ml (Fig. 9). In contrast, 30 patients with symptoms resembling angina and a positive exercise test, but with normal coronary arteries by angiography, had active TGF-β concentrations between 2 and 10 ng/ml (mean 4.5 ng/ml). The approximately fivefold difference in the mean active TGF-β concentration between the two groups corresponded to a much stronger correlation with advanced atherosclerosis than any of the conventional risk factors assayed for the same patients. However, significant inverse correlations ($p < .05$) were obtained for the patient groups between the proportion of TGF-β in the serum in the active form and the concentration of Lp(a) and of PAI-1. These correlations were very similar for the patient groups

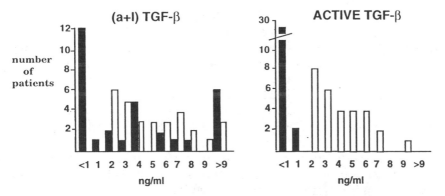

**Figure 9**   Distribution of (a+1)TGF-β and active TGF-β concentrations in serum for groups of patients with advanced atherosclerosis (filled bars) or normal coronary arteries (open bars) by angiography.

and for the age-and sex-matched volunteer group described above. As in the volunteer group, the proportion of TGF-$\beta$ in the active form was also substantially higher for the women than the men in the patient groups. Thus similar factors apparently regulate the activation of TGF-$\beta$ in the circulation for the patient groups selected by their coronary artery status and the general population.

Two further studies have confirmed the very low levels of active TGF-$\beta$ concentration for patients with advanced atherosclerosis and have also shown that the active TGF-$\beta$ concentrations for this group and for patient groups with normal coronary arteries by angiography overlap by ~15%.

## B.   Effects of Aspirin and Tamoxifen

Of the medications taken by the patient groups with advanced atherosclerosis and with normal coronary arteries by angiography, antianginals and calcium channel blockers had no effect on the concentrations of active TGF-$\beta$ and (a+1)TGF-$\beta$ (71). However, for the normal coronary artery group, taking aspirin was correlated with a ~70% increase in both active and (a+1)TGF-$\beta$. For the patients with advanced atherosclerosis aspirin did not elevate the active TGF-$\beta$ concentration into the range detectable by the ELISA (i.e., >1 ng/ml). Aspirin was also the only drug taken by the patient groups which stimulated the production of TGF-$\beta$ by human VSMCs in culture (see above). A more extensive study confirmed these effects of aspirin on the patient groups (44). For patients with advanced atherosclerosis (n = 44) or with normal coronary arteries (n = 42), the dose of aspirin was significantly correlated with the circulating concentration of (a+1)TGF-$\beta$ (Fig. 10a and b). For the normal coronary artery group, aspirin therapy was also associated with an increase in the circulating concentration of active TGF-$\beta$, but there was no detectable effect in the patient group with advanced atherosclerosis. These data suggest that if active TGF-$\beta$ protects against the development of advanced atherosclerosis, aspirin therapy is only likely to be beneficial by this mechanism for individuals who still retain detectable levels of active TGF-$\beta$.

In contrast to the observations for aspirin, tamoxifen is effective at stimulating detectable increases in active TGF-$\beta$ in patients with advanced atherosclerosis (79). Fifteen male patients with advanced atherosclerosis (at least 50% stenoses of all three major coronary arteries by angiography) were given 40 mg of tamoxifen daily for 10 days (see Fig. 10c). The (a+1)TGF-$\beta$ concentration in plasma increased throughout the treatment period (+22% at day 10; $p = .02$) and active TGF-$\beta$ was elevated by day 3 (+23%; $p = .05$) and was nearly threefold higher by day 10 (+169%; $p < .01$). Since tamoxifen therapy increases the active TGF-$\beta$ concentration relative to

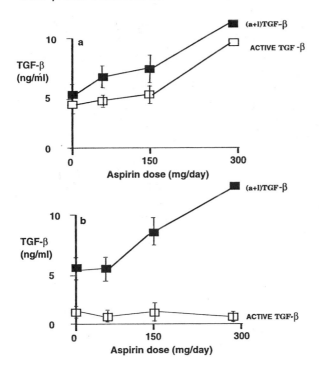

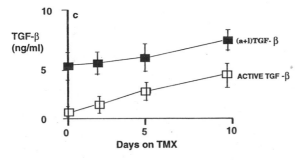

**Figure 10** Effect of aspirin dose on the plasma concentration of active TGF-β (□) and (a+1)TGF-β (■) in (a) patients with normal coronary arteries and (b) with advanced atherosclerosis. Note that aspirin stimulates similar increases in (a+1)TGF-β for both groups of patients but only causes a detectable increase in active TGF-β for patients with normal coronary arteries, not in patients with advanced atherosclerosis. (c) Effect of a dose of 40 mg of tamoxifen per day for 9 days on active TGF-β (□) and (a+1)TGF-β (■) for patients with advanced atherosclerosis. Unlike aspirin, tamoxifen causes a substantial increase in active TGF-β concentration for this group into the range associated with normal coronary arteries (see [a] and Fig. 9).

$(a+1)$TGF-$\beta$, we examined whether tamoxifen affected the known inhibitors of TGF-$\beta$ activation, Lp(a) and PAI-1. Tamoxifen markedly decreased Lp(a) levels ($-31\%$ by day 10; $p = .01$) but increased PAI-1 levels ($+17\%$ by day 10; $p = .05$). Furthermore, tamoxifen decreased the proportion of TGF-$\beta$ in the lipoprotein fraction, which would also be expected to increase the active TGF-$\beta$ concentration available in the plasma. The data suggest that tamoxifen has a complex set of effects on the control of TGF-$\beta$ which result in a substantial increase in the plasma concentration of active TGF-$\beta$ in patients with advanced atherosclerosis.

Any cardioprotective effect from tamoxifen treatment mediated by an increase in active TGF-$\beta$ concentration will depend on chronic elevation of TGF-$\beta$ activity during continuing therapy. In mice, TGF-$\beta$ activity remained elevated 3 months after beginning tamoxifen treatment, although maximal elevation was obtained 7 days after treatment began (56). Furthermore, active TGF-$\beta$ levels in circulation were similar at 28 days and 3 months after beginning treatment, suggesting that a new equilibrium had been established during chronic tamoxifen treatment. The effects of chronic treatment of men with tamoxifen remain to be determined, but the results of this pilot study are encouraging in that short-term treatment with tamoxifen for 10 days increased the circulating concentration of active TGF-$\beta$ into the range associated with cardiovascular protection.

Previous data from the Scottish trial of tamoxifen as adjuvant therapy for women after operable breast cancer showed a significant 60% reduction in the incidence of fatal myocardial infarct (80), although a much less marked reduction in the incidence of nonfatal myocardial infarctions in the same group of patients has recently been reported (81). The cardioprotective effect of tamoxifen in the Scottish trial was tentatively attributed to the effect of tamoxifen in lowering the total serum cholesterol concentration by about 10%. However, it is also plausible that the effect was due, at least in part, to the modulation of TGF-$\beta$ activity, and further studies will address this.

## C.  Predictive Value of TGF-$\beta$ Activity

If the very low active TGF-$\beta$ activity associated with advanced atherosclerosis is a causative mechanism rather than a response to the disease, then the absence of significant TGF-$\beta$ activity may indicate the presence of clinically silent disease or an enhanced risk of developing atherosclerosis. Small-scale pilot studies of two matched volunteer groups from Toulouse, France, and Belfast, Northern Ireland (approximately 100 in each group), where the incidence of cardiovascular disease is greater by at least two-fold in Belfast, showed that 25% of the Belfast group had active TGF-$\beta$ concentrations of 1 or <1 ng/ml, as in the patient groups with advanced atherosclerosis, compared with 14% of the Toulouse group (82). These observations suggest that a prospective study of the predictive value of TGF-β activity is worth considering. Also of interest was the observation that a far higher proportion of the Belfast group had (a+1)TGF-β levels of 1 or <1 ng/ml than the Toulouse group. Since the production of (a+1)TGF-β is mainly genetically determined, it is possible that significant differences in the genes determining (a + 1)TGF-β levels contribute to the differences in cardiovascular disease between the two groups in addition to any lifestyle factors which may affect TGF-β production and activation. It is therefore possible that high-risk genetic profiles for low TGF-β activity may be identified, which define either an inability to produce latent TGF-β and/or inability to activate it.

## D.  TGF-β and Other Vascular Diseases

The properties of smooth muscle cells associated with atherosclerosis which are antagonized by TGF-β are similar to the properties of smooth muscle cells associated with other vascular diseases involving migration and/or intimal hyperplasia. We have therefore examined the relationship between accelerated intimal hyperplasia after cardiac transplant, active TGF-β, and (a+1)TGF-β in the sera of 36 patients (30 men, 5 women) who had undergone cardiac transplant surgery more than 5 years earlier (83). The presence of coronary occlusive disease in 21 of 36 of the patients was determined by angiography. The coronary arteries were normal by angiography in the remaining 15 patients. There was no significant difference in the serum concentration of either active TGF-β, (a+1)TGF-β, or the proportion of TGF-β in the active form between the groups with or without coronary occlusive disease. However, the active TGF-β concentration in the serum of the patients who had originally received a cardiac transplant for cardiovascular disease were lower by 38% than the patients who had received a transplant for dilated cardiomyopathy.

These observations show that serum TGF-β levels do not correlate with the development of coronary occlusive disease following cardiac transplantation. Coronary arteries of cardiac allografts with prolonged survival often present with a distinct angiographic appearance. Although proximal focal stenoses similar to those of naturally occurring atherosclerosis are common, extensive diffuse obliterative lesions that are unlike those of nontransplant coronary artery disease are also seen (84). It has been concluded that the mechanisms underlying atherosclerosis and accelerated vascular cell hyperplasia are different (20), and these differences may well account for the lack of correlation of TGF-β activity with accelerated vascular cell hyperplasia.

It is unlikely that restenosis of coronary arteries following angioplasty will be strongly correlated with TGF-β activity to the extent that the rapid process of restenosis is more similar to the accelerated hyperplasia after cardiac transplant than to the development of atherosclerotic lesions. The limited evidence from animal models of intimal hyperplasia following balloon-induced injury suggest that TGF-$\beta$ does not inhibit lesion development (85,86). Furthermore, treatment with tamoxifen did not restrict vascular lesion development in the balloon-injured rat carotid artery (87). More effective inhibitors of VSMC proliferation or direct inhibition of the growth factors may be required to block the strong mitogenic and migratory stimuli to which the VSMCs are exposed in these animal models and in human restenosis. Important differences between the response to therapeutic agents (e.g., heparin), which are effective in some of the animal models but not in humans, have complicated the development of effective agents to prevent restenosis.

## IX. CONCLUSIONS

The protective cytokine hypothesis is based on the following evidence:

1. TGF-$\beta$ actively maintains the normal physiological phenotype of endothelial cells and smooth muscle cells in vivo as well as in vitro. Maintenance of phenotype is presumed to protect the vascular cells against a wide range of atherogenic stimuli and their inflammatory effects on the vessel wall.
2. Protection against atherosclerosis in humans is associated with significant levels active TGF-$\beta$ in the circulation and advanced atherosclerosis is associated with loss of TGF-$\beta$ activity in the circulation. A variety of disparate risk factors for atherosclerosis inhibit the production, activation, or bioavailability of TGF-$\beta$. TGF-$\beta$ also regulates the production of a variety of risk factors for atherosclerosis.

Together these observations provide a set of correlations between TGF-$\beta$ and protection from development of the disease. They do not demonstrate a causal relationship between maintenance of phenotype, protection against atherogenic stimuli, and the development of disease. However, the hypothesis provides a unifying explanation for a very broad set of observations which have not previously been incorporated in a coherent framework. It is therefore likely that the hypothesis is either correct, at least in broad outline, or that TGF-$\beta$ activity is a surrogate measure of a dominant protective mechanism which remains to be identified.

The hypothesis makes major predictions about atherogenesis which can, in principle, be tested experimentally. For example, the development of lesions in mouse models of atherosclerosis should be blocked by crossing each susceptible strain with mice overexpressing TGF-$\beta$ in the same genetic background, assuming the overexpressed TGF-β can be appropriately localized to exert protection on the vessel wall. Conversely, dominant inhibitor forms of TGF-β receptors expressed on vascular cells would be expected to promote atherogenesis in transgenic mice.

Direct tests of the hypothesis in the human population are less accessible. A phase III trial of the effects of tamoxifen therapy for men with advanced atherosclerosis is justified by the available data. However, a significant protective effect against myocardial infarct, as demonstrated for women of unknown cardiovascular status in the Scottish adjuvant trial, would not unambiguously demonstrate that the protective effect was exerted via TGF-β, given the spectrum of pharmacological activities of tamoxifen. Indirect evidence, for example, from the additive effects of tamoxifen with other cardioprotective agents (e.g., the statins, vitamin E) which may or may not affect TGF-β, would be indicative of a different mechanism for tamoxifen but would not identify TGF-β as the protective agent. Clearer evidence may be obtained from studies of the predictive value of TGF-β measurements for the development of clinically significant disease. If loss of TGF-β is the major determinant of risk, the predictive value of TGF-β measurements should be far greater than for any other single risk factor. However, it is uncertain whether TGF-β activity in plasma or activity in the arterial wall is the more relevant parameter or whether they are so closely linked that the plasma TGF-β activity is a sufficient indicator. Perhaps the most powerful evidence to test the hypothesis will come from identifying the genetic haplotypes which determine the ability to produce TGF-β. Haplotypes which determine constitutively low TGF-β production should define a strong predisposition to atherosclerosis if the hypothesis is correct. An identified population of constitutively low TGF-β producers would also enable the additional risk factor profiles needed for overt disease to be identified.

## ACKNOWLEDGMENTS

This work was supported by grants from the British Heart Foundation, the Wellcome Trust, Glaxo Wellcome Research and Development Limited, and the NeoRx Corporation. D.J.G. is a Royal Society University Research Fellow.

## REFERENCES

1.  Grainger DJ, Metcalfe JC. A pivotal role for TGF-beta in atherogenesis? Biol Rev 1995; 70:571–596.

2.  Metcalfe JC, Grainger DJ. TGF-beta and the protection from cardiovascular injury hypothesis. Biochem Soc Trans 1995; 23:403–406.
3.  Hogan BLM, Blessing M, Winnier GE, Suzuki N, Jones CM. Growth factors in development—the role of TGF-beta related polypeptide signaling molecules in embryogenesis. Development 1994; SS:53–60.
4.  Graycar JL, Miller DA, Arrick BA, Lyons RM, Moses HL, Derynck R. Human transforming growth factor-beta-3-recombinant expression, purification, and biological activities in comparison with transforming growth factor-beta-1 and factor-beta-2. Mol Endocrinol 1989; 3:1977–1986.
5.  Robinson SD, Silberstein GB, Roberts AB, Flanders KC, Daniel CW. Regulated expression and growth inhibitory effects of transforming growth-factor-beta isoforms in mouse mammary-gland development. Development 1991; 113:867–878.
6.  Lyons RM, Gentry LE, Purchio AF, Moses HL. Mechanism of activation of latent recombinant transforming growth factor beta 1 by plasmin. J Cell Biol 1990; 110:1361–1367.
7.  Lawrence DA, Pircher R, Kryceve-Martinerie, C, Jullien P. Normal embryo fibroblasts release transforming growth-factors in a latent form. J Cell Physiol 1984; 121:184–188.
8.  Kim SJ, Glick A, Sporn MB, Roberts AB. Characterization of the promoter region of the human transforming growth factor-beta gene. J Biol Chem 1989; 264:402–408.
9.  Kanzaki T, Olofsson A, Morén A, Wernstedt C, Hellman U, Miyazono K, Claesson-Welsh L, Heldin C-H. TGF-beta binding protein: a component of the large latent complex of TGF-beta1 with multiple repeat sequences. Cell 1990; 61:1051–1061.
10. Grainger DJ, Kemp PR, Lui AC, Lawn RM, Metcalfe JC. Activation of transforming growth factor beta is inhibited in transgenic apolipoprotein(a) mice. Nature 1994; 370:460–462.
11. Grainger DJ, Kemp PR, Metcalfe JC, Liu AC, Lawn RM, Williams NR, Grace AA, Schofield PM, Chauhan A. The serum concentration of active transforming growth factor beta is severely depressed in advanced atherosclerosis. Nature Med 1995; 1:74–79.
12. Dennis PA, Rifkin DB. Cellular activation of latent transforming growth factor beta requires binding of the cation-independent mannose 6-phosphate/insulin-like growth factor type II receptor. Proc Natl Acad Sci USA 1991; 88:580–584.
13. Grainger DJ, Metcalfe, JC, Kemp PR, Spector TD, Carter ND, Heathcote K. Unpublished data.
14. Grainger DJ, Wakefield LM, Metcalfe JC. Unpublished data.
15. Grainger DJ, Mosedale DE, Metcalfe JC, Weissberg PL, Kemp PR. Active and acid-activatable TGF-beta in human sera, platelets and plasma. Clin Chim Acta 1995; 235:11–31.
16. Wakefield LM, Smith DM, Flanders KC, Sporn MB. Latent transforming growth factor beta from human platelets. J Biol Chem 1988; 263:7646–7654.
17. Grainger DJ, Wakefield LM, Bethel HW, Farndale RW, Metcalfe JC. Release

and activation of platelet latent TGF-beta in blood clots during dissolution with plasmin. Nature Med 1995; 1:932–937.

18. Wakefield LM, Winokur TS, Hollands RS, Christopherson K, Levinson AD, Sporn MB. Recombinant latent transforming growth factor beta1 has a longer plasma half-life in rats than active transforming growth factor beta1, and a different tissue distribution. J Clin Invest 1990; 86:1976–1984.

19. Lamarre J, Hayes MA, Wollenberg GK, Hussaini I, Hall SW, Gonias SL. An alpha2-macroglobulin receptor dependent mechanism for the plasma clearance of transforming growth factor beta1 in mice. J Clin Invest 1991; 87:39–44.

20. Ross R. The pathogenesis of atherosclerosis: a perspective for the 1990s. Nature 1993; 362:801–809.

21. Gamble JR, Khewgoodall Y, Vadas MA. Transforming growth factor beta inhibits E-selectin expression on human endothelial cells. J Immunol 1993; 150:4494–4503.

22. Chen CC, Manning AM. TGF-beta1, 1L-10 and 1L-4 differentially modulate the cytokine expression of 1L-6 and 1L-8 in human endothelial cells. Cytokine 1996; 8:58–65.

23. Phan SH, Gharaeekermani M, McGarry B, Kunkel SL, Wolber FW. Regulation of rat pulmonary artery endothelial cell transforming growth factor-beta production by 1L-1beta and tumor necrosis factor alpha. J Immunol 1992; 149:103–106.

24. Schwartz SM, Foy L, Bowen-Pope DF, Ross R. Derivation and properties of platelet-derived growth factor independent rat smooth muscle cells. Am J Physiol 1990; 136:1417–1428.

25. Grainger DJ, Hesketh TR, Metcalfe JC, Weissberg PL. A large accumulation of non-muscle myosin occurs at first entry into M phase in rat vascular smooth muscle cells. Biochem J 1991; 277:145–151.

26. Kemp PR, Grainger DJ, Shanahan CM, Weissberg PL, Metcalfe JC. The Id gene is activated by serum but is not required for de-differentiation in rat vascular smooth muscle cells. Biochem J 1991; 277:285–288.

27. Grainger DJ, Kemp PR, Witchell CM, Weissberg PL, Metcalfe JC. TGF-beta decreases the rate of proliferation of rat vascular smooth muscle cells by extending the $G_2$ phase of the cell cycle and delays the rise in cAMP before entry into M phase. Biochem J 1994; 299:227–235.

28. Morisaki N, Kawano M, Koyama N, Koshikawa T, Umemiya K, Saito Y, Yoshida S. Effects of transforming growth factor-beta1 on growth of aortic smooth muscle cells. Atherosclerosis 1991; 88:227–234.

29. Owens GK, Geisterfer AA, Yang YW, Komoriya A. Transforming growth factor-beta induced growth inhibition and cellular hypertrophy in cultured vascular smooth muscle cells. J Cell Biol 1988; 107:771–780.

30. Björkerud S. Effects of transforming growth factor-beta1 on human arterial smooth muscle cells in vitro. Atheroscler Thromb 1991; 11:892–902.

31. Battegay EJ, Raines EW, Seifert RA, Bowen-Pope DF, Ross R. TGF-beta induces bimodal proliferation of connective tissue cells via complex control of an autocrine PDGF loop. Cell 1990; 63:515–524.

32. Sato Y, Rifkin DB. Inhibition of endothelial cell movement by pericytes and smooth muscle cells: activation of a latent transforming growth factor beta1-like molecule by plasmin during co-culture. J Cell Biol 1989; 109:309–315.
33. Kojima S, Harpel PC, Rifkin DB. Lipoprotein(a) inhibits the generation of transforming growth factor beta: an endogenous inhibitor of smooth muscle cell migration. J Cell Biol 1991; 113:1439–1445.
34. Majesky MW, Benditt EP, Schwartz SM. Expression and developmental control of platelet-derived growth factor A-chain and B-chain/Sis genes in rat aortic smooth muscle cells. Proc Natl Acad Sci USA 1988; 85:1524–1528.
35. Giachelli CM, Majesky MW, Schwartz SM. Developmentally regulated cytochrome p450IA1 expression in cultured rat vascular smooth cells. J Biol Chem 1991; 266:3981–3986.
36. Benditt EP, Benditt JM. Evidence for a monoclonal origin of human atherosclerotic plaques. Proc Natl Acad Sci USA 1973; 70:1753–1756.
37. Grainger DJ, Witchell CM, Ho LK, Weissberg PL, Shanahan CM, Watson JV, Metcalfe JC. Interconversions of vascular smooth muscle cell clones: in vitro evidence for a smooth muscle cell lineage. Submitted.
38. Schwartz SM. Vascular growth and development. The molecular biology of the cardiovascular system. Keystone Symposium, CO, Jan 29–Feb 4, 1996.
39. Grainger DJ. Unpublished observations.
40. Ho LK. Regulation of Differentiation and Proliferation of Vascular smooth Muscle Cells. PhD dissertation, University of Cambridge, UK, 1994.
41. Grainger DJ, Witchell CM, Watson JV, Metcalfe JC, Weissberg PL. Heparin decreases the rate of proliferation of rat vascular smooth muscle cells by releasing TGF-beta like activity from serum. Cardiovasc Res 1993; 27: 2238–2247.
42. McCaffrey TA, Falcone DJ, Brayton CF, Agawal LA, Welt FG, Wesker BB. Transforming growth factor-beta activity is potentiated by heparin via dissociation of the transforming growth factor beta/alpha2 macroglobulin inactive complex. J Cell Biol 1989; 109:441–448.
43. Hoover RL, Rosenberg RD, Haering W, Karnovsky MJ. Inhibition of rat arterial smooth muscle cell proliferation by heparin. II in vitro studies. Circ Res 1980; 47:578–583.
44. Grainger DJ, Witchell CM, Crook JR, Leatham EW, Salomone OA, Ireson N, Kaski J-C. Aspirin elevates production of TGF-beta by cultured human smooth muscle cells and is associated with increased circulating TGF-beta in vivo. Submitted.
45. Grainger DJ, Weissberg PL, Metcalfe JC. Tamoxifen decreases the rate of proliferation of rat vascular smooth muscle cells in culture by inducing production of transforming growth factor-beta. Biochem J 1993; 294:109–112.
46. Kirschenlohr HL, Metcalfe JC, Weissberg PL, Grainger DJ. Proliferation of human aortic vascular smooth muscle cells is modulated by active TGF-beta. Cardiovasc Res 1995; 29:848–855.
47. Butta A, MacLennan K, Flanders KC, Sacks NPM, Smith I, McKinna A, Dowsett M, Wakefield LM, Sporn MB, Baum M, Colletta AA. Induction of

transforming growth factor-beta1 in human breast cancer in vivo following tamoxifen treatment. Cancer Res 1992; 52:4261–4264.

48. Grainger DJ, Kirschenlohr HL, Metcalfe JC, Weissberg PL, Wade DP, Lawn RM. Proliferation of human smooth muscle cells promoted by lipoprotein(a). Science 1993; 260:1655–1658.

49. Kirschenlohr HL, Metcalfe JC, Weissberg PL, Grainger DJ. Adult human aortic smooth muscle cells in culture produce active TGF-beta. Am J Physiol 1993; 265:C571–C576.

50. Martin JS, Dickson MC, Cousins FM, Kulkarni AB, Karlsson S, Akhurst RJ. Analysis of homozygous TGF-beta1 null mouse embryos demonstrates defects in yolk-sac vasculogenesis and hematopoiesis. Ann NY Acad Sci 1995; 752:300–308.

51. Kulkarni AB, Ward JM, Yaswen L, Mackall CL, Bauer SR, Huh CG, Gress RE, Karlsson S. Transforming growth factor-beta1 null mice—an animal model for inflammatory disorders. Am J Pathol 1995; 146:264–275.

52. Boivin GP, O'Toole BA, Orsmby IE, Diebold RJ, Eis MJ, Doetschman T, Kier AB. Onset and progression of pathological lesions in transforming growth factor-beta-1 deficient mice. Am J Pathol 1995; 146:276–288.

53. Lefer AM, Tsao P, Aoki N, Palladino MA. Mediation of cardioprotection by transforming growth factor-beta. Science 1990; 249:61–64.

54. Lefer AM, Tsao PS, Lefer DJ, Ma XL. Role of endothelial dysfunction in the pathogenesis of reperfusion injury after myocardial ischaemia. FASEB J 1991; 5:2029–2034.

55. Kirschenlohr HL, Mosedale DE, Metcalfe JC, Grainger DJ. Unpublished observations.

56. Grainger DJ, Witchell CM, Metcalfe JC. Tamoxifen elevates transforming growth factor-beta and suppresses diet-induced formation of lipid lesions in mouse aorta. Nature 1995; 1:1067–1073.

57. Giachelli C, Bae N, Lombardi D, Majesky M, Schwartz SM. Molecular cloning and characterization of 2B7, a rat mRNA which distinguishes smooth muscle cell phenotypes in vitro and is identical to osteopontin. Biochem Biophys Res Commun 1991; 177:867–873.

58. Shanahan CM, Weissberg PL, Metcalfe JC. Isolation of gene markers of differentiated and proliferating smooth muscle cells. Cir Res 1993; 73:193–204.

59. Giachelli CM, Bae N, Almeida M, Denhardt DT, Alpers CE, Schwartz SM. Osteopontin is elevated during neointima formation in rat arteries and is a novel component of human atherosclerotic plaques. J Clin Invest 1993; 92:1686–1696.

60. Shanahan CM, Cary NRB, Metcalfe JC, Weissberg PL. High expression of genes for calcification—regulating proteins in human atherosclerotic plaques. J Clin Invest 1994; 93:2393–2402.

61. Furr BJA, Jordan VC. The pharmacology and clinical uses of tamoxifen. Pharmacol Ther 1984; 25:127–205.

62. Bertelli G, Pronzato P, Amoroso D, Cusimano MP, Conte PF, Montagna G, Bertolini S, Rosso R. Adjuvant tamoxifen in primary breast cancer: Influence

on plasma lipids and antithrombin III levels. Breast Can Res Treat 1988; 12:307–310.

63. Caleffi M, Fentiman IS, Clark GN, Warj DY, Neidham J, Clark K, Laville A, Levis B. Effect of tamoxifen on estrogen binding, lipid and lipoprotein concentrations and blood clotting parameters in premenopausal women with breast pain. J Endocrinol 1988; 119:335–339.

64. Love RR, Newcomb PA, Wiebe DA, Surawics TS, Jordan VC, Carbone PP, Demets DL. Effects of tamoxifen therapy on lipid and lipoprotein levels in postmenopausal patients with node-negative breast cancer. J Natl Cancer Inst 1990; 82:1327–1332.

65. Plump AS, Smith JD, Hayek T, Aalto-Setala K, Walsh A, Verstuyft JG, Rubin EM, Breslow JL. Severe hypercholesterolemia and atherosclerosis in apolipoprotein E deficient mice created by homologous recombination in ES cells. Cell 1992; 71:343–353.

66. Zhang SH, Reddick RL, Piedrahita JA, Maeda N. Spontaneous hypercholesterolemia and arterial lesions in mice lacking apolipoprotein E. Science 1992; 258:468–471.

67. Reddick RL, Zhang SH, Maeda N. Atherosclerosis in mice lacking apo E. Arterioscler Thromb 1994; 14:141–147.

68. Reckless J, Metcalfe JC, Grainger DJ. Tamoxifen decreases cholesterol sevenfold and abolishes lipid lesion development in apolipoprotein E knock-out mice. Submitted.

69. Lawn RM, Wade DP, Hammer RE, Chiesa G, Verstuyft JG, Rubin EM. Atherogenesis in transgenic mice expressing human apolipoprotein(a). Nature 1992; 360:670–672.

70. Lawn RM, Pearl JR, Rubin EM, Metcalfe JC, Grainger DJ. Unpublished observations.

71. Liu AC, Lawn RM, Verstuyft JG, Rubin EM. Human apolipoprotein-A-1 prevents atherosclerosis associated with apolipoprotein(a) in transgenic mice. J Lipid Res 1994; 35:2263–2267.

72. Ploplis VA, Carmeliet P, Vazirzadeh S, van Vlaenderen I, Moons L, Plow EF, Collen D. Effects of disruption of the plasminogen gene on thrombosis, growth and health in mice. Circulation 1995; 9:2585–2593.

73. Carmeliet P, Schoonjans L, Kieckens L, Ream B, Degen J, Bronson R, De Vos R, van den Oord JJ, Collen D, Mulligan RC. Physiological consequences of loss of plasminogen activator gene function in mice. Nature 1994; 368:419–424.

74. Wald NJ, Law M, Watt HC, Wu TS, Bailey A, Johnson AM, Graig WY, Ledue TB, Haddow JE. Apolipoproteins and ischemic heart disease—implications for screening. Lancet 1994; 343:75–79.

75. Grainger, DJ, Byrne CD, Witchell CM, Gilmore WS, Wallace JMW, Metcalfe JC. Transforming growth factor-beta is sequestered into an inactive pool by lipoprotein particles. Submitted.

76. Schectman G, Kaul S, Kissebah AH. Effect of fish oil concentrate on lipoprotein composition in NIDDM. Diabetes 1988; 37:1567–1573.

77. Goodnight SH. The effects of omega-3-fatty acids on atherosclerosis and the vascular response to injury. Arch Pathol Lab Med 1993; 117:102–106.
78. Byrne CD, Wareham NJ, Clark PMS, Martensz ND, Metcalfe JC, Grainger DJ. The decrease in active transforming growth factor beta concentrations during a fat tolerance test is predicted by the increase in plasminogen activator inhibitor levels. Submitted.
79. Grainger DJ, Metcalfe JC, Grace AA, Petch MC, Bethel HW. Tamoxifen elevates the concentration of active TGF-beta in plasma from patients with advanced atherosclerosis. Submitted.
80. McDonald CC, Stewart HJ. Fatal myocardial infarction in the Scottish adjuvant tamoxifen trial. Br Med J 1991; 303:435–437.
81. McDonald CC, Alexander FE, Whyte BW, Forrest AP, Stewart HJ. Cardiac and vascular morbidity in women receiving adjuvant tamoxifen for breast cancer in a randomized trial. Br Med J 1995; 311:977–980.
82. Williams NR, Metcalfe JC, Grainger DJ. Unpublished observations.
83. Chauhan A, Schofield PM, Metcalfe JC, Grainger DJ. Serum levels of active TGF-beta do not correlate with the development of coronary occlusive disease following cardiac transplantation. Submitted.
84. Johnson DE, Gao SZ, Schroeder JS, DeCampli WM, Billingham ME. The spectrum of coronary artery pathologic findings in human cardiac allografts. J Heart Transplant 1989; 8:349–359.
85. Wolf YG, Rasmussen LM, Ruoslahti E. Antibodies against transforming growth factor-beta-1 suppress intimal hyperplasia in a rat model. J Clin Invest 1994; 93:1172–1178.
86. Nabel EG, Shum L, Pompili VJ, Yang ZY, San H, Shu HB, Liptay S, Gold L, Gordon D, Derynck R, Nabel GJ. Direct transfer of transforming growth factor beta1 gene into arteries stimulates fibrocellular hyperplasia. Proc Natl Acad Sci USA 1993; 90:10759–10763.
87. Kunz L, Schroff RW, Modedale DE, Metcalfe JC, Grainger DJ. Unpublished observations.

# 8

# Coagulation Factors

**Michael Kalafatis, Jack O. Egan, and Kenneth G. Mann**

*University of Vermont, Burlington, Vermont*

## I. INTRODUCTION

The endothelium forms a continuous lining throughout the vascular system and maintains a selective barrier between the components of the blood and the subendothelium. Blood coagulation is initiated following damage to the vascular endothelium. Vessel damage exposes matrix tissues beneath the endothelial lining of the blood vessel to which blood platelets adhere and become activated. A multitude of proteins participate in the reactions which regulate blood coagulation and behave in a concerted manner to generate $\alpha$-thrombin. This enzyme acts on the soluble blood protein fibrinogen to create the insoluble fibrin clot. $\alpha$-Thrombin also triggers platelet activation and initiates a variety of vascular processes ranging from activation/inhibition of coagulation and activation of fibrinolysis to cell growth. Most of the enzymes that participate in the blood-clotting process circulate in blood as inactive zymogens and procofactors. The coagulation process is initiated by injury of the vessel wall, and the resulting exposure of the cell-associated protein, tissue factor. Exposure of tissue factor initiates a series of enzymatic reactions which are localized on cellular surfaces. Cell-associated membrane sites are expressed and regulated in the physiological system which provides appropriate and adequate expression of the coagulation complexes which support normal hemostasis. The $\gamma$-

carboxyglutamic and residues (gla) of each protein are required for $Ca^{2+}$ binding and exposure of the membrane binding sites(s) to the cell bilayer. The absence of γ-carboxylation of one or more of the critical glutamic acid residues in one of the blood-clotting proteins results in an impaired coagulation/anticoagulation process which may lead to a bleeding diathesis or thrombosis.

Two pathways for the generation of thrombin have been proposed: the *intrinsic* pathway initiated by the "surface" contact activation of factor XII and the *extrinsic* pathway initiated by the exposure of the non-enzymatic cell-associated protein, tissue factor (1). However, the primary proteins involved in blood clotting have been defined owing to their association with bleeding syndromes or thrombotic diatheses. Patients who lack factor VIII or factor IX have life-threatening bleeding disorders that require prophylactic therapy. This fact led researchers to believe that the *intrinsic* pathway of blood clotting is the primary pathway for normal hemostasis. However, although individuals with deficiencies of prekallikrein (2), high molecular weight kininogen (3), and factor XII have been identified (4), these laboratory-described congenital "defects" are not associated with bleeding disorders and do not require prophylactic therapy following a hemostatic challenge. Thus, it has been concluded that the most likely event for the initiation of hemostasis is the exposure of tissue factor on the surface of the injured vascular tissue (5–7).

Tissue factor is an integral membrane, single-chain glycoprotein which when exposed to circulating blood following vascular injury binds circulating factor VIIa and initiates the coagulation process (8). Although most factor VII circulates as a single-chain zymogen, 1–2% of the molecules are cleaved and possess a incompletely formed active site which is not a target for the circulating plasma serine protease inhibitors (9,10). Following binding to tissue factor, the catalytic efficiency of factor VIIa increases (11). The factor VIIa/tissue factor complex localized at the cell surface then initiates the series of enzymatic reactions which lead to thrombin generation and fibrin clot formation.

The participants of the normal blood-coagulation cascade are assembled complexes, each composed of a vitamin K–dependent enzyme and a protein cofactor. All of these multiprotein vitamin K–dependent reaction complexes are located at the site of vascular damage (Fig. 1). The binding of all zymogens and their subsequent activation are dependent on the correct orientation of the proteins on the membrane surface, which in turn depends on membrane site expression and proper γ-carboxylation of each protein.

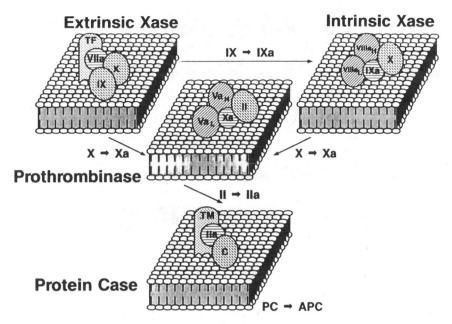

**Figure 1** Schematic representation of the vitamin K–dependent complexes that are required for normal clot formation (Extrinsic tenase, Intrinsic tenase, and prothrombinase), and clot elimination (protein C*ase*). (From ref. 73.)

## II.  THE VITAMIN K–DEPENDENT ZYMOGENS

### A.  Plasma Coagulation Factors

1.  Prothrombin

Prothrombin is a single-chain zymogen of $M_r$=72,000 which circulates in plasma at a concentration of 1.4 $\mu$M (Fig. 2) (12). The NH$_2$-terminal portion of the molecule contains the $\gamma$-carboxyglutamate residues which are necessary for membrane interaction. Factor Xa in the presence of its cofactor, factor Va, and Ca$^{2+}$ catalyzes the activation of prothrombin following cleavage at Arg$^{320}$ and Arg$^{284}$ to yield $\alpha$-thrombin. Several other thrombin-feedback cleavages (on prothrombin and/or thrombin) produce intermediates with lower catalytic properties.

2.  Factor X

Factor X ($M_r$=59,000 (13)) is composed of a heavy chain ($M_r$=42,000) and a light chain ($M_r$=16,500) which are associated through a disulfide bond

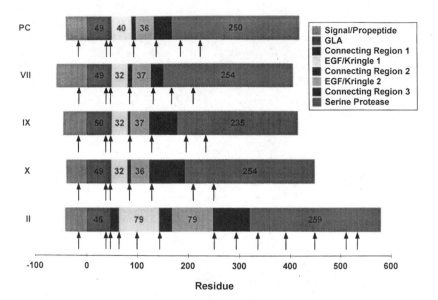

**Figure 2** Linear representation of the vitamin K–dependent products. The preprosequences are identified to the left of 0. The specific domains are identified in different shading that is indicated in the inset box. The intron-exon junctions are also shown by the arrows. (From ref. 74.)

(see Fig. 2) (14). The light chain contains the $\gamma$-carboxyglutamate residues which are necessary for the metal ion interaction of the protein (15). Factor X is converted to its active form, factor Xa, following cleavage of the heavy chain by either the intrinsic factor *tenase* (factor IXa in complex with its cofactor, factor VIIIa) (16,17) or by the extrinsic factor *tenase* (factor VIIa bound to tissue factor) at a single peptide bond ($Arg^{194}$-$Ile^{195}$). Factor Xa ($M_r=48,000$) is composed of a heavy chain ($M_r=30,000$) and a light chain ($M_r=16,500$) associated through a disulfide bond (13).

## 3.  Factor VII

Factor VII ($M_r=50,000$) is an inactive zymogen (18,19). The amino terminal part of the molecule contains the $\gamma$-carboxyglutamate residues which are involved in the metal binding properties of the protein (see Fig. 2) (20). Factor VII is converted to factor VIIa by thrombin (21), factor IXa (22), factor Xa (21), factor VIIa (11), and factor XIIa (23) following cleavage at $Arg^{152}$. Factor VIIa ($M_r=50,000$) is composed of a light chain ($M_r=20,000$) and a heavy chain ($M_r=30,000$) associated through a disulfide bond (18). It is noteworthy that a small portion of factor VII ($\sim$1–2% of the total factor

VII) circulates in plasma as factor VIIa, as it is thought to be responsible for the initiation of coagulation when tissue factor is exposed to the blood flow.

## 4. Factor IX

Factor IX ($M_r$=55,000) (see Fig. 2) is converted to factor IXa following two cleavages at $Arg^{145}$ and $Arg^{180}$ (24,25). Factor XIa or the extrinsic factor tenase (factor VIIa in the presence of tissue factor) can catalyze these cleavages which result in the release of the active enzyme, factor IXa ($M_r$=45,000), which is composed of a heavy chain ($M_r$=28,000) and a light chain ($M_r$=18,000) associated through a disulfide bond (26). The light chain, which is the $NH_2$-terminal part of the molecule, contains the $\gamma$-carboxyglutamate residues which are involved in the metal binding properties of the protein (27).

## 5. Protein C

Human protein C ($M_r$=62,000) is composed of a heavy chain ($M_r$=41,000) and a light chain ($M_r$=21,000) which are associated through a disulfide bond (28) (see Fig. 2). The $NH_2$-terminal part of the molecule, which is represented by the light chain, contains nine $\gamma$-carboxyglutamate residues which are involved in the metal binding properties of the protein. Protein C is converted to activated protein C (APC) after cleavage of the heavy chain at $Arg^{169}$ by the $\alpha$-thrombin–thrombomodulin complex. APC is the anticoagulant enzyme of the blood-clotting process, and it inactivates the cofactors of *prothrombinase* and intrinsic tenase, factor Va, and factor VIIIa, respectively (29,30). Cleavage of membrane-bound factor Va at $Arg^{506}$ is necessary for optimum exposure of the inactivating cleavage site at $Arg^{306}$ (29), whereas cleavage of membrane-bound factor VIIIa by APC at $Arg^{336}$ is solely responsible for inactivation (30). The function of activated protein C toward its substrates, factor Va and factor VIIIa, is clearly anionic membrane dependent. The essential inactivating cleavages of factor VIIIa and factor Va in the peptide regions between the A1 and A2 domains, at $Arg^{336}$ and $Arg^{306}$, respectively, only occur in the presence of anionic phospholipids. The importance of $\gamma$-carboxylation and binding to a lipid bilayer is illustrated by the $APC^{\gamma 20A}$ mutant molecule. This APC molecule that has a alanine at position 20 instead of a $\gamma$-carboxyglutamic acid, has impaired membrane binding capabilities, and thus cannot inactivate factor Va (31), which is the major substrate for APC.

## B. Soluble Cofactors

### 1. Factor V and Factor VIII

Factor V and factor VIII are two high molecular weight protein procofactors which circulate in plasma. There is approximately 40% sequence identity between factor V and factor VIII. Both cofactors can be activated by $\alpha$-thrombin and/or factor Xa into their active forms, factor Va and factor VIIIa, which are necessary for optimum catalytic efficiency of the prothrombinase and intrinsic tenase complexes, respectively.

*Factor V.* Factor V circulates in plasma (at a concentration of 20 nM) as a single-chain glycoprotein ($M_r$=330,000). The procofactor consists of three A domains (A1, A2, A3), two C domains (C1, C2) and a connecting B region (1) (Fig. 3). $\alpha$-Thrombin cleaves of factor V at $Arg^{709}$ and $Arg^{1545}$ to generate the factor Va molecule (32–34) (Fig. 3). Both subunits of factor Va are noncovalently associated via calcium bridges (35,36). Factor Va is inactivated by APC following three cleavages of the heavy chain at $Arg^{506}$, $Arg^{306}$, and $Arg^{679}$. We have previously shown that cleavage at $Arg^{506}$ is necessary for complete exposure of the inactivating cleavage sites at $Arg^{306}$ and $Arg^{679}$ (29). We have also demonstrated that cleavage at $Arg^{306}$ only occurs when the cofactor is bound to a membrane surface containing anionic phospholipid and is responsible for the loss of approximately 70–80% of factor Va cofactor activity. Further, cleavage at $Arg^{679}$ appears membrane independent and is responsible for the loss in the remaining 20–30% of cofactor activity. Elimination of the potential cofactor activity of factor V by APC also requires the presence of a membrane surface and is associated with four cleavages: at $Arg^{306}$, $Arg^{506}$, $Arg^{679}$, and $Lys^{994}$. Our data demonstrated that the first cleavage at $Arg^{306}$ is the inactivating cleavage site. The role of the three other cleavages remains to be identified.

*Factor VIII.* Human factor VIII circulates in plasma (0.7 nM) as a series of metal ion–dependent heterodimers in association with von Willebrand

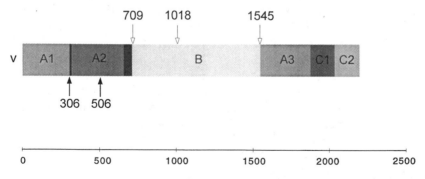

**Figure 3** Diagram of the organization of the human factor V molecule. The arrows on the top represent activation cleavages by $\alpha$-thrombin, whereas the arrows at the bottom indicate APC inactivation cleavage sites. (From ref. 74.)

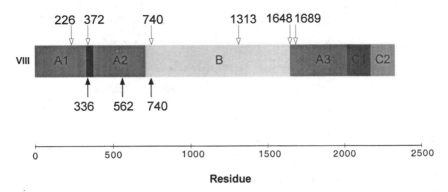

**Figure 4** Diagram of the organization of the human factor VIII molecule. The arrows on the top represent activation cleavages by $\alpha$-thrombin whereas the arrows at the bottom indicate APC inactivation cleavage sites. (From ref. 74.)

factor (vWF) and shares a number of structural and functional similarities with factor V (Fig. 4). Activation of factor VIII by $\alpha$-thrombin following cleavages at $\text{Arg}^{372}$, $\text{Arg}^{740}$, $\text{Arg}^{1689}$, and $\text{Arg}^{1648}$ yields an heterotrimer composed of fragments of $M_r = 50,000$ (A1 domain) and $M_r = 40,000$ (A2 domain), representing the heavy chain of the cofactor, and a light chain ($M_r = 74,000$) containing the A3-C1-C2 domains (37,38) (Fig. 4). The three subunits are noncovalently associated via divalent metal ion bridges. On $\alpha$-thrombin activation, factor VIIIa loses most of its cofactor activity spontaneously following dissociation of the A2 subunit (33,37–44). The remaining cofactor activity is lost following cleavage at $\text{Arg}^{336}$.

### 2. Protein S

Protein S is a nonenzymatic vitamin K–dependent glycoprotein (45,46). Protein S is composed of an $\text{NH}_2$-terminal "Gla" domain, a thrombin-sensitive region, four epidermal growth factor (EGF)–like structures, and a C-terminal portion containing 60% of the whole molecule (47,48) (Fig. 5). Protein S was initially identified because of the presence of $\gamma$-carboxy-glutamic acid (49). Protein S is synthesized in the liver and endothelial cells, testicular lining cells, and megakaryocytes. Plasma protein S exists in two states: free protein S and in complex with the C4B binding protein of complement. The anticoagulant properties of protein S are only observed for the fraction of the protein, which is not bound to C4BP. Cleavage of protein S by thrombin at the $\text{NH}_2$-terminal thrombin-sensitive region results in the inhibition of its cofactor activity. The cofactor activity of protein S is manifested by the acceleration of the inactivation of factor Va and factor VIIIa by APC. All

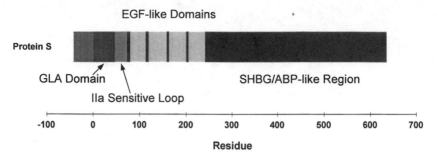

**Figure 5** Diagram of the organization of the preproprotein S molecule. The specific domains are indicated with different shadings.

functions of protein S require its interaction with a membrane surface that contains anionic phospholipid.

## III. COAGULATION FACTORS EXPRESSED IN VASCULAR TISSUES

### A. Tissue Factor

Tissue factor is a 263–amino acid ($M_r$=29,600) membrane-bound glycoprotein composed of three domains (Fig. 6): an extracellular domain containing amino acid residues 1–219 (soluble tissue factor), a hydrophobic membrane-spanning region composed of residues 220–242, and a cytoplasmic domain consisting of residues 243–263. The cytoplasmic domain

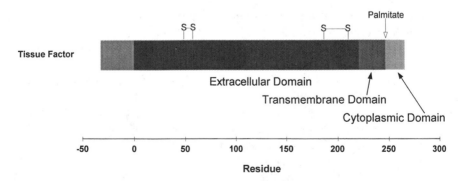

**Figure 6** Diagram of the organization of the preproprotein S molecule. The specific domains are indicated with different shadings. (From ref. 74.)

contains a potential glycosylation site (50,51) and a cysteine residue which is covalently associated with a palmityl-stearyl thioester (52).

Tissue factor is expressed in extravascular tissue and is selectively expressed by a variety of vascular and blood cells, including monocytes, macrophages, and endothelial cells. Endothelial cells contain very low levels of constitutively expressed tissue factor. Induction of tissue factor transcription occurs as a result of the expression of a variety of transcription factors which are constitutively expressed in differentiated cells or in response to activation by growth factors, bacterial lipopolysaccharide (LPS), or inflammatory cytokines such as tumor necrosis factor-$\alpha$ (TNF-$\alpha$) and interleukin-1$\beta$ (IL-1$\beta$), resulting in the establishment of a procoagulant environment. Transcriptional expression of the tissue factor gene is constitutively regulated in extravascular and vascular cells by three Sp1 binding sites in the minimal tissue factor promoter ($-111$ to $+14$ bp) (53). Transient induction of tissue factor gene expression is regulated by a distal enhancer ($-227$ to $-172$ bp) containing two AP-1 binding sites and a $\kappa$B binding site. The distal enhancer mediates LPS and cytokine induction of tissue factor expression in cultured monocytes and endothelial cells (54,55). A proximal enhancer element ($-111$ to $+14$ bp) controls transcription following phorbol myristate acetate (PMA) or serum induction of cultured epithelial cells. This enhancer element contains overlapping Egr-1/Sp-1 binding sites (54).

Vascular injury resulting in tissue factor exposure to plasma proteins allows formation of the tissue factor–factor VIIa complex resulting in initiation of the coagulation cascade.

## B.  Thrombomodulin

Thrombomodulin is composed of 559 amino acids and has a molecular weight of approximately 100,000 (Fig. 7). The protein is arranged in five domains: an $NH_2$-terminal lectin-like domain (residues 1–224) containing a potential binding site for $\alpha$-thrombin, a region containing six EGF-like domains (residues 225–461), a 34–amino acid region which is rich in serine and threonine residues and contains several potential O-linked glycosylation sites (residues 462–496), a hydrophobic membrane-spanning domain (residues 497–520), and a cytoplasmic region (residues 521–559). Expression of thrombomodulin, in contrast to tissue factor, is downregulated by exposure of endothelial cells to IL-1, TNF-$\alpha$, endotoxins, or hypoxia; thus also contributing to the establishment of a procoagulant environment.

Thrombomodulin is a thrombin binding anticoagulant molecule which is synthesized and constitutively expressed on the surface of endothelial cells (56). Formation of a thrombomodulin—$\alpha$-thrombin complex via the

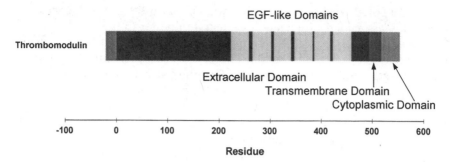

EGF-like Domains

Thrombomodulin

Extracellular Domain
Transmembrane Domain
Cytoplasmic Domain

-100      0      100      200      300      400      500      600

**Residue**

**Figure 7**   Diagram of the organization of the preprothrombomodulin molecule. The specific domains are indicated with different shadings.

fifth EGF-like domain of thrombomodulin causes a conformational alteration which makes thrombin unable to cleave fibrinogen, activate factor V, or activate platelets but allows efficient cleavage and activation of the zymogen protein C. Formation of the thrombin-thrombomodulin complex does not require $Ca^{2+}$. However, activation of protein C is $Ca^{2+}$ dependent (57). The phospholipid dependence of the thrombin-thrombomodulin complex appears to be somewhat species specific. With rabbit thrombomodulin, the presence of anionic phospholipids decreases the Km for protein C from 0.7 to 0.1 $\mu$M. However, with human thrombomodulin, negatively charged phospholipids have been reported to have a dramatic effect on the catalytic rate. Activated protein C can inactivate factors V(Va) and VIII(VIIIa), thereby downregulating coagulation by inhibiting the formation of the prothrombinase and intrinsic tenase complexes and thus inhibiting the generation of $\alpha$-thrombin.

## C.   von Willebrand Factor

von Willebrand factor (vWF), in addition to binding and stabilizing coagulation factor VIII in plasma, is the primary cofactor required for efficient platelet adhesion. Circulating levels of vWF are a result of constitutive expression and secretion by endothelial cells. Expression of vWF occurs in endothelial cells as a result of a positive regulatory region located in the first exon which relieves the effect of a negative regulatory region located upstream of the core promoter. This positive regulatory region contains potential SP1, GATA, and octamer binding sites and is active only in endothelial cells. vWF is differentially transcribed in endothelial cells based on the location of the cells within the vascular system. Cellular levels of vWF in vitro can be modulated in response to phorbol esters and steroid hormones. Granular stores of vWF (Weibel-Palade bodies) in endothelial cells can be secreted by exocytosis in response to agonists such as thrombin, histamine, vasopressin, adrenaline, phorbol esters, fibrin, and vascular endothelial growth factor (VEGF) (58,59).

## D.  Tissue Factor Pathway Inhibitor

Tissue factor pathway inhibitor (TFPI) inhibits the intrinsic pathway of coagulation through the formation of a quaternary complex with factor Xa, factor VIIa, and tissue factor (60–62) (Fig. 8). Although originally cloned from a hepatoma cell line, TFPI is synthesized primarily by endothelial cells and can be located bound to their surface in the circulation. TFPI is also secreted by platelets following stimulation with thrombin or the calcium ionophore A23187 (63). TFPI is present in blood at fairly low concentrations (2.4 nM) but is a very rapid inhibitor of the coagulation reaction. Increased levels of circulating TFPI found following endotoxin treatment may be a result of increased synthesis or release from the endothelium. A model of the organization of the overall protein is illustrated in Figure 8. TFPI can directly inhibit factor Xa activity; most likely through the second Kunitz domain which contains Arg at the $P_1$ site. In addition, in the presence of tissue factor and factor Xa, TFPI can inhibit factor VIIa; most likely through the first Kunitz domain which contains Lys at $P_1$. Thus, the inhibitor is bivalent in its interaction. It has been hypothesized to be a major regulator of the initiating events in blood clotting, since these events involve factor X activation by the factor VIIa–tissue factor complex. The bivalent interaction of TFPI with the newly formed factor Xa and the factor VIIa–tissue factor complex may provide an efficient mechanism to shut

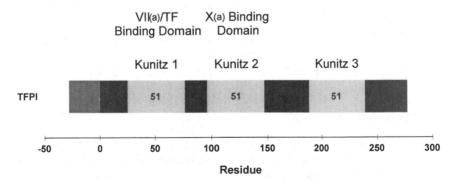

**Figure 8**  Diagram of the organization of the preproTFPI molecule. The specific domains are indicated with different shadings. The VIIa-tissue factor as well as the factor Xa binding domains are also indicated.

down factor Xa generation. No major changes in TFPI expression have been detected in response to cytokine exposure of endothelial cells.

## IV.  PLASMA INHIBITORS OF BLOOD COAGULATION

Although repair of vascular damage is vital to normal hemostasis, so too is the inactivation of the coagulation response. The sequestering of the enzyme complexes on the same membrane surface and channeling of intermediate enzyme products between them is potentially advantageous in vivo in providing a protected environment for enzyme function as well as enhancing the overall rate of $\alpha$-thrombin formation. From a mechanistic standpoint, the surface dependence of blood coagulation reduces the possibility that an intermediate enzyme product would be lost in the blood flowing past the wound site.

Two inhibitors are present in blood: TFPI (see above) and antithrombin III (see below). Both of these proteins circulate as active inhibitors which have the capacity to inhibit various coagulation enzymes. Their inhibitory capacity is directly related to their plasma concentrations on a stoichiometric basis.

### A.  Antithrombin III

Antithrombin III is found in plasma at a concentration of 3 $\mu$M (64). It is a member of the Serpin inhibitor family. Antithrombin III inhibits the majority of the serine proteases of the coagulation system (65). Inhibition of thrombin and factor Xa are of most significance in regulating the coagulation process (66). In the inhibition of factor Xa, the principal influence of heparin is associated with its ability to induce a conformational change in the antithrombin III protein, which makes it a better inhibitor of factor Xa. The endothelial cells are the source of the natural biological equivalent of "heparin." The target reaction site on antithrombin III for cleavage by blood clotting serine proteases corresponds to Arg[393] (Fig. 9). Following cleavage of the inhibitor at this site, there is a substantial rearrangement of the molecule.

### B.  Heparin Cofactor II

Heparin cofactor II is a circulating inhibitor that inhibits chymotrypsin-like proteases and is highly homologous to antithrombin III (67). Although this inhibitor can inhibit $\alpha$-thrombin in the presence of heparin, it is a poor inhibitor of other trypsin-like plasma proteases.

The pathology of thrombosis in association with diminished levels of antithrombin III has been clearly established. A relationship between TFPI

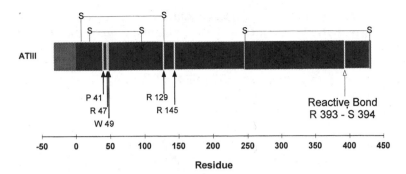

**Figure 9** Diagram of the organization of the preproATIII molecule. The specific domains are indicated with different shadings.

deficiency and an associated clinical pathology has not yet been established. However, interventive studies using TFPI in models of thrombosis suggests that this protein indeed is an important physiological regulator of coagulation.

The formation of a hemostatic plug involves the interactions of blood and vascular elements with tissue and plasma proteins. $\alpha$-Thrombin converts soluble plasma fibrinogen to insoluble fibrin (68). Concurrently, thrombin activates the plasma transglutaminase, factor XIII, which covalently cross links the fibrin polymers. Other plasma proteins bind onto the surface of the fibrin meshwork during the polymerization process, including vWF. Fibrinogen is also responsible for platelet aggregation. The importance of fibrinogen is emphasized by the bleeding diatheses associated with afibrinogenemia and some dysfibrinogenemias. However, in the latter cases, vWF can be substituted for fibrinogen and promote platelet aggregation.

## V. SURFACE–DEPENDENT REACTIONS DURING BLOOD CLOTTING

In vitro studies have shown that a membrane surface is essential for the function of the enzyme complexes of coagulation. In vivo, the lipid component is contributed by the cellular surfaces of the vasculature. However, the complex membrane composition of cells in vivo make it difficult to maintain the native character of the membrane in vitro. Therefore, the use of synthetic phospholipid vesicles has facilitated modeling and analyses of the kinetics of assembly and function of the enzyme-cofactor complexes in coagulation. There is substantial evidence for the association of the enzymes and cofactors of these complexes with naturally occurring cell membranes of the vasculature. The intricacies of the culmination of coagulation events at the lipid surface are still being appreciated by many investigators and studies have been greatly accelerated through the use of defined, purified systems employing synthetic phospholipid vesicles. The limitation for the comparison of the in vitro results with an in vivo situation is that binding sites available on synthetic phospholipid vesicles are not subject to regulation as they are on the cell surface.

Many studies have focused on understanding how the coagulation process is initiated, propagated, regulated, and terminated and how the resulting clot is eliminated. The prothrombinase complex has been the primary model system from which many hypotheses have been formulated. This complex, composed of factor Xa and factor Va resident on a membrane surface, catalyzes the activation of prothrombin approximately 300,000 times more efficiently than factor Xa alone. Much of the research has focused on the kinetics of the formation of the prothrombinase complex utilizing homogeneous preparations of factor Va, factor Xa, prothrombin, and synthetic phospholipid vesicles. The presence of anionic phospholipid within the mixture was found to be required for optimum procoagulant activity (69–71).

Analysis of the assembly of the components of the prothrombinase complex on phospholipid membranes has led to the hypothesis that all the enzymatic reactions which lead to the formation of $\alpha$-thrombin may interact on a membrane surface, since two-dimensional transfer of factor Xa between enzyme complexes would be many orders of magnitude faster than dissociation of factor Xa from one surface and reassociation on a second surface location. Hence, the individual protein-lipid complexes must be formed on separate sites on the same membrane and constitute the rate-limiting steps of prothrombinase assembly. This mechanism of assembly establishes the importance of the initial protein-lipid interactions in prothrombinase complex formation.

The serine proteases, factor IXa and factor Xa, and the cofactor proteins, factor VIIIa and factor Va, of the intrinsic factor tenase and the prothrombinase complexes share many structural and functional similarities. The assembly of the intrinsic factor tenase (factor VIIIa–factor IXa complex) is also a lipid-dependent process. Deficiencies of the components of the intrinsic factor tenase complex are well established (hemophilias A and B). It is also well documented that individuals with factor VIII deficiency have severe bleeding disorders. Factor VIII deficiency (hemophilia A) is an X chromosome–linked bleeding disorder, whereas factor V deficiency (parahemophilia) is an autosomal-linked bleeding disorder. There is a considerable amount of data concerning factor VIII deficiency when compared with factor V deficiency. This is most likely related to the severity of the deficiency and the survival of the patients with factor VIII deficiency, since very few patients with factor V deficiency were studied. Although the factor VIIIa–factor IXa complex has not been characterized as thoroughly as the prothrombinase complex, the assembly of the constituent components on a membrane surface increases the rate of factor Xa generation approximately 250,000-fold over that of factor IXa alone (72).

Similar to the intrinsic factor tenase and prothrombinase complexes, complex formation between the serine protease factor VIIa and its membrane-associated cofactor induces an alteration in the active site of factor VIIa. The tissue factor–factor VIIa complex activates factors IX and X. Evaluation of the activation of the individual factors IX and X by the extrinsic factor tenase in purified systems initially showed that factor X was the preferred substrate. However, if this complex could provide a significant amount of factor Xa in vivo, the bleeding disorders associated with deficiencies in the intrinsic factor tenase complex (i.e., hemophilia A and B) should not logically exist. Studies have shown that in mixtures containing both zymogens, factor IX, not factor X, is the preferred substrate for the factor VIIa–tissue factor complex. In this model of the coagulation response, the tissue factor–factor VIIa complex first activates small amounts of both factor IX and factor X. The factor Xa that is generated assists in the conversion of factor IX to the intermediate product, factor IX$\alpha$. The inactive factor IX$\alpha$ can then be converted to factor IXa by the tissue factor–factor VIIa complex. Factor IXa then forms the intrinsic factor tenase with its cofactor, factor VIIIa, and accelerates factor Xa generation more than 50-fold. Thus the role for the tissue factor–factor VIIa complex is in triggering the hemostatic response through activation of small quantities of factor X. The two membrane-bound enzymes, factor Xa and factor VIIa, then activate factor IX. Propagation of the formation of factor Xa would then be accomplished by the factor VIIIa–factor IXa complex.

The interaction of the different enzyme complexes of the procoagulant and anticoagulant pathways on a membrane surface warrant against disruption of the network of the vascular system either through injury and bleeding or through uncontrolled clot formation. The assembly of the enzyme complexes, procoagulant and anticoagulant, on a membrane surface fills the physiological requirement for rapid, localized, and regulated expression of procoagulant activity. The membrane surface thus provides a protected environment for the sequential procoagulant enzyme reactions which lead to the generation of $\alpha$-thrombin and hence the polymerized fibrin clot.

*260*        *Kalafatis et al.*

# REFERENCES

1. Davie EW, Ratnoff OD. Waterfall sequence for intrinsic blood clotting. Science 1964; 145:1310–1312.
2. Hathaway WE, Belhasen LP, Hathaway HS. Evidence for a new plasma thromboplastin factor. I. Case report, coagulation studies and physiochemical properties. Blood 1965; 26:521–532.
3. Colman RW, Bagdasarian A, Talamo RC, et al. Williams trait: human kininogen deficiency with diminished levels of plasminogen proactivator and prekallikrein associated with abnormalities of the Hageman factor–Dependent pathways. J Clin Invest 1975; 56:1650–1662.
4. Hoak JC, Swanson LW, Warner ED, Connor WE. Myocardial infarction associated with severe factor XII deficiency. Lancet 1966; 2:884–886.
5. Nemerson Y. Tissue factor and Hemostasis. Blood 1988; 71:1–8.
6. Edgington TS, Mackman N, Brand K, Ruff W. The structural biology of expression and function of tissue factor. Thromb Haemost 1991; 66:67–79.
7. Nakagaki T, Foster DC, Berkner KL, Kisiel W. Initiation of the extrinsic pathway of blood coagulation: Evidence for the tissue factor-dependent autoactivation of human coagulation factor VII. Biochemistry 1991; 30:10819–10824.
8. Drake TA, Morrissey JH, Edgington TS. Selective cellular expression of tissue factor in human tissues: implications for disorders of hemostasis and thrombosis. Am J Pathol 1989; 134:1087–1097.
9. Morrissey JH, Macik BG, Neuenschwander PF, Comp PC. Quantitation of activated factor VII levels in plasma using a tissue factor mutant selectively deficient in promoting factor VII activation. Blood 1993; 81:734–744.
10. Lawson JH, Butenas S, Ribarik N, Mann KG. Complex-dependent inhibition of factor VIIa by antithrombin III and heparin. J Biol Chem 1993; 268:767–770.
11. Lawson JH, Butenas S, Mann KG. The evaluation of complex-dependent alterations in human factor VIIa. J Biol Chem 1992; 267:4834–4843.
12. Lundblad RL, Kingdon HS, Mann KG. Thrombin. In: Lorand L, ed. Methods in Enzymology, Proteolytic Enzymes, Part B. New York: Academic Press, 1976:156–176.
13. Fujikawa K, Legaz ME, Davie EW. Bovine factors $X_1$ and $X_2$ (Stuart factor). Isolation and characterization. Biochemistry 1972; 11:4882–4891.
14. Davie EW, Fujikawa K. Basic mechanisms in blood coagulation. Ann Rev Biochem 1975; 44:799–829.
15. DiScipio RG, Hermodson MA, Yates SG, Davie EW. A comparison of human prothrombin, factor IX (Christmas factor), factor X (Stuart factor), and protein S. Biochemistry 1977; 16:698–706.
16. Lundblad RL, Davie EW. The activation of anti-hemophilic factor (factor VIII) by activated Christmas factor (activated factor IX). Biochemistry 1964; 3:1720–1725.
17. Osterud B, Rapaport SI. Synthesis of intrinsic factor X activator. Inhibition of the function of formed activator by antibodies to factor VIII and to factor IX. Biochemistry 1970; 9:1854–1861.

18. Kisiel W, Davie EW. Isolation and characterization of bovine factor VII. Biochemistry 1975; 14:4928–4934.
19. Bajaj SP, Rapaport SI, Brown SF. Isolation and characterization of human factor VII. J Biol Chem 1981; 256:253–259.
20. McMullen BA, Fujikawa K, Kisiel W. The occurrence of b-hydroxyaspartic acid in the vitamin K–dependent blood coagulation zymogens. Biochem Biophys Res Commun 1983; 115:8–14.
21. Radcliffe R, Nemerson Y. Activation and control of factor VII by activated factor X and thrombin. J Biol Chem 1975; 250:388–395.
22. Seligsohn U, Osterud G, Brown SF, Griffin JH, Rappaport SI. Activation of human factor VII in plasma and in purified systems: roles of activated factor IX, kallikrein and activated factor XII. J Clin Invest 1979; 64:1056–1065.
23. Kisiel W, Fujikawa K, Davie EW. Activation of bovine factor VII (proconvertin) by factor XIIa (activated Hageman factor). Biochemistry 1977; 16:4189–4194.
24. Braunstein KM, Noyes CM, Griffith MJ, Lundblad RL, Roberts HR. Characterization of the defect in activation of factor $IX_{Chapel\ Hill}$ by human factor XIa. J Clin Invest 1981; 68:1420–1426.
25. Griffith MJ, Breitkreutz L, Trapp H, et al. Characterization of the clotting activities of structurally different forms of activated factor IX. J Clin Invest 1985; 75:4–10.
26. Lawson JH, Mann KG. Cooperative activation of human factor IX by the human extrinsic pathway of blood coagulation. J Biol Chem 1991; 266: 11317–11327.
27. Kurachi K, Davie EW. Isolation and characterization of a cDNA coding for human factor IX. Proc Natl Aca Sci USA 1982; 79:6461–6464.
28. Kisiel W. Human plasma protein C. J Clin Invest 1979; 64:761–769.
29. Kalafatis M, Rand MD, Mann KG. The mechanism of inactivation of human factor V and human factor Va by activated protein C. J Biol Chem 1994; 269:31869–31880.
30. Eaton D, Rodriguez H, Vehar G. Proteolytic processing of human FVIII. Correlation of specific cleavages by thrombin FXa and activated protein C with activation and inactivation of Factor VIII coagulant activity. Biochemistry 1986; 25:505–512.
31. Lu D, Kalafatis M, Mann KG, Long GL. Loss of membrane-dependent factor Va cleavage: a mechanistic interpretation of the pathology of protein $C_{Vermont}$. Blood 1995; 84:687–690.
32. Katzmann JA, Nesheim ME, Hibbard LS, Mann KG. Isolation of functional human coagulation factor V by using a hybridoma antibody. Proc Natl Acad Sci USA 1981; 78:162–166.
33. Nesheim ME, Mann KG. Thrombin-catalyzed activation of single chain bovine factor V. J Biol Chem 1979; 254:1326–1334.
34. Kane WH, Majerus PW. Purification and characterization of human coagulation factor V. J Biol Chem 1981; 256:1002–1007.
35. Esmon CT. The subunit structure of thrombin-activated factor V. Isolation of

activated factor V, separation of subunits and reconstitution of biological activity. J Biol Chem 1979; 254:964–973.

36. Krishnaswamy S, Russell GD, Mann KG. The reassociation of factor Va from its isolated subunits. J Biol Chem 1989; 264:3160–3168.

37. Toole JJ, Knopf JL, Wozney JM, et al. Molecular cloning of a cDNA encoding human antihaemophilic factor. Nature 1984; 312:342–347.

38. Vehar G, Keyt B, Eaton D, et al. Structure of human factor VIII. Nature 1984; 312:337–342.

39. Kane WH, Davie EW. Cloning of a cDNA coding for human factor V, a blood coagulation factor homologous to factor VIII and ceruloplasmin. Proc Natl Acad Sci USA 1986; 83:6800–6804.

40. Jenny R, Pittman D, Toole J, et al. Complete cDNA and derived amino acid sequence of human FV. Proc Natl Acad Sci USA 1987; 84:4846.

41. Foster PA, Fulcher CA, Marti T, Titani K, Zimmerman TS. A major factor VIII binding domain resides within the amino-terminal 272 amino acid residues of von Willebrand factor. J Biol Chem 1987; 262:8443–8446.

42. Vehar G, Davie E. Preparation and properties of bovine FVIII (antihemophilic factor). Biochemistry 1980; 19:401–410.

43. Wood WI, Capon DJ, Simonsen CC, et al. Expression of active human factor VIII from recombinant DNA clones. Nature 1984; 312:330–336.

44. Gitschier J, Wood WI, Goralka TM, et al. Characterization of the human factor VIII gene. Nature 1984; 312:326–330.

45. Walker FJ. Regulation of activated protein C by a new protein: a possible function for bovine protein S. J Biol Chem 1980; 255:5521–5524.

46. Walker FJ. Regulation of activated protein C by protein S. J Biol Chem 1981; 256:11128–11131.

47. Baker ME, French FS, Joseph DR. Vitamin D–dependent protein S is similar to rat androgen binding protein. Biochemistry 1987; 243:293–296.

48. Gershagen S, Lundwall A, Fernlund P. Characterization of the human sex hormone binding globulin (SHBG) gene and demonstration of two transcripts in both liver and testis. Nucleic Acids Res 1989; 17:9245–9258.

49. Scharfstein J, Ferreira A, Gigli I, Nussenzweig V. Human C4b-binding protein. I. Isolation and characterization. J Exp Med 1978; 148:207–222.

50. Spicer EK, Horton R, Bloem L, et al. Isolation of cDNA clones coding for human tissue factor: primary structure of the protein and cDNA. Proc Natl Acad Sci USA 1987; 84:5148–5152.

51. Morrissey JH, Fakhrai H, Edgington TS. Molecular cloning of the cDNA for tissue factor, the cellular receptor for the initiation of the coagulation protein. Cell 1987; 50:129–135.

52. Bach R, Konigsberg W, Nemerson Y. Human tissue factor contains thioester-linked palmitate and stearate on the cytoplasmic half cysteine. Biochemistry 1988; 27:4227–4231.

53. Mackman N, Fowler BJ, Edgington TS, Morrissey JH. Functional analysis of the human tissue factor promoter and induction by serum. Proc Nat Acad Sci USA 1990; 87:2254–2258.

54. Donovan-Peluso M, George LD, Hassett AC. Lipopolysaccharide induction of tissue factor expression in THP-1 monocytic cells. J Biol Chem 1994; 269:1361–1369.
55. Mackman N, Brand K, Edgington TS. Lipopolysaccharide-mediated transcriptional activation of the human tissue factor gene in THP-1 monocytic cells requires both activator protein 1 and nuclear factor kb binding sites. J Exp Med 1991; 174:1517–1526.
56. Owen WG, Esmon CT. Functional properties of an endothelial cell cofactor for thrombin-catalyzed activation of protein C. J Biol Chem 1981; 256:5532–5535.
57. Esmon NL, Owen WG, Esmon CT. Isolation of a membrane-bound cofactor for thrombin-catalyzed activation of protein C. J Biol Chem 1982; 257:859.
58. Ferreira V, Assouline Z, Schwachtgen JL, Bahnak BR, Meyer D. The role of the 5'-flanking region in the cell-specific transcription of the human von Willebrand factor gene. Biochem J 1993; 293:641–648.
59. Jahroudi N, Lynch DC. Endothelial-Cell specific regulation of von Willebrand factor gene expression. Mol Cell Biol 1994; 14:999–1008.
60. Wun T, Kretzmer KK, Girard TJ, Miletich JP, Broze GJ, Jr. Cloning and characterization of cDNA coding for the lipoprotein-associated coagulation inhibitor shows that it consists of three tandem Kunitz-type inhibitory domains. J Biol Chem 1988; 263:6001–6004.
61. Novotny WF, Girard TJ, Miletich JP, Broze GJ, Jr. Purification and characterization of the lipoprotein-associated coagulation inhibitor from human plasma. J Biol Chem 1989; 264:18832–18837.
62. Girard TJ, Broze GJ. Tissue Factor Pathway Inhibitor. In: Lorand L. Mann KG, eds. Methods in Enzymology Part A. 222th ed. San Diego: Academic Press, 1993:195–209.
63. Novotny WF, Girard TJ, Miletich JP, Broze GJ, Jr. Platelets secrete a coagulation inhibitor functionally and antigenically similar to the lipoprotein-associated coagulation inhibitor. Blood 1988; 72:2020–2025.
64. Jesty J. The inhibition of activated bovine coagulation factors X and VII by antithrombin III. Arch Biochem Biophys 1978; 185:165–173.
65. Casu B, Oreste P, Torri G, Zoppetti G. The structure of heparin oligosaccharide fragments with high anti-(factor Xa) activity containing the minimal antithrombin III–binding sequence. Biochem J 1981; 197:599–609.
66. Olson ST, Shore JD. Demonstration of a two step reaction mechanism for inhibition of $\alpha$-thrombin by antithrombin III and identification of the step affected by heparin. J Biol Chem 1982; 257:14891–14895.
67. Blinder MA, Marasa JC, Reynolds CH, Deaven LL, Tollefsen DM. Heparin cofactor II: cDNA sequence, chromosome localization, restriction fragment length polymorphism, and expression in *Escherichia coli*. Biochemistry 1988; 27:752–759.
68. Doolittle RF. Fibrinogen and fibrin. Ann Rev Biochem 1984; 53:195.
69. Mann KG, Bovill EG, Krishnaswamy S. Surface-dependent reactions in the propagation phase of blood coagulation. Ann NY Acad Sci 1991; 614:63–75.

70. Krishnaswamy S, Mann KG. The binding of factor Va to phospholipid vesicles. J Biol Chem 1988; 263:5714–5723.
71. Krishnaswamy S, Jones KC, Mann KG. Prothrombinase complex assembly: kinetic mechanism of enzyme assembly on phospholipid vesicles. J Biol Chem 1988; 263:3823–3834.
72. van Dieijen G, Tans G, Rosing J, Hemker HC. The role of phospholipid and factor VIIIa in the activation of bovine factor X. J Biol Chem 1981; 256: 3433–3442.
73. Mann KW, Lorand L. Methods Enzymol 1993; 222:1–21.
74. Mann KG, Gaffney D, Bovill EG. Molecular biology, biochemistry and life-span of plasma coagulation factors. In: Beutler E, Lichtman MA, Coller BS, Kipps TJ, eds. Williams Hematology, 5th ed. New York: Mc-Graw Hill, 1995.

# 9

# Endothelial Dysfunction and Vascular Disease

## Paul M. Vanhoutte

*Institut de Recherches Internationales Servier, Courbevoie, France*

## Louis P. Perrault and Jean Paul Vilaine

*Institut de Recherches Servier, Suresnes, France*

## I. INTRODUCTION

The normal endothelium contributes to the local regulation of vasomotor tone and the maintenance of a nonthrombogenic surface; acts as a selective barrier controlling permeability and transport of solutes and macromolecules to help metabolize many factors circulating in the blood or generated locally; and helps to control the proliferation of underlying vascular smooth muscle cells and to regulate the adhesion and extravasation of neutrophils, monocytes, and lymphocytes. These properties are due to the ability of endothelial cells to sense humoral and hemodynamic stimuli and are underlain by three basic mechanisms: the secretion of endothelium-derived factors; the expression at the cell membrane surface of binding proteins, adhesive molecules, and metabolizing enzymes (e.g., converting enzyme); and shape changes. The discovery by Furchgott and Zawadzki of the obligatory role played by the endothelial cells in relaxations of isolated arteries in response to acetylcholine (1) has initiated a major scientific inquiry into the pivotal role of the endothelium in contributing to the normal physiological function of the vascular wall. It soon became obvious that endothelium-dependent responses are mediated by the release of several diffusible substances (endothelium-derived relaxing factor [EDRF] and contracting factor [EDCF]) from the endothelial cells. This chapter focuses on how the secretion by endothelial cells of vasoactive substances brings about moment to moment changes in the tone of the underlying vascular smooth muscle cells, and on why dysfunction of the endothelial cells may underly or accompany several major vascular diseases. It updates similar overviews to which the reader is referred for more exhaustive references (2–13).

## II.  ENDOTHELIUM-DERIVED VASOACTIVE FACTORS

Endothelial cells produce several substances which cause either relaxation or contraction of the underlying vascular smooth muscle.

### A.  Endothelium-Derived Nitric Oxide

The labile diffusible, nonprostanoid substance that mediates the endothelium-dependent relaxation response to acetylcholine described by Furchgott and Zawadzki (1) has been identified as nitric oxide (NO) or a closely related compound (3,14–16). NO is formed from the guanidine-nitrogen terminal of L-arginine by an enzyme called NO-synthase, which is constitutive (NO synthase III [17]) in normal endothelial cells. The activation of this NO synthase depends of the intracellular concentration of calcium ions in the endothelial cells, is calmodulin dependent, and requires reduced nicotinamide adenine dinucleotide phosphate (NADPH) and 5,6,7,8-tetrahydrobiopterin (BH4) for optimal activity. The enzyme can be inhibited competitively by L-arginine analogues such as $N^G$-monomethyl-L-arginine or $N^G$-nitro-L-arginine (Fig. 1). In addition to the constitutive NO synthase present in endothelial cells, two other isoforms of this enzyme are currently known: a neuronal (type I) and an inducible (type II) form which is calcium independent and can be observed in numerous cell types (including vascular smooth muscle) after exposure to endotoxin, tumor necrosis factor, and other cytokines. NO diffuses to the vascular smooth muscle cells and relaxes them by stimulating a cytosolic enzyme, soluble guanylate cylase, that leads to an increase in cyclic $3',5'$-guanosine monophosphate (cyclic GMP). The latter increase is associated with inhibition of the contractile apparatus (Fig 1). The production of NO is a major contributor to endothelium-dependent relaxations in large isolated arteries, including coronary, systemic, mesenteric, pulmonary, and cerebral arteries. Its significance in vivo is suggested by the observations that inhibitors of NO synthase cause vasoconstriction in most vascular beds and an increase in systemic arterial pressure both in animals and in humans (12,14).

The endothelial cell secretes NO not only toward the underlying vascular smooth muscle but also in the lumen of the blood vessel. Under normal conditions, the presence of oxyhemoglobin in the erythrocytes immediately

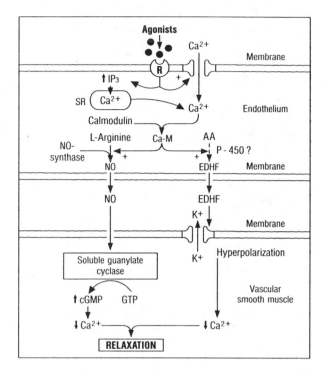

**Figure 1.** Role of the increase in cytosolic calcium concentration in the release of EDRF(s). Endothelial receptor activation induces an influx of calcium into the cytoplasm of the endothelial cell; following interaction with calmodulin, this activates NO synthase and leads to the release of endothelium-derived hyperpolarizing factor (EDHF). NO causes relaxation by activating the formation of cyclic GMP (cGMP) from GTP. EDHF causes hyperpolarization and relaxation by opening $K^+$ channels. Any increase in cytosolic calcium (including that induced by the calcium ionophore A23187) causes the release of relaxing factors. When agonists activate the endothelial cells, an increase in inositol phosphate (IP3) may contribute to the increase in cytoplasmic $Ca^{2+}$ by releasing it from the sarcoplasmic reticulum (SR). (From Vanhoutte et al. 1995, by permission.)

neutralizes NO, which only has a physiological role at the interface between the endothelial cells and the blood content. Thus, NO inhibits the adhesion of platelets and leukocytes to the endothelium. It acts (synergistically with prostacyclin) to inhibit platelet aggregation (3,4,10,14,18). NO also inhibits the growth of the vascular smooth muscle cells (19,20).

The release of NO is modulated by physical and humoral stimuli. Among the physical stimuli, the shear stress exerted by the blood on the arterial wall is one of the main factors regulating the local release of NO.

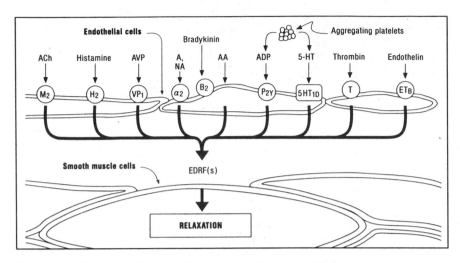

**Figure 2.** Some of the neurohumoral mediators which cause the release of endothelium-derived relaxing factors (EDRFs) through activation of specific endothelial receptors (circles). In addition, EDRFs can be released independently of receptor-operated mechanisms by the calcium ionophore A23187 (not shown). A, adrenaline (epinephrine); AA, arachidonic acid; ACh, acetylcholine; ADP, adenosine diphosphate; $\alpha$, $\alpha$-adrenergic receptor; AVP, arginine vasopressin; B, kinin receptor; ET, endothelin receptor; H, histaminergic receptor; 5-HT, serotonin (5-hydroxytryptamine), serotoninergic receptor; M, muscarinic receptor; NA, noradrenaline (norepinephrine); P, purinergic receptor; T, thrombin receptor; VP, vasopressinergic receptor. (From Vanhoutte et al. 1995, by permission.)

Indeed, flow-induced vasodilatation is endothelium-dependent in vivo (21,22). Bioassay studies show that increases in flow or the introduction of pulsatile flow stimulates the release of NO and prostacyclin from the endothelium of perfused arteries (23). Vasoconstriction of perfused arteries induced by the elevation of intraluminal pressure can be prevented by removal of the endothelium and is in part dependent on a reduced release of NO (24,25).

Several neurotumoral mediators cause the release of NO through activation of specific endothelial receptors (Fig. 2). The endogenous substances stimulating this release are either circulating hormones (e.g., catecholamines, vasopressin), autacoids generated within the vascular wall (e.g., bradykinin, histamine), or mediators released by platelets (serotonin, adenosine diphosphate [ADP]) or formed during coagulation (thrombin) (2–13). The receptors for these substances are connected to the production of NO by different coupling proteins (Fig. 3). For exam-

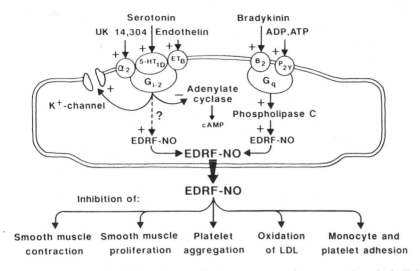

**Figure 3.** Postulated signal transduction processes in a normal endothelial cell. Activation of the cell causes the release of EDRF-NO, which has important protective effects in the vascular wall. $\alpha$, $\alpha$-adrenergic; 5-HT, serotonin-receptor; ET, endothelin receptors; B, bradykinin receptor; P, purinoceptor; G, coupling proteins; cAMP, cyclic adenosine monophosphate; NO, nitric oxide; LDL, low-density lipoproteins. (From Vanhoutte and Boulanger 1995, by permission.)

ple, in porcine endothelial cells, $\alpha_2$-adrenergic receptors, serotonin receptors, and thrombin receptors are coupled to pertussis toxin–sensitive $G_{i2}$ proteins, whereas for ADP or bradykinin, receptors mediate the production of NO by activation of pertussis toxin–insensitive $G_q$ protein (see 26,27).

From the physiological point of view, the substances produced during platelet aggregation are important releasers of NO. This conclusion is based on the findings that in various species, including humans, platelet aggregation induces endothelium-dependent relaxations and that the presence of endothelial cells substantially inhibits the vasoconstriction induced by thromboxane $A_2$ and platelet-derived serotonin. There are two major mediators of the endothelial response to platelets: serotonin and adenosine diphosphate (ADP), which act on 5-HT$_{1D}$-serotonin and P$_{2y}$-purinergic receptors, respectively (see Fig. 3). The endothelial action of thrombin and platelet products is crucial for the protective role played by the normal endothelium against unwanted coagulation (Fig. 4). Thus, local platelet aggregation, with the inevitable release of serotonin and ADP as well as the production of thrombin (because of the local activation of the coagula-

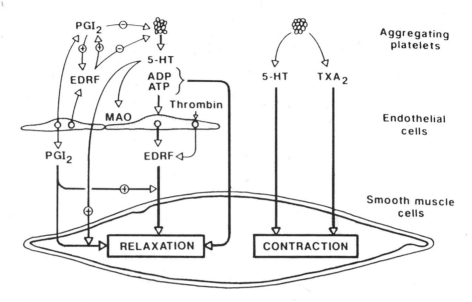

**Figure 4.** Interaction between platelet products, thrombin, and endothelium. If the endothelium is intact, several of the substances released from the platelets (in particular, the adenine nucleotides [ADP and ATP] and serotonin [5-HT]) cause the release of EDRF and prostacyclin ($PGI_2$). The same is true for any thrombin formed. The released EDRF will relax the underlying vascular smooth muscle, opening up the blood vessel, and thus flushing the microaggregate away; it will also be released toward the lumen of the blood vessel to brake platelet adhesion to the endothelium and, synergistically with prostacyclin, inhibit platelet aggregation. In addition, monoamine oxidase (MAO) and other enzymes will break down the vasoconstrictor serotonin, limiting the amount of the monoamine that can diffuse toward the smooth muscle. Finally, the endothelium acts as a physical barrier that prevents the access to the smooth muscle of the vasoconstrictor platelet products serotonin and thromboxane $A_2$ ($TXA_2$). These different functions of the endothelium play a key role in preventing unwanted coagulation and vasospastic episodes in blood vessels with a normal intima. If the endothelial cells are removed (e.g., by trauma), the protective role of the endothelium is lost locally, platelets can adhere and aggregate, and vasoconstriction follows; this contributes to the vascular phase of hemostasis. +, activation; −, inhibition. (From Vanhoutte et al. 1995, by permission.)

tion cascade) leads to massive local release of NO, which diffuses toward the underlying vascular smooth muscle, induces its relaxation, and thus dilatation of the artery. This reaction helps to eliminate the microaggregate. The release of NO toward the blood vessel lumen also inhibits platelet adhesion at the endothelium-blood interface and (in synergy with prostacyclin), exerts a major feedback on platelet aggregation, thereby eliminating the imminent danger of vascular occlusion. In addition, the endothelial barrier prevents the platelet-derived vasoconstrictor substances (mainly thromboxane $A_2$ and serotonin) from reaching the smooth muscle. Conversely, if the endothelial barrier has been removed, for example, as a result of trauma, there is a breakdown in the feedback control of platelet aggregation by NO (and prostacyclin). Aggregation proceeds with the continuous release of serotonin and thromboxane $A_2$, both of which, in the absence of the endothelial barrier, have unrestricted access to smooth muscle. Hence, the smooth muscle contracts and the blood vessel closes down to constitute the vascular phase of hemostasis (Fig. 4) (3,8,10,28).

## B. Prostacyclin

Prostacyclin, a major product of vascular cyclooxygenase, is formed primarily in endothelial cells but also in the media and adventitia in response to shear stress, hypoxia, and several mediators that also release NO. Prostacyclin causes relaxation of vascular smooth muscle by activating adenylate cyclase and increasing the production of cyclic $3',5'$-adenosine monophosphate (cyclic AMP). In most blood vessels, the contribution of prostacyclin to endothelium-dependent relaxation is negligible, and its effect is essentially additive to that of NO. However, the two substances act synergistically to inhibit platelet aggregation (Fig. 4) (18,29).

## C. Endothelium-Dependent Hyperpolarizing Factor

Electrophysiological studies in various arteries, including the human coronary artery, demonstrate that acetylcholine and other endothelium-dependent dilators cause endothelium-dependent hyperpolarizations and relaxations which are due to a diffusible endothelium-derived hyperpolarizing factor (EDHF) different from NO and prostacyclin (30,34). The chemical nature of EDHF remains speculative. In some blood vessels, epoxyeicosatrienoic acids (EETs), formed from arachidonic acid by the action of cytochrome P-450, may correspond to EDHF (31,34,35).

The hyperpolarization of smooth muscle cells induced by EDHF is mediated by an increased movement of potassium ions. The type of potassium channels involved has not been definitively established, but these channels are more likely to be calcium-dependent rather than ATP-dependent potassium channels (34,36). The release of EDHF, like that of NO, requires an increase in the intracellular calcium concentration of the endothelial cells (see Fig. 1).

The contribution of hyperpolarization in endothelium-dependent vascular relaxation varies in function according to the size of the arteries and is prominent in resistance vessels (33,35). In large arteries, both mediators can contribute to endothelium-dependent relaxations, but the role of NO predominates under normal circumstances. Nevertheless, in these arteries, EDHF can mediate near normal endothelium-dependent relaxations when the synthesis of NO is inhibited (34,37). This preservation may be important for the regulation of vascular tone in disease when the production and/or the activity of NO are reduced.

## D.   Endothelium-Derived Contracting Factors

Under certain conditions, the endothelium can initiate vasoconstriction through the release of diffusible substances (38,40). Endothelium-dependent contractions can be explained either by the withdrawal of the release of EDRFs or by the production of diffusible vasoconstrictor substances (EDCFs) (3,5,9,41). The EDCFs identified to date include superoxide anions (which presumably act by scavenging NO [42]), endoperoxides, thromboxane $A_2$, and the peptide endothelin-1 (Fig. 5). The latter is more

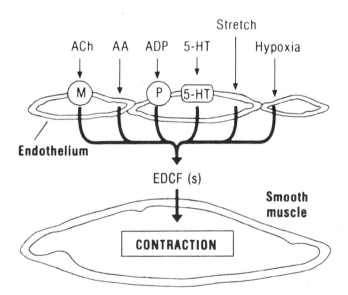

**Figure 5.**   A number of physicochemical stimuli, neurohumoral mediators, and the calcium ionophore A23187 can evoke endothelium-dependent contractions in certain blood vessels, presumably because they evoke the release of endothelium-derived contracting factor(s) (EDCF). AA, arachidonic acid; ACh, acetylcholine; ADP, adenosine diphosphate; 5-HT, serotonin (5-hydroxytryptamine), serotoninergic receptor; M, muscarinic receptor; P, purinergic receptor. (From Vanhoutte and Boulanger 1995, by permission.)

likely to play a role, if any, in the long-term modulation of vascular tone and structure than in moment to moment changes in the degree of contraction of vascular smooth muscle (43–47). The stimuli for endothelium-dependent contraction include hypoxia, physical stimuli such as pressure and stretch, and several neurohumoral mediators (see Fig. 4).

## III. ENDOTHELIAL DYSFUNCTION

In several types of vascular diseases, the endothelial cells become dysfunctional (3,4,8,10–13). Usually this dysfunction expresses itself as an impairment in endothelium-dependent relaxations either due to a reduced release (or action) of EDRFs and/or a greater propensity to evoke endothelium-dependent contractions.

### A. Regenerated Endothelium

The normal aging process induces a turnover and regeneration of endothelial cells resulting in an abnormal function. Indeed, the normal life span of an adult human endothelial cell has been estimated to be around 30 years. After this time, cells tend to disappear and are replaced by regenerated endothelium. However, these regenerated cells have lost some of their ability to release EDRF, in particular in response to platelet aggregation and thrombin. This conclusion is based on in vivo animal studies in which regeneration and the characteristics of endothelium-dependent responses were monitored following the removal of the coronary endothelium (48,49). Endothelial regrowth was satisfactory, but the regenerated endothelium was no longer able to prevent aggregating platelet-induced contraction. Indeed, the regenerated endothelium responds poorly to serotonin and other substances using the pertussis toxin–sensitive pathway controlling the release of EDRF (see Fig. 3). In cultured regenerated endothelial cells, pertussis toxin–sensitive $G_i$ proteins are expressed normally, but they have a reduced activity (50). The loss of the pertussis toxin–sensitive response is selective and does not apply to endothelium-dependent responses induced by ADP or bradykinin. The area of regenerated endothelium becomes a site of predilection for triggering exaggerated vasoconstriction in response to serotonin or ergonovine (51).

### B. Hypercholesterolemia and Atherosclerosis

#### 1. Animal Data

In experimental animals, hypercholesterolemia induced by high-fat and/or high-cholesterol diets impairs endothelium-dependent relaxations in the rabbit (3,7,10,52,53). By contrast, endothelium-independent relaxations to nitroglycerin, sodium nitroprusside, or adenosine are normal or only slightly impaired. A progressive deterioration of endothelium-dependent relaxations is also observed in genetically hyperlipidemic rabbits (54). Endothelium-dependent relaxations are reduced also in the coronary microcirculation of hypercholesterolemic animals and primates (55,56).

### 2.  Clinical Data

Endothelium-dependent relaxations are impaired also in humans with atherosclerosis and/or hypercholesterolemia. This conclusion rests on experiments with isolated coronary arteries from heart transplant recipients, in whom endothelium-dependent relaxations are reduced in atherosclerotic segments in comparison with segments without atherosclerosis (57,58). Coronarographic studies show that coronary arteries with atherosclerotic lesions constrict to injections of acetylcholine, whereas acetylcholine produces either vasodilatation or no change in the coronary diameter in normal patients (59). Studies with inhibitors of the L-arginine–NO pathway (methylene blue, free hemoglobin, and $N^G$-monomethyl-L-arginine) suggest that acetylcholine-induced coronary dilatation in humans is mediated mainly by NO (60–62). These arteries are capable of dilating in response to nitroglycerin. Thus, the paradoxical constriction of atherosclerotic arteries to acetylcholine suggests the occurrence of endothelial dysfunction with a loss of the dilator effect of NO to offset the direct constrictor action of acetylcholine on vascular smooth muscle.

The endothelial dysfunction occurs in the absence of intimal thickening and may be an early and pathogenic event in atherosclerosis (74). Abnormal coronary responses to acetylcholine are linked directly to the risk factors for coronary artery disease, and the degree of vasoconstriction (or vasodilatation) to acetylcholine varies linearly with the level of plasma cholesterol (70). Endothelial dysfunction occurs predominantly at coronary branching points, which may explain the propensity of these sites of disturbed flow to develop atherosclerosis (75).

In peripheral blood vessels, hypercholesterolemia and other risk factors of atherosclerosis are associated with endothelial dysfunction, as evidenced by abnormal responses to endothelium-dependent vasodilators. The latter can be detected before the development of vascular lesions and even during the first decade of life (76,77). The endothelium is also dysfunctional in microvessels of patients with atherosclerosis both in the coronary and peripheral circulations (78,79).

### 3.  Mechanism(s)

Because of the predominance of NO in endothelium-dependent relaxations, particularly in large arteries, many studies have focused on potential alterations of the L-arginine–NO pathway to explain the reduced response to acetylcholine and other endothelial agonists in atherosclerosis. Possible interferences include a reduced intracellular availability of L-arginine, alterations in signaling mechanisms, modification of the expression or the activity of NO synthase, or increased destruction of NO (3,80). A reduced availability of L-arginine appears unlikely, as endothelial cells contain concentrations of this substrate a thousand times greater (millimolar range) than those optimal for constitutive NO synthase activity (micromolar range). Nevertheless, L-arginine supplementation can normalize endothelium-dependent relaxation to acetylcholine in the microcirculation and the aorta of rabbits with an enriched cholesterol diet (81,82). In hypercholesterolemic patients, L-arginine improves the response to acetylcholine in coronary microvessels but not in large coronary arteries (78).

In the early stage of the atherosclerotic process, the endothelial dysfunction appears to be limited to the pertussis toxin–sensitive, $G_i$ protein–dependent pathway which leads to NO formation (Fig. 6). Thus, the ability

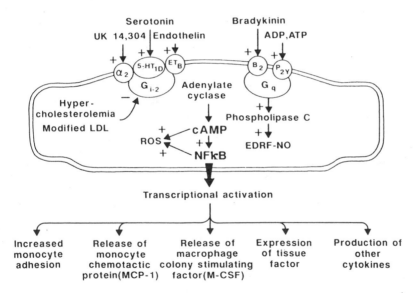

**Figure 6.** Postulated signal transduction processes in a dysfunctional endothelial cell. There is impairment in $G_{i-2}$ protein–dependent signaling with a subsequent decrease in the release of EDRF-NO. Furthermore, the resulting increase in cyclic AMP (cAMP) activates the transcription factor NFKB, which induces proatherogenic activity in the endothelial cell (ROS, reactive oxygen species; R, membrane-bound receptors) $\alpha$, $\alpha$-adrenergic; 5-HT, serotonin-receptor; ET, endothelin receptors; B, bradykinin receptor; P, purinoceptor; G, coupling proteins; NO, nitric oxide; LDL, low-density lipoproteins (Modified from Flavahan and Vanhoutte, 1995.)

of regenerated endothelial cells, chronically exposed to high cholesterol levels, to ADP-ribosylate pertussis toxin is reduced (83). Consequently, in coronary arteries from hypercholesterolemic pigs, endothelium-dependent relaxations evoked by agents that activate the pertussis toxin–sensitive $G_i$ protein (e.g., serotonin, $\alpha_2$-adrenergic agonists, aggregating platelets, thrombin) are depressed, whereas those induced by ADP, bradykinin, or the $Ca^{2+}$ ionophore A23187 are preserved (26,27,48,49,53,54,83). Oxidized low-density lipoproteins (LDL), which are considered to be more atherogenic than native LDL, in vitro, induce, a similar selective endothelial dysfunction for stimuli activating the pertussis-sensitive $G_i$ protein pathway, whereas at higher concentrations, they also inhibit endothelium-dependent responses evoked by receptor-independent stimuli (A23187) (3,80,84).

The most important mechanism in the reduction in endothelium-dependent responses is a lesser release of NO. Nevertheless, as the disease progresses and the artery thickens and stiffens, it becomes increasingly difficult for NO-EDRF to reach smooth muscle that is still able to relax. Endothelial dysfunction is probably a fundamental initial step in the progression of atherosclerosis (Fig. 7). This hypothesis argues that aging and prolonged exposure to shear stress, coupled with risk factors such as hypertension, smoking, and stress, accelerate endothelial aging and hence the process of endothelial regeneration. As a result, larger and larger sections of the endothelium become unable to resist platelet adhesion and aggregation and respond less well to thrombin formation. The feedback effect of NO (together with prostacyclin) on platelet aggregation decreases steadily, whereas vasoconstrictor factors (serotonin and thromboxane $A_2$) are released in increasingly greater amounts together with growth factors such as platelet-derived growth factor (PDGF), which is probably responsible for initiating the characteristic morphological changes in atherosclerosis (3,7,8,10,26–28).

## C.   Hypertension

### 1.   Endothelium-Dependent Relaxations

Endothelium-dependent relaxations are reduced in arteries from different animal models of the disease (3,6,11). Similarly, in the forearm circulation of hypertensive patients, the vasodilator response to the intra-arterial injection of acetylcholine is blunted (e.g., 86–87). These findings concur to suggest that the release of EDRF can be reduced in hypertensive blood vessels.

Inhibitors of NO synthases cause a sustained increase in arterial pressure in the intact animal and peripheral vasoconstriction in normotensive hu-

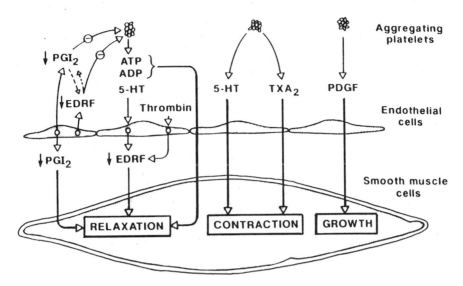

**Figure 7.** Endothelium-dependent responses under pathological conditions. The endothelium is dysfunctional in the regenerated state, hypercholesterolemia, and atherosclerosis, releasing less EDRF, whereas the ability of vascular smooth muscle to contract is unaltered. As a result, the contractions predominate. In atherosclerosis, the production of endothelium-derived relaxing factors and prostacyclin ($PGI_2$) is reduced, and their synergistic action against aggregating platelets decreases over time. Because of this reduced ability to inhibit platelet aggregation, the endothelium cannot prevent the release of platelet-derived growth factor (PDGF) and the stimulation of smooth muscle cell growth which it induces. ADP, adenosine diphosphate; ATP, adenosine triphosphate; 5-HT, serotonin; MAO, monoamine oxidase; $TXA_2$, thromboxane $A_2$; $-$, inhibition.(From Vanhoutte et al, 1995, by permission.)

mans (6,14). Since inhibitors of NO synthases cause less vasoconstriction in the forearm of hypertensive than normotensive subjects (88–90), a reduced efficiency of the L-arginine–NO pathway may contribute to the increased peripheral resistance characteristic of chronic hypertension. A similar conclusion may explain the blunted response to endothelium-dependent vasodilators in isolated blood vessels from hypertensive animals. Thus, for example, in the aorta of the hypertensive salt-sensitive Dahl rat, the endothelium-dependent relaxation to acetylcholine is diminished, suggesting a reduced release of NO. However, the response of the vascular smooth muscle to exogenous donors of NO is also reduced, which implies that the lesser response to acetylcholine is due in part to an impaired responsiveness of the hypertensive vascular smooth muscle to the endothelial mediator (3,6).

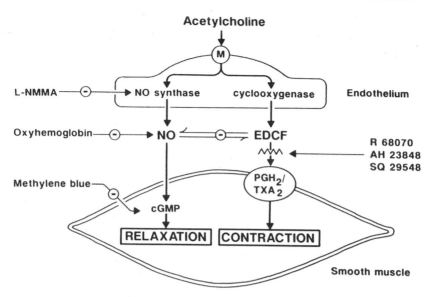

**Figure 8.** Stimulation of the thromboxane/endoperoxide receptor ($PGH_2/TXA_2$) is involved in endothelium-dependent contractions to acetylcoline in the aorta of the SHR. M, muscarinic receptor; NO, nitric oxide; EDCF, endothelium-derived contracting factor; cGMP, cyclic GMP; L-NMMA, $N^G$-methyl-L-arginine. The compounds R 68070, AH 23848, and SQ 29548 are antagonists of thromboxane receptors.

Not all reduced endothelium-dependent relaxations to acetylcholine (and other agonists) observed in arteries from hypertensive animals and humans can be attributed to abnormalities in the L-arginine–NO pathway. Indeed, in arteries of the spontaneously hypertensive rat (SHR), the blunted responses are observed despite a normal release of EDRF. A normal responsiveness to endothelium-dependent vasodilators can be restored by inhibitors of cyclooxygenase (79). Thus, in this model of hypertension, the reduced endothelium-dependent relaxations are explained best by the concommitant release of NO and EDCF, with the latter "scavenging" the former (Fig. 8); (3,6,91). Likewise, a reduced release of EDHF may contribute to the abnormal endothelium-dependent responses (34).

Since the abnormalities in endothelium-dependent relaxations are reversed by appropriate antihypertensive therapy (84), the reduced endothelium-dependent relaxation must be viewed as a consequence rather than a cause of the high blood pressure (3,6). Likewise, in hypertensive patients, the peripheral vasoconstrictor response to inhibitors of NO synthases is normalized by antihypertensive agents (90,92). In the arteries of the young SHRs, the relaxation to acetylcholine becomes progressively impaired as the arterial blood pressure increases (3,6). This suggests that the partial loss in endothelium-dependent relaxation may result from premature aging of the blood vessel wall exposed chronically to the higher distending pressure. If this were so, the curtailment of endothelium-dependent relaxations is not likely to play a primary role in the initiation of hypertension. However, at the later stages of the disease, it could contribute to the maintenance of an elevated peripheral vascular resistance or favor the occurrence of complications such as atherosclerosis (3,6,39). Premature aging also would help to explain the reduction in endothelium-dependent hyperpolarization observed in hypertensive arteries, as this type of response decreases markedly with age even in normotensive animals (34).

2.   Endothelium-Dependent Contractions

In quiescent rings of SHR aortas, acetylcholine causes endothelium-dependent contractions. Similar endothelium-dependent contractions have been obtained in response to arachidonic acid, serotonin, endothelin, and adenine nucleotides (3,6). The release of EDCF caused by serotonin and ADP presumably helps to explain why the presence of the endothelium does not reduce the contractions to aggregating platelets in the aorta of the SHR, as it does in blood vessels from normotensive controls. A cyclooxygenase-dependent EDCF is involved, since these responses can be prevented by indomethacin. The release of this EDCF explains the abnormal relaxations to acetylcholine observed in the aorta and small resistance arteries (3,6) of the SHR. The same may hold for certain types of human hypertension, as in essential hypertensive patients, the local administration of indomethacin normalizes the vasodilator response to intra-arterial acetylcholine (87).

The endothelium-dependent contractions of the SHR aorta are augmented by inhibitors of nitric oxide synthase and by oxyhemoglobin (which scavenges NO) but not by methylene blue (which inhibits soluble guanylate cyclase and the relaxations caused by NO). The logical interpretation from those findings is that the EDCF released from the hypertensive endothelium interacts chemically with NO and that both mediators inactivate each other (91). Such a chemical interaction (see Fig. 8) certainly would explain the blunting of endothelium-dependent relaxations despite a normal release of EDRF and a normal responsiveness of the smooth muscle of the SHR aorta to exogenous NO donors in the absence of endothelium (3,6).

The responses to acetylcholine, arachidonic acid, and adenine nucleotides are not prevented by inhibitors of thromboxane synthase but are abolished by antagonists of endoperoxide/thromboxane receptors (3,6). Thus, the EDCF involved is an endoperoxide. The larger release of prostaglandin $H_2$ in the SHR may result from a greater cyclooxygenase expression (92) and/or an altered metabolism of the endoperoxide into prostanoids. In addition to a larger production of endoperoxides, an altered responsiveness of the hypertensive vascular smooth muscle contributes to endothelium-dependent contractions (92). In the case of endothelium-dependent contractions evoked by endothelin, the endothelial mediator involved appears to be thromboxane $A_2$ (93).

## D.  Heart Failure

### 1.  Endothelium-Dependent Relaxations

An initial study (94) reported a decrease in acetylcholine-induced relaxation of isolated canine femoral arteries after pacing-induced congestive heart failure. However, impairment of endothelium-dependent vasodilatation in congestive heart failure depends on the vascular bed studied, the species, and the time of assessment after congestive heart failure has been induced or diagnosed (13). Considering the heterogeneity among results between ex vivo animal experiments and in vivo animal and human studies, there is not always perfect concordance. Animal studies usually refer to large conduit vessels, whereas resistance vessels are targetted in clinical studies. In addition, the impact on endothelium-dependent responses depends on the mode of induction of congestive heart failure and the vascular region studied (13,95).

In the conscious dog with pacing-induced heart failure, dilatation of large and small coronary vessels in response to acetylcholine is impaired. This is associated with a significant decrease in the production of nitrites (96). In dogs with congestive heart failure, the vasoconstrictor response to $N^G$-monomethyl-L-arginine (inhibitor of nitric oxide synthesis) is reduced (97). In the resistance vessels of anesthetized dogs with pacing-induced heart failure, the vasodilator response to both acetylcholine and to adenosine diphosphate is depressed, suggesting that the decreased responsiveness is not restricted to activation of muscarinic receptors (97). Thus, in the dog with congestive heart failure, a blunting of the endothelial release of nitric oxide occurs. However, this conclusion does not necessarily apply to other animal models of the disease (13).

In patients with congestive heart failure, the acetylcholine-induced vasodilatation is reduced in the forearm as well as in the skeletal muscles of the lower limbs (98,99). Normal vasodilatations can be restored by L-arginine (100). In the forearm resistance vessels of patients with congestive heart failure, the blunted response to acetylcholine is associated with an exaggerated decrease in blood flow induced by inhibitors of NO synthases (101,102). These observations suggest strongly that the released NO is reduced in human heart failure. In conduit vessels of these patients, both the endothelium-dependent (increased flow) and independent (nitroglycerine) responses are impaired. Thus, structural alterations in the vasculature could complicate the endothelial dysfunction. Since a reversal of the inability of peripheral vessels to dilate occurs with long-term treatment with angiotensin-converting enzyme inhibitor in patients with mild to moderate congestive heart failure (103), the endothelial defect seems to be a consequence rather than a cause of the disease process.

A decreased release of nitric oxide in congestive heart failure can also help to explain a reduced arterial compliance observed in patients with congestive heart failure (104–106). The mechanisms, the significance, and the etiological impact of the endothelial dysfunction in congestive heart failure are not clear. Various diseases coexist with congestive heart failure, including coronary disease, hypertension, and diabetes, all of which may result in impairment of endothelium-dependent relaxations.

2.  Endothelium-Derived Vasoconstrictors

In addition to the impaired endothelium-dependent vasodilatation, the increase in circulating endothelin-1 levels that occurs in congestive heart failure may have a determinant role. Indeed, the changes in plasma endothelin-1 are closely related to the alterations of the levels of other neurohormones such as vasopressin or norepinephrine which the in vitro release of endothelin (107). Thus, depending on the associated pathologies, the plasma level of endothelin increases from twofold to fivefold in patients with congestive heart failure (108).

A cyclooxygenase-dependent EDCF (3) may also be released in heart failure. Indeed, both in dogs and in patients with congestive heart failure, the vasodilator response to acetylcholine is enhanced after inhibition of cyclooxygenase with indomethacin (94,109). The restoration of the response to acetylcholine by angiotensin-converting enzyme inhibition in patients with mild heart failure probably is also related to cyclooxygenase (110,111).

The enhanced release of endothelium-derived vasoconstrictors probably is a consequence rather than a cause of the heart failure. The reduction in shear stress induced by a lower cardiac output in congestive heart failure must lead to chronic downregulation of the release of nitric oxide (3). Shear stress modulates not only the production of nitric oxide but also that of endothelin-1 (3,112,113). Under physiological conditions, nitric oxide would be continuously released with resulting depression of the release of endothelin-1 (3,114). Thus, the modulation of the production of these two endothelial mediators observed in congestive heart failure can be explained in part by the chronic reduction in cardiac output.

## ACKNOWLEDGMENT

The authors thank Marie Palumbo for superb secretarial assistance.

## REFERENCES

1. Furchgott RF, Zawadzki JV. The obligatory role of the endothelial cells in relaxation of arterial smooth muscle by acetylcholine. Nature 1980; 288: 373–376.
2. Furchgott RF, Vanhoutte PM. Endothelium-derived relaxing and contracting factors. FASEB J 1989; 3:2007–2018.
3. Lüscher TF, Vanhoutte PM. The Endothelium: Modulator of Cardiovascular Function. CRC Press, Boca Raton, FL, 1990:1–228.
4. Vanhoutte PM. The endothelium—modulator of vascular smooth-muscle tone. N Engl J Med 1988; 319:512–513.
5. Vanhoutte PM. The other endothelium-derived vasoactive factors. Circulation 1993; 87(suppl V):V-9–V-17.
6. Vanhoutte PM, Boulanger CM. Endothelium-dependent responses in hypertension. Hypertens Res Clin Exp 1995; 18:87–98.
7. Vanhoutte PM, Scott-Burden T. The endothelium in health and disease. Texas Heart Inst J 1994; 21:62–67.
8. Vanhoutte PM, Shimokawa H. Endothelium-derived relaxing factor(s) and coronary vasospasm. Circulation 1989; 80:1–9.
9. Vanhoutte PM, Gräser T, Lüscher TF. Endothelium-derived contracting factors. In: Rubanyi G, ed. Endothelin. Oxford, UK: Oxford University Press, 1992:3–16.
10. Vanhoutte PM. Hypercholesterolaemia, atherosclerosis and release of endothelium-derived relaxing factor by aggregating platelets Eur Heart J 1991; 12(suppl E):25–32.
11. Vanhoutte PM. State of the art lecture: endothelium and control of vascular function. Hypertension 1989; 13:658–667.
12. Vanhoutte PM., Boulanger CM, Mombouli JV. Endothelium-derived relaxing factors and converting enzyme inhibition. Am J Cardiol 1995; 76:3E–12E.
13. Vanhoutte PM. Endothelium-dependent responses in congestive heart failure. J Mol Cell Cardiol. In press.
14. Moncada S, Palmer RMJ, Higgs EA. Nitric oxide: physiology, pathophysiology, and pharmacology. Pharmacol Rev 1991; 43:109–142.
15. Pearson PJ, Vanhoutte PM. Vasodilator and vasoconstrictor substances produced by endothelium. Rev Physiol Biochem Pharmacol 1993; 122:1–67.
16. Schini-Kerth VB, Vanhoutte PM. Nitric oxide synthases in vascular cells. Exp Physiol 1995; 80:885–905.

17. Nishida K, Harrison DG, Navas JP, et al. Molecular cloning and characterization of the constitutive bovine aortic endothelial nitric oxide synthase. J Clin Invest 1992; 90:2092–2096.

18. Vane JR. The Croonian Lecture, 1993. The endothelium: maestro of the blood circulation. Phil Trans R Soc Lon B 1994; 348:225–246.

19. Scott-Burden T, Vanhoutte PM. Regulation of smooth muscle cell growth by endothelium-derived factors. Texas Heart Inst J 1994; 21:91–97.

20. Scott-Burden T, Vanhoutte PM. The endothelium as a regulator of vascular smooth muscle proliferation. Circulation 1993; 87(suppl V):V-51–V-55.

21. Holtz F, Fostermann U, Pohl U, et al. Flow-dependent, endothelium-mediated dilation of epicardial coronary arteries in conscious dogs: effects of cyclooxygenase inhibition. J Cardiovasc Pharmacol 1984; 6:1161–1169.

22. Bassenge E, Heuch G. Endothelial and neuro-humoral control of coronary blood flow in health and disease. Rev Physiol Biochem Pharmacol 1990; 116:79–163.

23. Rubanyi GM, Romero JC, Vanhoutte PM. Flow-induced release of endothelium-derived relaxing factor. Am J Physiol 1986; 250:H1145–H1149.

24. Rubanyi GM. Endothelium-dependent pressure-induced contraction of isolated canine carotid arteries. Am J Physiol 1988; 255:H783–H788.

25. Rubanyi GM, Freay AD, Johns A, et al. Elevated transmural pressure inhibits the release of EDRF by mechanism(s) similar to high $K^+$ and barium. In: Mulvany MJ, ed. Resistance Arteries, Structure and Function. New York: Elsevier, 1991:226–232.

26. Flavahan NA, Vanhoutte PM. G-protein and endothelial responses. Blood Vessels 1990; 27:218–229.

27. Flavahan NA, Vanhoutte PM. Endothelial cell signaling and endothelial dysfunction. Am J Hypertens 1995; 8:28S–41S.

28. Houston DS, Vanhoutte PM. Platelets and endothelium-dependent responses. In: Vanhoutte PM, ed. Relaxing and Contracting Factors: Biological and Clinical Research. Clifton, NJ: Humana Press, 1988:425–449.

29. Moncada S, Vane JR. Pharmacology and endogenous roles of prostaglandin endoperoxides, thromboxane $A_2$ and prostacyclin. Pharmacol Rev 1979; 30:293–331.

30. Feletou M, Vanhoutte PM. Endothelium-dependent hyperpolarization of canine coronary smooth muscle. Br J Pharmacol 1988; 93:515–524.

31. Komori K, Vanhoutte PM. Endothelium-derived hyperpolarizing factor. Blood Vessels 1990; 27:238–245.

32. Nagao T, Vanhoutte PM. Endothelium-derived hyperpolarizing factor and endothelium-dependent relaxations. Am J Respir Cell Mol Biol 1993; 8:1–6.

33. Nakashima M, Mombouli JV, Taylor AA, Vanhoutte PM. Endothelium-dependent hyperpolarization caused by bradykinin in human coronary arteries. J Clin Invest 1993; 92:2867–2871.

34. Vanhoutte PM. Endothelium-Derived Hyperpolarizing Factor. Harwood Academic Publishers, The Netherlands, 1996. In press.

35. Campbell WB, Gebremedhin D, Pratt PF, Harder DR. Identification of ep-

oxyeicosatrienoic acids as endothelium-derived hyperpolarizing. Circ Res 1996; 78:415–423.

36. Taylor SG, Weston AH. Endothelium-derived hyperpolarizing factor: a new endogenous inhibitor from the vascular endothelium. Trends Pharmacol Sci 1988; 9:272–274.

37. Kilpatrick EV, Cocks TM. Evidence for differential roles of nitric oxide (NO) and hyperpolarization in endothelium-dependent relaxation of pig isolated coronary artery. Br J Pharmacol 1994; 112:557–565.

38. De Mey JG, Vanhoutte PM. Heterogeneous behavior of the canine arterial and venous wall: importance of the endothelium. Circ Res 1982; 5:439–447.

39. Lüscher TF, Vanhoutte PM. Dysfunction of the release of endothelium-derived relaxing factor. In: Simionescu N, Simionescu M, eds. Endothelial Cell Dysfunction. New York: Plenum Press, 1992:65–102.

40. Rubanyi GM, Vanhoutte PM. Hypoxia releases a vasoconstrictor substance from the canine vascular endothelium. J Physiol 1985; 364:45–56.

41. Vanhoutte PM, Rubanyi GM, Miller VM, Houston DS. Modulation of vascular smooth muscle contraction by the endothelium. Ann Rev Physiol 1986; 48:307–320.

42. Rubanyi GM, Vanhoutte PM. Superoxide anions and hyperoxia inactivate endothelium-derived relaxing factor(s). Am J Physiol 1986; 250:H822–H827.

43. Yanagisawa M, Kurihara H, Kimura S, Tomobe Y, Kobayashi M, Mitsui Y, Yasaki Y, Goto K, Masaki T. A novel potent vasoconstrictor peptide produced by vascular endothelial cells. Nature 1988; 332:411–415.

44. Masaki T, Yanagisawa M, Goto K. Physiology and pharmacology of endothelins. Med Res Rev 1992; 12:391–421.

45. Sakurai S, Goto K. Endothelins. Vascular actions and clinical implications. Drugs 1993; 46:795–804.

46. Schini VB, Vanhoutte PM. Endothelin-1: A potent vasoactive peptide. Pharmacol Toxicol 1991; 69:1–7.

47. Vanhoutte PM. Is endothelin involved in the pathogenesis of hypertension? Hypertension 1993; 21:747–751.

48. Shimokawa H, Aarhus LL, Vanhoutte PM. Porcine coronary arteries with regenerated endothelium have a reduced endothelium-dependent responsiveness to aggregating platelets and serotonin. Circ Res 1987; 61:256–270.

49. Shimokawa H, Flavahan NA, Vanhoutte PM. Natural course of the impairment of endothelium-dependent relaxations after balloon endothelial removal in porcine coronary arteries. Possible dysfunction of a pertussis toxin-sensitive G protein. Circ Res 1989; 65:740–753.

50. Borg-Capra C, Fournet-Bourguignon MP, Janiak P, Villeneuve N, Bidouard JP, Vilaine JP, Vanhoutte PM. Morphological heterogeneity with normal expression but altered function of Gi proteins in cultured regenerated porcine coronary endothelial cells. In press.

51. Shimokawa H, Vanhoutte PM. Angiographic demonstration of hyperconstriction induced by serotonin and aggregating platelets in porcine coronary arteries with regenerated endothelium. J Am Coll Cardiol 1991; 17:1197–1202.

52. Shimokawa H, Vanhoutte PM. Impaired endothelium-dependent relaxation to aggregating platelets and related vasoactive substances in porcine coronary arteries in hypercholesterolemia and atherosclerosis. Circ Res 1989; 64: 900–914.

53. Shimokawa H, Flavahan NA, Vanhoutte PM. Loss of endothelial pertussis toxin–sensitive G protein function in atherosclerotic porcine coronary arteries. Circulation 1991; 83:652–660.

54. Kolodgie FD, Virmani R, Rice HE, et al. Vascular reactivity during the progression of atherosclerotic plaque. A study of Watanabe heritable hyperlipidemic rabbits. Circ Res 1990; 66:1112–1126.

55. Kuo L, Davis MJ, Cannon MS, et al. Pathophysiological consequences of atherosclerosis extend into the coronary microcirculation. Circ Res 1992; 70: 465–476.

56. Sellke FW, Armstrong ML, Harrison DG. Endothelium dependent vascular relaxation is abnormal in the coronary microcirculation of atherosclerotic primates. Circulation 1990; 81:1586–1593.

57. Bossaller C, Habib GB, Yamamoto H, et al. Impaired muscarinic endothelium-dependent relaxation and cyclic guanosine 5′ monophosphate formation on an atherosclerotic human coronary artery and rabbit aorta. J Clin Invest 1987; 79:170–174.

58. Föstermann U, Mügge A, Alheid U, et al. Selective attenuation of endothelium-mediated vasodilation in atherosclerotic human coronary arteries. Circ Res 1988; 62:185–190.

59. Ludmer PL, Selwyn AP, Shook TL, et al. Paradoxical vasoconstriction induced by acetylcholine in atherosclerotic coronary arteries. N Engl J Med 1986; 315:1046–1051.

60. Hodgson JM, Marshall JJ. Direct vasoconstriction and endothelium-dependent vasodilation: mechanisms of acetylcholine effects on coronary flow and arterial diameter in patients with nonstenotic coronary arteries. Circulation 1989; 79: 1043–1051.

61. Collins P, Burman J, Chung HI, et al. Hemoglobin inhibits endothelium-dependent relaxation to acetylcholine in human coronary arteries in vivo. Circulation 1993; 87:80–85.

62. Lefroy DC, Crake T, Uren NG, et al. Effect of inhibition of NO synthesis on epicardial coronary artery caliber and coronary blood flow in humans. Circulation 1993; 88:43–54.

63. Gollino P, Piscione F, Willerson JT, et al. Divergent effects of serotonin on coronary artery dimensions and blood flow in patients with coronary atherosclerosis and control patients. N Engl J Med 1991; 324:641–648.

64. Nabel EG, Ganz P, Gordon JB et al. Dilation of normal and constriction of atherosclerotic coronary arteries caused by the cold pressor test. Circulation 1988; 77:43–52.

65. Nabel EG, Selwyn AP, Ganz P. Large coronary arteries in humans are responsive to changing blood flow: an endothelium-dependent mechanism that fails in patients with atherosclerosis. J Am Coll Cardiol 1990; 16:349–356.

66. Drexler H, Zeiher AM, Wollschlager H, et al. Flow-dependent coronary artery dilatation in humans. Circulation 1989; 80:466–474.
67. Gordon JB, Ganz P, Nabel EG, et al. Atherosclerosis influences the vasomotor response of epicardial coronary arteries to exercise. J Clin Invest 1989; 83: 1946–1952.
68. Cox DA, Vita JA, Treasure CB, et al. Atherosclerosis impairs flow-mediated dilation of coronary arteries humans. Circulation 1989; 80:458–465.
69. Vita JA, Treasure CB, Ganz P, et al. Control of shear stress in the epicardial coronary arteries of humans: impairment by atherosclerosis. J Am Coll Cardiol 1989; 14:1193–1199.
70. Vita JA, Treasure CB, Nabel EG, et al. Coronary vasomotor response to acetylcholine relates to risk factors for coronary artery disease. Circulation 1990; 81:491–497.
71. Zeiher AM, Drexler H, Wollschlaeger H, et al. Coronary vasomotion in response to sympathetic stimulation in humans: importance of the functional integrity of the endothelium. J Am Coll Cardiol 1989; 14:1181–1190.
72. Yeung AC, Vekshtein VI, Krantz DS, et al. The effect of atherosclerosis on the vasomotor response of coronary arteries to mental stress. N Engl J Med 1991; 325:1551–1556.
73. Mc Lenachan JM, Williams JK, Fish RD, et al. Loss of flow-mediated endothelium-dependent dilation occurs early in the development of atherosclerosis. Circulation 1991; 84:1273–1278.
74. Reddy KG, Nair R, Sheehan HM, et al. Evidence that selective endothelial dysfunction may occur in the absence of angiographic or ultrasound atherosclerosis in patients with risk factors for atherosclerosis. J Am Coll Cardiol 1994; 23:833–843.
75. Mc Lenachan JM, Vita J, Fish DR, et al. Early evidence of endothelial vasodilator dysfunction at coronary branch points. Circulation 1990; 82: 1169–1173.
76. Creager MA, Cooke JP, Mendelsohn ME, et al. Impaired vasodilation of forearm resistance vessels in hypercholesterolemic humans. J Clin Invest 1990; 86:228–234.
77. Celermajer DS, Soresnsen KE, Gooch VM, et al. Noninvasive detection of endothelial dysfunction in children and adults at risk of atherosclerosis. Lancet 1992; 340:1111–1115.
78. Drexler H, Zeiher AM, Meinzer K, et al. Correction of endothelial dysfunction in coronary microcirculation of hypercholesterolemic patients by L-arginine. Lancet 1991; 338:1546–1550.
79. Creager MA, Roddy MA, Coleman SM, Dzau VJ. The effect of ACE inhibition on endothelium-dependent vasodilatation in hypertension. J Vasc Res 1992; 29:97–98.
80. Harrison DG. Alteration of vasomotor regulation in atherosclerosis. Cardiovasc Drugs Ther 1995; 9:55–63.
81. Cooke JP, Andon NA, Girerd XJ, et al. Arginine restores cholinergic relaxation of hypercholesterolemic rabbit aorta. Circulation 1991; 83:1057–1062.

82. Girerd XJ, Hirsch AT, Cooke JP, et al. Arginine augments endothelium-dependent vasodilatation in cholesterol-fed rabbit. Circ Res 1990; 67:1301–1308.

83. T. Shibano, J. Codina, L. Birnbaumer, and P.M. Vanhoutte. Pertussis toxin-sensitive G-proteins in regenerated endothelial cells after balloon denudation of porcine coronary artery. Am J Physiol 1994; 267:H979–H981.

84. Cox DA and Cohen ML. Effects of oxidized low-density lipoprotein on vascular contraction and relaxation: clinical and pharmacological implications in atherosclerosis. Pharmacol Rev 1996; 48:3–19.

85. Linder L, Kiowski W, Buhler FR, Luscher TF. Indirect evidence for release of endothelium-derived relaxing factor in human forearm circulation in vivo: blunted responses in essential hypertension. Circ Res 1990; 81:1762–1767.

86. Panza JA, Quyyumi AA, Brosh JE Jr, et al. Abnormal endothelium-dependent vascular relaxation in patients with essential hypertension. N Engl J Med 1990; 323:22–27.

87. Taddei S, Vordos A, Mattei P, et al. Vasodilatation to acetylcholine in primary and secondary forms of human hypertension. Hypertension 1993; 21:929–933.

88. Calver A, Collier J, Moncada S, Vallance P. Effect of local intraarterial $N^G$-monomethyl-L-arginine in patients with hypertension: the nitric oxide dilator mechanism appears abnormal. J Hypertens 1992; 10:1025–1031.

89. Panza JA, Casino PR, Kilcoyne CM, et al. Role of endothelium-derived nitric oxide in the abnormal endothelium-dependent vascular relaxation of patients with essential hypertension. Circulation 1993; 87:1468–1474.

90. Lyons D, Webster J, Benjamen N. The effect of antihypertensive therapy on responsiveness to local intra-arterial $N^G$-monomethyl-L-arginine in patients with essential hypertension. J Hypertens 1994; 12:1047–1052.

91. Auch-Schwelk W, Katusic ZS, Vanhoutte PM. Nitric oxide inactivates endothelium-derived contracting factor in the rat aorta. Hypertension 1992; 19:442–445.

92. Ge T, Hughes H, Junquero DC, Wu KK, Vanhoutte PM, Boulanger CM. Endothelium-dependent contractions are associated with both augmented expression of prostaglandin H synthase-1 and by sensitivity to prostaglandin $H_2$ in the SHR aorta. Circ Res 1995; 76:1003–1010.

93. Taddei S, Vanhoutte PM. Endothelium-dependent contractions to endothelin in the rat aorta are mediated by thromboxane $A_2$. J Cardiovasc Pharmacol 1993; 22(suppl 8):S328–S331.

94. Kaiser L, Spickard RC, Olivier NB. Heart failure depresses endothelium-dependent responses in canine femoral artery. Am J Physiol 1989; 256:H962–967.

95. Buikema H, Van Gilst WH, Van Veldhuisen DJ, de Smet BJ, Scholtens E, Lie KI, Wesseling H. Endothelium-dependent relaxation in two different models of chronic heart failure and the effect of ibopamine. Cardiovasc Res 1993; 27:2118–2124.

96. Wang J, Seyedi N, Xu XB, Wolin MS, and Hintze TH. Defective endothelium-mediated control of coronary circulation in conscious dogs after heart failure. Am J Physiol 1994; 266:H670–H680.

97. Ueno M, Kawashima S, Tsumoto S, Morita M, Iwasaki T. Impaired endothelium-dependent vasodilatory responses in hindlimb blood flow in dogs with congestive heart failure. Jpn Circ J 1994; 58:778–786.

98. 25. Kubo SH, Rector TS, Bank AJ, Williams RE, Heifetz SM. Endothelium-dependent vasodilation is attenuated in patients with heart failure. Circulation 1991; 84:1589–1596.

99. Katz SD, Biasucci L, Sabba C, Strom JA, Jondeau G, Galvao M, Solomon S, Nikolic SD, Forman R, Le Jemtel TH. Impaired endothelium-mediated vasodilation in the peripheral vasculature of patients with congestive heart failure. J Am Coll Cardiol 1992; 19:918–925.

100. Hirooka Y, Imaizumi T, Tagawa T, Shiramoto M, Endo T, Ando S, Takeshita A. Effects of L-arginine on impaired acetylcholine-induced and ischemic vasodilation of the forearm in patients with heart failure. Circulation 1994; 90:658–668.

101. Drexler H, Hayoz D, Munzel T, Just H, Zelis R, Brunner HR. Endothelial function in congestive heart failure. Am Heart J 1993; 126:761–764.

102. Drexler H, Hayoz D, Munzel T, Just H, Zelis R, Brunner HR. Endothelium dysfunction in chronic heart failure. Experimental and clinical studies. Arznei-mittelforschung 1994; 44:455–458.

103. Drexler H. Endothelial dysfunction in heart failure and potential for reversal by ACE inhibition. Br Heart J. 1994; 72:S11–S14.

104. Hayoz DH, Drexler T, Munzel B, Hornig AH, Zeiher H, Just HR, Brunner R, Zelis R. Flow mediated arterial dilation is abnormal in congestive heart failure. Circulation 1993; 87:92–96.

105. Ramsey MW, Goodfellow J, Jones CJH, Luddington LA, Lewis MJ, Henderson AH. Endothelial control of arterial distensibility is impaired in chronic heart failure. Circulation 1995; 92:3212–3219.

106. Giannattasio C, Failla M, Stella ML, Mangoni AA, Carugo S, Pozzi M, Grassi G, Mancia G. Alterations of radial artery compliance in patients with congestive heart failure. Am J Cardiol 1995; 76:381–385.

107. Stewart DJ. Endothelin in cardiopulmonary disease: factor paracrine vs neurohumoral. Eur Heart J 1993; 14:48–54.

108. Stevenson LW, Fonarow GC. Endothelin and the vascular choir in heart failure. J Am Coll Cardiol 1992; 20:854–857.

109. Katz SD, Schwartz M, Yuen J, Le Jemtel TH. Impaired acetylcholine-mediated vasodilation in patients with congestive heart failure. Role of endothelium-derived vasodilating and vasoconstricting factors. Circulation 1993; 88:55–61.

110. Nakamura M, Ishikawa M, Funakoshi T, Hashimoto K, Chiba M, Hiramori K. Attenuated endothelium-dependent peripheral vasodilation and clinical characteristics in patients with chronic heart failure. Am Heart J 1994; 128:1164–1169.

111. Nakamura M, Funakoshi T, Arakawa N, Yoshida H, Makita S, Hiramori K. Effect of angiotensin-converting enzyme inhibitors on endothelium-dependent peripheral vasodilation in patients with chronic heart failure. J Am Coll Cardiol 1994; 24:1321–1327.

112. Kanai AJ, Strauss HC, Truskey GA, Crews AL, Grunfeld S, Malinski T, Shear stress induces ATP-independent transient nitric oxide release from vascular endothelial cells, measured directly with a porphyrinic microsensor. Circ Res 1995; 77:284–293.
113. Noris M, Morigi M, Donadelli R, Aiello S, Foppolo M, Todeschini M, Orisio S, Remuzzi G, Remuzzi A. Nitric oxide synthesis by cultured endothelial cells is modulated by flow conditions. Circ Res 1995; 76:536–543.
114. Boulanger C, Lüscher TF. Release of endothelin from the porcine aorta. Inhibition by endothelium-derived nitric oxide. J Clin Invest 1990; 85:587–590.

# 10

# Complement and Endothelium: Novel Complement-Inhibitory Therapeutics

## Una S. Ryan

*T Cell Sciences, Inc., Needham, Massachusetts*

## I.  INTRODUCTION

The role of inflammatory mechanisms in vascular disease is becoming increasingly well recognized, whereas the role of immunological processes is only beginning to be uncovered. In fact, inflammatory and immune processes form a continuum, and whether one looks at acute inflammatory or ischemic damage to the vasculature, or longer term proliferative and remodeling events, it is clear that complement is a key culprit and that endothelium is a key target.

Activation of complement triggers a plethora of cellular and molecular interactions resulting in cell and tissue damage as well as inducing inflammatory responses. Activation of the endothelium leads to the release of mediators, growth factors, and upregulation of adhesion molecules. The downstream consequences represent a vast amplification of the original injurious stimuli and set in motion all of the major blood enzyme cascades resulting in thrombosis, coagulation, and ultimately loss of endothelial integrity. Thus, activation of complement and activation of the endothelium provide critical targets for therapeutic intervention in a wide variety of life-threatening disorders.

## II. ROLE OF COMPLEMENT IN THE HUMORAL IMMUNE SYSTEM

The complement system is an integral part of the body's humoral defense mechanism and also a primary mediator of the inflammatory process. The complement system consists of approximately 30 proteins, most of which circulate in the plasma in an inactive form and some of which are membrane-bound regulators. Activation of complement results in a cascade of interactions between the various protein components of the system, leading to the generation of products that possess important biological activities. Certain components of the activated system serve an opsonic function, coating bacteria and immune complexes and thereby facilitating their ingestion by phagocytic cells such as neutrophils or macrophages. Other products of the complement cascade promote leukocyte activation and chemotaxis through receptor-mediated mechanisms. Finally, the late-acting components of the activated system form a macromolecular complex that is cytotoxic to bacteria, fungi, parasites, virus-infected cells, and tumor cells. However, the ability of the complement system to recognize foreignness or nonself can unfortunately also turn it against innocent bystander host cells. When inappropriately or chronically activated, the complement system can be as powerful in promoting injury as it is when acting in the body's defense.

## III. ROLE OF COMPLEMENT IN VASCULAR INJURY AND DISEASE

Complement activation is a critical event in many acute inflammatory responses that subsequently lead to cellular and tissue damage. Products of complement activation cause degranulation of phagocytic cells, mast cells, and basophils, smooth muscle contraction, and increases in vascular permeability. C1q, a component of C1, the first step in the classical pathway, promotes cell adhesion and activation. C4, the second component to be activated in the classical pathway, influences antigen clearance and antibody responses. Activation of the complement cascade by either the classical or alternative pathways leads to the cleaving of C3 and then of C5 into their biologically active cleavage products. The smaller cleavage products, C3a and C5a, are extremely potent proinflammatory mediators. Both C3a and C5a cause histamine release from mast cells and basophils, contraction of smooth muscle, and increased permeability of vessels. C5a also activates endothelial cells and amplifies the inflammatory response by its ability to act as a chemoattractant and by its ability to induce oxygen radical formation. Activation of C3 and C5 via their respective convertases leads to the completion of the complement cascade and generation of C5b-9, the cytolytic membrane attack complex. Nonlytic amounts of C5b-9 can also activate proinflammatory cell functions. All of these actions of complement are described in more detail below in terms of their specific effects on individual cell types.

Any tissue of organ subjected to critical ischemia is at risk for increased tissue damage upon reperfusion with oxygenated whole blood. Although reperfusion of ischemic tissue is vital for the maintenance of cellular viability, it may also contribute to the extension of tissue injury. This phenomenon, referred to as reperfusion injury, may occur in a variety of clinical situations in which blood flow is restored after a period of ischemia. These conditions occur in the myocardium following coronary thrombolysis or coronary angioplasty and also during coronary artery bypass grafting and myocardial transplant procedures. Many efforts to eleviate reperfusion injury have focused on the role of reactive oxygen species and neutrophil-dependent inflammatory processes. Evidence also suggests that activation of the complement system contributes significantly to myocardial tissue damage induced by ischemia-reperfusion. For example, deposition of the terminal complement components is found to a greater degree in infarcted versus noninfarcted areas of the myocardium (1). Depletion of circulating complement components reduces neutrophil infiltration into the ischemic tissue and reduces ischemia induced myocardial injury in experiment animals (2–4). It is now widely accepted that three major components can be recognized as contributing to the phenomenon of reperfusion injury: molecular oxygen, neutrophils, and components of the activated complement system. All three probably act in concert, since complement components such as C5a activate neutrophils causing them to release proteases and generate toxic metabolites of oxygen. In fact, activation of complement has been shown in a number of in vitro and in vivo models to be the initiating event leading to release of toxic oxygen metabolites and recruitment of neutrophils.

The contribution of the complement system to myocardial injury is multifaceted. Generation of the anaphylatoxins is intimately related to the activation of neutrophils and the release of oxygen radicals. However, the potential exists for the complement system to induce tissue destruction directly via the formation of the cytolytic membrane attack complex (MAC, C5b-9) independent of oxygen metabolite production and neutrophil activation. Thus, effective inhibitors of complement activation should be able to reduce both inflammatory events and their sequelae as well as to reduce direct myocardial cell killing and thus attenuating both infarct size and area at risk (penumbra). The failure to consider the direct cytotoxic effects of complement activation may explain some of the controversy surrounding the efficacy of antioxidants (5–11). Thus, it is not surprising that myocardial infarction provides opportunities for investigating the use of complement inhibitions in animal models and in the clinic.

There is now abundant evidence that complement is involved in the rejection of vascularized organs following transplantation in addition to the contributions of complement activation and specific complement components to inflammation and ischemia-reperfusion, both of which processes accompany organ transplantation. The most striking examples of complement-mediated contributions to the rejection process are seen in the rejection of hypersensitized organs and in the hyperacute rejection of xenografts between discordant species. The role of complement in organ transplantation has been reviewed extensively elsewhere, including the detrimental effects of complement on both allografts and xenografts (12–16).

## IV.    COMPLEMENT EFFECTS ON ENDOTHELIAL CELLS AND PLATELETS

In the resting situation, normal endothelial cells maintain a barrier between cells and molecules of the vascular lumen and those of the organ parenchyma. Resting endothelial cells actively resist thrombosis via molecules such as thrombomodulin, antithrombin-III, tissue factor pathway inhibitor, and ADPase. Heparan sulfate on the endothelial surface binds endothelial cell superoxide dismutase, thus promoting antioxidant activities of the endothelium. Following injury, the situation changes dramatically. Inflammation, ischemia-reperfusion, and hyperacute rejection represent examples of injuries to the vasculature that lead to major, often irreversible, cell and tissue injury initiated via complement-mediated mechanisms. As shown in Figure 1, activation of complement in turn activates the endothelium, which causes disruption of endothelial junctions resulting in edema and hemorrhage and upregulation of adhesion molecules, leading to exacerbated inflammatory processes. This process also exposes subendothelial procoagulant surfaces to platelets which adhere by the interaction of platelet receptor gpIb and von Willebrand factor (vWF). Platelet binding to C1q or vWF associated with the exposed subendothelial matrix could result in the activation of the platelet receptor gpIIbIIIa with expression of P-selectin and procoagulant activity on the platelets (17). Surface expression of the adhesion molecule P-selectin promotes the interaction of platelets and leukocytes (18) resulting in tissue factor expression on monocytes following direct adhesive contact (19). The production of superoxide anion and other reactive oxygen species could be enhanced through the interaction of P-selectin and sialyl-Lewis$^x$ (sLeX) carbohydrate antigen, as has been demonstrated in vitro (20). In turn, these events would result in

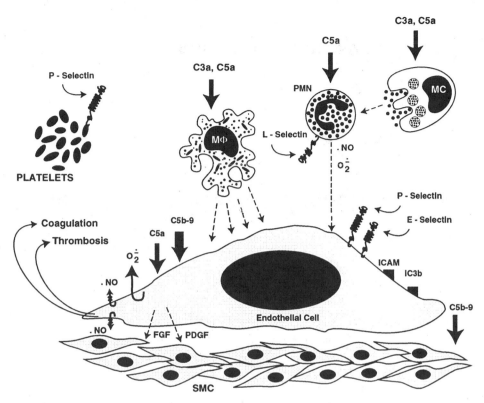

**Figure 1** Complement-mediated responses that are inhibited by soluble complement receptor type 1 (sCR1). Active fragments released during complement activation, such as anaphylatoxins C3a and C5a, lead to the release of cytokines and other
inflammatory mediators (dashed lines) from leukocytes and endothelial cells, as
well as upregulation of adhesion molecules. The terminal complex (C5b-9) also has
prelytic, agonist-like, effects on endothelial cells leading to procoagulant and
prothrombotic states and downregulation or destruction of nitric oxide. C5b-9–
stimulated release of growth factors, such as basic fibroblast growth factor (bFGF)
and platelet-derived growth factor (PDGF), might be expected to mediate longer
term responses such as smooth muscle and fibroblast hyperplasia. All these effects
of prolonged or inappropriate complement activation are injurious; all are amelio-
rated by treatment with sCR1. New complement inhibitors currently being developed, such as soluble complement receptor type 1—sialyl Lewis$^x$ (sCR1sLe$^x$) (see
Fig. 2), bind to selectins, thus targeting complement inhibition to sites where it is
most needed (e.g., activated endothelium), and blocking endothelial-neutrophil
and neutrophil-platelet adhesive interactions. (From ref. 16.)

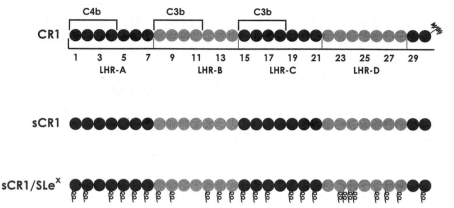

**Figure 2** (Top) Erythrocyte-bound complement receptor 1 (CR1) with its four long homogolous repeats (LHR) binds to immune complexes bearing C3b and C4b, thereby clearing them from the circulation in a process known as immune adherence. (Center) The therapeutic drug candidate TP10 (soluble complement receptor 1, sCR1) has been truncated before the transmembrane portion. Like CR1, sCR1 inhibits both complement pathways by binding to C4b and C3b (see Fig. 3). (Bottom)-sLe$^x$/sCR1, a version of sCR1 bearing sialylated Lewis$^x$ glycosylation (β), binds selectively to sites of selectin upregulation (i.e., activated endothelial cells and platelets) to inhibit complement and prevent neutrophil adhesion. (From ref. 15.)

further endothelial activation and consequent thrombosis (21). Thus, the immediate effects of complement activity on the endothelial surface result in the loss of barrier function and an upregulation of procoagulant and prothrombotic mechanisms as well as the initiation of downstream inflammatory amplification loops.

Activation of the complement cascade by either the classical or alternative pathway first leads to cleavage of C3 and then of C5 into biologically active products. The smaller cleavage products (anaphylatoxins C3a and C5a) are extremely potent proinflammatory mediators. Both C3a and C5a dramatically increase vascular permeability, trigger the release of histamine from mast cells and basophils, and stimulate smooth muscle contraction. C5a activates endothelial cells (22,23), although C5a receptors on endothelial cells are expressed at low density (24). Endothelial activation results in the release of heparan sulfate (22), synthesis of tissue factor (25), secretion of vWF from Weibel-Palade bodies, and transient expression of P-selectin (24). The acute consequences of endothelial cell activation, in the context of inflammation, ischemia-reperfusion, or transplant rejection, are dire. Fibrin deposition and augmented thrombin-mediated platelet aggrega-

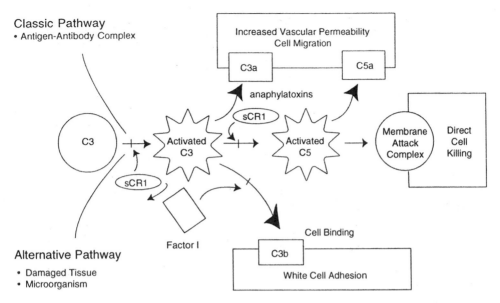

**Figure 3** TP10 (sCR1) inhibits both classical and alternative pathways of complement inhibition. The mechanism of action of TP10 is via inhibition of the C3 and C5 convertases preventing assembly of the MAC and release of C3a and C5a. It also acts as a cofactor for factor I and prevents deposition of C3b (see text). Thus, sCR1 inhibits the tissue-damaging and proinflammatory actions of complement and is not consumed in the process. (From ref. 15.)

tion together with edema and hemorrhage all serve to limit the function and viability of the affected organ or tissue.

The terminal effector phase of complement activation results in the formation and deposition of the membrane attack complex (MAC, C5b-9), a pore-forming complex of multiple complement components (C5b, C6, C7, C8, and C9). C5b-9 assembly on cell membranes causes ion and water fluxes that ultimately lead to cell death by lysis. Sublytic deposition of C5b-9 and consequent cytosolic ionic changes may initiate signaling cascades that activate a variety of proinflammatory responses (26), including the release of reactive oxygen metabolites, the production of prostaglandins and leukotrienes, and the secretion of cytokines, including interleukin-1 (IL-1) and IL-6. Insertion of C5b-9 causes a rapid fusion of cytoplasmic granules with the endothelial cell membrane exposing P-selectin to interact with platelets, neutrophils, and monocytes in the circulation (27). In addition, the vesiculation of the plasma membrane exposes a catalytic surface on vascular endothelial cells for assembly of the prothrombinase enzyme complex that can contribute to fibrin deposition associated with acute immune endothelial injury (28). Platelet aggregation and activation can be augmented by C5b-9 deposition on platelets (29). C5b-9–activated platelets also increase thromboxane synthesis, secrete storage granule contents, and express procoagulant activity. The involvement of platelets in vascular injury has been demonstrated in association with hyperacute rejection phenomena (30), and the contribution of platelets to accelerated atherosclerosis and chronic rejection is widely accepted. Through the action of C5b-9, complement activates a wide range of cell types, circumventing any requirement for a specific receptor-ligand interaction. Thus, the formation of the terminal complement complex can lead to endothelial cell destruction and at sublytic levels can trigger responses which mimic the effects of endothelial cell and platelet agonists.

## V.  COMPLEMENT EFFECTS ON LEUKOCYTES

Anaphylatoxin C5a is a powerful chemoattractant for granulocytes (eosinophils and basophils as well as neutrophils) and monocytes. C5a activates these cells and causes enzyme release by granulocytes (31,32), cytokine (IL-1, IL-6, IL-8, and [TNFα]) production by monocytes (33–35), and upregulation of the complement receptor type 1 (CR1) and type 3 (CR3) (36,37). C3a activates basophils (38) and eosinophils which may in turn activate neutrophils (39). The release of proinflammatory cytokines amplifies downstream adhesion and activation events, augments the proliferative responses of T lymphocytes, and enhances antibody production by B lymphocytes. The role of T cells in vascular disease is not fully understood, but the presence of T cells in vascular lesions has been well documented (40). C3b and its inactive product, iC3b, can serve as accessory adhesion molecules strengthening the contact between target and effector cells expressing CR1 and CR3 (41). CR3 (CD11b/CD18) is a member of the leukocyte integrin family and binds to fibrinogen, factor X, and β-glucan as well as iC3b (42,43). C5a activation of neutrophils and monocytes not only enhances CR1 and CR3 attachment to fixed C3b and iC3b but also exposes a binding site in CR3 for intracellular adhesion molecule-1 (ICAM-1) (44); the latter is known to be upregulated by inflammation, reperfusion following ischemia, and during transplant rejection (45–50). C5a also upregulates the leukocyte adhesion molecules CR4 (CD11c/CD18) and LFA-1 (CD11a/CD18) that bind to iC3b and ICAM-1, ICAM-2, and ICAM-3. Thus, C5a promotes adherence to endothelial cells and extravasation of monocytes and neutrophils.

Fc receptors (FcR) are coexpressed with receptors for iC3b, C3b, and C1q on monocytes, macrophages, neutrophils, platelets, and some lymphocytes. C5a upregulates monocyte expression of both CR1 and FcR (51), further increasing their potential contribution to target cell destruction. Engagement of FcR on macrophages increases their secretion of C3 at the site of inflammation (52). Thus, the activation of complement augments inflammatory injury. For example, allograft infiltrates containing large numbers of macrophages expressing both FcR and complement receptors have been correlated with severe rejection episodes in clinical biopsies (53) and animal models (54).

## VI. EFFECTS OF COMPLEMENT ON VASCULAR CELL PROLIFERATION

When allowed to proceed to completion, activation of the complement system can inflict severe damage to endothelial cells (in fact to cells and tissues in general) via insertion of C5b-9 and subsequent induction of cell lysis. At sublytic levels of C5b-9, the effects of complement activation can target a wide range of cells without the need for specific receptor-ligand interactions. Taken together, components of the complement system trigger or amplify numerous inflammatory processes largely mediated via the actions of the anaphylatoxins, C3a and C5a, in adherence and activation reactions (see Fig. 1). Similar recruitment and activation of key cellular components to damaged vascular wall cells are mediated by C1q, C3b, and C5b-9. The activation of platelets and the coagulation cascade are constant features of injured blood vessels and frequently are the final step contributing to irreversible organ failure. Ongoing complement activation would tend to perpetuate these responses. Whether acute inflammation leads to chronic inflammatory problems or how the acute effects of ischemia-reperfusion damage might predict a chronic outcome in the transplant situation is not known.

Assembly of C5b-9 on cell membranes can induce reversible changes in membrane permeability resulting in transient intracellular ionic changes in the absence of cell lysis. Ion fluxes and cytosolic ionic changes are integral steps in the signaling cascade initiated when growth factors bind to their receptors. It has been shown that C5b-9 induces reversible changes in membrane permeability that stimulate cell proliferation in 3T3 cells and also in vascular smooth muscle cells and fibroblasts (55). C5b-9 can stimulate cell proliferation in the absence of other exogenous growth factors, but it also can enhance the mitogenic effects of serum and platelet-derived growth factor (PDGF). Thus, the induction of mitogenesis represents a novel effect of the terminal complement complex that could contribute to focal tissue repair or pathological cell proliferation locally at sites of complement activation (55). Furthermore, insertion of C5b-9 into the endothelial cell membrane leads to the release of PDGF and basic fibroblast growth factor (bFGF) (56). These potent mitogens may contribute to chronic proliferative changes in vascular wall cells. Thus, complement activation, in particular the effects of sublytic C5b-9 on endothelial cells, leads to the proliferation of smooth muscle cells and fibroblasts in ways that could cause or contribute to the accelerated atherosclerosis seen in successful heart transplants and could contribute to restenosis following angioplasty (57). Furthermore, fibroblasia is a common outcome of chronic inflammation, and similar processes could contribute to the obliterative broncholitis that is a common problem following lung transplantation.

In view of the multiplicity of the effects of complement activation and the downstream amplification of these effects, an inhibitor of complement activation likely to be useful in the clinical arena should be able to block the proinflammatory consequences of complement activation driven by the anaphylatoxins, C3a and C5a, as well as the tissue-damaging and procoagulant effects of complement, largely driven by C5b-9. Whether the longer term proliferative responses to C5b-9 could be inhibited by blocking acute responses remains to be evaluated.

## VII. COMPLEMENT INHIBITION BY sCR1

Human complement receptor 1 (CR1) (C3b/C4b receptor; CD35) is a single-chain, cell surface glycoprotein found on erythrocytes, some T lymphocytes, all mature B lymphocytes, neutrophils, eosinophils, basophils, monocytes/macrophages, glomerular podocytes, and follicular dendritic cells (58). CR1 is also found circulating as a soluble form in plasma at low concentrations (59). Most CR1 is found at low levels on erythrocytes where it serves to clear immune complexes bearing C3b and C4b from the circulation in a process known as immune adherence (60). CR1 on neutrophils and macrophages mediates phagocytosis of opsonized immune complexes, particles, or cells (61). CR1 on lymphocytes and follicular dendritic cells appears to facilitate antibody responses and antigen presentation (62). In some cases, the interaction of the C3b or C4b with CR1 may be involved in cellular activation (63,64).

Soluble complement receptor 1 (sCR1) is a soluble form of the most common allotype of CR1 which lacks the transmembrane and cytoplasmic protein domains (65; Fig. 2). The resulting soluble complement receptor type 1 (sCR1) was expressed by Chinese hamster ovary cells and shown to retain all the known activities of the native, cell surface receptor. sCR1 was demonstrated in vitro to be a potent and selective inhibitor of both the classical and alternative complement pathways and to block proinflammatory consequences of complement activation; namely, the generation of

**Table 1** TP10 in Animal Models of Lung Injury

| Induced By | Species | Reference |
|---|---|---|
| Burns | Rat | 72 |
| Burns, CVF or IgG-IC | Rat | 73 |
| IgA-IC | Rat | 74 |
| Immune complexes | Guinea pig | 75 |
| Intestinal ischemia | Rat | 76 |
| Hindlimb ischemia | Rat | 30 |
| PAF/LPS | Rat | 77 |
| IL-2 | Rat | 78 |
| Cardiopulmonary bypass | Pig | 79 |

**Table 2** TP10 in Models of Ischemia-Reperfusion Injury

| Ischemic organ | Species | Reference |
|---|---|---|
| Heart | Rat | 80 |
| | | 65 |
| | | 81 |
| | | 82 |
| Skeletal muscle | Rat | 30 |
| Skeletal muscle | Mouse | 83 |
| Kidney | Rat | 84 |
| Liver | Rat | 85 |
| Intestine | Rat | 76 |
| Brain (trauma) | Rat | 86 |

C3a, C5a, and C5b-9. Furthermore, by serving as a cofactor for factor I, sCR1 facilitates the degradation of C3b and C4b to inactive forms which no longer bind sCR1, releasing it to recycle in the inhibitory process (66; Fig. 3).

The cofactor activity of sCR1, like the soluble regulatory protein factor H, makes possible the factor I cleavage of C3b to iC3b and of C4b to iC4b. Unlike factor H, however, sCR1 can also serve as a cofactor for the further cleavage by factor I of iC3b to C3dg and iC4b to C4d. Thus, sCR1 is capable of degrading the ligands for CR1 and CR3 expressed on macrophages and neutrophils which may mitigate cellular inflammatory responses. Like CR1, sCR1 possesses both convertase decay-accelerating activity and factor I cofactor activity in both the classical and alternative complement pathways.

The sequence homology of complement proteins has by and large been well conserved throughout evolution. The fact that sCR1, which is derived

**Table 3**  TP10 in Animal Models of Transplantation

| Graft | Recipient | Reference |
|---|---|---|
| Syngeneic rat lung | Rat | 87 |
| Allogeneic rat kidney | Rat | 88 |
| Allogeneic rat heart sensitized | Rat | 89 |
| Guinea pig heart | Rat | 90 |
| | | 91 |
| | | 92 |
| | | 93 |
| | | 94 |
| | | 95 |
| | | 96 |
| | | 97 |
| Guinea pig kidney | Rat | 98 |
| Pig heart | Monkey | 99 |
| | | 100 |
| | | 101 |

from a human gene product, retains significant regulatory activity for many nonhuman complement systems has allowed the evaluation of complement inhibition by sCR1 in a wide variety of animal species, including rats, guinea pigs, mice, pigs, and monkeys.

sCR1 has now been shown to ameliorate structural or functional damage in a wide variety of animal models of disease. These fall into the broad categories of inflammation, especially lung injury (Table 1); models of ischemia and reperfusion (Table 2); models of organ transplant rejection, especially hyperacute rejection (Table 3); and in a variety of other animal models, including cardiopulmonary bypass, reverse passive arthus, glomerulonephritis, rheumatoid arthritis, hemodialysis, traumatic brain injury, and aspiration-induced lung injury.

## VIII.  CLINICAL OPPORTUNITIES FOR COMPLEMENT–INHIBITOR THERAPEUTICS

Studies of the role of complement in disease models are no longer dependent on complement depletion using cobra venom factor, the use of animals deficient in one or more complement components, or complement knockout mice (67). sCR1 provides the first opportunity to examine C inhibition in the clinic, and it has been given the product name TP10 (T Cell Sciences, Inc.). The list of specific complement inhibitors now reported, in addition to sCR1, includes soluble decay-accelerating factor (68), anti-C5 monoclonal antibody (69), and C1-INH. In addition, complement inhibitors with specific targeting abilities and added function (sCR1/sLe$^x$) or with the ability to inhibit either the classical or alternative pathway C1-INH and (sCR1-desLHRa) (70), respectively, are becoming available.

The need for a clinically useful complement inhibitor is great. For many acute indications, inhibitors of both pathways will be required, whereas for certain diseases, inhibitors of one pathway (e.g., the classical pathway in Alzheimer's disease) may be ideal. In the future, small molecule complement inhibitors with possibilities for chronic dosing and the ability to access specific sites may be desirable.

Clinical trials of TP10 designed to assess safety and pharmacokinetics have demonstrated that in patients at risk of adult respiratory disease syndrome (ARDS), there were no adverse events attributed to TP10, and the half-life of the drug was over 30 hr. Complement inhibition was reduced in a dose-dependent fashion. Thus, TP10 appears to be safe and well tolerated in this group of patients (71). Similarly, a phase I safety trial of TP10 in patients with first-time myocardial infarction indicated a safety and pharmacokinetic profile well suited for administration to this group of patients. The trial included patients receiving thrombolytics and those scheduled for angioplasty (percutaneous transluminal coronary angioplasty [PTCA]). It will now be necessary to assess whether TP10, the first of the complement-inhibitor therapeutics to be used in the clinic, will provide benefits to patients with these and other complement-mediated disorders.

## REFERENCES

1. Hugo F, Hamdoch T, Mathey D, Schafer H, Bhakdi S. Quantiative measurement of SC5b-9 and C5b-9(m) in infarcted areas of human myocardium. Clin Exp Immunol 1990; 81:132–136.
2. Maroko PR, Carpenter CB, Chiariello M, Fishbein MC, Radvany P, et al. Reduction by cobra venom factor of myocardial necrosis after coronary artery occlusion. J Clin Invest 1978; 61:661–670.
3. Pinckard RN, O'Rourke RA, Crawford MH, Grover FS, McManus LM, et al. Complement localization and mediation of ischemic injury in baboon myocardium. J Clin Invest 1980; 66:1050–1056.
4. Crawford MH, Grover FL, Dolb WP, McMahan CA, O'Rourke RA, et al. Complement and neutrophil activation in the pathogenesis of ischemic myocardial injury. Circulation 1988; 78:1449–1458.
5. Lucchesi BR, Mullane KM. Leukocytes and ischemia-induced myocardial injury. Annu Rev Pharmacol Toxicol 1986; 26:201–224.
6. McCord JM. Oxygen-derived free radicals in postischemic tissue injury. N Engl J Med 1996; 312:159–163.

7. Lucchesi BR. Modulation of leukocyte-mediated myocardial reperfusion injury. Annu Rev Physiol 1990; 52:561–576.

8. Lucchesi BR, Werns SW, Fantone JC. The role of neutrophil and free radicals in ischemic myocardial injury. J Mol Cell Cardiol 1989; 12:1241–1251.

9. Reimer KA, Murray CE, Richard VJ. The role of neutrophils and free radicals in the ischemic-reperfused heart: why the confusion and controversy? J Mol Cell Cardiol 1989; 211:1225–1239.

10. Richard VJ, Murry CE, Jennings RB, Reimer KA. Oxygen-derived free radicals and postischemic myocardial reperfusion: therapeutic implications. Fundam Clin Pharmacol 1990; 4:85–103.

11. Hearse DJ, Bolli R. Reperfusion induced injury; manifestations, mechanisms, and clinical relevance. Cardiovasc Res 1992; 26:101–108.

12. Baldwin WM, III, Pruitt SK, Brauer RB, Daha MR, Sanfilippo F. Complement in organ transplantation. Transplantation 1995; 59:797–808.

13. Marsh HC, Ryan US. The therapeutic effect of soluble complement receptor type 1 (sCR1) in xenotransplantation. In: Cooper DKC, ed. Xenotransplantation. 2nd ed. New York: Springer-Verlag, 1996. In press.

14. Thomas LJ, Ryan US. Immunological consequences of organ transplantation: implications for therapeutic development. J Heart Lung Transplant 1995; 14: 938–944.

15. Ryan US. Complement inhibition: the sine qua non of xenotransplantation? Xeno 1994; 2:19–22.

16. Ryan US. Complement inhibitory therapeutics and xenotransplantation. Nature Med 1995; 1:967–968.

17. Peerschke El, Reid KB, Ghebrehiwet B. Platelet activation by C1q results in the induction of alpha IIb/beta 3 integrins (GPIIb-IIIa) and the expression of P-selectin and procoagulant activity. J Exp Med 1993; 178:579–587.

18. Ryan US, Worthington RE. Cell-cell contact mechanisms. Curr Opin Immunol 1992; 4:33–37.

19. Celi A, Pelligrini G, Lorenzet R, De Blaise A, Ready N, Furie BC, Furie B. P-selectin induces the expression of tissue factor on monocytes. Proc Natl Acad Sci 1994; 91:8767–8771.

20. Tsuji T, Nagata K, Koike J, Todoroki N, Irimura T. Induction of superoxide anion production from monocytes and neutrophils by activated platelets through the P-selectin-sialyl Lewis X interaction. J Leukoc Biol 1994; 56: 583–587.

21. Esmon CT. Cell mediated events that control blood coagulation and vascular injury. Annu Rev Cell Biol 1993; 9:1–26.

22. Platt JL, Dalmasso AP, Lindman BJ, Ihrcke NS, Bach FH. The role of C5a and antibody in the release of heparin sulfate from endothelial cells. Eur J Immunol 1991; 21:2887–2890.

23. Murphy HS, Shayman JA, Till GO, Mahrougui M, Owens CB, Ryan US, et al. Superoxide responses of endothelial cells to C5a and TNF-alpha: divergent signal transduction pathways. Am J Physiol 1992; 263:L51–L59.

24. Foreman KE, Vaporciyan AA, Bonish BK, Jones ML, Johnson KJ, Glovsky

MM, et al. C5a-induced expression of P-selectin in endothelial cells. J Clin Invest 1994; 94:1147–1155.

25. Carson SD, Johnson DR. Consecutive enzyme cascades: complement activation at the cell surface triggers increased tissue factor activity. Blood 1990; 76:361–367.

26. Morgan BP. Complement membrane attack on nucleated cells: resistance, recovery and nonlethal effects. Biochem J 1989; 264:1–14.

27. Hattori R, Hamilton KK, McEver RP, Sims PJ. Complement proteins C5b-C9 induce secretion of high molecular weight multimers of endothelial von Willebrand factor and translocation of granule membrane protein GMP-140 to the cell surface. J Biol Chem 1989; 264:9053–9060.

28. Hamilton KK, Hattori R, Esmon CT, Sims PJ. Complement proteins C5b-9 induce vesiculation of the endothelial plasma membrane and expose catalytic surface for assembly of the prothrombinase enzyme complex. J Biol Chem 1990; 265:3809–3814.

29. Sims PJ, Wiedmer T. The response of human platelets to activated components of the complement system. Immunol Today 1991; 12:338–342.

30. Lindsay TF, Hill J, Ortiz F, Rudolph AR, Valeri CR, Hechtman HB, et al. Blockade of complement activation prevents local and pulmonary albumin leak after lower torso ischemia-reperfusion. Ann Surg 1992; 216:677–683.

31. Konteatis ZD, Siciliano SJ, van Riper G, et al. Development of C5a receptor antagonists: differential loss of functional responses. J Immunol 1994; 153: 4200–4205.

32. Gulbins E, Schlottmann K, Rauterberg EW, Steinhausen M. Effects of rC5a on the circulation of normal and split hydronephrotic rat kidneys. Am J Physiol 1993; 265:F96–103.

33. Ember JA, Sanderson SD, Hugli TE, Morgan EL. Induction of interleukin-8 synthesis from monocytes by human C5a anaphylatoxin. Am J Pathol 1994; 144:393–403.

34. Morgan EL, Ember JA, Sanderson SD, Scholz W, Buchner R, Ye RD, et al. Anti-C5a receptor antibodies: characterization of neutralizing antibodies specific for a peptide, C5aR-(9-29), derived from the predicted aminoterminal sequence of the human C5a receptor. J Immunol 1993; 151:377–388.

35. Barton PA, Warren JS. Complement component C5 modulates the systemic tumor necrosis factor response in murine endotoxic shock. Infect Immunol 1993; 61:1474–1481.

36. Fearon DT, Collins LA. Increased expression of C3b receptors on polymorphonuclear leukocytes induced by chemotactic factors and by purification procedures. J Immunol 1983; 130:370–375.

37. Arnaout MA, Spits H, Terhorst C, Pitt J, Todd RF, III. Deficiency of a leukocyte surface glycoprotein (LFA-1) in two patients with Mo1 deficiency: effects of cell activation on Mo1/LFA-1 surface expression in normal and deficient leukocytes. J Clin Invest 1984; 74:1291–1300.

38. Glovsky MM, Hugli TE, Ishizaka T, Lichtenstein LM, Erickson BW. Anaphyla-

toxin-induced histamine release with human leukocytes. Studies of C3a leukocyte binding and histamine release. J Clin Invest 1979; 64:804–811.

39.  Daffern PJ, Pfeifer PH, Ember JA, Hugli TE. C3a is a chemotaxin for human
eosinophils but not for neutrophils. 1. C3a stimulation of neutrophils is secondary to eosinophil activation. J Exp Med 1995; 181:2119–2127.

40.  Libby P, Hansson GK. Involvement of the immune system in human atherosclerosis: current knowledge and unanswered questions. Lab Invest 1991; 64:5–15.

41.  Wahlin B, Perlmann H, Perlmann P, Schreiber RD, Muller-Eberhard HJ. C3
receptors on human lymphocyte subsets and recruitment of ADCC effector
cells by C3 fragments. J Immunol 1983; 130:2831–2836.

42.  Diamond MS, Garcia-Aguilar J, Bickford JK, Corbi AL, Springer TA. The I
domain is a major recognition site on the leukocyte integrin Mac-1 (CD11b/
CD18) for four distinct adhesion ligands. J Cell Biol 1993; 120:1031–1043.

43.  Rosen H, Law SK. The leukocyte cell surface receptor(s) for the iC3b product
of complement. Curr Top Microbiol Immunol 1990; 153:99–122.

44.  Diamond MS, Staunton DE, Marlin SD, Springer TA. Binding of the integrin
Mac-I (CD11b/CD18) to the third immunoglobulin-like domain of ICAM-1
(CD54) and its regulation by glycosylation. Cell 1991; 65:961–971.

45.  Bechtel U, Scheuer R, Landgraft R, Konig A, Feucht HE. Assessment of soluble adhesion molecules (sICAM-1, sVCAM-1, sELAM-1) and complement
cleavage products (sC4d, sC5b-9) in urine. Transplantation 1994; 58:905–911.

46.  Bishop GA, Hall BM. Expression of leucocyte and lymphocyte adhesion molecules in the human kidney. Kidney Int 1989; 36:1078–1085.

47.  Taylor PM, Rose ML, Yacoub MH, Pigott R. Induction of vascular adhesion
molecules during rejection of human cardiac allografts. Transplantation 1992;
54:451–457.

48.  Brockmeyer C, Ulbrecht M, Schendel DJ, Weiss EH, Hillebrand G, Burkhardt
K, et al. Distribution of cell adhesion molecules (ICAM-1, VCAM-1 ELAM-
1) in renal tissue during allograft rejection. Transplantation 1993; 55:610–615.

49.  Fuggle SV, Sanderson JB, Gray DW, Richardson A, Morris PJ. Variation in
expression of endothelial adhesion molecules in pretransplant and transplanted
kidneys—correlation with intragraft events. Transplantation 1993; 55:117–123.

50.  Hancock WW, Whitley WD, Tullius SG, Heemann WW, Wasowska B, Baldwin WM, 3d, et al. Cytokines, adhesion molecules, and the pathogenesis of
chronic rejection of rat renal allografts. Transplantation 1993; 56:643–650.

51.  Yancey KB, O'Shea J, Chused T, Brown E, Takahashi T, Frank MM, et al.
Human C5a modulates monocyte Fc and C3 receptor expression. J Immunol
1985; 135:465–470.

52.  Bajtay Z, Falus A, Erdei A, Gergely J. Fc gamma R-dependent regulation of
the biosynthesis of complement C3 by murine macrophages: the modulatory
effect of IL-6. Scand J Immunol 1992; 35:195–201.

53.  Svalander C, Nyberg G, Blohme I, Eggertsen G, Nilsson B, Nilsson U. Acute
early allograft failure and the C3/macrophage phenomenon. Transplant Proc
1993; 25:903–904.

54.  Hayry P, von Willebrand E, Parthenais E, Nemlander A, Soots A, Lauten-

schlager I, et al. The inflammatory mechanisms of allograft rejection. Immunol Rev 1984; 77:85–142.

55. Ogawa S, Gerlach H, Esposito C, Pasagian-Macaulay A, Brett J, Stern D. Hypoxia modulates the barrier and coagulant function of culture bovine endothelium. J Clin Invest 1990; 85:1090–1098.
56. Benzaquen LR, Nicholson-Weller A, Halperin JA. Terminal complement proteins C5b-9 release basic fibroblast growth factor and platelet-derived growth factor from endothelial cells. J Exp Med 1994; 179:985–992.
57. Zavoico GB, Ryan US. Complement and Mechanisms of Restenosis. In: Catravas JD, Callow AD, Ryan US, eds. Vascular Endothelium. New York: Plenum Press, 1996:61–68.
58. Ahearn JM, Fearon DT. Structure and function of the complement receptors, CR1 (CD35) and CR2 (CD21). Adv Immunol 1989; 46:183–219.
59. Yoon SH, Fearon DT. Characterization of a soluble form of the C3b/C4b receptor (CR1) in human plasma. J Immunol 1985; 134:3332–3338.
60. Nelson RA. The immune-adherence phenomenon. Science 1953; 118:733–737.
61. Gigli I, Nelson RA, Jr. Complement dependent immune phagocytosis. I. Requirements for C'1, C'4, C'2, C'3. Exp Cell Res 1968; 51:45–67.
62. Thorton BP, Vetvicka V, Ross GD. Natural antibody and complement-mediated antigen processing and presentation by B lymphocytes. J Immunol 1994; 152:1727–1737.
63. Fallman M, Andersson R, Andersson T. Signaling properties of CR3 (CD11b/CD18) and CR1 (CD35) in relation to phagocytosis of complement-opsonized particles. J Immunol 1993; 151:330–338.
64. Bacle F, Haeffner-Cavaillon N, Laude M, Couturier C, Kazatchkine MD. Induction of IL-1 release through stimulation of the C3b/C4b complement receptor type one (CR1, CD35) on human monocytes. J Immunol 1990; 144:147–152.
65. Weisman HF, Bartow T, Leppo MK, Marsh HC, Jr., Carson GR, Concino MF, et al. Soluble human complement receptor type 1: *In vivo* inhibitor of complement suppressing post-ischemic myocardial inflammation and necrosis. Science 1990; 249:146–151.
66. Mardiney MR, Muller-Eberhard HJ, Feldman JD. Ultrastructural localization of the third and four components of complement on complement-cell complexes. Am J Pathol 1968; 53:253–262.
67. Wessels MR, Butko P, Ma M, Warren HB, Lage AL, Carroll MC. Studies of group B streptococcal infection in mice deficient in complement component C3 or C4 demonstrate an essential role for complement in both innate and acquired immunity. Proc Natl Acad Sci USA 1995; 92:11490–11494.
68. Moran P, Beasley H., Gorrell A, Martin E, Gribling P, Fuchs H, et al. Human soluble decay accelerating factor inhibits complement activation in vitro and in vivo. J Immunol 1992; 149:1736–1743.
69. Wang Y, Rollins SA, Madri JA, Matis LA. Anti-C5 monoclonal antibody therapy prevents collagen-induced arthritis and ameliorates established disease. Proc Natl Acad Sci USA 1995; 92:8955–8959.

70. Scesney SM, Makrides SC, Gosselin ML, Ford PJ, Andrews BM, Hayman EG, et al. A soluble deletion mutant of the human complement receptor type 1, which lacks the C4b binding site, is a selective inhibitor of the alternative complement pathway. Eur J Immunol 1996. In press.

71. Ryan US. Role of complement and complement inhibitory therapies in ARDS. Am Coll Chest Physicians, Oct. 30, 1995; 25.

72. DiMartino MJ, Wolfe CE, Slivjak MJ, Minthorn EA, Feuerstein G. Effects of soluble complement receptor (sCR1, BRL55730) on thermal skin injury induced hemoconcentration and lung inflammation in rats. Pharmacol Commun 1993; 3:249–256.

73. Mulligan MS, Yeh CG, Rudolph AR, Ward PA. Protective effects of soluble CR1 in complement- and neutrophil-mediated tissue injury. J Immunol 1992; 148:1479–1485.

74. Mulligan MS, Warren JS, Smith CW, Anderson DC, Yeh CG, Rudolph AR, et al. Lung injury after deposition of IgA immune complexes. Requirements for CD18 and L-arginine. J Immunol 1992; 148:3086–3092.

75. Regal JF, Frase DG, Toth CA. Role of the complement system in antigen-induced bronchoconstriction and changes in blood pressure in the guinea pig. J Pharm Exp Ther 1993; 267:979–988.

76. Hill J, Lindsay TD, Oritz F, Yeh CG, Hechtman HB, Moore FD. Soluble complement receptor type 1 ameliorates the local and remote organ injury after intestinal ischemia-reperfusion in the rat. J Immunol 1992; 149:1723–1728.

77. Rabinovici R, Yeh CG, Hillegass LM, Griswold DE, DiMartino JJ, Vernick J, et al. Role of complement in endotoxin/platelet-activating factor-induced lung injury. J Immunol 1992; 149:1744–1750.

78. Rabinovici R, Sofronski MD, Borboroglu P, Spirig AM, Hellegas LM, Levin J, et al. Interleukin-2–induced lung injury: the role of complement. Circ Res 1994; 74:329–335.

79. Gillinov AM, DeValeria PA, Winklestein JA, Wilson I, Curtis WE, Shaw D, et al. Complement inhibition with soluble complement receptor type 1 in cardiopulmonary bypass. Ann Thorac Surg 1993; 55:619–624.

80. Weisman HF, Bartow T, Leppo MK, Boyle MP, Marsh HC, Carson GR, et al. Recombinant soluble CR1 suppressed complement activation, inflammation, and necrosis associated with reperfusion of ischemic myocardium. Trans Assoc Am Physicians 1990; 103:64–72.

81. Smith EF, III, Griswold DE, Egan JW, Hillegass LM, Smith RAG, Hibbs MJ, et al. Reduction of myocardial reperfusion injury with soluble complement receptor 1 (BRL 55730). Eur J Pharmacol 1993; 236:477–481.

82. Shandelya SML, Kuppusamy P, Herskowitz A, Weisfeldt ML, Zweier JL. Soluble complement receptor type 1 inhibits the complement pathway and prevents contractile failure in the postischemic heart: evidence that complement activation is required for neutrophil mediated reperfusion injury. Circulation 1993; 88:2812–2826.

83. Pemberton M, Anderson G, Vetvicka V, Justus DE, Ross GD. Microvascular effects of complement blockade with soluble recombinant CR1 on ischemia/reperfusion injury in skeletal muscle. J Immunol 1993; 150:5104–5113.

84. Chavez-Cartaya RE, Desola GP, Wright L, Jamieson NV, White DJG. Regulation of the complement cascade by soluble complement receptor type 1—protective effect in experimental liver ischemia and reperfusion. Transplantation 1995; 59:1047–1052.

85. Jaeschke H, Farhood A, Bautista AP, Spolarics Z, Spitzer JJ. Complement activates Kupffer cells and neutrophils during reperfusion after hepatic ischemia. Am J Physiol 1993; 264:G801–G809.

86. Kaczorowski SL, Schiding JK, Toth CA, Kochanek PM. Effect of soluble complement receptor-1 on neutrophil accumulation after traumatic brain injury in rats. J Cerebral Blood Flow Metab 1995; 15:860–864.

87. Naka Y, Roy DK, Marsh HC, Scesney SM, Ryan US, Stern DM, Liao H, Michler RE, Oz MC, Pinsky DJ. Protective effects of complement blockade in an isograft model of lung preservation and transplantation. Presented at the American College of Cardiology meeting, Orlando, FL, March 24–27, 1996.

88. Pratt JR, Hibbs MJ, Laver AJ, Smith RAG, Sacks SH. Allograft immune response with sCR1 intervention. Transplant Immunol 1995.

89. Pruitt SK, Bollinger RR. Allograft immune response with sCR1 intervention. J Surg Res 1991; 50:350–355.

90. Candinas D, Lesnikoski BA, Robson SC, Scesney SM, Otsu I, Myiatake T, et al. Soluble complement receptor type 1 and cobra venom factor in discordant xenotransplantation. Transplant Proc 1996; 28(2):581.

91. Candinas D, Lesnikoski BA, Robson SC, Scesney S, Otsu I, Marsh HC, et al. The effect of repetitive high dose treatment with soluble complement receptor type 1 and cobra venom factor on discordant xenograft survival. Transplantation 1996 in press.

92. Fujiwara I, Arakawa K, Akami T, Okamoto M, Akioka K, Takeshita K, et al. Prolongation of xenograft survival by soluble complement receptor type 1 (sCR1) and anti-thrombin-III (AT-III) combination therapy. Transplant Proc 1996; 28:685–686.

93. Pruitt SK, Baldwin WM, Marsh HC, Jr., Lin SS, Yeh CG, Bollinger RR. The effect of soluble complement receptor type 1 on hyperacute xenograft rejection. Transplantation 1992; 52:868–873.

94. Pruitt SK, Baldwin WM, Marsh HC, Lin SS, Yeh CG, Bollinger RR. Effect of soluble complement receptor type 1 on natural antibody levels during xenograft rejection. Transplant Proc 1992; 24:477–478.

95. Xia W, Fearon DT, Moore FD, Schoen FJ, Ortiz F, Kirkman RL. Prolongation of guinea pig cardiac xenograft survival in rats by soluble human complement receptor type 1. Transplant Proc 1992; 24:479–480.

96. Xia W, Fearon DT, Kirkman RL. Effect of repetitive doses of soluble human complement receptor type 1 on survival of discordant cardiac xenografts. Transplant Proc 1993; 25:410–411.

97. Zehr KJ, Herskowitz A, Lee PC, Kumar P, Gillinov AM, Baumgartner WJ. Neutrophil adhesion and complement inhibition prolongs survival of cardiac xenografts in discordant species. Transplantation 1994; 57:900–906.

98. Chrupcala M, Pomer S, Staehler G, Waldherr R, Kirschfink C. Prolongation of discordant renal xenograft survival by depletion of complement. Compara-

tive effects of systemically administered cobra venom factor and soluble complement receptor type 1 in a guinea-pig to rat model. Transpl Int 1994; 7:S650–S653.

99. Pruit, SK, Bollinger, RR, Collins, BH, Marsh, HC, Levin, JL, Rudolph, AR, Baldwin, WM and Sanfilippo, F. Continuous complement inhibition using soluble complement receptor type 1: effect on hyperacute rejection of pig-to-primate cardiac xenografts. Third International Congress for Xenotransplantation, Boston, Sept. 27–Oct. 1, 1995; OR-27:215.

100. Pruitt, SK, Kirk, AD, Bollinger, RR, Marsh HC, Jr., Collins, BH, Levin, JL, et al. The effect of soluble complement receptor type 1 on hyperacute rejection of porcine xenografts. Transplantation 1994; 57:363–370.

101. Sanfilippo, F. Effects of complement inhibitors on discordant rodent and pig-to-primate cardiac xenograft rejection. Third International Congress for Xenotransplantation, Boston, Sept. 27–Oct. 1, 1995; PL-26.

# 11

# The Receptor for Advanced Glycation Endproducts: Implications for the Development of Diabetic Vascular Disease

**Osamu Hori, Shi Du Yan, and Ann Marie Schmidt**

*Columbia University College of Physicians and Surgeons, New York, New York*

## I. INTRODUCTION

Proteins or lipids exposed to aldose sugars undergo nonenzymatic glycation and oxidation (1–7). The ultimate products of these interactions are called the advanced glycation endproducts (AGEs). Earlier, however, reversible adducts known as Schiff bases/Amadori products form in the course of exposure to aldoses. These products, distinct from AGEs, are reversibly formed and can dissociate to the native proteins on restoration of normoglycemia (4). Clinically, the reversible products have been used to assess the adequacy of glycemic control. The best known of these moieties used in this setting is hemoglobin $A_{1c}$ (8). In contrast, AGEs are irreversibly formed. Although a heterogeneous group of compounds, they nevertheless share in common certain characteristics such as yellow-brown color, the tendency to form cross links, the ability to generate reactive oxygen intermediates, fluorescence, and the ability to recognize specific receptors on cellular surfaces (9–13). AGEs accumulate in the plasma and vessel wall during normal aging, but they form to an accelerated degree in patients with diabetes.

A number of groups have developed specific reagents (both polyclonal and monoclonal antibodies) to detect the presence of AGEs in vivo (14–17). For example, we have identified increased immunoreactivity for AGEs in the vasculature of diabetic patients versus that in age-matched, nondiabetic control individuals (18). Similarly, others have found increased immunoreactivity for AGEs in the vessel wall and skin of diabetic patients (19–22). The results of these studies are consistent with the hypothesis that formation of AGEs correlates with the development of diabetic complications. As well, previous studies have suggested a possible link between the accumulation of AGEs in the vasculature and the development of vascular disease which occurs to an accelerated extent in diabetic individuals. For example, Nakamura and colleagues demonstrated increased immunoreactivity for AGEs in coronary atheromas of patients with diabetes (22).

It should be noted that in addition to normal aging (1,2,4) and diabetes (1–8), the development of proteins/lipids modified by irreversible nonenzymatic glycation may occur under other conditions which favor their generation. For example, AGEs may form on long-lived proteins, particularly in the setting of renal failure. In this context, under physiological conditions, the plasma protein $\beta_2$-microglobulin is readily cleared from the circulation. However, in the presence of its markedly delayed clearance characteristic of renal failure, $\beta_2$-microglobulin may undergo AGE formation (23), presumably as a consequence of its prolonged half-life in the setting of renal failure. In marked contrast to the native form, AGE–$\beta_2$-microglobulin is postulated to be important in the pathogenesis of the inflammatory disorder dialysis-related amyloidosis (DRA) that is associated with chronic renal failure and dialysis (24).

Another condition in which amyloid deposition may predispose to the development of AGE formation is in Alzheimer's disease (25). In this disorder, AGE formation may form on the components of intracellular neurofibrillary tangles (26–28) as well as in extracellular amyloid–$\beta$-peptide accumulations (29). The presence of these AGE-modified moieties has been postulated to be an important component of enhanced oxidant stress, which is likely involved, at least in part, in the pathogenesis of this disorder (26,28).

Taken together, these data suggest that AGEs may form under conditions of hyperglycemia, normal aging, delayed protein turnover (such as in renal failure), or extensive protein accumulation (such as in amyloidoses). In this chapter, we detail some of the biological properties of these structures with respect to their likely contributory role in the development of vascular/cellular pathology.

## II.  IDENTIFICATION OF CELLULAR RECEPTORS FOR AGEs

Earlier studies identified the ability of AGE-modified ligands to bind to cellular surfaces (4,30) in a specific and saturable manner. Although a number of cellular binding sites for AGEs have been identified (11,31,32), the

best characterized of these to date is the receptor for advanced glycation endproducts (RAGE) (11). By sequential chromatography on hydroxylapatite,
fast-pressure liquid chromatography (FPLC) Mono S, and FPLC gel filtra-
tion media, RAGE was purified to homogeneity from detergent extracts of
bovine lung. At the same time, another AGE binding polypeptide,
lactoferrin-like polypeptide (LF-L) was also described (11). This chapter is
confined to consideration of RAGE.

Molecular cloning studies (13) have revealed that RAGE is a newly identified member of the immunoglobulin superfamily of cell surface molecules.
The predicted hydropathy plot of the bovine cDNA for RAGE (Fig. 1)
suggests that RAGE contains a 332–amino acid extracellular domain with
one "V"-type immunoglobulin domain followed by two "C"-type domains.
This is followed by a hydrophobic transmembrane spanning domain and a
highly charged cytosolic tail. Preceding the above domains is a putative
signal sequence of 22 amino acids. Of note, the bovine, murine, rat, and
human counterparts of RAGE are remarkably similar. Critical to the hypothesis that RAGE was an AGE binding protein was the demonstration of
binding of $^{125}$I-AGE albumin to 293 cells transfected with the cDNA for
RAGE but not to cells transfected with irrelevant cDNA (13). Binding to
RAGE-transfected 293 cells was similar to that of radiolabeled AGE albumin to immobilized RAGE, endothelial cells, or mononuclear phagocytes
(11,13,16) with $K_d \approx 50–100$ nM and inhibitable in the presence of anti-
RAGE IgG (11,13,16).

Given the fact that RAGE was a member of the immunoglobulin superfamily, we postulated that under physiological conditions, RAGE might

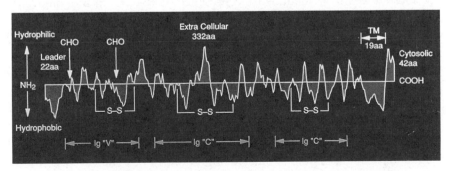

**Figure 1** Hydropathy plot of bovine RAGE. As generated by the Hopp and
Woods program of intelligenetics, this hydrophilicity plot of RAGE was generated.
NH$_2$, amino terminus; COOH, carboxyl-terminus; CHO, N-linked glycosylation
sites; TM, transmembrane domain; S–S, disulfide-linked cysteine residues; IgV
and IgC, immunoglobulin-like variable and constant domains, respectively.

function as a cell-cell adhesion molecule or receptor for cytokine(s) or growth factor(s). In this context, we have demonstrated that under the specific condition of perinatal development, RAGE is highly expressed in the developing central nervous system of the rat. Its specific interaction with the polypeptide amphoterin appears to mediate neurite outgrowth in in vitro assays designed to study this phenomenon (33). Another recently identified putative ligand of RAGE, a molecule with $M_r \approx 12$ kD, is a newly identified member of a family of proinflammatory cytokines (33). Detailed analysis of the consequences of its interaction with RAGE are in progress.

In addition to the presence of RAGE on endothelial cells and mononuclear phagocytes, a survey of normal tissue has identified its presence on other cell types such as mesangial cells and certain neurons (34). In addition, RAGE is also present in the vascular smooth muscle (34). As stated above, RAGE is also present to a significant degree in the developing nervous system in embryonic and postnatal (through P17) cortical neurons (33). These data lend further support to the hypothesis that AGEs may in fact be pathological ligands of this receptor, which under homeostatic conditions, act to mediate such functions as normal development and, potentially, other not yet identified phenomena.

In this chapter, we concentrate on the implications of AGE-RAGE interaction on mononuclear phagocytes and endothelial cells.

## III. INTERACTION OF AGEs WITH MONONUCLEAR PHAGOCYTE RAGE: INITIATION OF MONONUCLEAR PHAGOCYTE MIGRATION AND ACTIVATION

Previous studies have identified the presence of RAGE on mononuclear phagocytes by immunohistochemistry (16) and by in situ hybridization (S.D. Yan and A.M. Schmidt, unpublished observation). Radioligand binding studies with $^{125}$I-AGE albumin demonstrated specific saturable binding, with $K_D \approx 80$ nM, comparable to that observed on immobilized RAGE (11). Consistent with the concept that RAGE was important in mediating the interaction of AGEs with mononuclear phagocytes (MPs), binding was largely blocked in the presence of anti-RAGE IgG.

We hypothesized that soluble AGEs, such as those found circulating on modified plasma proteins or on the surface of diabetic red blood cells (35), for example, might initiate monocyte migration. In this context, when soluble AGEs (either AGE albumin or AGEs immunoisolated from diabetic plasma using affinity-purified anti-AGE IgG) were placed in the lower compartment of microchemotaxis chambers, monocyte migration was promoted in a dose-dependent manner (16). In contrast, native albumin was without effect. Furthermore, that this was true chemotaxis was demonstrated by further studies with checkerboard analysis. Similar results were observed with AGE–$\beta_2$ microglobulin with respect to true monocyte chemotaxis (24). Migration of monocytes in response to soluble AGE albumin was inhibited in the presence of anti-RAGE IgG (or F[ab']$_2$ fragments) or in the presence of soluble RAGE (sRAGE, the extracellular two thirds of the molecule [16]). In contrast, blockade of RAGE was without effect on monocyte migration initiated by the chemotactic peptide F-met-leu-phe (FMLP).

In addition to soluble AGEs, AGEs may also form on the long-lived proteins of the subendothelium, an area postulated to have an important role in the development of vascular lesions, such as atherosclerosis (36). In order for the AGEs formed/deposited in this area to be of pathological significance, they would likely need to attenuate monocyte migration. To study this hypothesis, we immobilized either AGE albumin or native albumin on the upper membranes of microchemotaxis chambers and tested monocyte migration in response to the chemotactic peptide FMLP placed in the lower compartment. When the upper surface was coated with native albumin, monocyte migration in response to increasing doses of FMLP was increased, as expected. However, when AGE albumin was immobilized on the upper surface, monocyte migration in response to FMLP in the lower compartment was attenuated in a dose-dependent manner (16). The central role of monocyte RAGE in mediating these interactions was demonstrated in studies employing RAGE blockade. When monocytes were preincubated with anti-RAGE F(ab')$_2$, monocyte migration in response to FMLP was restored despite the presence of immobilized AGE on the upper surface. In contrast, nonimmune fragments were without effect. Similarly, when the AGE-coated surface was pretreated with sRAGE, monocyte migration in response to FMLP in the lower compartment was restored (16).

To further test the hypothesis that when migrating MPs encounter immobilized RAGE, their migration is slowed, we performed phagokinetic track assays directly to visualize monocyte migration on either AGE albumin or native albumin–coated surfaces. When MPs were placed on coverslips coated with native albumin that had been overlaid by colloidal gold, their migration was evident with long paths of migration demonstrated (Fig. 2, left panel). In marked contrast, when MPs were placed on coverslips coated with AGE albumin, their migration was slowed, as evidenced by short paths of migration (Fig. 2, right panel).

Analogous experiments were performed in vivo to further demonstrate this concept. Polytetrafluoroethylene (PTFE) tubes were impregnated with either native rat serum albumin or AGE rat serum albumin and then implanted subcutaneously onto the backs of rats. When removed after 4 days, the tissue of rats treated with PTFE tubes to which had been absorbed

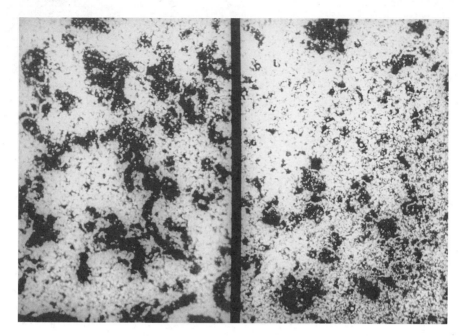

**Figure 2** Phagokinetic track assay. MPs were allowed to migrate for 6 hr on matrices of native albumin (left panel) or AGE albumin (right panel) which had been coated with colloidal gold particles. The dark tracks made by locomoting MPs are visualized by darkfield microscopy. ×125

native albumin revealed minimal inflammatory infiltrate except at the tissue-tube interface (Fig. 3, left panel). In contrast, however, tissue from rats treated with AGE-impregnated PTFE tubes revealed a considerable inflammatory infiltrate, with mononuclear cells observed moving through the interstices of the tubes (Fig. 3, right panel). Many of the monocytes appear to have undergone activation, as evidenced by leukocytoclastic changes.

These data are consistent with the concept that AGEs may promote monocyte activation. In fact, previous studies have shown that AGE-monocyte interaction results in their activation (37–38), as manifested by production of cytokines such as tumor necrosis factor-$\alpha$ (TNF-$\alpha$) and interleukin-1 (IL-1) as well as the growth factor platelet-derived growth factor (PDGF).

Taken together, these data suggest a model in which soluble AGEs, such as those circulating in modified plasma proteins or those on the surface of diabetic red blood cells, may attract monocytes and mediate their migra-

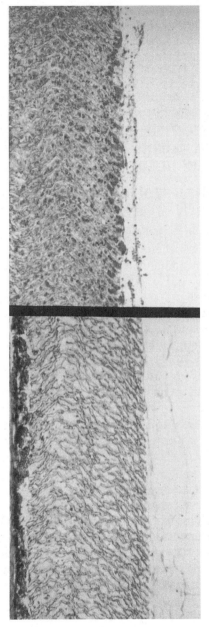

**Figure 3** Implantation of PTFE tubes with absorbed AGE albumin into rats. PTFE tubes were impregnated with either native albumin (left panel) or AGE albumin (right panel), implanted subcutaneously into the backs of rats, and removed after 4 days and stained with hematoxylin and eosin. ×110.

tion. In contrast, immobilized AGEs, such as those formed/deposited in the vascular wall, may retard the migration of monocytes, a process which may ultimately lead to their activation, a process which may predispose to the development of vascular lesions.

## IV. INTERACTION OF AGEs WITH ENDOTHELIAL CELL RAGE: CLEARANCE OF AGEs BY ENDOTHELIAL CELLS, INDUCTION OF CELLULAR OXIDANT STRESS, AND ENHANCED EXPRESSION OF VASCULAR CELL ADHESION MOLECULE-1

### A. Endothelial Cell Handling of AGEs: Clearance Studies and Experiments Assessing Cellular Activation

Previous studies have identified the presence of RAGE in the vascular endothelium by immunohistochemistry using anti-RAGE IgG and by in situ hybridization (34). The endothelium is in a critical position to mediate the effects of circulating AGEs, either those that form on circulating plasma proteins or those that deposit/form on the surface of diabetic red blood cells with the rest of the cell. In addition to its potential role in processing/removing AGEs from the intravascular space, the endothelium may also function to mediate certain perturbations that are a consequence of their interaction with AGEs, all of which may alter the cellular phenotype, thereby predisposing to vascular dysfunction. In this context, our earliest studies on AGE-endothelial interaction demonstrated that when cultured endothelial cells (ECs) were exposed to AGEs, critical cellular properties were altered resulting in a procoagulant and more permeable phenotype (30). Specifically, we observed suppression of thrombomodulin, sustained induction of low levels of tissue factor, and increased diffusional transit of macromolecular solutes across the EC monolayer (30). The central role of RAGE in mediating the interaction of AGEs with the endothelium is suggested by studies which demonstrated blockade of binding of radiolabeled AGEs to cultured ECs (11) by anti-RAGE IgG(11).

It was therefore most important in this context to study the effects of AGEs infused into animals. Extensive studies with $^{125}$I-AGE albumin administered intravenously into mice revealed that in contrast to radiolabeled native albumin, radiolabeled AGE albumin demonstrated an initial rapid phase of clearance, with greater than 50% of the protein being cleared from the vascular space within minutes after administration (39). Studies assessing tracer accumulation in the organs demonstrated that AGEs accumulated in the most vascular organs (39). Studies utilizing pretreatment of the animals with either anti-RAGE IgG or sRAGE resulted in a marked delay in AGE clearance, suggesting that these reagents were capable of interfering with the interaction of circulating AGEs with EC RAGE (39).

Electronmicroscopic studies utilizing AGE albumin linked to colloidal gold revealed that in a murine coronary vasculature model, AGEs quickly interact with the EC surface, are subsequently endocytosed, and traverse the EC layer, in part by transcytosis, ultimately being released at the abluminal surface (39). As with the radiolabeled AGE clearance studies, this process was significantly inhibited in the presence of anti-RAGE IgG, whereas nonimmune IgG was without effect.

The importance of these results is stressed by studies in which infused, nonradioactive AGEs into mice resulted in increased mRNA for interleukin-6, again a process inhibited in the presence of RAGE blockade (39). Taken together, these studies suggest that AGEs are capable of interacting with EC RAGE, with potential consequences, including activation of cytokines, which may predispose to the development of vascular lesions. The central role of RAGE in mediating these effects is demonstrated by studies in which blockade of RAGE—either by blocking access to cell surface RAGE with anti-RAGE IgG or by binding to AGEs in the intravascular space thereby limiting their interaction with cell surface RAGE utilizing sRAGE—inhibits not only AGE clearance but, in this case, induction of, for example, mRNA for IL-6 transcripts.

## B.  Induction of Oxidant Stress in the Vasculature by Exposure to AGEs via a RAGE-Dependent Pathway

During the process of AGE formation, oxidation and generation of reactive oxygen intermediates are formed (9,10). We therefore postulated that, at least in part, one of the main mechanisms by which AGE-RAGE interaction might alter/perturb cellular properties is via generation of oxidant stress. Initial studies in tissue culture revealed that exposure of AGE albumin to cultured ECs resulted in the production of thiobarbituric acid–reactive substances (TBARS), induction of heme oxygenase mRNA, and activation of the transcription factor NFκB (17). In contrast, native albumin was without effect. All of these markers, indicative of enhanced oxidant stress, were inhibited in the presence of anti-RAGE IgG (17). Comparable results were obtained when diabetic red blood cells, not red blood cells isolated from normal individuals, were exposed to cultured ECs (35).

To better test the hypothesis that ligation of cell surface RAGE by AGEs delivered oxidant stress to the tissues, AGE albumin was infused into normal mice resulting in increased tissue TBARS, increased mRNA for heme oxygenase, and activation of NF-κB as assessed by electrophoretic mobility shift analysis of liver nuclear extracts (17,40). Again, native albumin was without significant effect, and these processes in AGE-treated animals were inhibited by preinfusion of anti-RAGE IgG.

To detect these malondialdehyde-reactive epitopes in the vasculature itself, AGE albumin or native albumin was administered intravenously into rats, and after 1 h, samples were taken for immunohistochemical analysis using antibody that specifically recognizes malondialdehyde epitopes (17). Analysis of the lungs revealed vascular staining (in the ECs and vascular smooth muscle) of AGE-treated animals (Fig. 4, left panel) suggestive of enhanced oxidant stress. In contrast, no staining was observed in the pulmonary vasculature of animals treated with native albumin (Fig. 4, right panel). In the former case, nonimmune IgG was similarly without effect (17).

These studies were important to identify the site(s) where AGEs deliver oxidant stress after their infusion. Taken together, the data suggest that

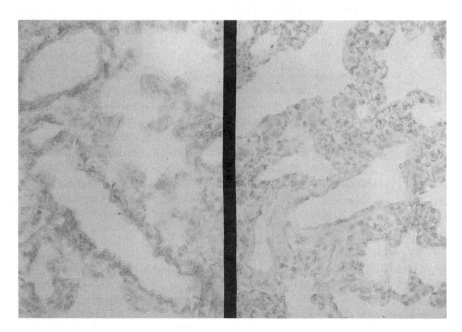

**Figure 4** Immunohistological detection of malondialdehyde-reactive epitopes in the vasculature of rats infused with AGE versus native rat serum albumin. Rats were infused with either AGE rat serum albumin (left panel) or native rat serum albumin (right panel). After 60 min, the animals were killed and lungs processed for the detection of malondialdehyde using indirect immunoalkaline phosphatase with antibody generously supplied by Dr. Joseph Witztum, University of California at San Diego. ×400.

AGEs interact with EC surface RAGE, and one of the consequences of this interaction is enhanced oxidant stress to the tissues, a process with multiple potential consequences. In this setting, one of the most important consequences may be activation of NFκB.

The implications of activation of the transcription factor NFκB are far reaching in this setting. Activation of this transcription factor has been linked to oxidant-sensitive mechanisms (40). Furthermore, its activation is probably important in the ultimate regulation of increased transcription of such entities as adhesion molecules, cytokines, or growth factors; all of which may be important in the pathogenesis of vascular lesions (41). In this context, we considered that enhanced expression of EC vascular cell adhesion molecule-1 (VCAM-1) might be a result of the interaction of AGEs with EC RAGE.

## C. AGE-RAGE Interaction Increases EC Expression of VCAM-1

It is likely that many factors contribute to the increased and accelerated course of vascular disease in diabetic individuals compared with normal controls. One of the critical steps in this process, however, is likely to be the enhanced expression of adhesion molecules on the vascular endothelium, which results in the adherence of circulating blood cells to the vessel wall. In this context, previous studies have indicated that, at least in part, the transcriptional regulation of VCAM-1 is controlled by oxidant-sensitive pathways (42). We, therefore, considered whether AGEs interacting with their cellular receptor RAGE might result in increased expression and functional activity of VCAM-1.

In the setting of diabetes, VCAM-1 is of particular interest, as its expression has been identified in the early phase of experimental hypercholesterolemia-induced atherosclerosis (43–44). Furthermore, enhanced VCAM-1 expression has been shown in the vessel wall of rabbits rendered diabetic with alloxan (45), as well as in human atherosclerotic lesions (46).

Our data indicated that when either AGE albumin or AGEs immuno-isolated from diabetic plasma were exposed to cultured human endothelial cells, ELISA of cellular extracts revealed increased cell-associated VCAM-1 compared with ECs treated with nonglycated proteins (47). In order to assess the functional implications of increased VCAM-1 on the cell surface, we treated ECs with either AGE or native albumin and subsequently performed binding assays using [51]chromium-labeled Molt-4 cells (cells which bear the counterligand for VCAM-1, VLA-4) and demonstrated significantly increased binding in the presence of AGEs (47). In both cases, the increased expression and function of cell-associated VCAM-1 was largely inhibited in the presence of RAGE blockade but not by control interventions (47). In addition, both processes were inhibited in the presence of antioxidants such as N-acetyl cysteine. Consistent with these data, Northern analysis and nuclear run-on analysis demonstrated increased transcription of VCAM-1 in the presence of AGE albumin, not native albumin, a process which is inhibited by anti-Rage IgG.

Since previous studies have identified binding sites for NF$\kappa$B in the promoter of VCAM-1, which have been shown to participate in the regulation of VCAM-1 in response to such factors as cytokines (48–49), at least in part, by oxidant-sensitive mechanisms. As demonstrated by electrophoretic mobility shift assay, in comparison with native albumin, nuclear extracts prepared from ECs exposed to AGE albumin resulted in an increased DNA binding activity for NF$\kappa$B site in the VCAM-1 promoter (Fig. 5, lanes 2 and 3, 6, and 10, respectively). This binding was blocked in a dose-dependent manner in the presence of anti-RAGE IgG (Fig. 5, lanes 11 and 12) but not in the presence of nonimmune IgG (Fig. 5, lane 13). Similarly, pretreatment with N-acetylcysteine resulted in inhibition of AGE-induced activation of NF$\kappa$B (Fig. 5, lane 14). Supershift studies using antibodies to p50 and p65 demonstrated that both members of the NF$\kappa$B are involved in binding to specific sites in the VCAM-1 promoter (Fig. 5, lanes 7–9). These data suggest that at least of the mechanisms by which AGEs induce enhanced expression of VCAM-1 is via activation of this transcription factor.

Consistent with these in vitro studies, infusion of AGE albumin into normal mice resulted in increased immunoreactivity for VCAM-1 in the lung vasculature (Fig. 6, right panel). In contrast, infusion of native albumin was without effect (Fig. 6, left panel).

In addition to increased expression of cell-associated VCAM-1 in the presence of AGEs, one of the further interesting findings in this setting was the detection of VCAM-1 antigen in the supernatants of AGE-treated (as well as TNF-$\alpha$–treated) ECs (47). We therefore inquired whether patients with diabetes had increased levels of soluble VCAM-1 (sVCAM-1) in their plasma compared with age-matched controls. In both cases, only patients with renal insufficiency were excluded from analysis. The level of sVCAM-1 in the plasma of diabetic patients was found to be 1,115 ng/ml compared with 632 ng/ml in the plasma of nondiabetic controls ($P < .05$). These data paralleled the changes in the levels of AGEs, as measured by AGE albumin equivalent in diabetic plasma compared with control plasma (244 ng/ml versus 157 ng/ml AGE albumin equivalents, $P < .05$) using an ELISA utilizing affinity-purified anti-AGE IgG (16,17,47).

Further analysis of sVCAM-1 in both AGE-treated EC supernatants and patient plasma demonstrated in immunoblotting studies that the immunoreactive material for VCAM-1 is intact, with an $M_r \approx 110$ kD. Fur-

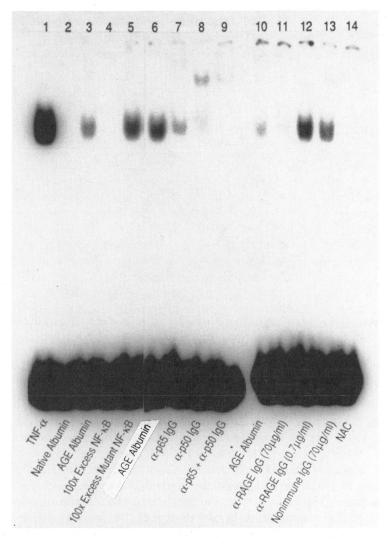

**Figure 5** Binding of endothelial cell nuclear proteins to NF-κB binding sites in the promoter of VCAM-1: analysis by electrophoretic mobility shift assay. All lanes contain labeled probe as follows: lane 1, ECs were incubated with TNF-α for 6 hr; lane 2, nonglycated albumin; lanes 3, 6, and 10, AGE albumin; lanes 7–9, nuclear extracts of AGE-treated cells with anti-p50 IgG, anti-p65 IgG, or both anti-p50 IgG and anti-p65 IgG together, respectively. In lanes 11 and 12, ECs were pretreated with anti-RAGE IgG (70 vs 7 μg/ml, respectively) prior to the addition of AGE. In lane 13, ECs were pretreated with nonimmune IgG prior to AGE, and in lane 14, ECs were pretreated with N-acetylcysteine prior to AGE albumin.

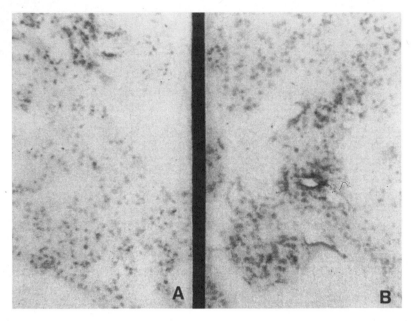

**Figure 6** Infusion of AGE albumin induces vascular expression of VCAM-1 in the pulmonary vasculature of mice. Mice were infused with either native albumin (left panel) or AGE mouse serum albumin (right panel). After 30 min, the animals were killed, lungs harvested, and immunostaining with antimurine VCAM-1 antigen performed. ×340.

thermore, no degradation was observed on the immunoblots (50), suggesting that VCAM-1 was released/cleaved from the cell surface in an intact form.

We hypothesized that elevation of sVCAM-1 might be, at least, a marker of endothelial perturbation in diabetic patients compared with control individuals and that its measurement might in fact be a marker of the effectiveness of therapeutic intervention. To further test this concept, we found that the levels of sVCAM-1 in diabetic patients with microalbuminuria were elevated compared with levels of sVCAM-1 in normoalbuminuric diabetic individuals (757 ng/ml vs 505 ng/ml, $P < 0.05$ [50]). The presence of microalbuminuria is of particular importance, since its presence in the diabetic patient has been linked to an increased incidence of cardiovascular morbidity and mortality, and it is considered a marker of diffuse vascular hyperpermeability (51–52). In fact, in our study, 5 of 12 patients with microalbuminuria had evidence of cardiovascular disease, whereas none of 8 patients with normoalbuminuria demonstrated abnormalities of the cardiovascular system, $P < .05$ (50). Taken together, these data suggest that the enhanced presence of VCAM-1 in diabetic vasculature may be, at least in part, a reflection of the interaction of AGEs interacting with cell surface RAGE. One of the consequences of this interaction may be the increased adherence of mononuclear cells to the vascular wall, which is a process likely pivotal in the development of diabetic vascular disease.

## V. BLOCKADE OF RAGE AS A POTENTIAL TARGET FOR INTERVENTION IN THE DEVELOPMENT OF VASCULAR COMPLICATIONS IN DIABETES

These data suggest that the interaction of AGEs with their cell surface receptor RAGE may be of central importance in the creation of an environment favorable to the development of vascular lesions. We have demonstrated that AGE-RAGE interaction is involved in the development of monocyte migration, as well as monocyte retention at sites of immobilized AGEs. Activation of monocytes is a likely sequela in this setting. RAGE has been demonstrated to be important in the clearance of AGEs from the intravascular space, and engagement of RAGE by AGEs results in the generation of enhanced oxidant stress in the vasculature. One of the consequences of this enhanced oxidant stress is likely to be the enhanced expression of cell-associated VCAM-1. These data further suggest that blockade of RAGE might ultimately be a target for therapeutic intervention in the setting of diabetic vascular disease. Indeed, recent findings have suggested that sVCAM-1 may have angiogenic properties, a situation to be of likely detriment in the diabetic vascular milieu, especially, for example, in such sites as the retina (53). Taken together, these findings suggest that blockade of AGE-RAGE interaction represents a logical target for therapeutic intervention in diabetic vascular disease.

In this context, our recent studies have demonstrated that infusion of sRAGE into diabetic rats reversed the increased tissue-blood isotope ratio (TBIR) observed in these animals, which is a marker of endothelial cell dysfunction (54–56).

In conclusion, these data suggest that further assessment of AGE-RAGE interaction and RAGE blockade in such models as wound healing and accelerated atherosclerosis will likely provide insight not only into the role of RAGE as a potential therapeutic target but will also aid in further dissecting the mechanisms set into motion on ligation of RAGE by AGEs or its other ligands.

# REFERENCES

1. Ruderman N, Williamson J, Brownlee M. Glucose and diabetic vascular disease. FASEB J 1992; 6:2905–2914.
2. Baynes J. Role of oxidative stress in development of complications in diabetes. Diabetes 1991; 40:405–412.
3. Sell D, Monnier V. Structure elucidation of senescence cross-link from human extracellular matrix: implication of pentoses in the aging process. J Biol Chem 1989; 264:21597–21602.
4. Brownlee M, Cerami A, Vlassara H. Advanced glycosylation endproducts in tissue and the biochemical basis of diabetic complications. N. Engl. J. Med. 1988; 318:1315–1320.
5. Bucala R, Makita Z, Koschinsky T, Cerami A, Vlassara H. Lipid advanced glycosylation: pathway for lipid oxidation in vivo. Proc. Natl. Acad. Sci. USA 1993; 90:6434–6438.
6. Hicks M, Delbridge L, Yue D, Reeve R. Catalysis of lipid peroxidation by glucose and glycosylated proteins. Biochem. Biophys. Res. Commun. 1988; 151:649–655.
7. Hunt J, Smith C, Wolff S. Autooxidative glycosylation and possible involvement of peroxides and free radicals in LDL modification by glucose. Diabetes 1990; 30:1420–1424.
8. Klein R, Klein B, Moss S, Davis M, DeMets DL. Glycosylated haemoglobin predicts the incidence and progression of diabetic retinopathy. JAMA 1989; 260:2864–2868.
9. Mullarkey C, Edelstein D, Brownlee M. Free radical generation by early glycation endproducts: a mechanism for accelerated atherogenesis in diabetes. Biochem. Biophys. Res. Commun. 1990; 173:932–939.
10. Sakurai T, Tsuchiya S. Superoxide production from nonenzymatically glycated protein. FEBS Lett. 1988; 236:406–410.
11. Schmidt AM, Vianna M, Gerlach M, et al. Isolation and characterization of binding proteins for advanced glycation endproducts from lung tissue which are present on the endothelial cell surface. J. Biol. Chem. 1992; 267:14987–14997.
12. Yang Z, Makita J, Horii Y, et al. Two novel rat liver membrane proteins that bind advanced glycosylation end products: relationship to macrophage receptor for glucose-modified proteins. J. Exp. Med. 1991; 174:515–524.
13. Neeper M, Schmidt AM, Brett J, Yan SD, Wang F, Pan YC, Elliston K, Stern D, Shaw A. Cloning and expression of RAGE: a cell surface receptor for advanced glycation endproducts of proteins. J. Biol. Chem. 1992; 267:14998–15004.
14. Nakayama H, Taneda S, Misuhashi T, Kuwajima S, Aoki S, Kuroda Y, Misawa K, Yanagisawa K, Nakagawa S. Characterization of antibodies to advanced glycosylation end products in vivo. J Immunol. Methods 1991; 140:119–125.
15. Makita Z, Vlassara H, Cerami A, Bucala R. Immunochemical detection of advanced glycosylation end products in vivo. J. Biol. Chem. 1992; 267: 5133–5138.
16. Schmidt AM, Yan SD, Brett J, Mora R, Nowygrod R, Stern D. Regulation of

human mononuclear phagocyte migration by cell surface binding proteins for advanced glycation endproducts. J. Clin. Invest. 1993; 92:2155–2168.

17. Yan S-D, Schmidt A-M, Anderson G, Zhang J, Brett J, Zou Y-S, Pinsky D, Stern D. Enhanced cellular oxidant stress by the interaction of advanced glycation endproducts with their receptors/binding proteins. J. Biol. Chem. 1994; 269:9889–9897.

18. Schmidt AM, Yan SD, Stern D. The Dark Side of Glucose. Nature Med. 1995; 1:1002–1004.

19. Beisswenger P, Moore L, Brinck-Johnsen T, Curphey T. Increased collagen-linked pentosidine levels and advanced glycosylation endproducts in early diabetic nephropathy. J. Clin. Invest. 1991; 92:212–217.

20. Dyer D, Dunn J, Thorpe S, Bailie K, Lyons T, McCance D, Baynes J. Accumulation of Maillard reaction products in skin collagen in diabetes and aging. J. Clin. Invest. 1993; 91:2463–2469.

21. McCance D, Dyer D, Dunn D, Bailie K, Thorpe S, Baynes J, Lyons T. Maillard reaction products and their relation to complications in insulin-dependent diabetes mellitus. J. Clin. Invest. 1993; 91:2470–2478.

22. Nakamura Y, Horii Y, Nishino T, Shiiki H, Sakaguch Y, Kagoshima T, Dohi K, Makita Z, Vlassara H, Bucala R. Immunohistochemical localization of advanced glycosylation end products in coronary atheroma and cardiac tissue in diabetes mellitus. Am. J. Pathol. 1993; 143:1649–1656.

23. Miyata T, Oda O, Inagi R, Iida Y, Araki N, Yamada N, Horiuchi S, Taniguchi N, Maeda K, Kinoshita T. $\beta_2$-Microglobulin modified with advanced glycation endproducts is a major component of hemodialysis-associated amyloidosis. J. Clin. Invest. 1993; 92:1243–1252.

24. Miyata T, Inagi R, Iida Y, Sato M, Yamada N, Oda O, Maeda K, Seo H. Involvement of $\beta_2$-microglobulin modified with advanced glycation endproducts in the pathogenesis of hemodialysis-associated amyloidosis. J. Clin. Invest. 1994; 93:521–528.

25. Harrington C, Colaco CALS. Alzheimer's disease: a glycation connection. Nature 1994; 370:247–248.

26. Smith M, Kutty R, Richey P, Yan SD, Stern D, Chader G, Wiggert B, Petersen R, Perry G. Heme oxygenase-1 is associated with the neurofibrillary pathology of Alzheimer disease. Am. J. Pathol. 1994; 145:42–47.

27. Smith M, Taneda S, Richey P, Miyata S, Yan SD, Stern D, Monnier V, Perry G. Advanced Maillard reaction end products are associated with Alzheimer disease pathology. Proc. Natl. Acad. Sci. USA 1994;91:5710–5714.

28. Yan SD, Chen X, Schmidt AM, et al. The presence of glycated tau in Alzheimer's disease: a mechanism for induction of oxidant stress. Proc. Natl Acad. Sci. USA 1994; 91:7787–7791.

29. Vitek M, Bhattacharya K, Glendening JM. AGEs contribute to amyloidosis in Alzheimer's disease. Proc. Natl. Acad. Sci. USA 1994; 91:4766–4770.

30. Esposito C, Gerlach H, Brett J, Stern D, Vlassara H. Endothelial receptor-mediated binding of glucose-modified albumin is associated with increased monolayer permeability and modulation of cell surface coagulant properties. J. Exp. Med. 1989; 170:13887–1407.

31. Vlassara H, Bucala R, Striker L. Pathogenic effects of AGEs: Biochemical, biologic, and clinical implications for diabetes and aging. Lab. Invest. 1994; 70:138–151.

32. Khoury J, Thomas C, Loike J, Hickman S, Cao L, Silverstein S. Macrophages adhere to glucose-modified basement membranes via their scavenger receptors. J. Biol. Chem 1994; 269:10197–10200.

33. Hori O, Brett J, Slattery T, Cao R, Zhang J, Chen J, Nagashima M, Nitecki D, Morser J, Stern D, Schmidt A.M. The receptor for advanced glycation endproducts (RAGE) is a cellular binding site for amphoterin: mediation of neurite outgrowth and coexpression of RAGE and amphoterin in the developing nervous system. J. Biol. Chem. 1995; 270:25752–25761.

34. Brett J, Schmidt A-M, Zou Y-S, Yan S-D, Weidman E, Pinsky D, Neeper M, Przysiecki M, Shaw A, Migheli A, Stern D. Tissue distribution of the receptor for advanced glycation endproducts (RAGE): expression in smooth muscle, cardiac myocytes, and neural tissue in addition to the vasculature. Am. J. Pathol. 1993; 143:1699–1712.

35. Wautier JL, Wautier MP, Schmidt AM, Anderson GM, Hori O, Zoukourian C, Capron L, Chappey O, Brett J, Guillausseau P.J, Stern D. AGEs on the surface of diabetic erythrocytes bind to the vessel wall via a specific receptor inducing oxidant stress in the vasculature: a link between surface-associated AGEs and diabetic complications. Proc Natl Acad Sci USA 1994; 91:7742–7746.

36. Ross R. The pathogenesis of atherosclerosis—an update. N. Engl. J. Med. 1986; 314:488–500.

37. Kirstein M, Brett J, Radoff S, Ogawa S, Stern D, Vlassara H. Advanced protein glycosylation induces transendothelial human monocyte chemotaxis and secretion of platelet-derived growth factor: role in vascular disease of diabetes and aging. Proc. Natl. Acad. Sci. USA 1990; 87:9010–9014.

38. Vlassara H, Brownlee M, Manogue K, Dinarello C, Pasagian A. Cachectin/TNF and IL-1 induced by glucose-modified proteins: role in normal tissue remodeling. Science 1990; 240:1546–1548.

39. Schmidt AM, Hasu M, Popov D, et al. The receptor for advanced glycation endproducts (AGEs) has a central role in vessel wall interaction and gene activation in response to AGEs in the intravascular space. Proc Natl Acad Sci USA 1994; 91:8807–8811.

40. Schreck R, Rieber P, Baeuerle P. Reactive oxygen intermediates as apparently widely used messengers in the activation of the NF-$\kappa$B transcription factor and HIV-1. EMBO J. 1991; 10:2247–2258.

41. Collins T. Endothelial nuclear factor $\kappa$B and the initiation of the atherosclerotic lesion. Lab Invest. 1993; 10:336–349.

42. Marui, N, Offerman M, Swerlick R, et al. VCAM-1 gene transcription and expression are regulated through an oxidant-sensitive mechanism in human vascular endothelial cells. J. Clin. Invest. 1993; 92:1866–1984.

43. Cybulsky M, Gimbrone M. Endothelial expression of a mononuclear leukocyte adhesion molecule during atherogenesis. Science 1991; 251:788–791.

44. Li H, Cybulsky M, Gimbrone M, Libby P. An atherogenic diet rapidly induces

VCAM-1: a cytokine-regulatable mononuclear leukocyte adhesion molecule in rabbit aortic endothelium. Arterioscler. Thromb. 1993; 13:197–204.

45. Richardson M, Hadcock S, DeReske, Cybulsky M. Increased expression in vivo of VCAM-1 and E-selectin by the aortic endothelium of normolipemic and hyperlipemic diabetic rabbits. Arterioscler. Thromb. 1994; 14:760–769.

46. O'Brien DK, Allen MD, McDonald TO, et al. Vascular cell adhesion molecule-1 is expressed in human coronary atherosclerotic plaques. Implications for the mode of progression of advanced coronary atherosclerosis. J. Clin. Invest. 1993; 92:945–951.

47. Schmidt A-M, Hori O, Chen J, Li J.F, Crandall J, Zhang J, Cao R, Yan S.D, Brett J, Stern D. Advanced glycation endproducts interacting with their endothelial receptor induce expression of vascular cell adhesion molecule-1 (VCAM-1): a potential mechanism for the accelerated vasculopathy of diabetes. J. Clin. Invest. 1995; 96:1395–1403.

48. Neish A, Williams H, Palmer H, Whitley M, Collins T. Functional analysis of the human VCAM-1 promoter. J. Exp. Med. 1992; 176:1583–1593.

49. Iademarco M, McQuillan J, Dean D. VCAM-1: contrasting transcriptional control mechanisms in muscle and endothelium. Proc. Natl. Acad. Sci. USA 1993; 90:3943–3947.

50. Schmidt AM, Crandall J, Cao R, Hori O, Lakatta E. Elevated plasma levels of vascular cell adhesion molecule-1 (VCAM-1) in diabetic patients with microalbuminuria: a marker of vascular dysfunction and progressive vascular disease. Br. J. Hematol. 1995; in press.

51. Messent J, Elliott T, Hill R, Jarrett R, Keen H, Viberti G. Prognostic significance of microalbuminuria in insulin-dependent diabetes mellitus: a twenty-three follow-up study. Kidney Int 1992; 41:836–839.

52. Nannipieri M, Rizzo L, Rapuano A, Pilo A, Penno G, Navelesi R. Increased transcapillary escape rate of albumin in microalbuminuric type II diabetic subject. Diabetes Care 1995; 18:1–9.

53. Koch AE, Halloran MM, Haskell CJ, Shah MR, Polverini PJ. Angiogenesis mediated by soluble forms of E-selectin and vascular cell adhesion molecule-1. Nature 1995; 376:517–519.

54. Wautier J-L, Zoukourian C, Chappey O, Wautier M-P, Guillausseau P-J, Cao R, Hori O, Stern D, Schmidt AM. Receptor-mediated endothelial cell dysfunction in diabetic vasculopathy: soluble receptor for advanced glycation endproducts blocks hyperpermeability. J. Clin. Invest. 1996; 97:238–243.

55. Williamson JR, Chang K, Tilton RG, Prater C, Jeffrey JR, Weigel C, Sherman WR. Increased vascular permeability in spontaneously diabetic BB/W rats and in rats with mild versus severe streptozocin-induced diabetes. Diabetes 1987; 36:813–821.

56. Albelda S, Sampson PM, Haselton FR, McNiff JM, Meller SN, Williams SK, Fishman AP. Permeability characteristics of cultured endothelial cell monolayers. J Appl. Physiol 1988; 64:308–322.

# 12

# Hypertension

**Pierre Moreau**

*Hôtel-Dieu de Montreal Research Center, Montreal, Quebec, Canada*

**Thomas F. Lüscher**

*University Hospital, Bern, Switzerland*

## I. INTRODUCTION

One of the hallmarks of hypertension is an elevation of peripheral vascular resistance. It is now clear that locally generated or transformed mediators are needed to determine the vascular tone and structure of arteries, capillaries, and veins (1). In that context, the dominant vasorelaxing properties of the endothelium may act as a compensatory mechanism in an attempt to limit vascular resistance. On the other hand, the vascular endothelium might be involved directly to increase the peripheral resistance via an enhanced release of constricting factors and/or a decreased release of relaxing factors. Furthermore, the endothelium may significantly contribute to the vascular complications of hypertension as it becomes dysfunctional. One has to consider, however, that not all functional changes occurring in the endothelium do occur in a similar fashion in all forms of hypertension, in all stages of the disease, or in all vascular beds (2) (Fig. 1). A better understanding of the endothelial dysfunction in several forms of genetic or acquired experimental hypertension may lead to more appropriate detection means of these alterations that could benefit the evaluation and the treatment of the endothelial function in essential hypertension. This chapter deals with modifications of endothelium-dependent vasodilatation and vasoconstriction in experimental models as well as in essential hypertension. In addition, the effect of

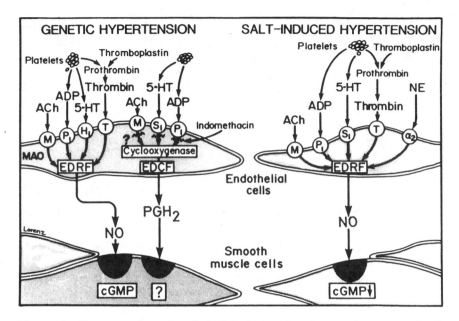

**Figure 1** Heterogeneity of endothelial dysfunction in spontaneous and salt-induced hypertension: Although in SHR the L-arginine nitric oxide pathway is overactive, NO seems to be inactivated either by oxygen-derived free radicals and/or fibrous tissue accumulating in the intima. In addition, a vasoconstrictor prostanoid (prostaglandin $H_2$/thromboxane $A_2$) if formed (left panel). In contrast, in Dahl rats, a deficient production of NO is most likely (right panel) (102).

currently available antihypertensive therapies on the endothelial function is discussed.

## II. ENDOTHELIAL ALTERATION IN EXPERIMENTAL MODELS OF HYPERTENSION

### A. Endothelium-Derived Relaxing Factors

One approach to determine the impact of an endogenous system on blood pressure regulation is to observe the hemodynamic changes following its inhibition. In that respect, the chronic blockade of nitric oxide (NO) synthase with an analogue of L-arginine, such as $N^\omega$-nitro-L-arginine methyl ester (L-NAME), leads to an increased vascular resistance (3,4) and, ultimately, to a marked and sustained increase in blood pressure (5,6). The cardiovascular system is therefore exposed to a continuous NO-dependent vasodilatory tone (5) and withdrawal of it mimics many features of human hypertension, including target organ damage (7,8). It is also of interest to note that an endogenous inhibitor of the L-arginine–NO pathway has been recently discovered: asymmetrical dimethyl-arginine (ADMA). This substance can regulate the activity of this pathway both locally and systemically, and it may have profound consequences on vascular tone when its production and/or clearance are altered, as it has been shown to occur in chronic renal failure (9).

Animals chronically treated with L-NAME usually suffer very early on from brain and spinal cord infarcts and die after only 7–11 weeks of treatment (7), reinforcing the belief that the L-arginine–NO pathway is very necessary to maintain a proper central nervous system perfusion and may be a major determinant of end-organ damage. Indeed, antihypertensive drugs that have been shown to lower blood pressure and to improve endothelium-dependent relaxations in this model of hypertension (10) also prevent the central nervous system complications (11) (Fig. 2). From most of the results obtained in L-NAME–induced hypertension, it is tempting to speculate that decreased production of NO by endothelial cells is responsible for the development of hypertension. However, the story seems far more complex when other models of hypertension are considered.

In spontaneously hypertensive rats (SHR), endothelial function becomes impaired as hypertension develops (12). This was reported in the aorta and mesenteric, skeletal muscle, carotid, and cerebral vessels (12–15). In contrast, in coronary and renal arteries, endothelial function does not seem to be affected by high blood pressure (15,16), at least in this model of hypertension. Although endothelium-dependent relaxations are either diminished of normal in SHR, the production of NO appears to be increased. Indeed, the release of NO from isolated coronary vessels is augmented in SHR (17). Furthermore, the activity of constitutive nitric oxide synthase (cNOS) is also enhanced in the heart left ventricle (Fig. 3) (18,19) and in small mesenteric arteries (21). These observations are consistent with the demonstration that pharmacologically induced elevations in blood pressure increase the release of NO in normotensive rats (20), suggesting that blood pressure per se is a stimulus for NO release in the rat. This interpretation is reinforced by the fact that cNOS activity is normal in prehypertensive 4-week-old SHR (19). Although its production is augmented in SHR, NO seems inefficient, probably due to increased inactivation (21). This could be due to an imbalance between superoxide production and superoxide dismutase (SOD) activity in the vessel wall and/or scavenging of NO by fibrous tissue which accumulates in the hypertensive intima. The direct measurement of NO (with a porphyrinic microsensor) diffusing from a mesenteric resistance artery segment lends support to this hypothesis. Indeed, SOD was effective to normalize the amount of NO

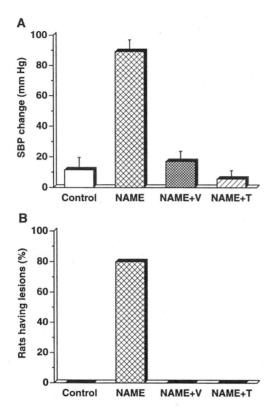

**Figure 2** (A) Net change of systolic blood pressure (tail cuff measurement) after 6 weeks of L-NAME–induced hypertension (50 mg/kg/day) alone or in combination with verapamil (NAME+V, a calcium antagonist) or trandolapril (NAME+T, an ACE inhibitor). (B) Brain parenchymal lesions in the same animals. Verapamil (NAME+V) and trandolapril (NAME+T) prevented these lesions that occured in four of 5 L-NAME–treated rats. Small infarcts were observed in two of five, focal glial proliferation in three of five, and a fresh hemorrhage was detected in one of five.

reaching the electrode that was blunted in untreated SHR arteries as compared to Wistar Kyoto rat arteries (22). This accentuated metabolism of NO may contribute to the impaired endothelium-dependent relaxations observed in this model of hypertension despite an increased activity of the L-arginine pathway (12). In addition, an increased production of endothelium-derived contracting factor(s) can explain the abnormal endothelial function of some vascular beds (see below). Other factors, such as sex steroid hormones, may also modulate the endolthelial function, as female SHR have a less severe endothelial dysfunction than male SHR (23).

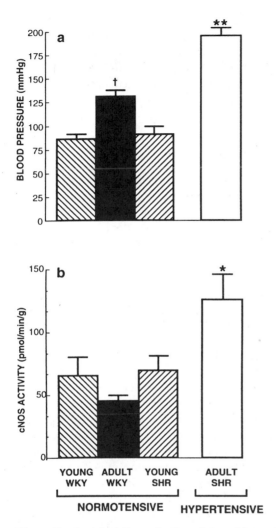

**Figure 3** Activity of constitutive nitric oxide synthase in the left ventricle of young and adult normotensive (WKY, Wistar Kyoto) and spontaneously hypertensive rats. Nitric oxide synthase activity increases as blood pressure increases in the SHR but not in the WKY (19).

Nitric oxide production and inactivation might be heterogenously affected in different forms of hypertension (24). For example, in Dahl salt-sensitive rats (24,25) and in two-kidney–one clip experimental hypertension (26), endothelium-dependent relaxations are impaired, but no release of vasoconstrictor prostanoids can be demonstrated. This suggests that a decreased NO production could contribute to the pathogenesis of this form of hypertension. Accordingly, following acetylcholine stimulation, the measurement of nitrite-nitrate (an index of NO production) in the perfusate of isolated kidneys was smaller in Dahl salt-sensitive rats than in controls (27). The same was demonstrated for deoxycorticosterone acetate (DOCA)–salt hypertensive rats with acetylcholine (27) and with $ET_B$-receptor stimulation (28).

## B.   Endothelium-Derived Contracting Factors

The vascular responses of hypertensive blood vessels to endothelin (ET) differ depending on experimental conditions, the model of hypertension, and the vascular bed studied (29). However, the majority of the studies have reported a depressed response to the peptide (30,31), including subcutaneous vessels from hypertensive patients (32). In contrast, in the renal circulation, which is important for long-term blood pressure regulation, the vasoconstrictor responses to ET are maintained (33) or even increased at least in the SHR model of hypertension (34).

The circulating levels of ET are not increased in most of experimental or human hypertension (29). However, they may not represent a good index of local vascular ET production, since more than twice as much ET is released abluminally by endothelial cells than luminally (35). It is reasonable to believe that very subtle increases in local ET levels that may not produce contraction, but that may facilitate the vascular contraction to other agonists, could be of some importance in hypertension. This hypothesis is strengthened by the observation that very low concentrations of ET, which by themselves exert no significant contraction, can amplify contractions to norepinephrine and serotonin in hypertensive rats (36) as well as in humans (37). These amplifying effects of ET are augmented with aging (38) and hypertension (36). Interestingly, in the mesenteric resistance circulation of the SHR, angiotensin II can produce enough ET of endothelial origin to amplify contractions to norepinephrine (36).

In DOCA-salt hypertensive rats, an increased production of ET in mesenteric arteries can be demonstrated even in the presence of normal circulating levels of the peptide (39). In contrast, however, in the same preparations taken from SHR, no increase in local ET production can be observed (39). These rats must be treated with a DOCA-salt regimen to overexpress ET in the vascular endothelium (40). However, in these animals, ET seems to mediate vascular hypertrophy rather than the elevation of blood pressure, since ET antagonists administered chronically have more profound effects on the vascular structure than on the blood pressure level (Fig. 4) (39,40). Cyclosporine-induced hypertension is also associated with

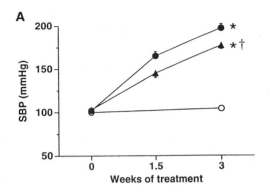

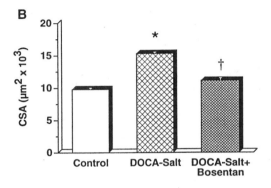

**Figure 4** Effect of chronic treatment with bosentan, a combined $ET_{A/B}$ receptor antagonist, on the evolution of systolic blood pressure (SBP, Panel A) and the structure of resistance arteries (CSA = Cross-Sectional Area, Panel B) in DOCA-salt hypertension. In panel A, ○ = Control; ● = DOCA-Salt; ▲ = DOCA-Salt + Bosentan. * $P < 0.05$ versus Control; † $P < 0.05$ versus DOCA-Salt. (Adapted from ref. 85.)

an increased expression of preproendothelin-1 and of the $ET_A$ receptor subtype (41). Studies with ET antagonists should be conducted to translate these changes in a more definitive role for ET in this form of hypertension.

Besides ET, the vascular endothelium can produce other constricting factors. In the aorta of SHR, the reduction of the endothelium-dependent relaxation produced by acetylcholine seems to be due to the enhanced production of a cyclooxygenase-dependent endothelium-derived contracting factor (EDCF), possibly prostaglandin $H_2$ (Fig. 5) (14,31). This observation does not seem to be limited to the use of acetylcholine, since ADP/ATP and serotonin also triggered an enhanced production of EDCF in the cerebral and coronary microcirculation of SHR (42,43). Platelet-derived substances

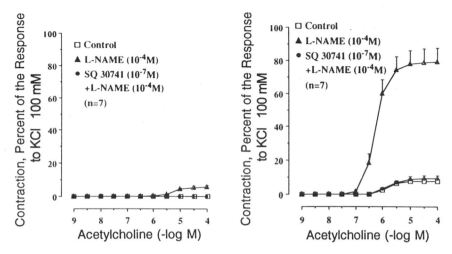

**Figure 5** Endothelium-dependent contractions in the aorta of normotensive Wistar Kyoto rats (WKY, left panel) and spontaneously hypertensive rats (SHR, right panel) at the age of 12 weeks. Note the marked endothelium-dependent contractions to acetylcholine after inhibition of nitric oxide production by L-NAME in SHR. The contractions can be prevented by the thromboxane receptor antagonist SQ30741 (31).

(ADP/ATP and serotonin) may therefore produce more contraction when aggregating in damaged vessels of hypertensive animals or individuals by a cyclooxygenase-dependent pathway, thus possibly contributing to the complications of hypertension. Part of the decreased endothelium-dependent relaxation observed in L-NAME–induced hypertension also has a thromboxane $A_2$/prostaglandin $H_2$ component (44), suggesting that a decreased production of NO can lead to an increased EDCF production and/or release, further altering the balance between the two pathways. However, this relationship may be different with aging, since the blunted endothelium-dependent relaxation was solely due to a decreased production or efficacy of NO in senescent SHR (31). It is not clear to which extent the increased production of a prostanoid EDCF really contributes to the elevation of blood pressure or only to complications of hypertension. Indeed, in SHR, the administration of a thromboxane $A_2$ receptor antagonist improved the endothelial function without lowering blood pressure, which argues against a significant effect of this mediator on blood pressure regulation (45).

The cyclooxygenase cascade is also the source of superoxide anions which can mediate endothelium-dependent contractions either by enhancing the breakdown of NO or by directly stimulating vascular smooth muscle cells (46). The cyclooxygenase pathway therefore produces multiple potentially constricting factors and the use of more specific inhibitors than indomethacin (such as the thromboxane $A_2$/prostaglandin $H_2$ receptor antagonists SQ 30741 or SQ 29548 and the superoxide anion scavenger superoxide dismutase) will help better to determine their importance in vascular function and in hypertension. Such a selective pharmacological approach has emphasized the important role of superoxide anions in the balance between endothelium-dependent contractions and relaxations (47).

## III. ENDOTHELIAL ALTERATION IN ESSENTIAL AND SECONDARY FORMS OF HYPERTENSION

The studies in animal models of hypertension, described above, helped to define the major alterations of the vascular endothelium in the disease process. Fewer studies are available in humans and, so far, most of the studies have evaluated the integrity of the vasodilatatory pathways (and mainly NO) of the endothelium in hypertensive subjects. The development of ET receptor antagonists should help to determine the influence of endothelium-mediated vasoconstriction on the vascular tone in primary or secondary forms of human hypertension.

### A. Endothelium-Derived Relaxing Factors

Pharmacological experiments in humans provided indirect evidence for a diminished basal and stimulated NO production (48,49). Indeed, the decrease in forearm blood flow induced by Nω-nitro-monomethyl-L-arginine (L-NMMA) is smaller in hypertensive than in normotensive patients (Fig. 6) (49). In addition, most studies, but not all, find a reduced endothelium-dependent vasodilatation in patients with primary or secondary hypertension (Table 1) (50–52). These first studies performed with acetylcholine were confirmed with bradykinin, another endothelium-dependent vasodilator (53). The impaired endothelial response in hypertensives can be improved (albeit not normalized) by indomethacin, suggesting that vasoconstrictor prostanoids also contribute to impaired endothelium-dependent relaxation in hypertensive patients (51). So far, it is not clear if an increased metabolism of NO is also present in human forms of hypertension. Reduced endothelium-dependent relaxations were also found in the coronary circulation of patients with atherosclerosis risk factors, including hypertension, implying such consequences as a limited microvascular coronary vasodilatation potentially contribute to myocardial ischemia (54–56).

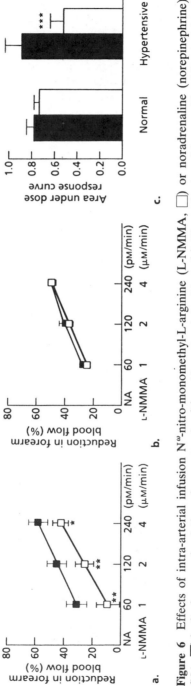

**Figure 6** Effects of intra-arterial infusion $N^{\omega}$-nitro-monomethyl-L-arginine (L-NMMA, □) or noradrenaline (norepinephrine) (NA, ■) in the forearm circulation of normotensive (b) and hypertensive subjects (a). The reduction of forearm blood flow produced by L-NMMA is blunted in hypertensive patients (a and c) (9).

**Table 1** Results of Studies Examining the Response of Intra-arterial Infusion of Acetylcholine in the Forearm Circulation of Patients with Essential Hypertension

| Investigators | NT | HT | Result |
|---|---|---|---|
| 1. Linder L, Kiowski W, Bühler FR, Lüscher TF. Circulation 1990; 81:1762–1767 | 8 | 8 | ↓ |
| 2. Panza JA, Quyyumi AA, Brush JE, Epstein SE. N Engl J Med 1990; 323:22–27 | 18 | 18 | ↓ |
| 3. Panza JA, Quyyumi AA, Callahan TS, Epstein SE. JACC 1993: 21:1145–1151 | 15 | 15 | ↓ |
| 4. Panza JA, Casino PR, Kilcoyne CM, Quyyumi AA. Circulation 1993: 87:1468–1474 | 11 | 11 | ↓ |
| 5. Panza JA, Casino PR, Badar DM, Quyyumi AA. Circulation 1993: 87:1475–1481 | 12 | 14 | ↓ |
| 6. Hirooka Y, Imazumi T, Masaki H, Ando S, Parada S, Momohara M, Takeshita A. Hypertension 1992; 20:175–180 | 14 | 12 | ↓ |
| 7. Creager MA, Roddy ME, Coleman SM, Dzau, VJ. Blood Vessels 1992; 29:97–98 | 15 | 21 | ↓ |
| 8. Taddei S, Virdis A, Mattei P, Salvetti A. Hypertension 1993; 21:929–933 | 24 | 28 | ↓ |
| 9. Cockcroft JR, Chowienczyk PJ, Benjamin, N, Ritter JM. N Engl J Med 1994; 330:1036–1040 | 37 | 58 | ⟷ |
| Total | 117 | 127 | ↓ |
|  | 37 | 58 | ⟷ |

NT = normative subjects.
HT = hypertensive patients.

Small arteries obtained from gluteal biopsies showed only a slight reduction in their relaxation to acetylcholine, but, in contrast to studies in the forearm, this impairment was not corrected by indomethacin (57). It must be pointed out, however, that these vessels seem to depend more on alternative vasorelaxing mechanisms than the L-arginine–NO pathway for endothelium-dependent relaxations (57).

Nitric oxide plays an important role in renal function, since the inhibition of NO synthesis primarily affects the renal excretion of sodium and water before any changes in blood pressure occur (58,59). Thus, deficient renal synthesis or efficacy of NO may constitute a primary factor in the development of hypertension (58,59). Accordingly, the administration of L-arginine, the precursor of NO, decreases mean blood pressure to the same extent in normotensive and hypertensive subjects, but the renal function is not improved as much in the latter group (60). Therefore, a local renal alteration may exist that could potentially lead to the development of hypertension. Moreover, it has been recently shown that renal failure is also associated with an accumulation of an endogenous inhibitor of NO synthesis, asymmetrical dimethylarginine (9), which could also explain the increase in peripheral resistance and hypertension observed in this condition.

## B.  Endothelium-Derived Contracting Factors

Owing to the very recent development of ET antagonists, fewer observations are available in essential hypertension than in animal models. As outlined above, plasma concentrations of ET are not increased in hypertension (29), although this is not a representative index of local ET activity. Indeed, plasma levels of ET-1 were related to blood pressure only in cases of hemangioendothelioma characterized by very high circulating ET-1 levels (61). However, this report suggests that high circulating ET-1 has a blood pressure–raising effect in humans. One study in the cutaneous hand veins of hypertensive subjects suggested an enhanced response to ET-1 (62), whereas studies in subcutaneous vessels demonstrated the opposite (32). The results of the first clinical trials with ET receptor antagonists will help better to define the role of ET in essential hypertension or in secondary forms of the disease.

The vasodilatation induced by acetylcholine is blunted in the forearm circulation of hypertensive patients (see above). In that context, indomethacin, an inhibitor of cyclooxygenase, partially restored the blunted relaxation produced by acetylcholine (Fig. 7) (51). This would suggest that these vessels are submitted to a greater vasoconstriction from endothelial origin, probably mediated by thromboxane $A_2$ or prostaglandin $H_2$. This avenue will have to be investigated with more selective antagonists working

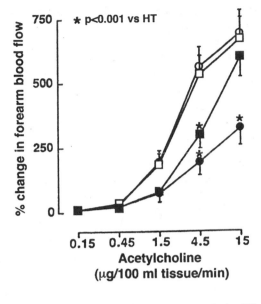

O Normotensives + Indomethacin (n=12)
□ Normotensives (n=12)
● Hypertensives (n=12)
■ Hypertensives + Indomethacin (n=12)

**Figure 7** Endothelium-dependent increases in forearm blood flow in normotensive and hypertensive patients during infusion of increasing dosages of acetylcholine. In the hypertensives, the response to acetylcholine is increased (albeit not normalized) by treatment with the cyclooxygenase inhibitor indomethacin (51).

at the level of the thromboxane $A_2$ receptor to confirm the nature of the EDCF involved in essential hypertension.

## IV.  ANTIHYPERTENSIVE THERAPY AND ENDOTHELIAL FUNCTION

Endothelial dysfunction seems to be a common feature of several pathological processes including hypertension, hyperlipidemia, and atherosclerosis. Drugs that could improve the endothelial function or enhance alternative pathways to substitute for the alterations of the release of endothelial mediators may have a potential advantage in the protection and treatment of these pathological conditions. Several antihypertensive agents can prevent and reverse the impaired endothelium-dependent relaxations in large conduit arteries (63,64) as well as in resistance arteries of hypertensive rats (65). Since diuretics, calcium antagonists, angiotensin-converting enzyme (ACE) inhibitors and angiotensin receptor antagonists are able to improve or normalize the endothelial dysfunction in hypertensive rats, the anti-hypertensive properties of the agents appear to be involved in this effect. However, additional important considerations cannot be ruled out and are described for each class of pharmacological agents.

## A.  Nitrates

Nitrovasodilators such as nitroglycerin, sodium nitroprusside, and linsido-mine exert their vasodilator effects by releasing NO from their molecule (66); therefore acting through a mechanism identical with that of endoge-nously produced NO. Hence, these drugs may be particularly useful at sites of reduced vascular formation of NO such as diseased coronary arteries. Of particular interest is the fact that the endogenous production of NO re-duces the sensitivity of the blood vessel wall to nitrates and nitrovaso-dilators (67). Inversely, in human arteries devoid of endothelium, the concentration-relaxation curve to linsidomine is shifted to the left (4,68). This could ensure a more selective action of these drugs to dysfunctional vascular beds.

   In addition, to be more effective at sites of reduced NO formation, the nitrovasodilators seem to be more effective in larger epicardial coronary arteries rather than in smaller coronary arteries (69). This may be due to the fact that small coronary arteries are unable to transform nitroglycerin into active molecules. Since adenosine, which primarily relaxes small ves-sels, may precipitate ischemia, this selective efficacy of nitrovasodilators may have important clinical implications. A clinically important drawback, however, is the fact that most nitrovasodilators are prone to tolerance.

## B.  Calcium Antagonists

Under acute conditions, calcium antagonists do not affect the release of endothelium-derived vasoactive substances, although the production of these factors in the endothelial cell is associated with an increase in in-tracellular calcium (70). Indeed, endothelial cells do not appear to possess voltage-operated calcium channels. During their chronic administration, however, these antihypertensive agents improve the endothelial function (10,44,64). Since this beneficial effect was present in L-NAME–induced hypertension, in which the synthesis of NO is inhibited, alternative path-ways of endothelium-dependent relaxation may be involved (10,44). Cal-cium antagonists may also facilitate the effects of endothelium-derived relaxing factors at the level of vascular smooth muscle, as it has been suggested by enhanced sodium nitroprusside–induced relaxations in certain conditions (71).

In addition, calcium antagonists seem to interfere with the vasoconstrictor effects of ET and cyclooxygenase-derived contracting factors (72). Accordingly, in the porcine coronary artery, ET receptors are linked to voltage-operated calcium channels via a G-protein and calcium antagonists attenuate ET-induced vasoconstriction in this blood vessel (73). Furthermore, in the human forearm circulation, ET-1 induces potent contractions which are prevented by nifedipine and verapamil, unmasking the vasodilator effects of the peptide (74). However, there may be regional differences, as calcium antagonists are ineffective to inhibit ET-induced contractions in some vessels, such as the internal mammary artery (75). It is not clear, however, if the usual clinical doses of calcium antagonists are sufficient to antagonize endogenous ET-induced contractions.

## C. Angiotensin-Converting Enzyme Inhibitors

ACE is mainly located on the endothelial cell membrane where it activates angiotensin I into angiotensin II and breaks down bradykinin, a potent stimulator of the L-arginine and cyclooxygenase pathways (76). Therefore, ACE inhibitors not only prevent the formation of a potent vasoconstrictor with proliferative properties but also increase the local concentration of bradykinin and, in turn, the production of NO and prostacyclin (77). This latter effect may participate in the protective effects of the ACE inhibitors by improving local blood flow and preventing platelet activation. Accordingly, pretreatment of human saphenous vein and coronary artery with an ACE inhibitor enhances endothelium-dependent relaxation to bradykinin (78,79). The decreased degradation of bradykinin could therefore explain the improved endothelial function observed with ACE inhibitors in normotensive and particularly in hypertensive rats (65,80,81). However, the improvement of the endothelial function by ACE inhibitors in L-NAME–induced hypertension suggest that they may also enhance other endothelium-dependent mechanisms, since the activity of the enzyme NOS is inhibited in this experimental model (10,44). The mechanism used by ACE inhibitors also seems to require some time to develop and cannot be reproduce in acute conditions, again suggesting that another mechanism than ACE inhibition, which is rapid, is involved (10). Endothelium-dependent hyperpolarization may be responsible for this effect, as suggested by one study (80).

In contrast to the striking improvements obtained in experimental models of hypertension, studies in hypertensive patients have failed to show any beneficial effect of this class of drug on the endothelial function (82).

The reasons for this discrepancy are not clear at the present time. This discrepancy may originate from the fact that endothelial dysfunction may be treated at a much later stage in patients than in the rat. Prolonged therapy may be required to restore the endothelial function in hypertensive patients.

## D. Angiotensin II Receptor Antagonists

The recently developed angiotensin receptor antagonists may have advantages, as they are more potent inhibitors of the angiotensin II vasoconstrictor axis than ACE inhibitors (83). These new drugs are also not associated with cough, which is a side effect of ACE inhibitors generally attributed to the diminished breakdown of bradykinin. However, if indeed the concomitant stimulation of the L-arginine NO pathway by bradykinin also proves to be an important property of ACE inhibitors, angiotensin II receptor antagonists would lack this beneficial effect.

## E. Endothelin Antagonists

The use of ET receptor antagonists, which are becoming increasingly available, will help to determine the role of ET in health and disease. In hypertension, the picture is still unclear. In most experimental models of hypertension, these molecules are not effective to lower blood pressure (84). As discussed above, they have a modest antihypertensive efficacy in DOCA-salt hypertensive rats, although they have a more profound effect on vascular hypertrophy (85). These antagonists administered for 6 weeks also showed very modest activity in L-NAME–induced hypertension (Moreau, Takase, and Lüscher, unpublished observation), although they would be expected to be effective if one considers the negative feedback exerted by NO on ET-1 release that is blocked in this model. This inhibition of the negative feedback was demonstrated in acute conditions by showing that ET receptor antagonists blunted the blood pressure rise induced by acute L-NAME administration (86). Endothelin receptor antagonists may therefore be effective to delay the onset of hypertension, but not to prevent its development. In the same line, one study in a canine model of hypertension reported a significant acute effect of bosentan, an $ET_{A/B}$ receptor antagonist (87). Studies in human hypertension will help to elucidate the contribution of ET, since there is evidence that ET may contribute to basal vascular tone as shown in the forearm circulation (88) and in the human skin microcirculation (89).

The type of antagonist ($ET_A$ receptor selective or combined $ET_{A/B}$ receptor antagonists) that would be more effective is still a matter of theoretical debate. Most of the first-generation molecules were specific $ET_A$ receptor

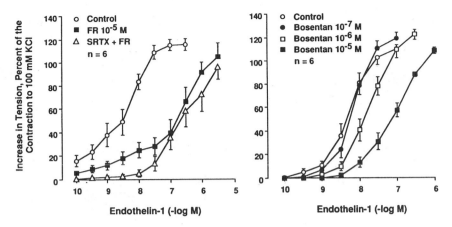

**Figure 8** Effects of endothelin and endothelin receptor antagonists in the human internal mammary artery: Although the $ET_A$-receptor antagonist FR139317 (left panel) causes a parallel shift of the concentration response curve to endothelin 1 at higher, but not at lower, concentrations of endothelin-1, the $ET_A/ET_B$ receptor antagonist bosentan (right panel) causes a parallel rightward shift of the concentration response curve (100).

antagonists (90–92). Combined $ET_{A/B}$ receptor antagonists are now also available (93–97), and they may prove to be better therapeutic agents, since in several blood vessels, including humans vessels, both $ET_A$ and $ET_B$ receptors mediate vasoconstriction (Fig. 8) (98–100). However, these nonselective antagonists also block the endothelium-dependent vasodilation of ET by blocking $ET_B$ receptors (93,101). Endothelin-converting enzyme inhibitors may also prove to be valuable therapeutic agents, although their development lags behind the receptor antagonists.

## V. CONCLUSIONS

The vascular endothelium, by the inappropriate synthesis, release, or metabolism of its mediators, is an important candidate for the development and maintenance of hypertension. The study of several models of hypertension have provided evidence for heterogeneity of endothelial dysfunction, suggesting that this may also be the case in essential as well as secondary forms of hypertension in humans. Some commonly used therapeutic agents such as calcium antagonists and ACE inhibitors seem to have favorable effects on the endothelial function. A better understanding of the mechanisms involved in the alterations of the endothelial properties in cardiovascular diseases, as well as of the interaction of antihypertensive drugs with the endothelium, will be a necessary step for the development of more specific and effective ways to interact with the vascular endothelium.

## REFERENCES

1. Lüscher. Endothelial regulation of vascular tone and growth. Am J Hypertens 1993; 6:283S–293S.
2. Lüscher TF. The endothelium in hypertension: Bystander, target or mediator? J Hypertens 1994; 12(suppl 10):105–116.
3. Vallance P, Collier J, Moncada S. Effects of endothelium derived nitric oxide on peripheral arteriolar tone in man. Lancet 1989; 2:997–1000.
4. Joannides R, Richard V, Haefeli WE, Linder L, Lüscher TF, Thuillez C. Role of basal and stimulated release of nitric oxide in the regulation of radial artery caliber in humans. Hypertension 1995; 26:237–331.
5. Rees DD, Palmer RMJ, Moncada S. Role of endothelium-derived nitric oxide in the regulation of blood pressure. Proc Natl Acad Sci USA 1989; 86: 3375–3378.
6. Arnal JF, Warin L, Michel JB. Determinants of arotic cyclic guanosine monophosphate in hypertension induced by chronic inhibition of nitric oxide synthase. J Clin Invest 1992; 90:647–652.
7. Blot S, Arnal J-F, Xu Y, Gray F, Michel J-B. Spinal cord infarcts during long term inhibition of nitric oxide synthesis in rats. Stroke 1994; 25:1666–1673.
8. Palmer RMJ, Bridge L, Foxwell NA, Moncada S. The role of nitric oxide in endothelial damage and its inhibition by glucocorticoids. Br J Pharmacol 1992; 105:11–12.
9. Vallance P, Leone A, Calver A, Collier J, Moncada S. Accumulation of an endogenous inhibitor of nitric oxide synthesis in chronic renal failure. Lancet 1992; 329:572–575.
10. Takase H, Moreau P, Küng CF, Nava E, Lüscher TF. Antihypertensive therapy improves the endothelial function of resistance arteries in nitric oxide deficient hypertension: effect of verapamil and trandolapril. Hypertension 1996; 27:25–31.
11. Moreau P, Takase H, Küng CF, van Rooijen M-M, Schaffner T, Lüscher TF. Structure and function of the rat vasilar artery during chronic nitric oxide synthase inhibition. Stroke 1995; 26:1922–1929.
12. Dohi Y, Thiel MA, Bühler FR, Lüscher TF. Activation of endothelial L-arginine pathway in pressurized resistance arteries. Effect of age and hypertension. Hypertension 1990; 16:170–179.
13. Koller A, Huang A. Shear stress-induced dilation is attenuated in skeletal muscle arterioles of hypertensive rats. Hypertension 1995; 25:758–763.
14. Lüscher TF, Vanhoutte PM. Endothelium-dependent contractions to acetylcholine in the aorta of the spontaneously hypertensive rat. Hypertension 1986; 8:344–348.
15. Lüscher TF. Endothelium-derived nitric oxide: the endogenous nitrova-

sodilator in the human cardiovascular system. Eur Heart J 1991; 12(suppl E):2–11.

16. Tschudi MR, Criscione L, Lüscher TF. Effect of aging and hypertension on endothelial function of rat coronary arteries. J Hypertens 1991; 9:164–165.

17. Kelm M, Feelisch M, Krebber T, Motz W, Strauer BE. The role of nitric oxide in the regulation of coronary vascular resistance in arterial hypertension: comparison of normotensive and spontaneously hypertensiv rats. J Cardiovasc Pharmacol 1992; 20:183–186.

18. Nava E, Noll G, Lüscher TF. Increased activity of constitutive nitric oxide synthase in hearts from spontaneously hypertensive rats. Circulation 1994; 90:I–299.

19. Nava E, Noll G, Lüscher TF. Increased activity of constitutive nitric oxide synthase in cardiac endothelium in spontaneous hypertension. Circulation 1995; 91:2310–2313.

20. Nava E, Leone AM, Wiklund NP, Moncada S. Detection of release of nitric oxide by vasoactive substances in the anaesthetized rat. In: Feelisch M, Busse R, Moncada S, eds. The Biology of Nitric Oxide. London: Portland Press, 1994:179–181.

21. Nava E, Moreau P, Lüscher TF. Basal production of nitric oxide is increased, but inefficaceous in spontaneous hypertension (abstract). Circulation 1995; 92 (suppl I):I–347.

22. Tschudi MR, Mesaros S, Lüscher TF, Malinski T. Direct in situ measurement of nitric oxide in mesenteric resistance arteries: increased decomposition by superoxide in hypertension. Hypertension 1996; 27:32–35.

23. Kauser K, Rubanyi GM. Gender difference in endothelial dysfunction in the aorta of spontaneously hypertensive rats. Hypertension 1995; 25:517–523.

24. Lüscher TF, Vanhoutte PM. Mechanisms of altered endothelium-dependent responses in hypertensive blood vessels. In: Vanhoutte PM, ed. Relaxing and Contracting Factors. Clifton, NJ: Humana Press, 1988:495–509.

25. Lüscher TF, Raij L, Vanhoutte PM. Endothelium-dependent vascular responses in normotensive and hypertensive Dahl rats. Hypertension 1987; 9: 157–163.

26. Lee JG, Choi KC, Yeum CH, et al. Impairment of endothelium-dependent vasorelaxation in chronic two-kidney, one clip hypertensive rats. Nephrol, Dialysis Transplant 1995; 10:619–623.

27. Hayakawa H, Hirata Y, Suzuki E, et al. Mechanisms for altered endothelium-dependent vasorelaxation in isolated kidneys from experimental hypertensive rats. Am J Physiol 1993; 264:H1535–H1541.

28. Hirata Y, Hayakawa H, Suzuki E, et al. Direct measurement of endothelium-derived nitric oxide release by stimulation of endothelin receptors in rat kidney and its alteration in salt-induced hypertension. Circulation 1995; 91:1229–1235.

29. Lüscher TF, Boulanger CM, Dohi Y, Yang Z. Endothelium-derived contracting factors. Hypertension 1992; 19:117–130.

30. Nguyen PV, Parent A, Deng LY, Fluckiger JP, Thibault G, Schiffrin EL. Endothelin vascular receptors and responses in deoxycorticosterone acetate-salt hypertensive rats. Hypertension 1992; 19(suppl):1198–1204.

31. Küng CF, Lüscher TF. Different mechanisms of endothelial dysfunction with aging and hypertension in rat aorta. Hypertension 1995; 25:194–200.
32. Schiffrin EL, Deng LY, Larochelle P. Blunted effects of endothelin upon small subcutaneous resistance arteries of mild essential hypertensive patients. J Hypertens 1992; 10:437–444.
33. Seo B, Lüscher TF. $ET_A$ and $ET_B$ receptors mediate contractions to endothelin-1 in renal artery of aging spontaneously hypertensive rats: effects of FR139317 and bosentan. Hypertension 1995; 25:501–506.
34. Tomobe Y, Miyauchi T, Saito A, et al. Effects of endothelin on the renal artery from spontaneously hypertensive and Wistar Kyoto rats. Eur J Pharmacol 1988; 152:373–374.
35. Wagner O, Christ G, Wojta J, et al. Polar secretion of endothelin-1 by cultured endothelial cells. J Biol Chem 1992; 267:16066–16068.
36. Dohi Y, Hahn AWA, Boulanger CM, Bühler FR, Lüscher TF. Endothelin stimulated by angiotensin II augments contractility of spontaneously hypertensive rat resistance arteries. Hypertension 1992; 19:131–137.
37. Yang Z, Richard V, Segesser Lv, et al. Threshold concentrations of endothelin-1 potentiate contractions to norepinephrine and serotonin in human arteries: A new mechanism of vasospasm? Circulation 1990; 82:188–195.
38. Dohi Y, Lüscher TF. Aging differentially affects direct and indirect actions of endothelin-1 in perfused mesenteric arteries of the rat. Br J Pharmacol 1990; 100:889–893.
39. Larivière R, Thibault G, Schiffrin EL. Increased endothelin-1 contents in blood vessels of deoxycorticosterone acetate-salt hypertensive rats but not in spontaneously hypertensive rats. Hypertension 1993; 21:294–300.
40. Schiffrin EL, Larivière R, Li J-S, Sventek P, Touyz RM. Deoxycorticosterone acetate plus salt induce overexpression of vascular endothelin-1 and severe vascular hypertrophy in spontaneously hypertensive rats. Hypertension 1995; 25 (pt 2):769–773.
41. Iwai J, Kanayama Y, Okamura M, Takeda T. Gene expression of endothelin receptors in aortic cells from cyclosporin-induced hypertensive rats. Clin Exp Pharmacol Physiol 1995; 22:404–409.
42. Lüscher TF, Rubanyi GM, Aarhus LL, Vanhoutte PM. Serotonin reduces coronary flow in isolated hearts of the spontaneously hypertensive rat. J Hypertens 1986; 4(suppl 5):148–150.
43. Mayhan WG, Faraci FM, Heistad DD. Responses of cerebral arterioles to adenosine diphosphate, serotonin and the thromboxane analogue U-46619 during chronic hypertension. Hypertension 1989; 12(suppl 6):556–561.
44. Küng CF, Moreau P, Takase H, Lüscher TF. L-NAME induced hypertension, impairs endothelial function in rat aorta: Reversal by trandolapril and verapamil. Hypertension 1995; 26:744–751.
45. Tesfamariam B, Ogletree ML. Dissociation of endothelial cell dysfunction and blood pressure in SHR. Am J Physiol 1995; 38:H189–H194.
46. Katusic ZS, Vanhoutte PM. Superoxide anion is an endothelium-derived contracting factor. Am J Physiol 1989; 257:H33–H37.

47. Cosentino F, Sill JC, Katusic ZS. Role of superoxide anions in the mediation of endothelium-dependent contractions. Hypertension 1994; 23:229–235.
48. Linder L, Kiowsky W, Bühler FR, Lüscher TF. Indirect evidence for the release of endothelium-derived relaxing factor in human forearm circulation in vivo: Blunted response in essential hypertension. Circulation 1990; 81: 1762–1767.
49. Calver A, Collier J, Moncada S, Vallance P. Effect of local intra-arterial $N^G$-monomethyl-L-arginine in patients with hypertension: the nitric oxide dilator mechanism appears abnormal. J Hypertens 1992; 10:1025–1031.
50. Panza JA, Casino PR, Kilcoyne CM, Quyyumi AA. Role of endothelium-dependent vascular relaxation of patients with essential hypertension. Circulation 1993; 87:1468–1474.
51. Taddei S, Virdis A, Mattei P, Salvetti A. Vasodilation to acetylcholine in primary and secondary forms of human hypertension. Hypertension 1993; 21:929–933.
52. Cockcroft JR, Chowienczyk PJ, Benjamin N, Ritter JM. Preserved endothelium-dependent vasodilation in patients with essential hypertension. N Engl J Med 1994; 330:1036–1040.
53. Panza JA, Garcia CE, Kilcoyne CM, Quyyumi AA, Cannon RO. Impaired endothelium-dependent vasodilation in patients with essential hypertension. Evidence that nitric oxide abnormality is not localized to a single signal transduction pathway. Circulation 1995; 91:1732–1738.
54. Antony I, Lerebours G, Nitenberg A. Loss of flow-dependent coronary artery dilatation in patients with hypertension. Circulation 1995; 91:1624–1628.
55. Nitenberg A, Antony I, Aptecar E, Arnoult F, Lerebours G. Impairment of flow-dependent coronary dilation in hypertensive patients. Demonstration by cold pressor test induced flow velocity increase. Am J Hypertens 1995; 8: S13–S18.
56. Quyyumi AA, Dakak N, Andrews NP, Gilligan DM, Panza JA, Cannon RO. Contribution of nitric oxide to metabolic coronary vasodilation in the human heart. Circulation 1995; 92:320–326.
57. Deng LY, Li JS, Schiffrin EL. Endothelium-dependent relaxations of small arteries from essential hypertensive patients. Mechanisms and comparison with normotensive subjects and with responses of vessels from spontaneously hypertensive rats. Clin Sci 1995; 88:611–622.
58. Salazar FJ, Alberola A, Pinilla JM, Romero JC, Quesada T. Salt-induced increase in arterial pressure during nitric oxide synthesis inhibition. Hypertension 1993; 22:49–55.
59. Lahera V, Salom MG, Miranda Guardiola F, Moncada S. Effects of $N^G$-nitro-L-arginine methyl ester on renal function and blood pressure. Am J Physiol 1991; 261:F1033–F1037.
60. Higashi Y, Oshima T, Ozono R, Watanabe M, Matsuura H, Kajiyama G. Effects of L-arginine infusion on renal hemodynamics in patients with mild essential hypertension. Hypertension 1995; 25:898–902.
61. Yokokawa K, Tahara H, Kohno M, et al. Hypertension associated with

endothelin-secreting malignant hemangioendothelioma. Ann Int Med 1991; 114:213–215.

62. Haynes WG, Hand WF, Webb DJ. Enhanced venoconstriction to endothelin-1 in essential hypertension (abstr). J Hypertens 1993; 11(suppl 5):S436.

63. Lüscher TF, Vanhoutte PM, Raij L. Antihypertensive therapy normalizes endothelium-dependent relaxations in salt-induced hypertension of the rat. Hypertension 1987; 9(suppl 3):193–197.

64. Tschudi MR, Criscione L, Novosel D, Pfeiffer K, Lüscher TF. Antihypertensive therapy augments endothelium-dependent relaxations in coronary arteries of spontaneously hypertensive rats. Circulation 1994; 89:2212–2218.

65. Dohi Y, Criscione L, Pfeiffer K, Lüscher TF. Angiotensin blockade or calcium antagonist normalize endothelial dysfunction in hypertension: studies in perfused SHR mesenteric resistance arteries. J Cardiovasc Pharmacol 1994; 24: 372–379.

66. Feelisch M, Noack EA. Correlation between nitric oxide formation during degradation of organic nitrates and activation of guanylate cyclase. Eur J Pharmacol 1987; 139:19–30.

67. Pohl U, Busse R. Endothelium-derived relaxant factor inhibits effects of nitrocompounds in isolated arteries. Am J Physiol 1987; 252:H307–H313.

68. Lüscher TF, Richard V, Yang Z. Interaction between endothelium-derived nitric oxide and SIN-1 in human and porcine blood vessels. J Cardiovasc Pharmacol 1990; 14(suppl 11):76–80.

69. Selke FW, Myers PR, Bates JN, Harrison DG. Influence of vessels size on the sensitivity of porcine coronary microvessels to nitroglycerin. Am J Physiol 1990; 258:H515–H520.

70. Vanhoutte PM. Vascular endothelium and Ca×+-antagonists. J Cardiovasc Pharmacol 1988; 12(suppl 6):21–28.

71. Küng C, Tschudi MR, Noll G, Clozel JP, Lüscher TF. Differential effects of the calcium antagonist mibefradil in epicardial and intramyocardial coronary arteries J Cardiovasc Pharmacol 1995; 26:312–318.

72. Noll G, Bühler FR, Lüscher TF. Different potency of endothelium-derived relaxing factors against thromboxane, endothelin and potassium chloride in porcine intramyocardial resistance arteries. J Cardiovasc Pharmacol 1991; 18: 120–126.

73. Goto K, Kasuya Y, Matsuki N, et al. Endothelin activates the dihydropyridine-sensitive, voltage-dependent Ca×+ channel in vascular smooth muscle. Proc Natl Acad Sci USA 1989; 86:3915–3918.

74. Kiowski W, Lüscher TF, Linder L, Bühler FR. Endothelin-1-induced vasoconstriction in humans: reversal by calcium channel blockade but not by nitrovasodilators or endothelin-derived relaxing factor. Circulation 1991; 83:469–475.

75. Yang Z, Bauer E, von SL, Stulz P, Turina M, Lüscher TF. Different mobilization of calcium in endothelin-1-induced contractions in human arteries and veins: effects of calcium antagonists. J Cardiovasc Pharmacol 1990; 16:654–60.

76. Palmer RMJ, Ferrige AG, Moncada S. Nitric oxide release accounts for the biological activity of endothelium-derived relaxing factor. Nature 1987; 327: 524–526.

77. Wiemer G, Scholkens BA, Becker RH, Busse R. Ramiprilat enhances endothelial autocoid formation by inhibiting breakdown of endothelial derived bradykinin. Hypertension 1991; 18:558–563.
78. Yang Z, Arnet U, von Segesser L, Siebenmann R, Turina M, Lüscher TF. Different effects of angiotensin-converting enzyme inhibition in human arteries and veins. J Cardiovasc Pharmacol 1993; 22(suppl 5):7–22.
79. Auch-Schwelk W, Bossaller C, Claus M, Graf K, Gräfe M, Fleck E. Endothelium-dependent relaxations to angiotensin-converting enzyme inhibitors in isolated coronary arteries stimulated with bradykinin. J Cardiovasc Pharmacol 1992; 20(suppl 9):S62–S67.
80. Kahonen M, Makynen H, Wu XM, Arvola P, Porsti I. Endothelial function in spontaneously hypertensive rats. Influence of quinapril treatment. Br J Pharmacol 1995; 115:859–867.
81. Bossaller C, Auch-Schwelk W, Weber F, et al. Endothelium-dependent relaxations are augmented in rats chronically treated with the angiotensin-converting enzyme inhibitor enalapril. J Cardiovasc Pharmacol 1992; 20(suppl 9):S91–S95.
82. Creager MA, Roddy MA, Coleman SM, Dzau VJ. The effect of ACE-inhibition on endothelium-dependent vasodilation in hypertension. J Vasc Res 1992; 29:97–101.
83. Timmermans PB, Wong PC, Chiu AT, et al. Angiotensin II receptors and angiotensin II receptor antagonists. Pharmacol Rev 1993; 45:205–251.
84. Li J-S, Schiffrin EL. Effect of chronic treatment of adult spontaneously hypertensive rats with an endothelin receptor antagonist. Hypertension 1995; 25:495–500.
85. Li JS, Larivière R, Schiffrin EL. Effect of a nonselective endothelin antagonist on vascular remodeling in deoxycorticosterone acetate-salt hypertensive rats: evidence for a role of endothelin in vascular hypertrophy. Hypertension 1994; 24:183–188.
86. Richard V, Hogie M, Clozel M, Löffler B-M, Thuillez C. In vivo evidence of an endothelin-induced vasopressor tone after inhibition of nitric oxide synthesis in rats. Circulation 1995; 91:771–775.
87. Donckier J, Stoleru L, Hayashida W, et al. Role of endogenous endothelin-1 in experimental renal hypertension in dogs. Circulation 1995; 92:106–113.
88. Haynes WG, Webb DJ. Contribution of endogenous generation of endothelin-1 to basal vascular tone. Lancet 1994; 344:852–854.
89. Wenzel RR, Noll G, Lüscher TF. Endothelin receptor antagonists inhibit endothelin in human skin microcirculation. Hypertension 1994; 23:581–586.
90. Ihara M, Fukuroda T, Saeki T, et al. An endothelin receptor ($ET_A$) antagonist isolated from *Streptomyces misakiensis*. Biochem Biophys Res Commun 1991; 178:132–137.
91. Itoh S, Sasaki T, Ide K, Ishikawa K, Nishikibe M, Yano M. A novel endothelin $ET_A$ receptor antagonist, BQ-485, and its preventive effect on experimental cerebral vasospasm in dogs. Biochem Biophys Res Commun 1993; 195:969–975.
92. Sogabe K, Nirei H, Shoubo M, et al. Pharmacological profile of FR139317, a

novel, potent endothelin ET$_A$ receptor antagonist. J Pharmacol Exp Ther 1993; 264:1040–1046.

93. Clozel M, Breu V, Gray GA, et al. Pharmacological characterization of bosentan, a new potent orally active non-peptide endothelin receptor antagonist. J Pharmacol Exp Ther 1994; 270:228–235.

94. Clozel M, Breu V, Burri K, et al. Pathophysiological role of endothelin revealed by the first orally active endothelin receptor antagonist. Nature 1993; 365:759–761.

95. Lüscher TF. Do we need endothelin antagonists? Cardiovasc Res 1993; 27: 2089–2093.

96. Ikeda S, Awane Y, Kusumoto K, Wakimasu M, Watanabe T, Fujino M. A new endothelin receptor antagonist, TAK-044, shows long-lasting inhibition of both ET$_A$- and ET$_B$-mediated blood pressure responses in rats. J Pharmacol Exp Ther 1994; 270:728–733.

97. Ohlstein EH, Nambi P, Douglas SA, et al. SB 209670, a rationally designed potent nonpeptide endothelin receptor antagonist. Proc Natl Acad Sci USA 1994; 91:8052–8056.

98. Ihara M, Saeki T, Funabashi K, et al. Two endothelin receptor subtypes in porcine arteries. J Cardiovasc Pharmacol 1991; 17(suppl 7):S119–S121.

99. Sumner MJ, Cannon TR, Mundin JM, White DG, Watts IS. Endothelin ET$_A$ and ET$_B$ receptors mediate vascular smooth muscle contraction. Br J Pharmacol 1992; 107:858–860.

100. Seo B, Oemar BS, Siebenmann R, von Ludwig S, Lüscher TF, Both ET$_A$ and ET$_B$ receptors mediate contraction to endothelin-1 in human blood vessels. Circulation 1994; 89:1203–1208.

101. Takase H, Moreau P, Lüscher TF. Endothelin receptors subtypes in small arteries: Studies with FR139317 and bosentan. Hypertension 1995; 25(part 2):739–743.

102. Lüscher TF, Noll G. The endothelium in coronary vascular control. In: Braunwald E, ed. Heart Disease. Update 3. W.B. Saunders Company, 1995: 1–10.

# 13

# Arterial Restenosis

**Michael A. Reidy and Stephen M. Schwartz**

*University of Washington, Seattle, Washington*

## I. INTRODUCTION

In this chapter, the processes involved in neointimal growth are reviewed, and at the same time, these findings are related to the events which occur in humans following angioplasty and subsequent restenosis. Until recently, most work in this field was based on the hypothesis of Ross (1,2) put forward over 20 years ago which emphasized smooth muscle proliferation as a dominant component of atherosclerosis, both in terms of lesion formation and progression. The same process was thought to occur in the accelerated narrowing of the lumen seen after angioplasty. In support of this concept were the data from experimental animals in which injury to arteries with balloon catheters caused dramatic changes in cell proliferation and formation of neointimal mass. Therefore, it seems reasonable to proceed on the assumption that the exuberant smooth muscle cell proliferation seen following injury to either normal or previously atherosclerotic animal vessels also occurs in human vessels following therapeutic angioplasty. As is discussed, however, this view may be erroneous.

## II. MECHANISM OF LUMEN OCCLUSION

It is commonly believed that neointimal formation is the principal cause of lumen narrowing in the restenosis that occurs after angioplasty (1). The experimental data supporting the assumption that new mass obstructs the lumen of large vessels, however, is not as clear as first supposed. Glagov, and more recently, Clarkson, noted that human vessels can undergo growth of atherosclerotic plaque without any narrowing of the lumen (3,4). In this case, the wall compensates for the lesion by remodeling and dilating to permit a normal level of blood flow (3). Compensatory structural change is a normal response which allows the vessel to maintain normal levels of blood flow and wall stress, and this can be seen in small muscular arteries as well as in large elastic arteries (5,6). Interestingly, when Langille and his colleagues studied the balloon-injured rabbit carotid artery, they found no narrowing of the lumen despite an increase in wall thickness (7). The same study, however, showed a significant (14%) narrowing in response to an experimental restriction of blood flow in the vicinity of the thyroid artery where endothelium had regenerated (6). The effect of the endothelium in an injured vessel was consistent with observations that structural adaptation to changes in flow requires the presence of an endothelium (7). Since reendothelialization generally correlates with a diminution of intimal thickening (8), these data may even imply a *negative* correlation of intimal mass with luminal narrowing. Conversely, the decrease in lumen size in areas where there was an intact endothelium is poorly understood, but this offers an important alternative mechanism to explain luminal narrowing, especially in human lesions where there may be extensive vascularization of the plaque by transmural vessels (9). Thus, endothelial-induced remodeling may be as important as intimal thickening in determining lumen size.

## III.  NEOINTIMAL FORMATION IN THE RAT CAROTID ARTERY

In contrast to the term *intima,* which may be defined as a normal structure that arises during development, the term *neointima* refers to new intimal tissue formed in response to injury. This distinction may be important, because most of our knowledge of the response to balloon injury comes from studies of the formation of the neointima in the rat carotid artery.

The rat carotid injury model is appealing, because this artery is a very simple vessel, consisting only of endothelium and media. Normally, no intima is found and there is no penetration of the media by vasa vasorum. Moreover, neointimal formation is a very simple process in the rat, involving only the cells of the injured wall and platelets (10,11). The simplicity of the rat model has greatly facilitated identification of molecular and pharmacological mechanisms involved in the formation of a neointima. We do not know, however, whether the processes involved in forming a neointima are also important in the response of lesions to angioplasty. Nevertheless, the rat model is an essential starting point useful in understanding the responses of more complex vessels.

Neointimal formation is a general response to a wide range of stimuli, including irradiation, application of turpentine to the adventitia, wrapping the vessel, and electrical stimulation, as well as mechanical injuries, including placement of a suture, scratching with a probe, or dilatation of the common carotid artery with an embolectomy balloon catheter (10–16). The best-studies procedure uses a balloon catheter to dilate the vessel. This procedure causes complete denudation of the endothelium over the length of the vessel as well as variable amounts of medial smooth muscle cell death (15–25%) due to stretching injury (17,18). During the first few hours after denudation, platelets adhere and form a monolayer on the exposed subendothelial surface (17). Although the subendothelium is exposed, accumulation of insoluble fibrin is rarely observed by scanning or transmission electron microscopy of injured rat arteries (19). This probably reflects the lack of tissue factor in the media of normal blood vessels (20,21) and the synthesis of tissue plasminogen activator (tPA) by the smooth muscle cells (22). The smooth muscle cells respond to balloon injury by replicating and then migrating into the intima, which ultimately culminates in the formation of a new layer of muscular tissue, the neointima, inside the internal elastic lamina.

The smooth muscle cell response to injury follows a pattern that conveniently can be broken down into three stages. The first stage is the onset of medial smooth muscle cell proliferation that peaks within a few days after injury and subsides within the next 10 days following repopulation of the media to the preinjury level (Fig. 1a). This proliferative response is caused by the synchronous entry into the cell cycle of 10–20% of the smooth muscle cells remaining in the media (17). Replication in the media 2 days after balloon injury is similar whether or not rats are rendered thrombocytopenic with an antibody against circulating platelets (23). This result suggests that platelet-derived products, such as platelet-derived growth factor (PDGF), do not play a major role in the initiation of smooth muscle cell proliferation in the media following injury. As will be discussed below, however, basic fibroblast growth factor (bFGF) appears to play a central role in the first stage.

The second stage of smooth muscle cell response to injury results from migration of smooth muscle cells across the internal elastic lamina to form the intima (Fig. 1b). Smooth muscle cells are readily observed on the luminal side of the internal elastic lamina 4 days after injury. The duration of the second stage in the rat injured carotid is not known, nor do we know whether replication is required before smooth muscle migration. It is clear, however, that migration can be greatly stimulated without any

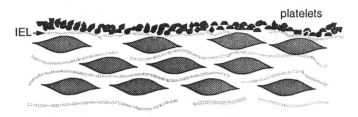

Features:
• loss of endothelium
• platelet adhesion
• injury to SMC and bFGF release
• replication due to bFGF is 10% -20% (48 hr)
• SMC replication can be inhibited by bFGF antibodies

**(a)**

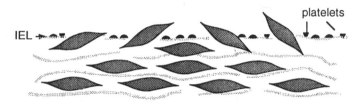

Features:
• cells migrate to intima by day 4
• stimulated by platelets, PDGF, and bFGF
• migrating cells show proteinase activity, i.e., uPA, tPA, MMP2, and MMP9 activity
• migrating is blocked with plasminogen activator and MMP inhibitors
• inhibition of migration does not permanently inhibit intimal lesion growth

**(b)**

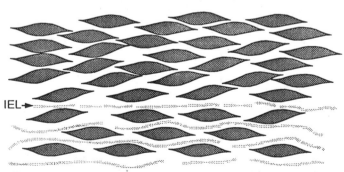

Features:
• SMC replication is high (>70%) and continues for approx. 4 weeks
• SMC replication is not blocked by antibodies to FGF or PDGF
• SMC respond weakly to bFGF and to PDGF
• By 12 weeks the intima is mainly matrix (70%) and quiescent SMC (30%)
• SMC on luminal surface are not thrombogenic

**(c)**

increase in smooth muscle cell replication (24). Smooth muscle cell migration is probably reduced once medial smooth muscle cells have stopped replicating, because cellular depletion of the media does not occur. Mural thrombosis may be an important contribution to the second stage. Elimination of circulating platelets, a treatment that does not affect the first stage, prevents the appearance of smooth muscle cells on the luminal side of the internal elastic lamina at day 4 after balloon injury (23). Depletion of circulating platelets also significantly reduces the size of the intimal lesion at day 7 after injury. A similar result was obtained when PDGF was blocked by administration of an antibody. Migration of cells into the intima was markedly suppressed at day 4 (22) and the intimal lesion was also reduced (25). This treatment had no effect on smooth muscle cell replication. Thus, it is apparent that migration is critical for intimal lesion development in an artery with no preexisting intimal smooth muscle cells, such as a rat carotid artery. This is very different from humans, in whom there is a well-developed intima even in normal arteries. Thus, any new growth in these arteries could be derived from intimal cell replication as well as cell migration into the intima. Until there is a reliable marker for detecting smooth muscle cell migration, we can only speculate if migration is a critical event in lesion growth in human arteries. This is important, because many of the agents which have worked well in preventing lesion growth in the rat do so by inhibiting cell migration.

The third stage of the smooth muscle cell response of the rat artery to injury is the proliferation of intimal smooth muscle cells and the formation of extracellular matrix which contributes to the rapid growth of the lesion during the first 4 weeks after injury (Fig. 1c). Proliferation is sustained for several weeks, and in all likelihood this cell replication is responsible for the ultimate size of the lesion. Chronic proliferation in the intima is particularly striking at the luminal surface of the lesion, where the number of

---

**Figure 1** The three waves. (a) First stage. Balloon catheter injury removes the endothelium and causes variable damage to the underlying medial cells. Within 48 hr, the replication rate of the medial smooth muscle cells of rat carotid artery is frequently increased to 10–20%. (b) Second stage. Within 4 days after balloon injury, medial smooth muscle cells migrate from the media into the intima and in the continued absence of the endothelium these cells form a pseudoendothelium. The precise duration of migration is not known, but our data with rat arteries would suggest that migration is completed after 2 weeks. (c) Third stage. Once intimal smooth muscle cells have migrated to the intima, they undergo extensive replication for the next 2 weeks. The increase in size of the intima is most probably due to this cell proliferation. After 2 weeks, some cells continue to replicate; however, the intima does not enlarge.

smooth muscle cells incorporating tritiated thymidine is consistently higher than in the deeper layers of the intima as late as 12 weeks after injury (26). The mechanisms important for this chronic cell growth are poorly understood. Treatment with an antibody to bFGF after injury does not affect intimal smooth muscle cell proliferation (27), suggesting that this process is not dependent on bFGF. The addition of bFGF, however, can stimulate intimal smooth muscle cell replication, although far less than observed with the medial cells immediately after injury and infusion of bFGF. Large doses of transforming growth factor-$\beta$ (TGF-$\beta$) given 2 weeks after injury produce a modest increase in the percentage of proliferating cells in the intima (28). PDGF antibodies do not influence this intimal cell replication, nor does the addition of PDGF influence this event.

Deposition of extracellular matrix by intimal smooth muscle cells also contributes to the growth of the intimal lesion until 3 months following injury, after which time the intima appears stable (17). During this time, there is a gradual loss of cells with an increase in the matrix component such that by 3 months, approximately 70–80% of the intima is made up of matrix, although this is not accompanied by any increase in lesion size. This change from a cellular lesion to one which comprises matrix is even less well understood than cell replication controls. Further, we have no data showing whether this increase in matrix is in any way related to the changes in smooth muscle cell proliferation.

## IV.   MOLECULES INVOLVED IN NEOINTIMAL FORMATION

### A.   FGF in Neointimal Formation

bFGF is perhaps the best understood mitogen active in the arterial wall (29,30). Basic, but not acidic, FGF is normally found in the rat vessel wall and appears to be stored in an intracellular compartment; not, as first thought, in the extracellular matrix. If a vessel is gently denuded to prevent injury to medial smooth muscle cells, the first wave of smooth muscle cell replication is largely averted. If, however, the artery is subjected to balloon injury, which is known to traumatize the medial cells, then replication can reach a level as high as 20%. Both injuries cause platelet adhesion to the denuded arterial wall. One early conclusion was that the degree of medial cell replication correlated to the severity of the injury, and this may reflect the release of bFGF from the traumatized smooth muscle cells. In this view, the greater the injury, the more bFGF released, and so the greater the replication. This concept was supported by the fact that infusion of FGF at the same time after injury caused significant increases in cell proliferation. Perhaps more conclusive in determining the role of bFGF in the injured artery was a study in which animals were pretreated with an antibody to FGF and then subjected to balloon injury. This had the effect of almost completely abolishing smooth muscle cell replication (30).

Central to the role of bFGF in the arterial wall is its displacement from an intracellular location to one where it can interact with the FGF high-affinity receptors on the extracellular side of the cell membrane. This was difficult to demonstrate directly, so the question was approached in an indirect manner (31). We exploited the well-known affinity of FGF to heparin, and the fact that adding heparin exogenously can release FGF bound to extracellular sites, to see if balloon injury caused a change in the location of $FGF_2$ in the artery. Our hypothesis was that injury caused the release of FGF from traumatized cells, thereby displacing it into the extracellular pool, where it could bind to heparin sulfate–rich matrix. Subsequent administration of soluble heparin would compete for binding of FGF to the matrix and so cause efflux of FGF from the arterial wall. Our results showed that a single bolus of heparin had no effect on bFGF concentration in an uninjured artery. However, if heparin was given immediately following balloon injury, then a dramatic loss of bFGF from the arterial wall was observed which coincided with a marked reduction in smooth muscle cell replication. We interpret these data as indicative of displacement of bFGF from its intracellular storage pool to the extracellular environment where it is bound to heparin and so transported away from the artery. Thus, FGF is present in the artery, is released from injured cells, and so stimulates the first wave of DNA synthesis by medial smooth muscle cells.

Intriguingly, using the FGF antibody to abolish the first stage of cell replication did not abolish intimal thickening (30). Thus, the other stages of lesion development, that is, migration and intimal cell proliferation, must be critical parts of lesion formation and would seem to be controlled by factors different from those important for the first wave (28,30,32). These data differ from experiments in which antisense has been used to block neointimal lesion growth, and in some circumstances, medial cell replication was reduced by this procedure (33,34). One possible explanation for this finding is that antisense treatment affects multiple targets in these injured arteries by some unknown mechanism.

## V.  PDGF IN NEOINTIMAL FORMATION

In vitro studies have emphasized the multiple roles of PDGF as a stimulant of smooth muscle proliferation, migration, and matrix synthesis. PDGF seems to play a more limited role in vivo, at least in the rat. We know, for example, that PDGF has very little mitogenic effect in the first stage of lesion growth, but it does appear to increase the numbers of cells that cross the internal elastic lamella (1,24). Other molecules, including FGF, also stimulate migration (35), although the relative contributions of different molecules remain to be explored. PDGF has little detectable effect on replication in the third stage, but overexpression of PDGF–A chain is prominent in areas of the neointima that show elevated replication (36). In contrast, PDGF is a consistent mitogen for smooth muscle in vitro, but is only a weak mitogen in vivo (24). The difference between observations in vivo and in vitro casts some doubt on the validity of in vitro assays of smooth muscle growth control. A recent report from Lindner et al. (37) indicates that a percentage of smooth muscle cells in both normal and injured arteries express PDGF–B chain as well as the β-receptor in vivo, which is consistent with an older report showing that intimal smooth muscle cells in vitro express PDGF–B chain (38). Unfortunately, these new data still do not suggest a role for PDGF in the injured artery, because, as stated above, PDGF is at best a weak mitogen. One possible action of PDGF is that its local release from these smooth muscle cells in the intima may stimulate chronic migration of cells into the intima; without a marker for migration, however, these data are difficult to obtain. Alternatively, the small increase in smooth muscle cell replication stimulated by PDGF is important, since even a 1–2% replication rate over several months can be responsible for a significant increase in smooth muscle cell numbers.

## VI.  TGF-β IN NEOINTIMAL FORMATION

The potential role of TGF-β in these processes is very intriguing. TGF-β is present in the neointima of balloon-injured rats. Infusion of TGF-β causes a restimulation of replication in the neointima (28). TGF-β may contribute to connective tissue accumulation as well as to cell proliferation (39). Moreover, when TGF-β is overexpressed within the vessel wall, the result is a remarkable increase in connective tissue matrix formation in the neointima (40). All of this suggests a possible central role for TGF-β in plaque progression or restenosis.

Most studies in vitro have argued for a role for TGF-β as an inhibitor of smooth muscle proliferation. In part, this set of studies may be confusing, because the ability of TGF-β to act as a mitogen appears to be complicated by the strain of smooth muscle cells studied and by their state of confluence (41,42). Gibbons and co-workers showed that the mitogenic effects of angiotensin II were enhanced by a TGF-β inhibitory antibody. These investigators noted the sometimes contradictory literature on angiotensin II as an in vitro mitogen and proposed that this variability had to do with the ability of these cells to synthesize and activate autocrine TGF-β (43).

An intriguing indication for a potential role for TGF-$\beta$ comes from a recent report that the activity of this growth factor in atherosclerosis may be influenced by a major risk factor, lipoprotein(a) (Lp[a]). Lp(a) levels in humans correlate highly with atherosclerosis risk (44). Moreover, a recent study suggests that apolipoprotein (Apo[a]) levels may also correlate with increased incidence of restenosis (44). The apoprotein for this lipoprotein, Apo(a), is highly homologous with plasminogen activator (PA) and is believed to have a procoagulant effect by inhibiting the formation of plasmin. Current theory suggests that the proatherosclerotic effect is the result of deficient clot lysis. Grainger and his colleagues, however, have pointed out that plasmin, besides its role as a thrombolytic enzyme, is essential to the activation of TGF-$\beta$. Apo(a) competes with PA for membrane sites required for the latter's activity. Grainger and his colleagues found that Apo(a) was mitogenic for smooth muscle cells in culture, but that this effect was due to the prevention of the activation of TGF-$\beta$ as an endogenous growth inhibitor (45). In this view, the predominant role of TGF-$\beta$ would be as an endogenous inhibitor of lesion formation at sites of active coagulation. Apo(a) would enhance lesion formation by diminishing the production of activated TGF-$\beta$.

## VII. PROTEASES IN NEOINTIMAL FORMATION

Much of the work on restenosis has focused on the early replication of smooth muscle cell replication and has shown that inhibition of smooth muscle cell replication will not inhibit growth of intimal lesions. Following replication of medial smooth muscle cells in the rat injured artery, there is a period when smooth muscle cells move to the intima and thus form the beginnings of an intimal lesion. As mentioned above, PDGF B–chain and bFGF stimulate smooth muscle cell migration in rat injured arteries and inhibition of either factor will significantly suppress migration (35,46). Critical to the process is the expression of proteases which digest matrix proteins and thereby permit cell movement. Study of the molecules which control this process in the arterial wall is in its infancy, but recent data have implicated both PA and certain matrix metalloproteinases (MMPs) in lesion development (22,47).

Balloon catheter injury induces expression of both urokinase-type plasminogen activator (uPA) and tPA in rat arteries, and a significant increase in plasmin activity can be detected in the artery by the third day, which is sustained for approximately another 10 days (48). This time sequence is interesting, because the earliest time smooth muscle cells are found in the intima is 4 days after injury and the rate of intimal lesion growth has slowed by 2 weeks. In situ hybridization of these arteries shows that almost all the smooth muscle cells which have migrated to the lumen of the injured artery express tPA, uPA, and the receptor for uPA (uPAR), but with the exception of tPA, no signal can be detected when the lesion is quiescent. tPA, however, is still expressed after 6 weeks by those luminal smooth muscle cells, and en face zymography shows this surface to be strongly antifibrinolytic. Thus, tPA may be involved both in the movement of cells into the intima and in preventing thrombosis on this deendo-thelialized surface. The importance of these PAs in the injured artery can best be understood by the study in which their active product, plasmin, was blocked in vivo with the inhibitor transexamic acid (22). The total number of cells which migrated through the internal elastic lamella into the intima was significantly reduced with no concomitant change in cell replication. These data illustrate that arterial lesion development may be inhibited by blocking cell movement. An interesting finding which relates to smooth muscle cell migration is that heparin, a well-documented inhibitor of intimal lesion growth, also inhibits arterial plasmin activity and cell migra-tion (49). Thus, the ability of heparin to inhibit intimal hyperplasia (50) may be due to an effect on migration as well as replication.

Another group of proteolytic enzymes, namely, the MMPs, are also im-portant for smooth muscle migration. MMPs have the ability to degrade a variety of matrix molecules found in the arterial wall (10–13,51). Recently, two gelatinases, MMP2 and MMP9, have been reported to be present in rat injured arteries. Within 6 hours after balloon injury, a significant increase in mRNA of an 88-kD gelatinase (MMP9) is observed, and it remains elevated for approximately 6 days (47). Expression of this MMP was not seen in the intima, nor was it correlated to smooth muscle cell replication. The tran-script for 72-kD gelatinase (MMP2) was present in normal arteries and showed little change after injury. The activity of MMP in balloon-injured rat arteries was assessed by zymography, and within 1 day, an increase in 88-kD activity was observed. Both inactive and active MMP2 were observed in control arteries, but by day 4, a marked increase in active MMP2 was noted. Thus, there is a correlation in balloon-injured arteries between the expres-sion of MMP9 and activities of MMP9 and MMP2 with the migration of smooth muscle cells into the intima. The importance of these proteases for the development of arterial lesions is not well understood currently, but using a metalloprotease inhibitor (15), the migration of smooth muscle cells into the intima was blocked and intimal lesion size was markedly reduced by day 10. These data illustrate that migration is a critical event in lesion growth in rat arteries and that proteases which facilitate the breakdown of matrix proteins are necessary for lesion development.

Although these data show that migration is critical for lesion growth in normal arteries, the question arises whether cell migration is necessary for lesion growth in arteries which already possess intimal smooth muscle cells. In such arteries, one possibility is that intimal lesion growth is due solely to replication of the existing intimal cells. Currently, there are no reliable markers for cell migration, and therefore we are unable to answer this question. It will be important to resolve this issue, because thus far many successful protocols for inhibiting intimal lesions in the rat use agents that inhibit smooth muscle cell migration (14). Both PDGF antibodies and the angiotensin-converting inhibitors fall into this category. These treatments were found to have no effect on intimal cell replication, yet they success-fully inhibit lesion growth in the rat. The process of smooth muscle cell migration, however, has not been shown thus far to be important in humans (52–54).

A final issue relates to the ability of proteases to digest a variety of matrix substrates and cause plaque instability. The premise is that excessive or chronic synthesis of the proteases will weaken the arterial wall and so initiate plaque ulceration or formation of aneurysms. Indeed, data now show that these enzymes are present in atherosclerotic plaques and aneu-rysms; thus far, however, the data are only anecdotal.

## VIII. PROLIFERATION IN HUMAN RESTENOTIC CORONARY ARTERY LESIONS

In contrast to the wealth of information available on the proliferation kinetics in animal models of arterial injury and repair, little is known about the proliferative profile of human restenotic coronary artery lesions. Most studies that have described proliferation in human restenotic coronary ar-teries have not used an objective measurement of replication. For example, Nobuyoshi et al. examined the histological findings in 39 dilated lesions from 20 patients who had undergone antemortem coronary angioplasty (55). These investigators defined proliferation by the presence of stellate cells and noted that there were more of these cells in lesions with evidence of medial or adventitial tears as compared with those without tears or with tears limited to the intima. Nobuyoshi assumed that cells with this morphol-ogy had recently proliferated. Unfortunately, these "proliferative-like" stellate cells are commonly seen in primary atherosclerotic coronary artery lesions that have never been exposed to an interventional device (56,57). Similar cellular morphology can be seen in normal intima of human arteries (58,59).

Since stellate cells are seen in normal arterial wall and in plaque, their apparent increase in number might be an artifact resulting from a change in the sampling of cells already in the wall as a result of the redistribution of cell types secondary to the dilatation. For example, it is conceivable that primary coronary atherectomy specimens may include more of the superficial luminal layer. Typically, this is the fibrous cap. With subsequent restenotic biopsies, deeper layers of the plaque may be removed. Alternatively, the stellate cells could represent a phenotypic change in preexisting cells. In either case, one must be careful not to assume that differences in histology between primary and restenotic coronary atherectomy specimens are necessarily due to a difference in vessel wall biology that occurred with the so-called restenotic process.

Two other approaches have been used to attempt to determine the role of proliferation in restenosis. Recently, we have used immunocytochemical labeling for the proliferating cell nuclear antigen (PCNA) to determine the proliferative profile of 100 restenotic coronary atherectomy specimens (60). PCNA is regulated at both the pretranscriptional and posttranscriptional levels, and the protein is expressed during S-phase (as well as $G_1$ and $G_2$) of the cell cycle (61). To our surprise, the vast majority of the restenotic specimens (74%) had no evidence of PCNA labeling. The majority of the remaining specimens had only a modest number of PCNA-positive cells per slide (typically <50 cells per slide). On the basis of the mean number of nuclei per slide, the majority of these specimens had ≤1% of all cells labeled PCNA positive. PCNA labeling was detected over a wide time interval after the initial procedure (3.g., 1–390 days) with no obvious proliferative peak. There was no difference in the proliferative profile of restenotic specimens collected in the first 3 months, 4–6 months, 7–9 months, or >9 months after the initial interventional procedure (Spearman rank correlation coefficient = 0.081, $P$ = .43). Furthermore, only 12 of 30 specimens obtained within 60 days of the initial coronary interventional procedure had one or more PCNA-positive nuclei per slide (including 9 specimens collected within 6 days of the initial procedure, only 3 of which had immunolabeling of 1, 7, and 20 cells per slide) (60). Moreover, a recent preliminary report of in vitro bromodeoxyuridine labeling of restenotic atherectomy specimens also found low levels of proliferation (62). Similarly, Strauss et al. found no PCNA-positive cells in four postmortem stented vessels (63). Pickering et al. detected high levels of proliferation in restenotic atherectomy tissue (64). Their data, however, are inconsistent with the animal models and probably represent an artifact. In Pickering's study, both primary and restenotic coronary specimens had surprisingly high percentages of cells that were considered PCNA positive as measured by either immunocytochemistry (15.2 ± 13.6%) or in situ hybridization (20.6 ± 18.2%). However, only 4 of the 19 restenotic atherectomy specimens were obtained from coronary artery lesions, and none were obtained within 1 month of the initial interventional procedure (e.g., 1.6, 5.2, 6.1, and 7.9 months). Overall, the labeling indices reported by Pickering et al.

seem exceptionally high (e.g., as high as 59% of cells being PCNA positive) and resemble those of malignant neoplasms (65). Furthermore, unlike our own study, which used intestinal crypt epithelium, the Pickering study lacked a reference tissue with a known replication rate, thereby making the subjective interpretation of PCNA positively difficult. Nonetheless, it is unlikely that mean PCNA labeling indices of 15–20% are physically possible in atherosclerotic coronary arteries where small changes in vessel wall mass can result in dramatic changes in residual luminal diameter.

The discrepancy in the proliferation data can likely be explained by assessing the adequacy of PCNA control experiments. Using immunocytochemistry, proliferating cells show increased PCNA labeling as compared with mitotically quiescent cells (61,66). Previous studies of injured arterial tissue using the same protocol as that used in our studies have shown good correlation of PCNA immunolabeling with thymidine or bromodeoxyuridine incorporation (67,68). The inclusion of rat small intestine as positive control tissue with each PCNA immunocytochemistry experiment in our study provided evidence that the antibody was routinely labeling the nuclei of highly proliferating crypt epithelium as PCNA positive. Moreover, our PCNA index for primary atherosclerotic tissue is in close agreement with the tritiated thymidine labeling index determined by incubating atherosclerotic tissue in vitro (69). Although these data show replication in primary and restenotic tissue as very low, using the same set of criteria, identical PCNA immunolabeling of rapidly stenosing human arteriovenous fistulas showed high levels of replication (70). Finally, one criticism of PCNA labeling relative to other proliferative measurements is that it is likely to be oversensitive in detecting proliferative cells, since PCNA is expressed through a broader period of cell cycle traverse (67). Therefore, if anti-PCNA antibodies are overlabeling proliferating cells, the degree of proliferation in these atherectomy specimens may actually be lower than the already minimal levels that we have measured.

It is also worth noting that PCNA does pick up replicating cells with a high labeling frequency in plaque. These cells, however, are not the expected smooth muscle cells. Using cell-specific immunohistochemical markers and a double-labeling technique, PCNA-positive cells were identified as smooth muscle cells, macrophages, and endothelial cells. The relative abundance of each cell type was studied in a selected number of specimens that were positive for PCNA immunolabeling. All fragments had evidence of PCNA-positive smooth muscle cells and macrophages, and approximately 50% of tissue fragments had PCNA-labeled endothelial cells. The percentage of PCNA-positive cells that were endothelial cells was surprisingly high (e.g., $14 \pm 15\%$).

Finally, independent clinical evidence suggests that hyperplasia is not a sufficient explanation of restenosis. Analysis of vessel wall growth has become possible as a result of advances in intravascular ultrasound (IVUS). Unlike angiography, IVUS images the full cross-sectional thickness of the vessel wall. Furthermore, IVUS can be performed serially, before and after an interventional procedure in vivo, to determine the mechanisms by which the intervention enlarges the vessel lumen. Recent preliminary information on vessel wall dimensions with IVUS before and after balloon dilatation, as well as crude measurements of vessel wall composition, are promising. Mintz et al. (71) report that increases in plaque area with restenosis are actually small (5–7%). The clinical significance of this small increase in plaque mass in an artery that is already severely diseased is unknown. The investigators speculate that intimal hyperplasia may not be a dominant factor in the restenotic lesion, and that instead, "chronic recoil" may account for most of the progressive luminal narrowing. The idea of "chronic recoil" is remarkably similar to the observations of remodeling described by Langille et al. (7) and by Folkow et al. (5). Given the modest and relatively infrequent proliferation that we have detected by PCNA immunolabeling in restenotic coronary atherectomy specimens, these imaging data provide complementary evidence that proliferation is only one of several important events in the biology of restenosis.

## IX.   ARE ANIMAL MODELS OF LESION GROWTH APPLICABLE TO HUMANS?

Despite the considerable data now accrued on the mechanisms of arterial lesions in animal models, almost all attempts to modify restenosis in humans have failed. This has led to the idea that data from these animal models is not applicable to humans and that other, more suitable animal models should be developed. In particular, since most of the work on smooth muscle cell proliferation has been carried out in the rat, this species is now considered by some to be inappropriate to the study of lesion growth in human arteries. We suggest that this is a misleading conclusion. The problem may not be the choice of species but the process being studied; that is, we simply do not know that intimal hyperplasia is critical to restenosis. On the other hand, it is difficult to argue that the formation of new intimal mass does not contribute to loss of lumen size. It is our belief that if smooth muscle cell growth is an important process in humans, then in all probability this growth occurs via the mechanisms listed above. This may not be an overly simplistic approach, since the restenotic lesions that form after angioplasty are comprised of smooth muscle–like cells and matrix not too dissimilar to that seen in rat lesions at late times after balloon injury.

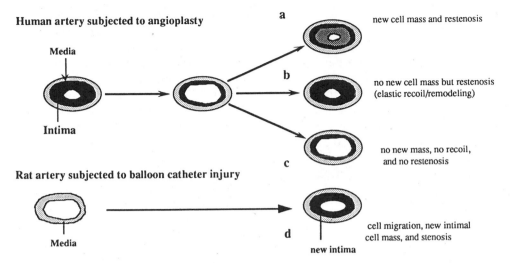

Human artery subjected to angioplasty

Media

Intima

a    new cell mass and restenosis

b    no new cell mass but restenosis
     (elastic recoil/remodeling)

c    no new mass, no recoil,
     and no restenosis

Rat artery subjected to balloon catheter injury

Media

d    cell migration, new intimal
     cell mass, and stenosis

new intima

**Figure 2** Proposed outcomes after angioplasty (PTCA) of human atherosclerotic coronary arteries (a, b, c). This is compared with the growth of intima lesion in rat artery after balloon catheter injury (d). With PTCA, the lumen of the diseased artery is increased in size. Following this acute change in lumen size, there are three possible outcomes: (a) Angioplasty stimulates new growth and restenosis—poor outcome. (b) Lumen returns to original size without new growth, restenosis—poor outcome. (c) Lumen stays dilated, no restenosis—successful outcome. This is contrasted with (d) balloon injury to rat artery where only new growth leads to stenosis of artery.

An insight as to potential differences in lesion growth in the arteries of rats and humans is illustrated in Figure 2. Critical to this discussion is the fact that human arteries with preexisting intimal lesions are subjected to angioplasty, whereas most animal studies subject a normal artery with no intima to balloon catheter injury. One immediate consequence of this fact is that unless vasospasm is an important issue in the ballooned rat artery, lumen narrowing will only occur because of new cell mass. There is a short period of arterial spasm in the first few days after injury, but it disappears soon after injury and is not thought to contribute to lumen narrowing. This is in contrast to the diseased human artery, in which remodeling and vasospasm as well as intimal cell growth after angioplasty will all have the effect of reoccluding the artery (Fig. 2a, 2b). It is also important to note that since angioplasty does not debulk the lesion, reocclusion can occur without synthesis of new mass; that is, cell replication or matrix synthesis. Clearly, this process is very different from that observed in rat arteries after injury. Given these facts, it is quite plausible that drugs designed to inhibit the processes of neointimal formation in any nonhuman species may have little effect in humans.

Study of the important events in lesion formation in humans is nascent and it is not yet clear which processes are most important. If restenosis in humans is due in part to remodeling or elastic recoil, then certain practical consequences must be considered. One is that lesion growth should be reexamined using animal arteries with preexisting intimal lesions. Intimal smooth muscle cells have unique properties which are not found in medial cells (see ref. 72 for a review) and so may well respond differently to injury in vivo. Indeed, preliminary studies in rats show that intimal smooth muscle cells from an established arterial lesion do not respond well to bFGF, and this relates to a significant downregulation of the FGFR1 in the these cells. The process of intimal cell growth is not well understood; although there are agents which can interrupt the first two stages of lesion growth, none have been identified which inhibit intimal cell proliferation. Furthermore, the fact that human atherectomy sections show little cell proliferation would suggest that the replication of these cells is not a key event. It would therefore be prudent to study other mechanisms of lumen reocclusion, such as vasoregulation of the intima and cell migration.

Another course of action will be to examine human tissue for signs of remodeling of the arterial wall. The term remodeling is frequently used without a clear understanding of its meaning; what we refer to is an alteration in the artery which leads to changes in its structure, such as lumen narrowing, loss of mass, cell death, or vasospasm, which is dictated by changes in its local environment. Since we do not know what is involved in this process, it would seem logical to study it in experimental models. Thus, we return again to the question of whether we can model the process of lumen narrowing in experimental animals. We contend that without sufficient knowledge of the mechanisms involved in restenosis in humans, it is not possible to predict if data from animal models is applicable to humans. It is equally clear that "lesions" can be induced by several processes, and that thus far, the majority of experiments have concentrated on only one. We now need to formulate hypotheses based on the new information collected from human tissue, and with this knowledge proceed to evaluate such processes in detail in experimental animal models.

## ACKNOWLEDGMENTS

This work was supported by NIH grants HL-03174 and HL-41103.

## REFERENCES

1. Marikovsky M, Breuing K, Yu Liu P, Eriksson E, Higashiyama S, Farber P, Abraham J, Klagsbrun M. Appearance of heparin-binding EGF-like growth factor in wound fluid as a response to injury. Proc Natl Acad Sci USA 1993; 90:3889–3893.
2. Ross R. The pathogenesis of atherosclerosis: an update. N Engl J Med 1986; 314:488–500.
3. Glagov S, Weisenberg E, Zarins CK, Stankunavicius R, Kolettis G. Compensatory enlargement of human atherosclerotic coronary arteries. N Engl J Med 1987; 316:1371–1375.
4. Clarkson TB, Prichard RW, Morgan TM, Petrick GS, Klein KP. Remodeling of coronary arteries in human and nonhuman primates. JAMA 1994; 271: 289–294.
5. Folkow B. Physiological aspects of primary hypertension. Physiol Rev 1982; 62:347–504.
6. Jamal A, Bendeck M, Langille BL. Structural changes and recovery of function after arterial injury. Arterioscler Thromb 1992; 12:307–317.
7. Langille BL, O'Donnell F. Reductions in arterial diameter produced by chronic decreases in blood flow are endothelium-dependent. Science 1986; 231:405–407.
8. Haudenschild CC, Schwartz SM. Endothelial regeneration. II. Restitution of endothelial continuity. Lab Invest 1979; 41:407–418.
9. Barger AC, Beeuwkes R, Lainey LL, Silverman KJ. Hypothesis: vasa vasorum and neovascularization of human coronary arteries. A possible role in the pathophysiology of atherosclerosis. N Engl J Med 1984; 310:175–177.
10. Clowes AW, Reidy MA, Clowes MM. Mechanisms of stenosis after arterial injury. Lab Invest 1983; 49:208–215.
11. Friedman RJ, Stemerman MB, Wenz B, Moore S, Gauldie J, Gent M, Tiell ML, Spaet TH. The effect of thrombocytopenia on experimental arteriosclerotic lesion formation in rabbits. Smooth muscle proliferation and re-endothelialization. J Clin Invest 1977; 60:1191–1201.
12. Bjorkerud S, Bondjers G. Arterial repair and atherosclerosis after mechanical injury. 2. Tissue response after induction of a total local necrosis (deep longitudinal injury). Atherosclerosis 1971; 14:249–268.
13. Schwartz SM, Stemerman MB, Benditt EP. The aortic intima. II. Repair of the aortic lining after mechanical denudation. Am J Pathol 1975; 81:15–32.
14. Betz E, Schlote W. Responses of vessel walls to chronically applied electrical stimuli. Basic Res Cardiol 1979; 74:10–20.
15. French JE. Atherosclerosis in relation to the structure and function of the arterial intima, with special reference to the endothelium. Int Rev Exp Pathol 1966; 5:253–353.
16. Stemerman M, Spaet TH, Pitlick F, Clinton J, Lejnick S, Tiell ML. Intimal healing: the pattern of re-endothelialisation and intimal thickening. Am J Pathol 1977; 87:125–142.
17. Clowes AW, Reidy MA, Clowes MM. Kinetics of cellular proliferation after

arterial injury. I. Smooth muscle growth in the absence of endothelium. Lab Invest 1983; 49:327–333.

18. Clowes AW, Clowes MM, Fingerle J, Reidy MA. Regulation of smooth muscle cell growth in injured artery. J Cardiovasc Pharmacol 1989; 14(suppl 6):S12–S15.

19. Clowes AW, Reidy MA. Prevention of stenosis after vascular reconstruction: pharmacologic control of intimal hyperplasia—a review. J Vasc Surg 1991; 13:885–891.

20. Wilcox JN, Smith KM, Schwartz SM, Gordon D. Localization of tissue factor in the normal vessel wall and in the atherosclerotic plaque. Proc Natl Acad Sci USA 1989; 86:2839–2843.

21. Marmur JD, Rossikhina M, Guha A, Fyfe B, Friedrich V, Mendlowitz M, Nemerson Y, Taubman MB. Tissue factor is rapidly induced in arterial smooth muscle after balloon injury. J Clin Invest 1993; 91:2253–2259.

22. Jackson CL, Raines E, Ross R, Reidy MA. Role of endogenous platelet-derived growth factor in arterial smooth muscle cell migration after balloon catheter injury. Arteriosclerosis 1993; 13:1218–1226.

23. Fingerle J, Johnson R, Clowes AW, Majesky MW, Reidy MA. Role of platelets in smooth muscle cell proliferation and migration after vascular injury in rat carotid artery. Proc Natl Acad Sci USA 1989; 86:8412–8416.

24. Jawien AD, Bowen-Pope DF, Lindner V, Schwartz SM, Clowes AW. Platelet-derived growth factor promotes smooth muscle migration and intimal thickening in a rat model of balloon angioplasty. J Clin Invest 1992; 89:507–511.

25. Ferns GAA, Raines EW, Sprugel KH, Montani AS, Reidy MA, Ross R. Inhibition of neointimal smooth muscle cell accumulation after angioplasty by an antibody to PDGF. Science 1991; 253:1129–1132.

26. Clowes AW, Clowes MM, Reidy MA. Kinetics of cellular proliferation after arterial injury. III. Endothelial and smooth muscle growth in chronically denuded vessels. Lab Invest 1986; 54:295–303.

27. Olson NE, Chao S, Lindner V, Reidy MA. Intimal smooth muscle cell proliferation after balloon catheter injury: the role of basic fibroblast growth factor. Am J Pathol 1992; 140:1017–1023.

28. Majesky MW, Lindner V, Twardzik DR, Schwartz SM, Reidy MA. Production of transforming growth factor-$\beta_1$ during repair of arterial injury. J Clin Invest 1991; 88:904–910.

29. Lindner V, Lappi DA, Baird A, Majack RA, Reidy MA. Role of basic fibroblast growth factor in vascular lesion formation. Circ Res 1991; 68:106–113.

30. Lindner V, Reidy MA. Proliferation of smooth muscle cells after vascular injury is inhibited by an antibody against basic fibroblast growth factor. Proc Natl Acad Sci USA 1991; 88:3739–3743.

31. Lindner V, Olson NE, Clowes AW, Reidy MA. Inhibition of smooth muscle cell proliferation in injured rat arteries. Interaction of heparin with basic fibroblast growth factor. J Clin Invest 1992; 90:2044–2049.

32. Daemen MJAP, Lombardi DM, Bosman FT, Schwartz SM. Angiotensin II

induces smooth muscle cell proliferation in the normal and injured rat arterial wall. Circ Res 1991; 68:450–456.

33. Morishita R, Gibbons GH, Ellison KE, Nakajima M, Zhang L, Kaneda Y, Ogihara T, Dzau VJ. Single intraluminal delivery of antisense cdc2 kinase and proliferating-cell nuclear antigen oligonucleotides results in chronic inhibition of neointimal hyperplasia. Proc Natl Acad Sci USA 1993; 90:8474–8478.

34. Simons M, Edelman ER, Rosenberg RD. Antisense proliferating cell nuclear antigen oligonucleotides inhibit intimal hyperplasia in a rat carotid artery injury model. J Clin Invest 1994; 93:2351–2356.

35. Jackson CL, Raines EW, Ross R, Reidy MA. Role of endogenous platelet-derived growth factor in arterial smooth muscle cell migration after balloon catheter injury. Arterioscler Thromb 1993; 13:1218–1226.

36. Majesky MW, Reidy MA, Bowen-Pope DF, Hart CE, Wilcox JN, Schwartz SM. PDGF ligand and receptor gene expression during repair of arterial injury. J Cell Biol 1990; 111:2149–2158.

37. Lindner V, Giachelli C, Schwartz SM, Reidy MA. A subpopulation of smooth muscle cells in rat arteries express PDGF-B chain mRNA. Circ Res 1995; 76:951–957.

38. Walker LN, Reidy MA, Bowyer DE. Morphology and cell kinetics of fatty streak lesion formation in the hypercholesterolemic rabbit. Am J Pathol 1986; 125:450–459.

39. Roberts AB, Sporn MB. Physiological actions and clinical applications of transforming growth factor-$\beta$ (TGF-$\beta$). Growth Factors 1993; 8:1–9.

40. Nabel EG, Shum L, Pompili VJ, Yang Z, San H, Shu HB, Liptay S, Gold L, Gordon D, Derynck R, Nabel GJ. Direct transfer of transforming growth factor-$\beta_1$ gene into arteries stimulates fibrocellular hyperplasia. Proc Natl Acad Sci USA 1993; 90:10759–10763.

41. Majack RA, Majesky MW, Goodman LV. Role of PDGF-A expression in the control of vascular smooth muscle cell growth by transforming growth factor-$\beta$. J Cell Biol 1990; 111:239–247.

42. Battegay EJ, Raines EW, Seifert RA, Bowen-Pope BF, Ross R. TGF-$\beta$ induces bimodal proliferation of connective tissue cells via complex control of an autocrine PDGF loop. Cell 1990; 63:515–524.

43. Gibbons GH, Pratt RE, Dzau VJ. Vascular smooth muscle cell hypertrophy vs. hyperplasia. Autocrine transforming growth factor-$\beta_1$ expression determines growth response to angiotensin II. J Clin Invest 1992; 90:456–461.

44. Hearn JA, Donohue BC, Ba'albaki H, Douglas JS, King SB, Lembo NJ, Roubin GS, Sgoutas DS. Usefulness of serum lipoprotein (a) as a predictor of restenosis after percutaneous transluminal coronary angioplasty (see comments). Am J Cardiol 1992; 69:736–739.

45. Grainger DJ, Kirschenlohr HL, Metcalfe JC, Weissberg PL, Wade DP, Lawn RM. Proliferation of human smooth muscle cells promoted by lipoprotein(a). Science 1993; 260:1655–1658.

46. Okada Y, Katsuda S, Matsui Y, Nakanishi I. The modulation of collagen

synthesis in cultured arterial smooth muscle cells by platelet-derived growth factor. Cell Biol Int Rep 1992; 16:1015–1022.

47. Bendeck MP, Zempo N, Clowes AW, Galardy RE, Reidy MA. Smooth muscle cell migration and matrix metalloproteinase expression after arterial injury in the rat. Circ Res 1994; 75:539–545.

48. Block PC, Myler RK, Stertzer S, Fallon JT. Morphology after transluminal angioplasty in human beings. N Engl J Med 1981; 305:382–385.

49. Clowes AW, Clowes MM, Kirkman TR, Jackson CL, Au YPT, Kenagy R. Heparin inhibits the expression of tissue-type plasminogen activator by smooth muscle cells in injured rat carotid artery. Circ Res 1992; 70:1128–1136.

50. Clowes AW, Karnowsky MJ. Supression by heparin of smooth muscle cell proliferation in injured arteries. Nature 1977; 265:625–626.

51. Fischell TA, Grant G, Johnson DE. Determinants of smooth muscle injury during balloon angioplasty. Circulation 1990; 82:2170–2184.

52. Galis ZS, Muszynski M, Sukhova GK, Simon-Morrissey E, Unemori EN, Lark MW, Amento E, Libby P. Cytokine-stimulated human vascular smooth muscle cells synthesize a complement of enzymes required for extracellular matrix digestion. Circ Res 1994; 75:181–189.

53. Newman KM, Ogata Y, Malon AM, Irizarry E, Gandhi RH, Nagase H, Tilson MD. Identification of metrix metalloproteinases 3 (stromelysin-1) and 9 (gelatinase b) in abdominal aortic aneurysm. Arterioscler Thromb 1994; 14:1315–1320.

54. Newman KM, Malon AM, Shin RD, Scholes JV, Ramey WG, Tilson MD. Matrix metalloproteinases in abdominal aortic aneurysm: characterization, purification, and their possible sources. Connect Tissue Res 1994; 30:265–276.

55. Nobuyoshi M, Kimura T, Ohishi H, Horiuchi H, Nosaka H, Hamasaki N, Yokoi H, Kim K. Restenosis after percutaneous transluminal coronary angioplasty: pathologic observations in 20 patients. J Am Coll Cardiol 1991; 17: 433–439.

56. Miller MJ, Kuntz RE, Friedrich SP, Leidig GA, Fishman RF, Schnitt SJ, Baim DS, Safian RD. Frequency and consequences of intimal hyperplasia in specimens retrieved by directional atherectomy of native primary coronary artery stenoses and subsequent restenoses. Am J Cardiol 1993; 71:652–658.

57. Schnitt SJ, Safian RD, Kuntz RE, Schmidt DA, Baim DS. Histologic findings in specimens obtained by percutaneous directional coronary atherectomy. Hum Pathol 1992; 23:415–420.

58. Orekhov AN, Karpova II, Tertov VV, Rudchenko SA, Andreeva ER, Krushinsky AV, Smirnov VN. Cellular composition of atherosclerotic and uninvolved human aortic subendothelial intima. Light-microscopic study of dissociated aortic cells. Am J Pathol 1984; 115:17–24.

59. Andreeva ER, Rekhter MD, Romanov YA, Antonova GM, Antonov AS, Mironov AA, Orekhov AN. Stellate cells of aortic intima: II. Arborization of intimal cells in culture. Tissue Cell 1992; 24:697–704.

60. O'Brien ER, Alpers CE, Stewart DK, Ferguson M, Tran N, Gordon D, Benditt EP, Hinohara T, Simpson JB, Schwartz SM. Proliferation in primary

and restenotic coronary atherectomy tissue: implications for antiproliferative therapy. Circ Res 1993; 73:223–231.

61. Fairman MP. DNA polymerase δ/PCNA. Actions and interactions. J Cell Sci 1990; 95:1–4.

62. Leclerc G, Kearney M, Schneider D, Rosenfield K, Losordo DW, Isner JM. Assessment of cell kinetics in human restenotic lesions by in vitro bromodeoxyuridine labeling of excised atherectomy specimens. Clin Res 1993; 41:343A.

63. Strauss BH, Umans VA, van Suylen R, De Feyter PJ, Marco J, Robertson GC, Renkin J, Heyndrickx G, Vuzevski VD, Bosman FT, et al. Directional atherectomy for treatment of restenosis within coronary stents: Clinical, angiographic and histologic results. J Am Coll Cardiol 1992; 20:1465–1473.

64. Pickering JG, Weir L, Jekanowski J, Kearney MA, Isner JM. Proliferative activity in peripheral and coronary atherosclerotic plaque among patients undergoing percutaneous revascularization. J Clin Invest 1993; 91:1469–1480.

65. Garcia RL, Coltrera MD, Gown AM. Analysis of proliferative grade using anti-PCNA/cyclin monoclonal antibodies in fixed, embedded tissues. Comparison with flow cytometric analysis. Am J Pathol 1989; 134:733–739.

66. Celis JE, Bravo R, Larsen PM, Fey SJ. Cyclin: a nuclear protein whose level correlates directly with the proliferative state of normal as well as transformed cells. Leukemia Res 1984; 8:143–157.

67. Gordon D, Reidy MA, Benditt EP, Schwartz SM. Cell proliferation in human coronary arteries. Proc Natl Acad Sci USA 1990; 87:4600–4604.

68. Zeymer U, Fishbein MC, Forrester JS, Cercek B. Proliferating cell nuclear antigen immunohistochemistry in rat aorta after balloon denudation. Comparison with thymidine and bromodeoxyuridine labeling. Am J Pathol 1992; 141:685–690.

69. Spagnoli LG, Villaschi S, Neri L, Palmieri G, Taurino M, Faraglia V, Fiorani P. Autoradiographic studies of the smooth muscle cells in human arteries. Paroi Arterielle 1981; 7:107–112.

70. Rekhter M, Nicholls S, Ferguson M, Gordon D. Cell proliferation in human arteriovenous fistulas used for hemodialysis. Arterioscler Thromb 1993; 13:609–617.

71. Mintz GS, Douek PC, Bonner RF, Kent KM, Pichard AD, Satler LF, Leon MB. Intravascular ultrasound comparison of de nova and restenotic coronary artery lesions. J Am Coll Cardiol 1993; 21:118A.

72. Schwartz SM, deBlois D, O'Brien RM. The intima. Soil for atherosclerosis and restenosis. Circ Res 1995; 77:445–465.

# 14

# Pathobiology and Clinical Consequences of Plaque Rupture

**Richard Gallo, Juan J. Badimon, James H. Chesebro, and Valentin Fuster**

*Cardiovascular Institute, Mount Sinai Medical Center, New York, New York*

**Lina Badimon**

*Cardiovascular Research Center, Barcelona, Spain*

## I. INTRODUCTION

Atherosclerosis is unarguably the most prevalent disease of modern society. Coronary atherosclerosis and its thrombotic complications are responsible for over one half million deaths annually and for countless other complications. Coronary plaques appear early in an individual's life. By the end of the second decade, asymptomatic atherosclerotic lesions are present in most people living in Western societies. As these lesions grow, they may eventually limit blood flow to the myocardium resulting in chronic ischemic syndromes. If progression is rapid, as in the case of plaque rupture accompanied by luminal thrombosis, an acute ischemic syndrome such as unstable angina, myocardial infarction, or sudden death may result from the sudden narrowing or occlusion of the artery. Identification and treatment of such vulnerable plaques that after years of indolent growth give rise to a life-threatening condition has become the cornerstone of modern coronary care (1,2).

The concept that atherosclerotic plaques undergo disruption or rupture leading to thrombus formation was proposed many years ago (3,4). The composition of an atherosclerotic plaque rather than its size (stenosis severity) has emerged as the most important determinant for the development of the thrombus-mediated acute coronary syndromes. Indeed clinical and pathological observations indicate that the most vulnerable, most thrombogenic plaques are more often soft and lipid rich than hard and collagen rich (1–3). This chapter first describes the pathoanatomical features of stable and vulnerable atherosclerotic plaques and then explores potential mechanisms for the sudden conversion of a slowly progressing atherosclerotic plaque to a life-threatening atherothrombotic lesion.

## II.  DEVELOPMENT OF ATHEROSCLEROSIS

The pathogenesis and etiology of atherosclerosis is elaborated in previous chapters. In this section, a framework is provided to allow a better understanding of the pathoetiology of plaque rupture.

The morphological studies by Stary (5) have provided many interesting answers about plaque evolution (Fig. 1). The first observation made by Stary was that all humans develop focal eccentric thickening of the intima due to smooth muscle cell proliferation. This lesion appears very early in life; in fact, by the end of the second decade, most people will have such lesions present. This initial atherosclerotic lesion (Stary type I) is only microscopi-

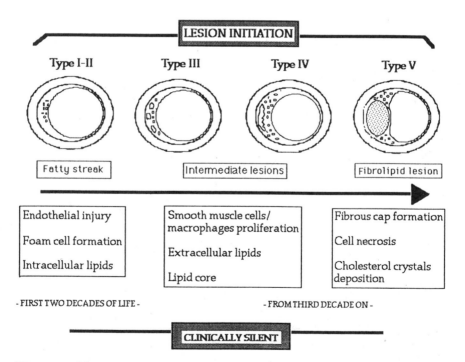

**Figure 1.**  The typical evolution and progression of coronary atherosclerosis, according to pathological findings.

cally and chemically perceivable, and it consists of isolated groups of macrophages and monocytes filled with lipid droplets (mainly cholesterol esters). Type II lesions, or fatty streaks, are composed of more lipid-laden cells than the initial lesions, and they are macroscopically visible as fatty dots or barely raised streaks (fatty streak). Each lesion is made up of one or more layers of lesion-filled foam cells within the intima and is accompanied by occasional scattered smooth muscle cells containing lipid droplets. There is evidence that such traits may be precursors of larger plaques. Transitional forms between fatty streaks and advanced plaques develop in sites where fatty streaks are more frequent. Progression beyond the fatty streak stage is associated with a sequence of changes starting with the appearance of extracellular lipid forming a more pronounced intimal layer (Stary type III lesion). Multiple scattered pools of extracellular lipids may progress to a large, confluent accumulation of extracellular lipid mainly as free cholesterol and its esters forming the lipid core characteristic of Stary type IV lesions. In Stary type V lesions, smooth muscle cells migrate into and proliferate within the plaque forming a layer over the luminal side of the lipid core. This lesion is also known as the fibroatheroma. As additional collagen is produced and the plaque increases in size, the lipid-rich core becomes avascular and almost totally acellular, consisting of pultaceous debris, including dead macrophages and mesenchymal cells along with abundant free cholesterol crystals (fatty gruel) (6,7). Lesions having visible thrombotic deposits and/or hemorrhage in addition to lipid and collagen are referred to as complicated fibroatheroma or complex lesions and are classified as Stary type VI lesions. Stary type VII lesions are reserved for advanced, mineralized lesions (calcific lesions). Finally, atherosclerotic lesions consisting almost entirely of fibrotic collagen, where the lipid may actually have regressed, are referred to as Stary type VIII lesions.

## A. Early Lesion (*Stary Types I, II, and III*)

Atherosclerotic lesions tend to develop in lesion-prone areas, as in arterial bifurcations, which are subject to repeated mechanical forces, such as oscillating shear forces (8,9). The *endothelium* at these sites is dysfunctional and is characterized by increased permeability leading to an influx of low-density lipoproteins (LDLs) and other plasma proteins into the intima (10,11).

Additionally, circulating monocytes stick to activated *endothelial cells* (expressing adhesive cell surface glycoproteins such as E-selectn, vascular cell adhesion molecule 1 (VCAM-1), or intracellular adhesion molecule 1 (ICAM-1) (12,13), pass between *endothelial cells,* and enter the intima where they differentiate into macrophages which can endocytose native and oxidized LDL. Lipids can also accumulate indirectly after death of lipid-rich foam cells (14).

Recent pathological evidence suggests that the lipid-rich core originates primarily from lipoprotein trapping and binding to matrix proteins such as glycosaminoglycans, collagen, and fibrinogen (15–18). This process results in focal collections of lipid-laden foam cells seen microscopically as yellow fatty clots or streaks raised above the intimal surface (Stary type II).

## B. Mature Plaques (*Stary Types III, IV, and V*)

The initial lipid- and macrophage-driven process is subsequently accompanied by smooth muscle cell activation, migration, and proliferation, which is followed by extracellular matrix deposition and further lipid accumulation. This gives rise to a more mature and clinically significant atherosclerotic plaque (Stary types III, IV, and V) (19,20). The endothelium is intact but dysfunctional in the early phases of atherosclerosis. Later the endothelium is often physically and functionally impaired by the further recruitment of monocytes and macrophages (21,22), compounded by the toxic effects of oxidized LDL, and degradation products such as oxygen-free radicals (14,192). Platelets and thrombi are often found adherent to areas of *endothelial denudation,* and they can become incorporated into the atherosclerotic plaque (2). Furthermore, platelet-derived growth factors and thrombin, generated by the intrinsic and extrinsic coagulating pathways, have been found to possess chemotactic and mitogenic properties (23,24) that can contribute to plaque growth by stimulating adjacent smooth muscle cells.

## C. Vulnerable Plaques (*Stary Types IV, V, and VI*)

Atherosclerosis is a multifocal disease in which the coronary arteries are generally diffusely involved with confluent plaques carpeting the vessel wall (25), but individual plaques vary greatly in composition and consistency even within the same coronary artery. However, in patients presenting with acute coronary syndromes, a significant atheromatous core is present in a significant majority of culprit lesion (26,27).

Plaques that are predominantly fibrous (Stary type VII) are hard, stable, and often resistant to rupture. Clinically, they are often innocuous but may give rise to stable angina when coronary blood flow is compromised (Fig. 2).

A vulnerable fibrolipid plaque consists of an lipid-rich core separated from the vascular lumen by a cap of fibrous tissue (Fig. 3). This atheromatous core is avascular (28,29), hypocellular (except at the periph-

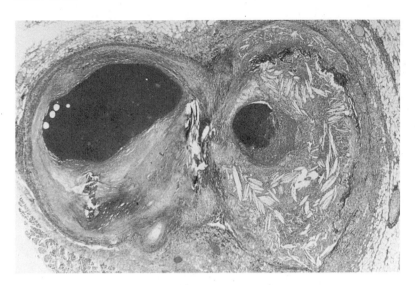

**Figure 2.** Photomicrograph illustrating a combined masson elastin stained left circumflex artery (left) and adjacent first marginal side branch (right). Note the differences in fibrous cap thickness. The plaque in the marginal artery has been disrupted and there is superimposed nonocclusive thrombus (darker shade). (Courtesy of Dr. Erling Falk, University of Odense).

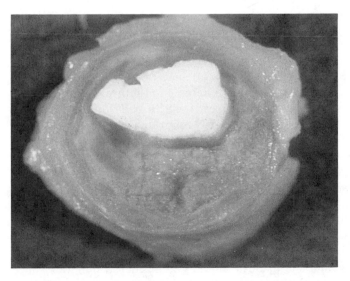

**Figure 3.** Coronary artery segment showing a vulnerable atheromatous plaque. Note the significant lipid-rich core "gruel" and thin fibrous plaque. (Courtesy of Dr. Erling Falk, University of Odense).

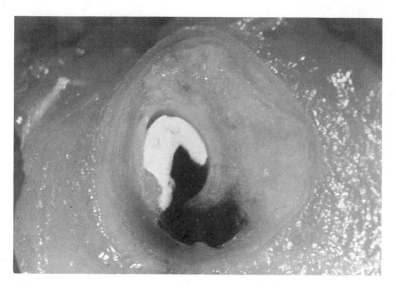

**Figure 4.** Photomicrograph of a disrupted plaque. The site of plaque rupture in this eccentric lesion occurred at the shoulder area, where the edge of the plaque meets the less diseased adjacent vessel wall. Plaque rupture is accompanied by an intraplaque hemorrhage and nonocclusive luminal thrombus.

ery where macrophage foam cells are frequently present [16,28,30]), devoid of supporting collagen (31), rich in free cholesterol esters, and very soft (32,33) (see Fig. 2). In postmortem studies, the atheromatous gruel has a toothpaste-like consistency at room temperature and is even softer at body temperature in vivo (32,33). It is no surprise, therefore, that these soft plaques are less stable and more vulnerable to rupture. Plaque rupture will most frequently occur at the weakest point; usually this site is where the fibrous cap is thinnest and most heavily infiltrated with foam cells. This also happens to be the site where the sum of all physical forces acting (see below) on the plaque are greatest. For eccentric plaques, this point is often the shoulder area, where the edge of the plaque meets the less diseased adjacent vessel wall (34–36) (Fig. 4).

The atheromatous gruel is the most thrombogenic component of an atherosclerotic plaque (37,38). Disruption of these vulnerable plaques results in exposition of highly thrombotic fatty gruel to flowing blood culminating in vessel narrowing and occlusion by thrombus (Fig. 5). Therefore, nonstenotic but vulnerable plaques should be considered ominous, since myocardial infarctions will often result from sudden occlusion of these lipid-laden lesion.

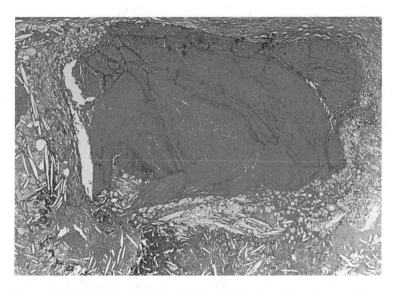

**Figure 5.** Microphotograph of a disrupted vulnerable plaque, with exposition of highly thrombotic fatty gruel (cholesterol crystals are clearly seen at the site of disruption), resulting in vessel occlusion by thrombus. (Courtesy of Dr. Erling Falk, University of Odense).

## III. PROGRESSION OF ATHEROSCLEROSIS

No obvious relationship between plaque size, stenosis severity, and plaque composition has been elucidated to date. Atherogenesis and lesion progression may be expected to be linear with time. However, angiographic studies show that progression of coronary artery disease in humans is neither linear nor predictable (39,40). New high-grade lesions often appear in segments of artery that appeared normal or near normal on previous angiographic examinations (41). Two thirds or more of the culprit lesions responsible for unstable angina or myocardial infarction were only mildly to moderately stenotic on prior angiograms (42). Giroud and colleagues (43) demonstrated that over three quarters of myocardial infarctions were in areas supplied by mildly stenosed (<50%) coronary arteries on a previous angiogram. Ambrose et al. (42) and Little et al. (44) further supported these observations by showing that the average degree of stenosis in lesions progressing to a later myocardial infarction was less than 50%.

### A. Risk Factors

Progression of early atherosclerotic lesions to larger or disrupted, clinically manifest lesions is variable and poorly understood. However, in persons at risk for coronary artery disease, this progression appears more rapid (2). The extent of atherosclerotic lesions or overall plaque burden found at autopsy was found to correlate well to age, male sex, hypercholesterolemia, hypertension, smoking, and diabetes (45–49). However, with the exception of data suggesting more extracellular oxidized lipids in smokers (50), no relation of specific risk factors to plaque composition has been identified.

## IV.  PLAQUE DISRUPTION

Rupture of the fibrous cap overlying an atheromatous core allows dissection into the intima by blood and exposing of the thrombogenic gruel (1,2). A mass of platelet-rich thrombus forms within the intima leading to plaque expansion. Ultimately the intraluminal thrombus may grow to become totally occlusive, or it is lysed and the plaque fissure reseals and becomes incorporated within the atheromatous plaque. Over the site of rupture, thrombus forms in the lumen but is not necessarily occlusive; it rather waxes and wares in size over hours or days (51).

Plaque tears run more often longitudinally than transversely (35), and most tears are microscopic, but when intraintimal thrombosis or luminal thrombosis is significant, the tear may be visible to the naked eye (35).

Plaque disruption is very important clinically. In early work by Constantinides, thrombi causing myocardial infarction (reconstructed from serial sections of coronary arteries) could be traced to cracks or fissures into a plaque (52). Further work by Davies and colleagues and Falk have convincingly shown that plaque rupture underlies the majority of thrombi responsible for acute coronary syndromes (51,53).

The risk of plaque disruption is essentially a function of two factors. The first factor is a reflection of the inherent pathoanatomical features and active disease processes of individual plaques–collectively referred as a plaques intrinsic vulnerability to rupture. The second factor is a sum of all external physical, hemodynamic, and pathophysiological forces acting on plaques, which can precipitate plaque rupture. We refer to the aggregate of these forces as triggering factors.

### A.  Vulnerability of Atherosclerotic Plaques

From direct pathological examination and computer-generated analysis, four intrinsic properties of an atherosclerotic plaque contribute to their vulnerability: (1) The size and consistency of the atheromatous core. (2) The structure and strength of the collagen-rich fibrous cap. (3) The active monocyte/macrophage–dependent inflammatory process. (4) The long-term repetitive cyclic mechanical forces acting on the plaque resulting in plaque fatigue or mechanical failure.

## 1. Atheromatous Core "Fatty Gruel"

The average coronary plaque is predominantly constituted of a sclerotic, collagen-rich component ($\geq 70\%$) (54,55). However, it is the size and consistency of the atheromatous core that determines lesion stability. By studying postmortem aortic plaques, Davies and colleagues (56) demonstrated that the greater the atheromatous core size, the more vulnerable the plaque was. In fact, they established an atheromatous core occupying more than 40% of total plaque area as a threshold above which the plaque was considered particularly at high risk for subsequent rupture and thrombosis (56). In an earlier study, Gertz and colleagues (57) examined 17 infact-related arteries postmortem and found larger atheromatous cores in 39 segments with plaque disruption (32% of total plaque area) compared with 229 segments with intact fibrous caps (5–12% of total plaque area). Richardson et al. (58) examined 85 coronary thrombi superimposed on fissured plaques. The majority (83%) of the thrombi occurred over a soft atheromatous core, whereas the rest had hard collagenous tissue beneath them.

Chemically, the atheromatous core is extremely rich in plasma-derived lipid; predominantly free cholesterol and its esters (32). The cholesterol ester composition of the atheromatous core is very similar to that of circulating plasma-LDL, with a high fraction of cholesterol linoleate. Cholesterol esters are less viscous at body temperatures and will soften plaques, whereas crystalline cholesterol has an opposite effect (32,59). Lipid-lowering therapy in humans is beneficial for reducing cardiovascular events. Presumably, they tilt the balance toward greater crystalline cholesterol and lesser cholesterol ester content of plaques; thus stabilizing the lesion and ultimately decreasing the incidence of plaque rupture (see below).

## 2. Fibrous Cap

Cap structure and strength are important determinants of plaque stability (60). Fibrous caps vary widely in thickness, cellularity, strength, and stiffness (31). Additionally, there are no blood vessels within the cap; therefore, all nutrients must be acquired by diffusion, which is a less efficient process (3,61).

Fibrous caps are thinnest at the shoulders of the lesion; that is, at the junction of the fibrous cap with adjacent, more normal intima (58). This region is often heavily infiltrated by macrophages and foam cells (21,58).

Early during cap development, smooth muscle cells are present in significant numbers (3,30), but as the lesion progresses, there is a steady decline in their presence (62,63). Smooth muscle cells could vanish as a result of programmed cell death or apoptosis (64–67). Lee and colleagues (68) have shown that cellular and calcified caps were one to two times and four to five times stiffer than hypocellular caps.

Ruptured caps have reduced mechanical strength. They contain less collagen and glycosaminoglycans, more extracellular lipids, less smooth muscle cells, and significantly more macrophages (31,36,69,70).

## 3.   Macrophage/Monocyte–Dependent Inflammation

Infiltration of disrupted fibrous caps by activated macrophage and foam cells has been known for some time (52,53,71,72). As mentioned above, the shoulder regions of eccentric plaques are sites of predilection for macrophage infiltration and plaque rupture (58). In vitro studies have also confirmed that foam cell infiltration reduces the tensile strength of fibrous caps (72). In a postmortem study of 71 disrupted atherosclerotic plaques, Richardson and colleagues (58) found that 53 (75%) of rupture site were infiltrated with foam cells. van de Wal et al. (72) identified superficial macrophage infiltration in plaques beneath all coronary thrombi examined. Further evaluation by immunohistochemistry confirmed the presence of activated macrophages and T lymphocytes, both markers of ongoing inflammation. A recent in vivo study (73) demonstrated that culprit lesions responsible for acute coronary syndromes (unstable angina, non–Q-wave myocardial infarction) contained significantly more macrophages than lesions responsible for stable angina (14 versus 3% of plaque tissue occupied by macrophages).

Macrophage and progressive extracellular lipid accumulation destabilizes plaques by destroying intimal tissue and fibrous caps (74). Macrophage and foam cell recruitment is associated with progressive tissue destruction eroding into and even through surrounding tissue (3,36,75,76). At the base beneath the core, the internal elastic membrane is often disrupted, and the adjacent media is frequently atrophic (77) and occasionally destroyed. Likewise the fibrous cap may be eroded from beneath thinning and weakening it. Macrophages and/or foam cells within the atheromatous core and fibrous cap are capable of degrading extracellular matrix by direct phagocytosis or by secreting numerous proteolytic enzymes such as plasminogen activators and a variety of matrix metalloproteinases (MMPs: collagenases, gelatinases, and stromelysins) (78,79). Together with the generation of toxic products (free radicals, products of lipid oxidation) they facilitate vessel wall damage and contribute to plaque instability. In recent years, a great deal of research has contributed to a better comprehension of the role of matrix metalloproteinases. MMPs are secreted in a proenzyme form requiring extracellular activation by a still undetermined activator (78) after which they are capable of degrading practically all components of the extracellular matrix. Additionally, MMPs are cosecreted with their natural inhibitors, being referred to collectively as tissue inhibitors of metalloproteinases (TIMPs). These inhibitors have been identified as participants in cell migration, tumor invasion, wound healing, inflammation, and vascular remodeling (78,79). A wide variety of cells, including monocytes and smooth muscle cells, can secrete MMPs (78). Human monocyte-derived macrophages grown in culture may express interstitial collagenase (MMP-1) and degrade collagen of aortic fibrous caps during incubation (80). Stromelysin and other MMPs capable of degrading extracellular matrix components have been identified in macrophages in human atherosclerotic plaques (81–85) and lipid-laden foam cells (86).

Other inflammatory cells found in disrupted plaques include mast cells and neutrophils (87–89). Mast cells are present in the shoulder regions of intact atherosclerotic plaques but at relatively low densities. They can secrete very powerful proteolytic enzymes such as tryptase and chymase which subsequently can activate the proenzymatic form of MMPs (88). The role of neutrophils is less clear. Their role in tissue destruction, especially in inflammatory diseases, is well established (90). However, they are rare in intact atherosclerotic plaques. It is postulated that they enter plaques shortly after disruption (71).

## 4. Cap Fatigue

After repeated normal loading, not only metals but also collagen-rich tissue such as bones (stress fractures) and bioprosthetic valves may tear suddenly (36). The cyclic stretching, compression, bending, flexing, shear, and pressure fluctuations encountered in a normal cardiac cycle may weaken and *fatigue* a fibrous cap leading to spontaneous rupture. Theoretically, lowering the number (heart rate) and magnitude (pressure) of the repetitive load should postpone the time to rupture. By reducing the physical strain on plaques could be one way $\beta$-blockers reduce the rate of reinfarctions.

## B. Extrinsic Triggers of Plaque Disruption

Acute coronary syndromes are not a random event. Nearly 50% of patients with an acute myocardial infarction report a triggering event (91). Muller and colleagues introduced the concept of an atherosclerotic plaque that may have been progressively weakened by prior internal processes (see above), and becomes susceptible to even minor everyday stresses that are now capable of triggering plaque rupture. It was also noticed that most myocardial infarctions occurred with increased frequency in the morning (92–94), particularly within the first hour after awakening (95). He referred to this phenomena as circadian triggering. Additional clinical observations indicate that the incidence of myocardial infarctions is higher on Mondays (96), during cold days (97), especially during the winter months (98), and during emotional stress (99–102) and physical exercise, especially in previously sedentary patients (103,104). In the following section, we briefly identify and review the extrinsic physical forces and patho-physiologic factors that may "trigger" plaque rupture.

## 1. Extrinsic Physical Forces

Atherosclerotic plaques will rupture when the sum of all external forces acting on it exceed its intrinsic tensile strength (36,105). Normally, blood pressure exerts two forces on the surrounding vessel wall. The first force is a circumferential (tensile) stress exerted to all components around the vessel wall. The second force is a radial (compressive) force exerted across the vessel wall (105). In order for the vessel wall to remain intact, both these forces must be counteracted by an equal and opposite force. In the case of plaque rupture, circumferential stress appears to be the predominant disruptive force (68,105).

Circumferential wall stress is described by the law of Laplace which relates luminal pressure and radius to wall tension: $\partial = p \cdot r/h$, where $\partial =$ circumferential wall stress; $r =$ vessel radius; and $h =$ wall thickness. Accordingly, the larger the vessel, the higher the blood pressure, or the thinner the vessel wall, the greater will be the force exerted on the vessel wall (105). Similarly, the tension created in fibrous caps of mildly or moderately stenotic plaques is greater than that created in caps of severely stenotic plaques if the pressure and cap thickness are similar.

In vessels with heterogeneous components, such as atherosclerotic plaques, the circumferential forces will be redistributed to those areas most capable of bearing the imposed forces, resulting in focal concentrations of circumferential stress at certain critical points within a plaque (58,106). The soft atheromatous gruel of a vulnerable plaque has almost no tensile strength; all the stress that should normally be borne by that region is displaced to the overlying fibrous cap (58). Using computer modeling for analysis of tensile strength, Richardson (58) and Cheng (107) both found high concentrations of stress at the ends of plaque caps overlying an area of lipid pool, especially when the atheromatous gruel exceeded 45% of the vessel circumference. The thickness of the fibrous cap is also an important determinant of tensile strength. Using computer modeling, Lorre and colleagues (108) demonstrated a fourfold increase in wall stress as plaque thickness was reduced from 250 to 50 $\mu$m for a constant vessel stenosis.

*Other Physical Forces.*

Compressive stress. As has been described, it is believed that most plaques rupture from forces exerted from the lumen into the plaque. However, certain forces can exert their pressure from the plaque out into the lumen. Collapse of high-grade, compliant stenosis caused by negative transmural pressures (caused by high-velocity jets or turbulent eddy currents through very tight stenoses) may produce highly concentrated compressive stresses from the buckling and deformation of the vessel wall (109). As an already weakened plaque bends and twists, it may ultimately rupture.

Vasospasm, plaque edema, or bleeding from vaso vasorum may also increase intraplaque pressures, "blowing out" the fibrous cap from the inside. They will be discussed in greater detail in the following section.

Bending stress.  Coronary arteries cyclically undergo changes in size and shape during each cardiac cycle. A normal coronary artery may vary as much as 10% in diameter throughout a cardiac cycle. The transmitted pulse pressure causes changes in the size and shape of atheromatous plaques, resulting in deformation and circumferential bending (110). Concentric plaques do not change as much as eccentric plaques during each systolic-diastolic cycle (111). Eccentric plaques typically bend most at their shoulder regions; that is, the site where the less compliant plaque meets with the more compliant vessel wall. Sudden accentuation of this bending may be a trigger for plaque rupture. Long-term repetitive bending may result in tissue fatigue with a similar outcome.

Flexing stress.  Similar to circumferential bending, coronary arteries undergo longitudinal or axial bending and stretching during each cardiac cycle. In an interesting angiographic study performed by Stein and colleagues (113), the angle of flexing correlated with subsequent lesion progression; however, the coefficient of correlation was rather low.

Hemodynamic stress.  Hemodynamic forces do not appear to be as important as the physical forces imposed on the plaque by blood pressure and pulse pressure. In normal coronary arteries, the response to increased shear stress is to vasodilate. This compensatory endothelium-dependent vasodilation does not occur in atherosclerotic segments (113). Shear stress can cause superficial endothelial damage (114). Whether this damage is sufficient to provoke plaque rupture is unlikely (56). If shears stress was a major factor in plaque rupture, we would expect to see more severely stenotic lesions rupture more frequently; however, as already mentioned, numerous angiographic studies do not prove this to be the case. Theoretically, shear stress may also contribute indirectly to plaque rupture by modulating the influx of monocytes/macrophages and plasma proteins into an atherosclerotic lesion (105).

2.  Pathophysiological Conditions

*Sympathetic Activity and Catecholamines.*  The sympathetic nervous system is enhanced and circulating catecholamines are elevated in the early morning, especially on arousal, during emotional stress, smoking, and exercise. Both can increase blood pressure, heart rate (pulse pressure), coronary flow, and coronary tone. This in turn causes surges in circumferential wall tension, radial stresses, and axial stresses which together may trigger rupture of an already vulnerable plaque (115–116). β-Blockade blunts the morning peak in onset of infarction, probably by limiting the sympathetic surge in the morning (117). Accordingly, the beneficial effects of β-blockers in secondary prevention (25% reduction in reinfarctions) has been attributed to the reduction in the heart rate (118). Similar, but less impressive, results were obtained with the heart rate–reducing calcium antagonists verapamil and diltiazem (119–121) but not with the heart rate–increasing calcium antagonist nifedipine (121).

*Thrombosis.* The thrombotic response to plaque rupture is influenced by the various components of the atherosclerotic plaque exposed following rupture. Our group has demonstrated that the most thrombogenic component of the atherosclerotic plaque is the atheromatous gruel (Fig. 6) (37). Therefore, lipid-rich plaques are not only the most vulnerable, but moreover, they are the most thrombogenic when their content is exposed to flowing blood. The atheromatous core is also a rich source of *tissue factor* (122,123). The source of this tissue factor is unknown at this time, but it may originate from disintegrating macrophages or be produced de novo by activated smooth muscle cells, macrophages/monocytes, and possibly acti-

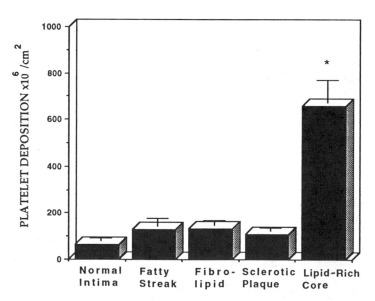

**Figure 6.** Graph showing the different levels of thrombogenicity of various atherosclerotic plaque components (*p < 0.05). (Adapted from reference 37.)

vated endothelial cells. We have recently shown a strong positive correlation between platelet thrombus formation on atheromatous core and the amount of tissue factor present (38).

The acute thrombotic response following plaque disruption also depends on the degree of stenosis and sudden geometrical changes following rupture. The greater the geometrical deformation, the greater the shear stress. Platelet and fibrinogen deposition increase directly with shear stress (124). With higher shear forces, circulating red blood cells displace platelets, monocytes, fibrinogen, and other plasma proteins to the periphery and enhance their deposition.

Recent experimental and clinical evidence suggests that a primary hypercoaguable or thrombogenic state of circulation can favor thrombosis. Platelet activation and the generation of thrombin may be enhanced by circulating catecholamines (125–127). Ruptured plaques may thrombose preferentially in the early morning; when the fibrinolytic activity is lowest (128,129) and platelet aggregability is highest (130–131). Additionally, plasma fibrinogen levels and blood viscosity are highest in the morning (132,133). Enhanced sympathetic tone can also stimulate $\alpha$-receptors, promoting platelet aggregation and vasoconstriction (134–140). Accordingly, aspirin blocks the morning increase in platelet activity (141) and, like $\beta$-blockers, blunts the morning increase in plaque rupture–associated events (142). Thus, the circadian variation in thrombogenic factors parallels variations in the sympathetic and catecholamine levels (see Fig. 6).

Platelet activation and generation of thrombin may also be enhanced by hypercholesterolemia, increased levels of lp(a) (143–145), smoking (138), and diabetes mellitus (146,147).

*Vasoconstriction.* Plaque disruption and vasoconstriction do frequently coexist (148,149), but spasm is not necessarily the causative factor (149–152). Proponents of vasospasm as a trigger of plaque rupture suggest that vessel constriction will result in a compression of an atheromatous core resulting in rupture of the fibrous cap into the lumen (152,153). However, spasm has been provoked in many patients with severely diseased coronary arteries without serious complications (154–156). Furthermore, spasmolytic agents (such as calcium antagonists) have not been proven to be effective in the prevention of myocardial infarctions. In a study by Nobuyoshi and colleagues, a positive correlation between ergonovine-induced vasospasm and plaque progression was found, but it was not clear whether this resulted in an increase in the incidence of myocardial infarctions (157).

*Vasa Vasorum.* Atherosclerosis is often accompanied by neovascularization (angiogenesis), resulting in the formation of a dense plexus of microvessels extending from the adventitia to the base of the plaque (158).

Transudation (edema) or small bleeds from these fragile vessels theoretically may increase the intraplaque pressure sufficient to blow out the cap from the inside (36).

## V.   CLINICAL CONSEQUENCES OF PLAQUE RUPTURE

The clinical manifestations of atherosclerotic plaques depend on several factors, including the degree and suddenness of blood flow obstruction, the duration of decreased myocardial perfusion, and the myocardial oxygen demand at the time of blood flow obstruction. The thrombotic response to the disrupted plaque is also a major determinant. Plaque rupture is accompanied by hemorrhage into the plaque and is accompanied by various amounts of luminal thrombosis. If the thrombus is small, plaque rupture probably proceeds unnoticed. If on the other hand the thrombus is large, compromising blood flow to the myocardium, the individual may experience an acute ischemic syndrome.

Plaque disruption is a common event, and in the majority of cases, it is asymptomatic (36,159) (Fig. 7). Plaque growth is also usually silent and the result of a dynamic thrombotic deposition (160). Most coronary thrombi (≥80%) have a layered structure indicating an episodic growth by repeated mural deposits (161). A ruptured plaque is found beneath almost all coronary thrombi, and displaced plaque fragments are frequently found buried deeply in the platelet thrombus, indicating that plaque growth involves repeated plaque ruptures followed by incorporation of luminal thrombus (161).

Autopsy data indicate that 9% of healthy persons dying of noncardiovascular deaths have asymptomatic disrupted plaques in their coronary arteries; this number increases to 22% in patients with diabetes mellitus (2,162). Numerous disrupted plaques are also found in patients who die of ischemic heart disease.

### A.   Unstable Angina

In unstable angina, a smaller fissure or disruption leads to an acute change in plaque structure, thrombus formation, and a reduction of blood flow resulting in an exacerbation of angina. Transient episodes of thrombotic vessel occlusion or near occlusion at the site of plaque injury may occur leading to angina at rest. The thrombus may be labile and result in temporary obstruction to flow that may last for minutes. In addition, the release of vasoactive substances by platelets and vasoconstriction secondary to endothelial vasodilator dysfunction contributes to further reduction of blood flow (163). The process may be sufficiently severe to cause total occlusion and myocar-

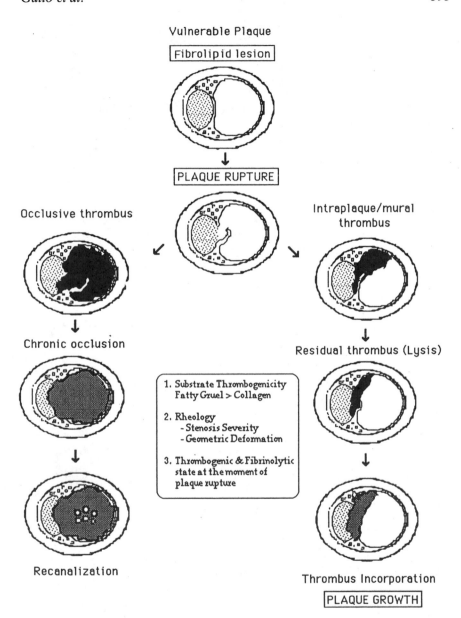

**Figure 7.** The thrombotic response after severe arterial injury (such as plaque rupture) is a function of three factors: (1) thrombogenicity of the exposed substrate; (2) rheological conditions of flowing blood (e.g., shear stress); (3) primary thrombogenic and fibrinolytic condition of the individual. (See text for details.)

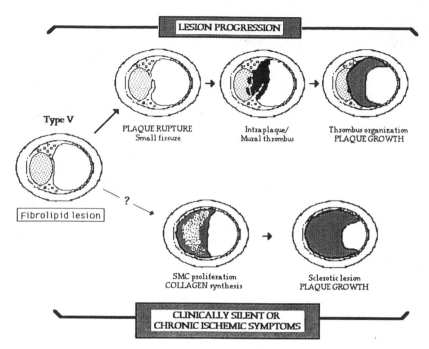

**Figure 8.** Dynamic evolution of plaque disruption. Plaque disruption is a common event, and in the majority of cases it is asymptomatic (36, 159).

dial infarction. Collateral vessels, however, may modify the outcome of a sudden coronary occlusion (164,165). Chronic ischemia may promote collateral development, and a severe stenosis can subsequently occlude silently (166). A total occlusion is found in 10% of patients with unstable angina (167,168) (Fig. 8).

## B. Non–Q-Wave Myocardial Infarction

In non–Q-wave myocardial infarction, the angiographic form of the responsible lesion is similar to that seen in unstable angina (167). More severe plaque damage would result in more persistent, but transient, thrombotic occlusion, which may last up to 1 hr. At early angiography, about one fourth of patients with non–Q-wave infarction have an infarct-related vessel that is completely occluded, with the distal territory usually being supplied by collaterals (168–173). Spontaneous thrombolysis, the resolution of arterial spasm, and the presence of collaterals limits the duration and extent of myocardial ischemia and prevents Q-wave infarction (1).

## C. Q-Wave Infarction

In Q-wave infarction, a larger plaque disruption may be associated with deep arterial injury or ulceration, resulting in the formation of a fixed and persistent thrombus. This leads to an abrupt cessation of myocardial perfusion, often for more than 1 hr, and subsequent necrosis of the involved myocardium. As discussed, the coronary lesion responsible for the infarction is frequently only mildly to moderately stenotic (42–44), which suggests that the severity of the underlying lesion is not the primary determinant of acute occlusion. In patients with long-standing coronary artery disease and severe coronary stenosis, well-developed collaterals prevent or reduce the extent of infarction. In a minority of patients, coronary thrombosis results from superficial injury or blood stasis in areas of high-grade stenosis (173).

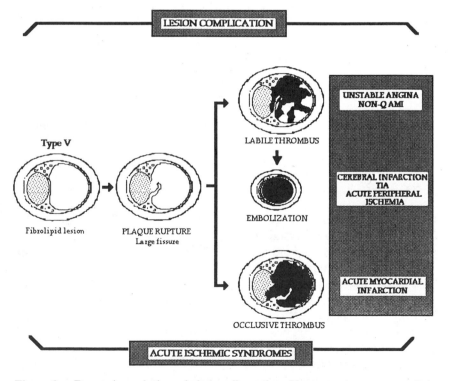

**Figure 9.** Dynamic evolution of plaque disruption. Plaque rupture may result in a labile luminal thrombus compromising coronary blood flow and resulting in unstable angina. If the thrombus is transiently occlusive a non–q-wave myocardial infarction may result. The persistence of an occlusive thrombus may result in a transmural q-wave myocardial infarction.

## D.   Sudden Death Related to Ischemia

Sudden death related to ischemia probably involves the disruption of a plaque that is rapidly obstructive resulting in acute occlusion generating a polymorphic arrhythmia. Absence of collateral flow, vasoconstriction, or platelet microthrombi to the microcirculation may contribute to the syndrome (1,173).

In patients with stable angina, coronary blood flow does not meet the myocardial oxygen demand. Usually the stenosis results in a $\geq 50\%$ reduction in luminal diameter. The atherosclerotic lesions can be of any type, but they are predominantly advanced fibrolipoid plaques (Stary type VI) or fibrotic lesions (Stary type VII). There is usually no plaque ulceration or thrombosis, but signs of previous plaque rupture with intraplaque hemorrhage or luminal thrombosis incorporated in the plaque are observed (174). The pattern of angina is not proportional to the severity of the underlying disease; mild or infrequent angina does not imply insignificant disease (1,2). The prognosis in stable angina is not accurately predicted by the extent and severity of individual obstructions (25) and by left ventricular function.

## VI.   PREVENTION OF PLAQUE DISRUPTION

A plaque's intrinsic vulnerability and extrinsic rupture triggers are the two principal determinants for plaque rupture. If we are to reduce or prevent the incidence of plaque rupture, both factors must be addressed.

## A.   Plaque Stabilization

Human atherosclerotic plaques can be stabilized against disruption by antiatherogenic therapy, including modifications of lifestyle and serum lipids (175–177). Numerous lipid-lowering trials with angiographic follow-up have independently demonstrated significant clinical benefits (reduction in the incidence of myocardial infarction, unstable angina, and death) can be obtained with little regression (175–182). For example, the Familial Atherosclerosis Treatment Study (FATS trial) (176) produced only a 1% mean regression of coronary stenoses with lipid-lowering agents. However, this was translated into a striking 73% reduction in cardiovascular events. This and other similar results are presumably because of increased plaque stability. Collectively, these trials did not demonstrate significant regression, but they did show a slowing of the progression of atherosclerotic lesions. One could speculate that this is because of a reduced incidence of asymptomatic plaque growth (cyclic plaque rupture and thrombosis).

The atheromatous core of most vulnerable plaques are rich in soft, semiliquid cholesterol esters. Theoretically, by reducing the liquid cholesteryl ester content and increasing the relative content of the remaining harder crystalline cholesterol and fibrous tissue, lipid-lowering therapy may result in stiffer, more stable lesions (59). Additionally, reduction in the level of circulating low-density lipoprotein (LDL) reduces the amount of bad cholesterol entering the plaque and permits increased cholesterol clearance from the plaque by high-density lipoprotein (HDL) (183).

Other approaches that may reduce the incidence of plaque rupture include angiotensin-converting enzyme (ACE) inhibitors. ACE inhibitors influence both plaque vulnerability and the triggering mechanisms responsible for disease onset. The latter will be discussed in the next section. ACE activity may contribute to the development of coronary artery disease (184). Results from the large Survival and Ventricular Enlargement (SAVE) (185–187) and Studies of Left Ventricular Dysfunction (SOLVD) (188,189) trials point to a reduction of 14–28% in the incidence of myocardial infarction and other ischemic events in patients with left ventricular dysfunction. The mechanisms for this reduction are uncertain. Angiotensin II is a growth factor for smooth muscle cells (190). ACE-inhibitors can reduce intimal hyperplasia after endothelial injury (191); however, there are no data that the prevention of infarction by these agents is due to the prevention of atherogenesis.

Oxidized LDL is a powerful activator of macrophages, and is a toxin for surrounding tissue (14,192–194). A plaque's content in oxidized LDL and macrophages can be theoretically reduced with the use of antioxidants (194,195). Initial experiments in a rabbit model of atherosclerosis showed a promising reduction in atherosclerosis with the powerful antioxidant probucol. However, a recent clinical trial failed to show a reduction in femoral artery atherosclerosis using the same agent (196).

Large epidemiological trials have reported up to a 50% reduction in the rate of cardiovascular mortality in postmenopausal women treated with estrogen-replacement therapy (198). Estrogens can increase a women's HDL cholesterol level and lower LDL cholesterol levels (199). Estrogens also have direct antiischemic effects such as coronary artery vasodilation (200,201). However, the effect of estrogens on coronary artery disease progression remains unknown.

## B. Trigger Reduction

Of all secondary risk factors, smoking is the most important preventable cause of morbidity and mortality from coronary artery disease (202,203). Smoking accelerates coronary artery disease (204–206), but fortunately this increased risk is rapidly reversible by cessation of the behavior (207). Smoking appears to impair endothelial function (208) and promote lipid oxidation (209). Furthermore, smoking is related to increases in catecholamine release (205,10), enhanced platelet aggregability (204,211), and thrombin generation (138).

$\beta$-Blockers and possibly heart rate-reducing calcium antagonists reduce the incidence of plaque rupture. The lower the heart rate, the better the protection against reinfarction and sudden death (212). $\beta$-Blockers reduce circumferential wall tension (by reduction in blood pressure and blunting of catecholamine surges) and both radial and axial stresses (by reduction in pulse pressure). By reducing the frequency and force of cyclic bending and stretching, $\beta$-blockers may reduce plaque cap fatigue.

The renin angiotensin system can interfere with endogenous fibrinolysis (213). Patients with high-renin hypertension are at a higher risk of myocardial infarction then patients with low-renin hypertension (214). ACE-inhibitors may indirectly enhance endogenous fibrinolysis, resulting in a reduced thrombotic response to plaque disruption (215).

## VII.  CONCLUSIONS

The mechanism responsible for the conversion of a stable atherosclerotic lesion to a life-threatening condition is plaque rupture with superimposed thrombosis. The risk of plaque rupture is a function of both plaque vulnerability (intrinsic disease) and rupture triggers (extrinsic forces). The major determinants of plaque vulnerability are size and consistency of the atheromatous core, structure and strength of the fibrous cap, and ongoing inflammation within the plaque. Plaque disruption occurs when the sum of all extrinsic forces acting on it are greater than its tensile strength. Plaque disruption occurs at points at which the plaque surface is weakest, which often coincides with points at which stresses from physical and hemodynamic forces are greatest.

The natural history of acute coronary syndromes mirrors that of the underlying plaque rupture and thrombosis. Stabilization corresponds to resealing and incorporation of the thrombus within the plaque; accentuation of symptoms to the development of a labile thrombus impinging on coronary blood flow; non–Q-wave myocardial infarction to the development of a transient occlusion; and transmural Q-wave infarction to the establishment of a persistent occlusive thrombus. Plaque disruption can be prevented by the stabilization of vulnerable plaques and by avoiding or reducing potential trigger mechanisms. To obtain maximum risk reduction against plaque disruption, both approaches should be pursued.

## REFERENCES

1. Fuster V, Badimon L, Badimon JJ, Chesebro JH. The pathogenesis of coronary artery disease and the acute coronary syndromes. N Engl J Med 1992; 326 (parts 1 and 2):242–250, 310–318.

2. Fuster V, Lewis A. Conner Memorial Lecture: Mechanisms leading to myocardial infarction: insights from studies of vascular biology. Circulation 1994; 90:2126–2146.
3. Falk E, Shah PK, Fuster V. Coronary plaque rupture. Circulation 1995; 92: 657–671.
4. Herrick JB. Clinical features of sudden obstruction of the coronary arteries. JAMA 1912; 59:2015–2020.
5. Stary HC. Composition and classification of human atherosclerotic lesions. Virchows Archiv A Pathol Anat 1992; 421:277–290.
6. Richardson PD, Davies MJ, Born GVR. Influence of plaque configuration and stress distribution on fissuring of coronary atherosclerotic plaques. Lancet 1989; 2:941–944.
7. Davies MJ, Woolf N, Rowles PM, Pepper J. Morphology of the endothelium over atherosclerotic plaques in human coronary arteries. Br Heart J 1988; 60:459–464.
8. Glagov Z, Zarins C, Giddens DP, Ku DN. Hemodynamics and atherosclerosis. Insights and perspectives gained from studies of human arteries. Arch Pathol Lab Med 1988; 112:1018–1031.
9. Stary HC, Blankenhorn DH, Chandler AB, Glagov S, Insull W, Richardson M, et al. A definition of the intima of human arteries and of its atherosclerosis-prone regions. A report from the committee on vascular lesions of the council on Atherosclerosis, American Heart Association. Circulation 1992; 85:391–405.
10. Ross R. The pathogenesis of atherosclerosis: a perspective for the 1990s. Nature 1993; 362:801–809.
11. Johnson-Tidey RR, McGregor JL, Taylor PR, Poston RN. Increase in adhesion molecule P-selectin in endothelium overlying atherosclerotic plaques. Am J Pathol 1994; 144:952–961.
12. Rosenfled ME, Pestel E. Cellularity of atherosclerotic lesions. Coron Artery Dis 1994; 5:189–197.
13. Navab M, Hama SY, Nguyen TB, Fogelman AM. Monocyte adhesion and transmigration in atherosclerosis. Coron Artery Dis 1994; 5:198–204.
14. Guyton JR, Klemp KF. Development of the lipid-rich core in human atherosclerosis. Thromb Vasc Biol 1996; 16:4–11.
15. Guyton JR, Klemp KF. Transitional features in human atherosclerosis. Intimal thickening, cholesterol clefts, and cell loss in human aortic fatty streaks. Am J Pathol 1993; 143:1444–1457.
16. Guyton JR, Klemp KF. Development of atherosclerotic core region. Chemical and ultrastructural analysis of microdiseased atherosclerotic lesions from human aorta. Arterioscler Thromb 1994; 14:1305–1314.
17. Berenson GS, Radhakrishnamurthy B, Srinivasan R, Vijayagopal P, Dalferes ER. Arterial wall injury and proteoglycan changes in atherosclerosis. Atherosclerosis 1988; 112:1002–1010.
18. Wright TN. Cell biology of arterial proteoglycans. Arteriosclerosis 1989; 9: 1–20.

19. Schwartz CJ, Valente AJ, Sprague EA, Kelley JL, Nerem RM. The pathogenesis of atherosclerosis: an overview. Clin Cardiol 1991; 14(suppl I):1–16.
20. Davies MJ, Woolf N. Atherosclerosis: What is it and why does it occur? Br Heart J 1993; 69(suppl):S3–S11.
21. Poston RN, Haskard DO, Coucher JR, Gall NP, Johnson-Tidey RR. Expression of intercellular adhesion molecule-1 in atherosclerotic plaques. Am J Pathol 1992; 140:665–673.
22. Hansson GK. Immune and inflammatory mechanisms of monocyte recruitment and accumulation. Br Heart J 1993; 69(suppl):9–S29.
23. Rabbani LE, Loscalzo J. Recent observations on the role of hemostatic determinants in the development of the atherothrombotic plaque. Atherosclerosis 1994; 105:1–7.
24. Falk E, Fernandez-Ortiz A. Role of thrombosis in atherosclerosis and its complications. Am J Cardiol 1995; 75:1B–7B.
25. Roberts WC. Diffuse extent of coronary atherosclerosis in fatal coronary artery disease. Am J Cardiol 1990; 90:1614–1621.
26. Falk E. Coronary thrombosis: pathogenesis and clinical manifestations. Am J Cardiol 1991; 68:28B–35B.
27. Falk E. Morphologic features of unstable atherothrombotic plaques underlying acute coronary syndromes. Am J Cardiol 1989; 63:114E–120E.
28. Friedman M. The coronary thrombus: its origin and fate. Hum Pathol 1971; 2:81–128.
29. Gertz SC, Roberts WC. Hemodynamic shear force in rupture of coronary arterial atherosclerotic plaques. Am J Cardiol 1990; 66:1368–1372.
30. Stary HC. Evolution and progression of atherosclerotic lesions in coronary arteries of children and young adults. Arteriosclerosis 1989; 9(suppl I):I19–I32.30.
31. Davies MJ. A macro and micro view of coronary vascular insult in ischemic heart disease. Circulation 1990; 82(Suppl II):II38–II46.
32. Small DM. Progression and regression of atherosclerotic lesions. Insights from lipid physical biochemistry. Arteriosclerosis 1988; 8:103–129.
33. Lundberg B. Chemical composition and physical state of lipid deposits in atherosclerosis. Atherosclerosis 1985; 56:93–110.
34. Falk E. Plaque rupture with severe preexisting stenosis precipitating coronary thrombosis: characteristics of coronary atherosclerotic plaques underlying fatal occlusive thrombi. Br Heart J 1983; 50:127–134.
35. Richardson PD, Davies MJ, Born GVR. Influence of plaque configuration and stress distribution on fissuring of coronary atherosclerotic plaques. Lancet 1989; 2:941–944.
36. Falk E. Why do plaques Rupture? Circulation 1992; 86(suppl III):III30–III42.
37. Fernandez-Ortiz A, Badimon J, Falk E, Fuster V, Meyer B, Mailhac A, Weng D, Shah PK, Badimon L. Characterization of the relative thrombogenicity of atherosclerotic plaque components: implications for consequences of plaque rupture. J Am Colil Cardiol 1994; 23:1526–1569.
38. Toschi V, Gallo R, Lettino M, Fallon JT, Fernandez-Ortiz A, Badimon L,

Chesebro JH, Nemerson Y, Fuster V, Badimon JJ. Tissue factor predicts the thrombogenicity of human atherosclerotic plaque components (abstr). Circulation 1995:I–112.

39. Moise A, L'Esperance J, Theroux P, Taeymans Y, Goulet C, Bourassa MG. Clinical and angiographic predictors of new total coronary occlusion in coronary artery disease: analysis of 313 nonoperated patients. Am J Cardiol 1984; 54:1176–1181.

40. Ambrose JA, Winters SL, Arora RR, Eng A, Riccio A, Gorlin R, Fuster V. Angiographic evolution of coronary artery morphology in unstable angina. J Am Coll Card 1988; 12:54–62.

41. Badimon L, Chesebro JH, Badimon JJ. Thrombus formation on ruptured atherosclerotic plaques and rethrombosis on evolving thrombi. Circulation 1992; 86(suppl III):III-74–III-85.

42. Ambrose JA, Tannenbaum MA, Alexopoulos D, et al. Angiographic progression of coronary artery disease and the development of myocardial infarction. J Am Coll Cardiol 1988; 12:56–62.

43. Giroud D, Li JM, Urban P, Meier B, Rutishauser W. Relation of the site of acute myocardial infarction to the most severe coronary arterial stenosis at prior angiography. Am J Cardiol 1992; 69:729–732.

44. Little WC, Constantinescu M, Applegate RJ, Kutcher MA, Burrows MT, Kahl FR, Santamore WP. Can coronary angiography predict the site of a subsequent myocardial infarction in patients with mild-to-moderate coronary artery disease? Circulation 1988; 78:1157–1166.

45. Solberg LA, Strong JP. Risk factors and atherosclerotic lesions: a review of autopsy studies. Atherosclerosis 1983; 3:187–198.

46. Reed DM, Strong JP, Resch J, Hayashi T. Serum lipids and lipoproteins as predictors of atherosclerosis: an autopsy study. Arteriosclerosis 1989; 9:560–564.

47. Robertson WB, Strong JP. Atherosclerosis in persons with hypertension and diabetes mellitus. Lab Invest 1968; 18:538–551.

48. Pathobiological Determinants of Atherosclerosis in Youth (PDAY) Research Group. Relationship of atherosclerosis in young men to serum lipoprotein cholesterol concentrations and smoking: a preliminary report. JAMA 1990; 264:3018–3024.

49. Pathobiological Determinants of Atheroscleroses in Youth (PDAY) Research Group. Natural history of aortic and coronary atherosclerotic lesions in youth: findings from the PDAY study. Arterioscler Thromb 1993; 13:1291–1298.

50. Wissier RW, the PDAY collaborating investigators. New insights into the pathogenesis of atherosclerosis as revealed by PDAY. Atherosclerosis 1994; 108(suppl):S3–S20.

51. Davies MJ, Thomas AC. Plaque fissuring—the cause of acute myocardial infarction, sudden ischaemic death, and crescendo angina. Br Heart J 1985; 53:363–373.

52. Constantinides P. Plaque fissures in human coronary thrombosis. J Atheroscl Res 1966; 6:1–17.

53. Falk E. Plaque rupture with pre-existing stenosis precipitating coronary throm-

bosis. Characteristics of coronary atherosclerotic plaques underlying fatal occlusive thrombi. Br Heart J 1983; 50:127–134.

54. Kragel AH, Reddy SG, Wittes JT, Roberts WC. Morphometric analysis of the composition of atherosclerotic plaques in the four major epicardial coronary arteries in acute myocardial infarction and in sudden coronary death. Circulation 1989; 80:1747–1756.

55. Kragel AH, Reddy SG, Wittes JT, Roberts WC. Morphometric analysis of the composition of coronary arterial plaques in isolated unstable angina pectoris with pain at rest. Am J Cardiol 1990; 66:562–567.

56. Davies MJ, Richardson PD, Woolf N, Katz DR, Mann J. Risk of thrombosis in human atherosclerotic plaques: role of extracellular lipid, macrophage, and smooth muscle cell content. Br Heart J 1993; 69:377–381.

57. Gertz SD, Roberts WC. Hemodynamic shear force in rupture of coronary arterial atherosclerotic plaques. Am J Cardiol 1990; 66:1368–1372.

58. Richardson PD, Davies MJ, Born GVR. Influence of plaque configuration and stress distribution on fissuring of coronary atherosclerotic plaques. Lancet 1989; 2:941–944.

59. Wagner WE, St Clair RW, Clarkson TB, Connor JR. A study of atherosclerosis regression in *Macaca mulatto,* III: chemical changes in arteries from animals with atherosclerosis induced for 19 months and regressed for 48 months at plasma cholesterol concentrations of 300 or 200 mg/di. Am J Pathol 1980; 100:633–650.

60. Loree HM, Kamm RD, Stringfellow RG, Lee RT. Effects of fibrous cap thickness on peak circumferential stress in model atherosclerotic vessels. Circ Res 1992; 71:850–858.

61. Bouch DC, Montgomery GL. Cardiac Lesions in fatal cases of recent myocardial ischemia from a coronary care unit. Br Heart J 1970; 32:795–803.

62. Davies MJ, Richardson PD, Woolf N, Katz DR, Mann J. Risk of thrombosis in human atherosclerotic plaques: role of extracellular lipid, macrophage, and smooth muscle cell content. Br Heart J 1993; 69:377–381.

63. Hangartner JRW, Charleston AJ, Davies MJ, Thomas AC. Morphological characteristics of clinically significant coronary artery stenosis in stable angina. Br Heart J 1986; 56:501–508.

64. Geng YJ, Libby P. Evidence for smooth muscle cell death via apoptosis in advanced human atherosclerotic lesions: implications for plaque destabilization and rupture. Circulation 1995; 92(suppl I):I–101.

65. Pollman MJ, Sherwood SW, Gibbons GH. Cell cycle arrest induces vascular smooth muscle cell programmed death: implications for antiproliferative therapies for restonsis. Circulation 1995; 92(suppl I):I–101.

66. Bennett MR, Gibson DF, Schwartz SM, Tait JF. Phagocytosis of apoptic vascular smooth muscle cells is mediated by exposure to phosphatidylserine. Circulation 1995; (suppl I):I–101.

67. Isner JM, Kearney M, Bortman S, Passeri J. Apoptosis in human atherosclerosis and restenosis. Circulation 1995; 91:2703–2711.

68. Lee RT, Grodzinsky AJ, Frank EH, Kamm RD, Schoen FJ. Structure-

dependent dynamic mechanical behavior of fibrous caps from human athero-sclerotic plaques. Circulation 1991; 83:1764–1770.

69. Davies MJ, Woolf N, Katz DR. Structure and cellular composition of aortic atherosclerotic plaques undergoing ulceration (abstr). Br Heart J 1991; 66:92.

70. Lendon CL, Davies MJ, Born GVR, Richardson PD. Atherosclerotic plaque caps are locally weakened when macrophage density is increased. Atherosclerosis 1991; 87:87–90.

71. Friedman M. The coronary thrombus: its origin and fate. Hum Pathol 1971; 2:81–128.

72. van der Wal AC, Becker AE, van der Loos CM, Das PK. Site of intimal rupture or erosion of thrombosed coronary atherosclerotic plaques is characterized by an inflammatory process irrespective of the dominant plaque morphology. Circulation 1994; 89:36–44.

73. Moreno PR, Falk E, Palacios IF, Newell JB, Fuster V, Fallon JT. Macrophage infiltration in acute coronary syndromes: implications for plaque rupture. Circulation 1994; 90:775–778.

74. Stary HC. The sequence of cell and matrix changes in atherosclerotic lesions of coronary arteries in the first forty years of life. Eur Heart J 1990; (suppl E):E-3–19.

75. Tracy RE, Devaney K, Kissling G. Characteristics of the plaque under a coronary thrombus. Virchows Arch A Pathol Anat Histopathol 1985; 405:411–427.

76. Guyton JR, Black BI, Seidel CL. Focal toxicity of oxysterols in vascular smooth muscle cell culture. A model of the atherosclerotic core region. Am J Pathol 1990; 137:425–434.

77. Isner JM, Donaldson RF, Fortin AH, Tischler A, Clarke RH. Attenuation of the media of coronary arteries in advanced atherosclerosis. Am J Cardiol 1986; 58:937–939.

78. Matrisian LM. The matrix degrading metalloproteinases. Bioessays 1992; 14: 455–463.

79. Libby P. Molecular bases of the acute coronary syndromes. Circulation 1995; 91:2844–2850.

80. Shah PK, Falk E, Badimon JJ, Fernandez-Ortiz A, Mailhac A, Levy G, Fallon JT, Regnstrom J, Fuster V. Human monocyte derived macrophages induce collagen breakdown in fibrous caps of atherosclerotic plaques: potential role of matrix degrading metalloproteinases and implications for plaque rupture. Circulation 1995; 91:657–671.

81. Henney AM, Wakeley PR, Davies MJ, Foster K, Hembry R, Murphy G, Humphries S. Localization of stromelysin gene expression in atherosclerotic plaques by in situ hybridization. Proc Natl Acad Sci USA 1991; 88:8154–8158.

82. Galis ZS, Sukhova GK, Lark MW, Libby P. Increased expression of matrix-metalloproteinases and matrix degrading activity in vulnerable regions of human atherosclerotic plaques. J Clin Invest 1994; 94:2493–2503.

83. Brown DL, Hibbs MS, Keamey M, Loushin C, Isner JM. Identification of 92-kD gelatinase in human coronary atherosclerotic lesions: association of active enzyme synthesis with unstable angina. Circulation 1995; 91:2125–2131.

84. Sukhova GS, Simon DI, Chapman HA, Libby P. Cytokines regulate the expression by vascular smooth muscle cells of cathepsin S, an elastase found in human atheroma. Circulation 1995; 92(suppl I):I–169.

85. Tyagi SC, Borders S, Kumar SG, Cassatt S, Parker JL. Expression of matrix metalloproteinase activity in coronary collateral arteries. Circulation 1995; 92(suppl I):I–169.

86. Rennick RE, Ling KLE, Humprhries SE, Henney AM. Effect of acetyl-LDL on monocyte/macrophage expression of matrix metalloproteinases (abstr). Atheroscierosis 1994; 109(suppl):192.

87. Kaartinen M, Penttil A, Kovanen PT. Accumulation of activated mast cells in the shoulder region of human coronary atheroma, the predilection site of atheromatous rupture. Circulation 1994; 90:1669–1678.

88. Atkinson JB, Harlan CW, Harlan GC, Virmani R. The association of mast cells and atherosclerosis: a morphologic study of early atherosclerotic lesions in young people. Hum Pathol 1994; 25:154–159.

89. Jonasson L, Holm J, Skalli O, Bondjers G, Hansson GK. Regional accumulations of T cells, macrophages, and smooth muscle cells in the human atherosclerotic plaque. Arteriosclerosis 1986; 6:131–138.

90. Weiss SJ. Tissue destruction by neutrophils. N Engl J Med 1989; 320:365–376.

91. Tofler GH, Stone PH, Maclure M, Edelman E, Davis VG, Robertson T, Antman EM, Muller JE, and the MILIS Study Group. Analysis of possible triggers of acute myocardial infarction (the MILIS Study). Am J Cardiol 1990; 66:22–27.

92. Muller JE, Toiler GH, Stone PH. Circadian variation and triggers of onset of acute cardiovascular disease. Circulation 1989; 79:733–743.

93. Willich SN, Collins R, Peto R, Linderer T, Sleight P, Schroder R, ISIS-2 (Second International Study of Infarct Survival) Collaborative Group. Morning peak in the incidence of myocardial infarction: experience in the ISIS-2 trial. Eur Heart J 1992; 13:594–598.

94. Gnecchi-Ruscone T, Piccaluga E, Guzzetti S, Contini M, Montano N, Nicolis E. Morning and Monday: critical periods for the onset of acute myocardial infarction: the GISSI 2 Study Experience. Eur Heart J 1994; 15:882–887.

95. Goldberg RJ, Brady P, Muller JE, Chen ZY, de Groot M, Zonneveld P, Dalen JE. Time of onset of symptoms of acute myocardial infarction. Am J Cardiol 1990; 66:140–144.

96. Willich SN, Lowel H, Lewis M, Hermann A, Arntz H, Keil U. Weekly variation of acute myocardial infarction: increased Monday risk in the working population. Circulation 1994; 90:87–93.

97. Merchant B, Ranjadayalan K, Stevenson R, Wilkinson P, Timmis AD. Circadian and seasonal factors in the pathogenesis of acute myocardial infarction: the influence of environmental temperature (abstr). Eur Heart J 1994; 25(suppl):473.

98. Ornato JP, Siegel L, Craren EJ, Nelson N. Increased incidence of cardiac death attributed to acute myocardial infarction during winter. Coron Artery Dis 1990; 1:199–203.

99. Trichopoulos D, Katsouyanni K, Zavitsanos X, Tzonou A, Dalla Vorgia P. Psychological stress and fatal heart attack: the Athens (1981) earthquake natural experiment. Lancet 1983; 1:441–444.

100. Meiset SR, Kutz I, Dayan KI, Pauzner H, Chetboun I, Arbel Y, David D. Effect of Iraqi missile war on incidence of acute myocardial infarction and sudden death in Israeli citizens. Lancet 1991; 338:660–661.

101. Gelernt MD, Hochman JS. Acute myocardial infarction triggered by emotional stress. Am J Cardiol 1992; 69:1512–1513.

102. Jacobs SC, Friedman R, Mittleman M, Maclure M, Sherwood J, Benson H, Muller JE. 9-fold increased risk of myocardial infarction following psychological stress as assessed by a casecontrol study (abstr). Circulation 1992; 86(suppl 1):I–198.

103. Mittleman MA, Maclure M, Toiler GH, Sherwood JB, Goldberg RJ, Muller JE. Triggering of acute myocardial infarction by heavy physical exertion: protection against triggering by regular exertion. N Engl J Med 1993; 329: 1677–1683.

104. Willich SN, Lewis M, Lowel H, Arntz H-R, Schubert F, Schröder R. Physical exertion as a trigger of acute myocardial infarction. N Engl J Med. 1993; 329:1684–1960.

105. MacIsaac AI, Thomas JD, Topol EJ. Toward the quiescent plaque. J Am Coll Cardiol 1993; 22:1228–1241.

106. Loree HM, Tobias BJ, Gibson U, Kamm RD, Small DM, Lee RT. Mechanical properties of model atherosclerotic lesion lipid pools. Arterioscler Thromb 1994; 14:230–234.

107. Cheng GC, Loree HM, Kamm RD, Fishbein MC, Lee RT. Distribution of circumferential stress in ruptured and stable atherosclerotic lesions: a structural analysis with histopathological correlation. Circulation 1993; 87:1179–1187.

108. Loree HM, Kamm RD, Stringfellow RG, Lee RT. Effects of fibrous cap thickness on peak circumferential stress in model atherosclerotic vessels. Circ Res 1992; 71:850–858.

109. Aoki T, Ku DN. Collapse of diseased arteries with eccentric cross section. J Biomech 1993; 26:133–142.

110. Mizushige K, Reisman M, Buchbinder M, Dittrich H, DeMaria AN. Atheroma deformation during the cardiac cycle: evaluation by intracoronary ultrasound (abstr). Circulation 1993; 88(suppl 1):I–550.

111. Alfonso F, Macaya C, Goicolea J, Hernandez R, Segovia J, Zamorano J, Baiiuelos C, Zarco P. Determinants of coronary compliance in patients with coronary artery disease: an intravascular ultrasound study. J Am Coll Cardiol 1994; 23:879–884.

112. Stein PD, Hamid MS, Shivkumar K, Davis TP, Khaja F, Henry JW. Effects of cyclic flexion of coronary arteries on progression of atherosclerosis. Am J Cardiol 1994; 73:431–437.

113. Rubanyi GM, Romero JC, Vanhoutte PM. Flow induced release of endothelium-derived relaxing factors. Am J Physiol 1986; 250:H1145–1149.

114. Gertz SD, Uretzky G, Wajnberg RS, Navot N, Gotsman MS. Endothelial cell damage and thrombus formation after partial arterial constriction: relevance to the role of coronary artery spasm in the pathogenesis of myocardial infarction. Circulation 1981; 63:476–486.

115. Gelernt MD, Hochman JS. Acute myocardial infarction triggered by emotional stress. Am J Cardiol 1992; 69:1512–1513.

116. Leren P. Ischaemic heart disease: how well are the risk profiles modulated by current beta blockers? Cardiology 1993; 82(suppl 3):8–12.

117. Willich SN, Linderer T, Wegsheider K, Leizorovicz A, Alamercery I, Schroder R, and the ISAM Study Group. Increased moming incidence of myocardial infarction in the ISAM Study: absence with prior P-adrenergic blockade. Circulation 1989; 80:853–858.

118. Kjekshus JK. Importance of heart rate in determining betablocker efficacy in acute and long-term acute myocardial infarction intervention trials. Am J Cardiol 1986; 57(suppl F):43F–49F.

119. The Danish Study Group on Verapamil in Myocardial Infarction. The effect of verapamil on mortality and major events after myocardial infarction: the Danish Verapamil Infarction Trial II (DAVIT II). Am J Cardiol 1990; 66:779–785.

120. Pahor MP, The CRIS Investigators. Secondary prevention of myocardial infarction with verapamil: Calcium Antagonist Reinfarction Italian Study (CRIS) (abstr). Eur Heart J 1994; 15(suppl):134.

121. Held PH, Yusuf S. Calcium antagonists in the treatment of ischemic heart disease: myocardial infarction. Coron Artery Dis 1994; 5:21–26.

122. Annex BH, Denning SM, Channon KM, Sketch MH, Stack RS, Morrissey JH, Peters KG. Differential expression of tissue factor protein in directional atherectomy specimens from patients with stable and unstable coronary syndromes. Circulation 1995; 91:619–622.

123. Wilcox JN, Smith KM, Schwartz SM, Gordon D. Localization of tissue factor in normal vessel wall and in the atherosclerotic plaque. Proc Natl Acad Sci USA 1989; 86:2839–2843.

124. Lassila R, Badimon JJ, Vallabhajosula S, Badimon L. Dynamic monitoring of platelet deposition on severely damaged vessel wall in flowing blood: effects of different stenosis on thrombus growth. Atherosclerosis 1990; 10:306–315.

125. Badimon L, Lasila R, Badimon JJ, Fuster V. An acute surge of epinephrine stimulates platelet deposition to severely damages vascular wall. J Am Coll Cardiol 1990; 15(suppl):181A.

126. Hjemdal P, Larsson PT, Waller NH. Effects of stress and β-blockade on platelet function. Circulation 1991; 84(suppl III):III-4–III-61.

127. Larsson PT, Wallen NH, Hjemdahl P. Norepinephrine-induced human platelet activation in vivo is only partially counteracted by aspirin. Circulation 1994; 89:1951–1957.

128. Andreotti F, DAvies MJ, Hackett DR, Knan MI, DeBart ACW, Aber VR, Maseri A, Kluft . Major circadian fluctuations in fibrinolytic factors and possible relevance to time of onset of myocardial infarction, sudden cardiac death and stroke. Am J Cardiol 1988; 62:635–637.

129. Angleton P, Chandler WL, Schmer G. Diurnal variation of tissue-type

plasminogen activator and its rapid inhibitor (PAI-1). Circulation 1989; 62: 635–637.

130. Tofler GH, Brezinski D, Schafer AL, Czeisler CA, Rutherford JD, Willilch SN, Gleason RE, Williams G, Muller JE. Concurrent morning increase in platelet aggregability and the risk of myocardial infarction and sudden death. N Engl J Med 1987; 316:1514–1518.

131. Brezinski D, Tofler GH, Muller JE, Pohjola-Sintonen S, Willich SN, Schafer AL, Czeisler CA, Williams G. Morning increase in platelet aggregability: Association with assumption of the upright posture. Circulation 1988; 78: 35–40.

132. Meade TW, Dyer S. Concurrent morning increase in platelet aggregability and the risk of myocardial infarction and sudden cardiac death. N Engl J Med 1987; 317:1737.

133. Ehrly AM, Jung G. Circadian rhythm of human blood viscosity. Biorheology 1973; 10:577–583.

134. Hjemdahl P, Chronos NA, Wilson DJ, Bouloux P, Goodall AH. Epinephrine sensitizes human platelets in vivo and in vitro as studied by fibrinogen binding and P-selectin expression. Arterioscler Thromb 1994; 14:77–84.

135. Quyyumi AA, Panza JA, Diodati JG, Lakatos E, Epstein SE. Circadian variation in ischemic threshold: a mechanism underlying the circadian variation in ischemic events. Circulation 1992; 86:22–28.

136. Kestin AS, Ellis PA, Barnard MR, Errichetti A, Rosner BA, Michelson AD. Effect of strenuous exercise on platelet activation state and reactivity. Circulation 1993; 88:1502–1511.

137. Larsson PT, Wallen HN, Hjemdahl P. Norepinephrine-induced human platelet activation in vivo is only partly counteracted by aspirin. Circulation 1994; 89:1951–1957.

138. Kimura S, Nishinaga M, Ozawa T, Shimada K. Thrombin generation as an acute effect of cigarette smoking. Am Heart J 1994; 128:7–11.

139. Winniford MD, Wheelan KR, Kremers MS, Ugolini V, van den Berg E Jr, Niggemann EH, Jansen DE, Hillis LD. Smoking-induced coronary vasoconstriction in patients with atherosclerotic coronary artery disease: evidence for adrenergically mediated alterations in coronary artery tone. Circulation 1986; 73:662–667.

140. Moliterno DJ, Willard JE, Lange RA, Negus BH, Boehrer JD, Glamann DB, Landau C, Rosen JD, Winniford MD, Hillis LD. Coronary-artery vasoconstriction induced by cocaine, cigarette smoking, or both. N Engl J Med 1994; 330:454–459.

141. McCall NT, Tofler GH, Schafer AI, Williams GH, Muller JE. The effect of enteric-coated aspirin on the morning increase in platelet activity. Am Heart J 1991; 65:177–178.

142. Ridker PM, Manson JE, Buring JE, Muller JE, Hennekens CH. Circadian variation of acute myocardial infarction and the effect of low-dose aspirin in a randomized trial of physicians. Circulation 1990; 82:897–902.

143. Liu AC, Lawn RM. Lipoprotein(a) and atherogenesis. Trans Cardvasc Med 1994; 1:40–44.

144. Berg K. Lp(a) lipoprotein: an overview. Chem Phy Lipids 1994; 68:9–16.
145. Anglés-Cano E, Hervio L, Rouy D, Fournier C, Chapman JM, Laplaud M, Koschinsky ML. Effects of lipoprotein (a) on the binding to fibrin and its activation by fibrin-bound tissue-type plasminogen activator. Chem Phy Lipids 1994; 67/68:369–380.
146. Schneider DJ, Sobel BE. Effect of diabetes on the coagulation and fibrinolytic-systems and its implications for atherogenesis. Coron Artery Dis 1992; 3:26–32.
147. Mautner SL, Lin F, Roberts WC. Composition of atherosclerotic plaques in the epicardial coronary arteries in juvenile (type 1) diabetes mellitus. Am J Cardiol 1992; 70:1264–1268.
148. Etsuda H, Mizuno K, Arakawa K, Satomura K, Shibuya T, Isojima K. Angioscopy in variant angina: coronary artery spasm andintimal injury. Lancet 1993; 342:1322–1324.
149. Bogaty P, Hackett D, Davies G, Maseri A. Vasoreactivity of the culprit lesion in unstable angina. Circulation 1994; 90:5–1 1.
150. Lam JY, Chesebro JH, Steele PM, Badimon L, Fuster V. Is vasospasm related to platelet deposition? Relationship in a porcine preparation of arterial injury in vivo. Circulation 1987; 76: 243–248.
151. Golino P, Ashton JH, Buja LM, Rosolowsky M, Taylor AL, McNatt J, Campbell WB, Willerson JT. Local platelet activation causes vasoconstriction of large epicardial canine coronary arteries in vivo: thromboxane A, and serotonin are possible mediators. Circulation 1989; 79:154–166.
152. Leary T. Coronary spasm as a possible factor in producing sudden death. Am Heart J 1934; 10:338–344.
153. Lin CS, Penha PD, Zak FG, Lin JC. Morphodynamic interpretation of acute coronary thrombosis, with special reference to volcano-like eruption of atheromatous plaque caused by coronary artery spasm. Angiology 1988; June:535–547.
154. Zeiher AM, Schnechinger V, Weitzel SH, Wolischlbger H, Just H. Intracoronary thrombus formation causes vasoconstriction of epicardial arteries in patients with coronary artery disease. Circulation 1991; 83:1519–1525.
155. Bertrand ME, LaBlanche JM, Tilment PY, Thieuleux FA, Delforge MR, Carre AG, Asseman P, Berzin B, Libersa C, Laurent JM. Frequency of provoked coronary artery spasm in 1089 consecutive patients undergoing coronary arteriography. Circulation 1982; 65:1299–1306.
156. Kaski JC, Tousoulis D, McFadden E, Crea F, Pereira WI, Maseri A. Variant angina pectoris: role of coronary spasm in the development of fixed coronary obstructions. Circulation 1992; 85:619–626.
157. Nobuyoshi M, Tanaka M, Nosaka H, Kimura T, Yokoi H, Hamasaki N, Kim K, Shindo T, Yimura K. Progression of coronary atherosclerosis: is coronary spasm related to progression? J Am Coll Cardiol 1991; 18:904–910.
158. Barger AC, Beeuwkes R, Lainey LL, Silverman KJ. Hypothesis: vaso vasorum and neovascularization of human coronary arteries: a possible role in the pathophysiology of atherosclerosis. N Engl J Med 1984; 310:175–177.
159. Frink RJ. Chronic ulcerated plaques: new insights into the pathogenesis of acute coronary disease. J Invasive Cardiol 1994; 6:173–185.

160. Gertz SD, Malekzadeh S, Dollar AL, Kragel A-H, Roberts WC. Composition of atherosclerotic plaques in the four major epicardial coronary arteries in patients *−90* years of age. Am J Cardiol 1991; 67:1228–1233.

161. Falk E. Unstable angina with fatal outcome: dynamic coronary thrombosis leading to infarction and/or sudden death. Autopsy evidence of recurrent mural thrombosis with peripheral embolization culminating in total vascular occlusion. Circulation 1985; 71:699–708.

162. Davies MJ, Bland JM, Hangartner JRW, Angeline A, Thomas AC. Factors influencing the presence or absence of acute coronary artery thrombi in sudden ischaemic death. Eur Heart J 1989; 10:203–208.

163. Chesebro JH, Fuster V. Thrombosis in unstable angina. N Engl J Med 1992; 327:192–194.

164. Cohen M, Sherman W, Rentrop KP, Gorlin R. Determinants of collateral filling observed during sudden controlled coronary artery occlusion in human subjects. J Am Coll Cardiol 1989; 13:297–303.

165. Rentrop KP, Feit F, Sherman W, Stecy P, Hosat S, Cohen M, Rey M, Ambrose J, Nachamie M, Schwartz W, Cole W, Pedroncin R, Thorton JC. Late thrombolytic therapy preserves left ventricular function in patients with collateralized total coronary occlusion: primary end point findings of the second Mount Sinai–New York University Reperfusion Trial. J Am Coll Cardiol 1989; 14:58–64.

166. Danchin N, Oswald T, Voiriot P, Juillière Y, Cherrier F. Significance of spontaneous obstruction of high degree coronary artery stenoses between diagnostic angiography and later percutaneous transluminal coronary angioplasty. Am J Cardiol 1989; 63:660–662.

167. Ambrose JA, Hjemdahl-Monsen CE, Borrico S, Gorlin R, Fuster V. Angiographic demonstration of a common link between unstable angina pectoris and non–Q-wave acute myocardial infarction. Am J Cardiol 1988; 61:244–247.

168. Ambrose JA, Alexopoulos D. Thrombolysis in unstable angina: will the beneficial effects of thrombolytic therapy in myocardial infarction apply to patients with unstable angina? J Am Coll Cardiol 1989; 13:1666–1671.

169. De Wood MA, Stifter WF, Simpson CS, et al. Coronary arteriographic findings soon after non–Q wave myocardial infarction. N Engl J Med 1986; 315:417–423.

170. Fuster V, Frye RL, Kennedy MA, Connolly DC, Mankin HT. The role of collateral circulation in the various coronary syndromes. Circulation 1979; 59:1137–1144.

171. Sasayama S, Fujita M. Recent insights into coronary collateral circulation. Circulation 1992; 85:1197–1204.

172. Little WC. Angiographic assessment of the culprit lesion before acute myocardial infarction. Am J Cardiol 1990; 66:44G–47G.

173. Fuster V, Frye RL, Kennedy MA, Connolly DC, Mankin HT. The role of collateral circulation in the various coronary syndromes. Circulation 1979; 59:1137–1144.

174. Sherman CT, Litvak F, Grundfest W, Lee M, Hickey A, Chaux A, Kass R, Blanche C, Matloff J, Morgenstern L, Ganz W, Swan HGC, Forrester J.

Coronary angioscopy in patients with unstable angina pectoris. N Engl J Med 1986; 315:913–919.

175. Ornish D, Brown SE, Scherwitz LW. Can lifestyle changes reverse coronary artery disease? The Lifestyle Heart Trial. Lancet 1990; 336:129–133.

176. Brown G, Albers JJ, Fischer LD, et al. Regression of coronary artery disease as a result of intensive lipid lowering therapy in men with high levels of apolipoprotei B. N Engl J Med 1990;336:129–133.

177. Scandinavian Simvastatin Survival Study Group. Randomised trial of cholesterol lowering in 4444 patients with coronary heart disease: the Scandinavian Simvastatin Survival Study (4S). Lancet 1994; 344:1383–1389.

178. Blankenhorn DH, Nessim SA, Johnson RL. Beneficial effects of combined colestipol-niacin therapy on coronary atherosclerosis and coronary venous bypass grafts. JAMA 1987; 257:3233–3240.

179. Cashin-Hemphill L, Mack, WJ, Pogoda JM, et al. Beneficial effects of colestipol-niacin on coronary atherosclerosis. JAMA 1978; 257:3233–3240.

180. Buchwald H, Varco RI, Matts JP, et al. Effect of partial ileal bypass surgery on mortality and morbidity from coronary heart disease in patients with hyperlipidemia. N Engl J Med 1990; 323:946–955.

181. Watts GF, Lewis B, Brunt JN, et al. Effects on coronary artery disease of lipid-lowering diet, or diet plus cholestyraminee, in the St Thomas Atherosclerosis Regression Study (STARS). Lancet 1992; 339:563–569.

182. Waters D, Higginson L, Gladstone P, Kimball B, Le May M, Boccuzzi SJ, L'Esperance J. Effects of monotherapy with an HMG-CoA reductase inhibitor on the progression of coronary atherosclerosis as assessed by serial quantitative arteriography. The Canadian Coronary Atherosclerosis Intervention Trial. Circulation 1994; 89:959–968.

183. Badimon JJ, Badimon L, Fuster V. Regression of atherosclerotic lesions by high density lipoprotein plasma fraction in the cholesterol-fed rabbit. J Clin Invest 1990; 85:1234–1241.

184. Cambien F, Costerousse O, Tiret L, Poirier L, Lecerf L, Gonzales MF, Evans A, Arveiler D, Cambou JP, Luc G, Rakotovao R, Ducimetiere P, Soubrier F, Alhenc-Gelas F. Plasma level and gene polymorphism of angiotensin-converting enzyme in relation to myocardial infarction. Circulation 1994; 90:669–676.

185. Yusuf S, Pepine CJ, Garces C, Pouleur H, Salem D, Kostis J, Benedict C, Rousseau M, Bourassa M, Pitt B. Effect of enalapril on myocardial infarction and unstable angina in patients with low ejection fractions. Lancet 1992; 340:1173–1178.

186. Pfeffer MA, Braunwald E, on behalf of SAVE investigators. Effect of captopril on mortality and morbidity in patients with left ventricular dysfunction after myocardial infarction. N Engl J Med 1992; 327:669–677.

187. Rutherford JD, Pfeffer MA, Moyé LA, Davies BR, Flaker GC, Kowey PR, Lamas GA, Miller HS, Packer M, Rouleau JL, Braunwaid E, on behalf of the SAVE Investigators. Effects of captopril on ischemic events after myocardial infarction: results of the Survival and Ventricular Enlargement trial. Circulation 1994; 90:1731–1738.

188. The SOLVD investigators. Effect of enalapril on survival in patients with reduced left ventricular ejection fractions and congestive heart failure. N Engl J Med 1991; 325:293–298.

189. The SOLVD investigators. Effects of enalapril on mortality and the development of heart failure in asymptomatic patients with reduced left ventricular ejection fractions. N Engl J Med 1992; 327:685–670.

190. Powell JS, Clozel J-P, Muller RKM, et al. Inhibitors of angiotensin converting enzyme prevent myocardial proliferation after vascular injury. Science 1989; 245:186–188.

191. Lonn EM, Yusuf S, Jha P, Montague TJ, Teo KK, Benedict CR, Pitt B. Emerging role of angiotensin-converting enzyme inhibitors in cardiac and vascular protection. Circulation 1994; 90:2056–2069.

192. Frei B. Reactive Oxygen Species and Antioxidant vitamins: mechanisms of action. Am J Med 1994; 97(suppl 3A):3A-5–3A-12.

193. Morel DW, DiCorleto PE, Chisolm GM. Endothelial and smooth muscle cells alter low density lipoprotein in vitro by free radical oxidation. Arteriosclerosis 1984; 4:357–364.

194. Hodis HN, Mack WJ, LaBree L, Hemphill LC, Azen SP. Natural antioxidant vitamins reduce coronary artery lesion progression as assessed by sequential coronary angiography (abstr). J Am Coll Cardiol 1994; 23(suppl A):481A.

195. Gaziano JM. Antioxidant vitamins and coronary artery disease risk. Am J Med 1994; 97(suppl 3A):3A-18–3A-21.

196. Walldius G, Erikson U, Olsson AG, Bergstrand L, Hadell K, Johansson J, Kaijser L, Lassvik C, Molgaard J, Nilsson S, SchäferElinder L, Stenport G, Holme I. The effect of probucol on femoral atherosclerosis: the Probucol Quantitative Regression Swedish Trial (PQRST). Am J Cardiol 1994; 75:875–883.

197. Stamper MJ, Colditz GA, Willett WC, Manson JE, Rosner B, Speizer FE, Hennekens CH. Postmenopausal estrogen therapy and cardiovascular disease: ten year follow-up from the nurses' health study. N Engl J Med 1991; 325:756–762.

198. Nabulsi AA, Folsom AR, White A, Patsch W, Heiss G, Wu KK, Szklo M. Association of hormone replacement therapy in various cardiovascular risk factors in postmenopausal women. N Engl J Med 1993; 28:1070–1075.

199. Grady D, Rubin SM, Petitti DB, Fox CS, Black D, Ettinger B, Ernster VL, Cummings SR. Hormone therapy to prevent disease and prolong life in postmenopausal women. Ann Intern Med 1992; 117:1016–1037.

200. Collins P, Rosano GMC, Jiang C, Lindsay D. Cardiovascular protection by estrogens—a calcium antagonist effect? Lancet 1993; 341:1264–1265.

201. Jonas MA, Oates JA, Ockene J, Hennekens CH. Statement on smoking and cardiovascular discase for health care professionals. American Heart Association Medical/Scientific Statement. Circulation 1992; 86:1664–1669.

202. Deckers JW, Agema WRP, Huijibrechts IPAM, Erdman RAM, Boersma H, Roelandt JRTC. Quitting of smoking in patients with recently established coronary artery disease reduces mortality by over 40%: results of a meta-analysis (abstr). Eur Heart J 1994; 15(suppl):171.

203. Shah PK, Helfant RH. Smoking and coronary artery disease. Chest 1988; 94:449–452.
204. Lichtlen PR, Nikutta P, Jost S, Deckers J, Wiese B, Rafflenbeul W, the INTACT Study Group. Anatomical progression of coronary artery disease in humans as seen by prospective, repeated, quantitated coronary angiography: relation to clinical events and risk factors. Circulation 1992; 86:828–838.
205. Waters D, Higginson L, Gladstone P, Boccuzzi S, Cook T, Lespérance J. Smoking accelerates the progression of coronary atherosclerosis as assessed by serial quantitative coronary arteriography (abstr). Circulation 1993; 88(suppl 1):I–344.
206. Rosenberg L, Kaufman DW, Helmrich SP, Shapiro S. The risk of myocardial infarction after quitting smoking in men under 55 years of age. N Engl J Med 1985; 313:1511–1514.
207. Celermajer DS, Sorensen KE, Bull C, Robinson J, Deanfield JE. Endothelium-dependent dilation in the systemic arteries of symptomatic subjects relates to coronary risk factors and their interaction. J Am Coll Cardiol 1994; 24:1468–1474.
208. Morrow JD, Frei B, Longmire AW, Gaziano JM, Lynch SM, Shyr Y, Strauss WE, Oates JA, Roberts LJ. Increase in circulating products of lipid peroxidation (F2-isoprostanes) in smokers: smoking as a cause of oxidative damage. N Engl J Med 1995; 332:1198–1203.
209. Winniford MD, Wheeland KR, Kremers MS, Ugolini V, van den berg S Jr, Niggemann EH, Jansen DE, Hillis LD. Smoking-induced coronary vasoconstriction in patients with atherosclerotic coronary artery disease: evidence for adrenergically mediated alterations in coronary artery disease. Circulation 1986; 73:662–667.
210. Hung J, Lam JY, Lacoste L. Cigarette smoking acutely increases platelet thrombus formation in patients with coronary artery disease taking aspirin. Circulation 1995; 92:2432–2436.
211. Kjekshus JK. Importance of heart rate in determining betablocker efficacy in acute and long-term acute myocardial infarction intervention trials. Am J Cardiol 1986; 57(suppl F):43F–49F.
212. Ridker PM, Gaboury CL, Conlin PR, Seely EW, Williams GH, Vaughan DE. Stimulation of plasminogen activator inhibitor in vivo by infusion of angiotensin 11: evidence of a potential interaction between the renin-angiotensin system and fibrinolytic function. Circulation 1993; 87:1969–1973.
213. Alderman MH, Madhaven S, Ooi WL. Association of the renin-sodium profile with the risk of myocardial infarction in patients with hypertension. N Engl J Med 1991; 324:1098–1104.
214. Wright RA, Flapan AD, Alberta KG, Ludlam CA, Fox KA. Effects of captopril therapy on endogenous fibrinolysis in men with recent, uncomplicated myocardial infarction. J Am Coll Cardiol 1994; 24:67–73.

# 15

# Isoprostanes and Antioxidant Therapy in Human Diseases

**Emma A. Meagher and Garret A. FitzGerald**

*The University of Pennsylvania, Philadelphia, Pennsylvania*

## I. INTRODUCTION

Free radicals are independent chemical species, having unpaired electrons (1). The simplest free radical is an atom of the element hydrogen with one proton and a single electron. Table 1 gives examples of other free radicals. The medical importance of free radicals is due to their high reactivity, through which they can denature biomolecules such as proteins, lipids, and nucleic acids resulting in tissue injury. Potentially harmful oxidative stresses may arise from exogenous sources such as the diet, environmental pollution, including cigarette smoke and exhaust fumes, or as products of ionizing radiation (2,3). Many oxidants are also generated endogenously during normal physiological processes such as mitochondrial respiration (4) and activation of phagocytic cells during the immune response (5).

Research in the area of free radical biology has grown at a rapid rate over the last decade. It is now recognized that nonradical moieties, which are highly reactive, also possess the ability to denature lipids, proteins, and DNA (6). This becomes important when one uses electron spin resonance (ESR), which is specific for the detection and measurement of free radicals only (7). Accompanying this growth in knowledge has been the evolution of confusing terminology as depicted in Table 2. Most of these terms are used interchangeably.

**Table 1**  Examples of Free Radicals

| Name | Formula | Comments |
| --- | --- | --- |
| Hydrogen atom | $H^{\cdot}$ | Simplest free radical |
| Superoxide | $O_2^{\cdot-}$ | Selectively reactive oxygen-centered radical |
| Hydroxyl | $OH^{\cdot}$ | Highly reactive oxygen-centered radical |
| Peroxyl, alkoxyl | $RO_2^{\cdot}$, $RO^{\cdot}$ | Breakdown products of organic peroxides |
| Nitric oxide | $NO^{\cdot}$ | "Beneficial" free radical—a vasodilator |
| Thiyl | $RS^{\cdot}$ | Sulfur-centered free radical |
| Trichloromethyl | $CCl_3^{\cdot}$ | Carbon-centered radical formed during the metabolism of $CCl_4$ in the liver contributing to the toxic effects of this solvent. Toxicity is enhanced by its rapid reaction with $O_2^{\cdot-}$, resulting in peroxyl radical generation. |

**Table 2**  Terminology

| Term | Example | Comments |
| --- | --- | --- |
| Free radical | $H^{\cdot}$, $CCl_3^{\cdot}$ $RS^{\cdot}$ $NO^{\cdot}$ | All differ in reactivity; not all have deleterious effects |
| Oxygen free radicals | $O_2^{\cdot-}$, $RO_2^{\cdot}$, $RO^{\cdot}$, $OH^{\cdot}$ | Oxygen-centered radicals only |
| Reactive oxygen species | $H_2O_2$, $O_3$, $HOCl$ | Includes radical and nonradical oxygen-derived species |
| Oxygen-derived species | $H_2O_2$, $O_3$, $O_2^{\cdot-}$, $NO^{\cdot}$ | *Reactive* is a relative term. Neither $O_2^{\cdot-}$ nor $H_2O_2$ are particularly reactive in aqueous solutions such as plasma. |
| Oxidants | $H_2O_2$, $O_3$, $O_2^{\cdot-}$, | Not an accurate term, because $H_2O_2$ and $O_2^{\cdot-}$ act as both oxidants and reductants in solution |
| Oxidative stress | | A disturbance in the prooxidant-antioxidant balance in favor of the former, leading to potential damage (8). |

The list of disorders in which free radical–mediated tissue injury has been implicated is extensive (Table 3). Many of these changes may be a consequence rather than a cause of damage. The direct association of free radicals with any specific toxicity or disease has been difficult to determine with very few exceptions. To establish a cause and effect relationship, it is essential that the parameter chosen to reflect injury is not merely an indication of normal biological adaptive processes, which in themselves are not detrimental to the integrity of cells or tissue. Conversely, it is important to appreciate that clearly deleterious phenomena, such as lipid peroxidation, may occur at the point of cell death and membrane lysis, events in which free radicals conceivably have played no role. The presence of lipid peroxide products in diseased tissues, therefore, does not provide evidence for a pathogenic role for free radicals in that disorder (9).

Protection against the deleterious effects of free radicals and other oxygen-derived species is provided by a number of antioxidant defense systems (10–13). These can be broadly categorized according to their method of action or by their location (Table 4). Antioxidants can be preventive by inactivating or scavenging free radicals before they interact with susceptible targets or they can act as "chain breakers" and thereby minimize free radical damage. Inactivating antioxidants include the enzymes superoxide dismutase (SOD), catalase and glutathione peroxidase, which all act intracellularly (14–16).

Endogenously derived oxidant stress is thought to arise largely from the incomplete reduction of molecular oxygen as it passes down the respiratory transport chain on the inner mitochondrial membrane. The single electron reduction creates the superoxide anion, which is thought to be a major player in the initiation of lipid peroxidation. SOD catalyzes the dismutation of two superoxide radicals to hydrogen peroxide. For this reason, it is referred to as an *incomplete* preventive antioxidant, because hydrogen peroxide is in itself a reactive species. Catalase, which is closely associated with SOD in vivo, then facilitates the breakdown of hydrogen peroxide to water and oxygen.

$$2O_2 \rightarrow 2HOOH + O_2 \qquad 2HOOH \rightarrow 2H_2O + O_2$$
$$\text{SOD} \qquad\qquad\qquad \text{catalase}$$

Extracellular antioxidant capacity is dependent on several reactions (17). A number of membrane-bound proteins are present to bind free transition metal ions and prevent their participation in the formation of the hydroxyl radical via the fenton reaction. The potential importance of transition metal ions in amplifying the threat from hydroxyl and peroxyl radical is well recognized (18). These antioxidants include the iron binding proteins, transferrin and lactoferrin, the copper binding proteins, ceruloplasmin and

**Table 3**  Clinical Conditions in Which Free Radicals Are Thought to Play a Role in Pathogenesis

| System/organ | Disease process | Disease process |
| --- | --- | --- |
| Cardiovascular | Atherosclerosis<br>Reperfusion injury<br>  (postinfarct / transplant) | Ethanol / doxorubicin induced<br>  cardiomyopathy Keshan disease (selenium deficiency) |
| Brain | Hyperbaric oxygen<br>Neurotoxins<br>Senile dementia<br>Parkinson's disease<br>Hypertensive cerebrovascular<br>  injury/ cerebral trauma | Ataxia-telangiectasia syndrome<br>Aluminum overload<br>Neuronal ceroid<br>  lipofuscinoses<br>Deyelinating syndromes |
| Kidney | Autoimmune nephrosis<br>Heavey metal nephrotoxicity | Aminoglycoside<br>  nephrotoxicity<br>Renal graft rejection |
| Liver | Reperfusion injury<br>Endotoxin-induced liver<br>  injury<br>$CCl_4$-induced toxicity<br>Alcohol-induced liver disease | Hemochromatosis<br>Wilson's disease<br>Acetaminophen-induced<br>  hepatitis |
| Lung | Hyperoxic injury<br>Bronchopulmonary dysplasia<br>Oxidant pollutants<br>Chemicals (paraquat, bleomycin) | Cigarette smoke<br>Asbestosis<br>Emphysema<br>Adult respiratory distress syndrome (ARDS)<br>Idiopathic pulmonary fibrosis |
| Skin | Solar/ionizing radiation<br>Thermal injury<br>Bloom's syndrome | Porphyria<br>Contact dermatitis<br>Photosensitive dyes / drugs<br>  (tetracyclines) |
| Eye | Retinopathy of prematurity<br>Cataracts | Photic retinopathy<br>Macular degernation |
| Blood | Malaria<br>Lead<br>Fanconi's anemia | Sickle cell disease<br>Favism<br>Drugs (primaquine,<br>  sulfonamides,<br>  phenylhydrazine) |
| Multiorgan diseases | Vasculitides<br>Autoimmune diseases<br>Ischemia-reflow states<br>Drug- and toxin-induced reactions<br>Nutritional deficiencies<br>  (kwashiorkor / vitamins E and C<br>  deficiencies) | Aging<br>Cancer<br>Radiation injury<br>Amyloid disease |

**Table 4** Antioxidant Systems

| Agent | Type, distribution, and comments |
|---|---|
| Catalase | Preventive, high in RBC but low in cardiac muscle and endothelium. Reacts very rapidly to convert $H_2O_2$ to $O_2 + H_2O$. Water soluble. Intracellular. |
| Superoxide dismutase | Preventive, ubiquitous. Rapidly converts $O_2^-$ to $H_2O_2$, which may be scavenged by catalase. Intracellular. |
| Glutathione peroxidase | Preventive or chain breaking. Water soluble. Levels maintained by NADPH. Activity is dependent on the presence of selenium. Increasing (GSH) amounts of oxidized form (GSSG) used as a marker of oxidative stress. Intracellular. |
| Hemoglobin/myoglobin | Preventive. Can convert $H_2O_2$ to $O_2 + H_2O$. Most effective in presence of ascorbate. Reaction is slow but compensated for by high concentrations of heme proteins in erythrocytes and monocytes. |
| Ascorbate | Water-soluble vitamin. Major antioxidant in plasma. Regenerates vitamin E by reducing the tocopherol radical that results when vitamin E scavenges a peroxyl radical. Vitamin C interaction with heme proteins may also be important. Vitamin C is deficient in smokers with ischemic heart disease. |
| Vitamin E | Lipid-soluble. Exists in the lipid bilayer of cell membranes and in lipoproteins. Chain-breaking antioxidant. |
| Uric acid | Obligatory endpoint of purine degradation in humans. It is a powerful extracellular chain-breaking antioxidant that is present in abundance. Its relative importance in vivo has yet to be established. |
| Sulfhydryl groups | Present in large numbers in all body fluids. Found on proteins and can be consumed by oxidants but may be damaged in the process. If protein is present in abundance and has a high turnover rate (albumin), the damage may be of little significance. |

albumin, the hemoglobin binding protein, haptoglobin, and the heme binding protein, hemopexin. Interestingly, hemoglobin and myoglobin are also thought to have weak antioxidant properties via their ability to convert hydrogen peroxide to oxygen and water (19,20).

Although these proteins will rapidly sequester ions that may participate in the formation of free radicals, they are virtually ineffective in mopping up free radicals once they are formed. This function is fulfilled by a variety of extracellular and membrane-bound molecules capable of reducing radicals that would otherwise initiate or propagate free radical chain reactions (21). These molecules are called chain-breaking antioxidants, and examples of these are also listed in Table 4.

The properties of an ideal antioxidant, according to Rose et al., are that it is present in adequate amounts in the body; that it is versatile, reacting with a wide variety of free radicals; that it can be compartmentalized, allowing it to build locally in response to need; that it is readily available to the body either through the diet or synthesized de novo in vivo; that it can be regenerated; that it could be conserved by the kidneys; and that it has tolerable toxicity (22). No ideal scavenger exists. Antioxidants vary enormously in their degree of reactivity and versatility. There is a considerable inter- and intraindividual variation in the concentration of antioxidants within the body at any given time. This is a function of both their intake or production and their rate of consumption during oxidative stress. A cause and effect relationship has been proposed between antioxidant deficiencies and disease (24–27).

## II.  ASSESSMENT OF OXIDANT STRESS

A variety of indices have been developed to assess free radical–mediated injury (Table 5). Most of these measure tissue changes that are consistent with an oxidative process but not always specific for free radicals. Increased free radical generation, however, may merely reflect homeostatic mechanisms or changes that are not toxic to the cell. In addition, the ability to detect elevated free radicals prior to or concomitant with injury is consistent with a role for these species in the damage, but it does not establish a cause and effect relationship (9). Substrates for free radical attack, as alluded to earlier, include DNA, proteins, and lipids. Lipids have been the most extensively studied because of their critical structural and functional role in membranes and because of the ease with which lipid peroxidation can be measured (28). Table 5 includes some of the methods used to measure lipid peroxidation. The technical simplicity of such methods has led to a large body of published research, which in many cases has not reflected the theoretical limitations of their application to clinical specimens. For example, membrane lipids become much more susceptible to peroxidation after cell death; thus, lipid peroxidation may be a marker rather than a mechanism of cell death (29). Other limitations include the difficulty in extrapolating measurements performed in vitro (e.g., light emmission, fluoresence, ESR spectroscopy) or *ex vivo* (e.g., low-density lipoprotein [LDL]) oxidizability) to *in vivo* situations. Oxidation of lipoproteins, primarily of LDL, is thought to play a major pathogenic role in atherosclerosis

**Table 5** Biochemical Endpoints Used to
Assess Radical-Induced Injury

---

Lipid peroxidation
  Isoprostanes
  Conjugated dienes
  TBARs
  Ethane/pentane
  Light emmission/fluorescence
  Fatty acid analyses
Protein carbonyl groups
Glutathione/glutathione disulfide
Protein thiols /protein mixed disulfide
Enzyme activities
  Those inhibited by radicals—e.g., calcium
  ATPase
  Those induced by radicals—e.g., SOD
Antioxidant contents/capacity
  Vitamin E
  Vitamin C
  Enhanced chemiluminescence
Oxidized oligonucleoside
  8-Hydroxydeoxyguanosine

---

(30–34). The role oxidative stress plays in the evolution of any disease remains unclear, partly owing to the limitation of the methodologies available to measure free radical generation *in vivo*. The measurement of oxidation products in tissues, plasma, or urine has been the most common method employed in clinical studies to reflect lipid peroxidation in vivo. Examples include measurement of conjugated dienes, thiobarbituric acid reactive substances (TBARS), serum lipid peroxides, exhalation of pentane and ethane gases, and cytotoxic aldehydes. Limitations as reviewed by Halliwell et al. exist with each of these methodologies (35).

Recently, interest has focused on a group of prostaglandin isomers, termed isoprostanes, which offer a potentially novel approach to the assessment of oxidative stress *in vivo*. These compounds will be considered below in some detail.

## A.  Isoprostanes

Arachidonic acid is a normal constituent of the phospholipid domain in cell membranes. Receptor-dependent and receptor-independent stimuli catalyze its release from the sn-2 position owing to the action of phosophlipases.

Free arachidonic acid is subject to enzymatic metabolism by (1) cyclooxygenases to form prostaglandins and related compounds; (2) epoxygenases to form epoxyeicosatrienoic acids and related compounds; and (3) lipoxygenases to form leukotrienes and related compounds. Recently, Morrow and Roberts have described a series of prostaglandin F isomers which are formed from arachidonic acid in an enzyme-independent manner following free radical attack, resulting in peroxyl radical formation (36). These isoprostanes are formed in situ esterified in the phospholipids and, once released, may exhibit biological activity (37). Analogous families of E and D isoprostanes have since been described (38) as have isothroboxanes and isoleukotrienes (39).

We have focused on 8-epi Prostaglandin $F_{2\alpha}$ ($PGF_{2\alpha}$) as a model isoprostane to explore the utility of this class of compounds as in vivo markers of oxidant stress. We have developed a quantitative assay for this compound using gas chromatography/mass spectrometry (GC/MS) and demonstrated its presence in human urine and plasma (40). Alternative approaches include the use of GC/MS to estimate "total" $F_2$ isoprostanes using a $PGF_{2\alpha}$ internal standard (36) and immunoassays for 8-epi $PGF_{2\alpha}$ (41).

Isoprostanes are chemically stable, and we have shown that 8-epi $PGF_{2\alpha}$ excretion does not change with posture or with moderate exercise in healthy volunteers. In addition, urinary 8-epi $PGF_{2\alpha}$ excretion undergoes no significant diurnal variation and does not differ in excretion between men and women. Studies in our laboratory have demonstrated urinary 8-epi $PGF_{2\alpha}$ is increased in a variety of clinical situations putatively associated with oxidant stress. These include patients poisoned with paraquat and paracetamol, chronic cigarette smokers, and patients suffering from ischemic syndromes who are reperfused after coronary artery bypass grafting, carotid reperfusion, or after administration of thrombolytic drugs (42–44).

## III.   ANTIOXIDANT DRUGS

### A.   Vitamin E

$\alpha$Tocopherol (vitamin E) is a lipid-soluble molecule that exists in the lipid bilayer of cell membranes and lipoproteins. Apart from its other important biological functions, vitamin E is also considered to be nature's most effective lipid-soluble, chain-breaking antioxidant; protecting cell membranes from peroxidative damage (45–47). It is thought to be the first line of defense against lipid peroxidation; protecting polyunsaturated fatty acid in cell membranes through its capacity to reduce the peroxyl radical to the much less reactive hydroperoxide, thus inhibiting the propagating step in lipid peroxidation (48). $\alpha$-Tocopherol appears to be highly efficient as an antioxidant because of it its ability to be "recycled." The tocopheroxyl radical may be regenerated to the native form of vitamin E by the action of a tocopheroxyl radical reductase enzyme (49). In addition, it can be reduced following oxidation by ascorbic acid and glutathione (22). Eight different forms of vitamin E exist which all differ in their biological and antioxidant activities. D-$\alpha$-tocopherol is the major biological dietary component with prominent antioxidant activity (50). The majority of both animal and human studies have used this form of vitamin E for supplementation. Several studies have shown that dietary supplements of vitamin E inhibit the oxidative modification of LDL *in vitro* and *ex vivo* (51–53). In addition, it has been demonstrated in vitro that LDL oxidation will only occur after depletion of endogenous vitamin E (54). Vitamin E is consumed when LDL is oxidized (55). The oxidizability of LDL ex vivo is reportedly enhanced in men with an increased risk for developing atherosclerosis such as diabetics, smokers, and patients with coronary heart disease (56). In addition, reduced plasma vitamin E and C levels and alterations in endogenous antioxidant status have been linked with disease and are thought to reflect consumption, secondary to free radical processes (57–59). Taken together, these data have suggested that antioxidant vitamins may play an important role in reducing the risk of developing atherosclerosis. However, definitive prospective data concerning a protective role for antioxidant vitamins have yet to be provided. Curiously, despite ongoing prospective studies, we do not know the dosing regimen, with this or other vitamins, which is optimal to achieve an antioxidant effect *in vivo*.

## B. Vitamin C (Ascorbic Acid)

Ascorbic acid is a water-soluble vitamin that provides the first line of defense against oxygen radicals in plasma. It reacts directly with superoxide and hydroxyl radicals, and it reduces the tocopheroxyl radical back to $\alpha$-tocopherol (60). In humans, ascorbic acid is highly concentrated in leukocytes, compartments of the eye, and the pituitary gland. More than 60% of the total vitamin C pool resides in skeletal muscle (22). The ease with which ascorbic acid can be oxidized has resulted in its commercial utility, as it is used to prevent oxidation in a wide variety of food products. Its versatility as a free radical scavenger has led to it being used also as an antioxidant in clinical trials. However, vitamin C may exhibit prooxidant properties *in vitro* (61,62). Ascorbate in the presence of iron will initiate lipid peroxidation and ascorbate with copper is a chemical system used to generate hydroxyl radicals. It is not known whether this vitamin exhibited prooxidant properties at the doses used *in vivo*. Although ascorbic acid is hydrophilic, it is synergistic with vitamin E *in vitro* in protecting LDL from oxidation (45,46). Recently, the confusion over the most appropriate dose of vitamin C has been highlighted (63).

## C.  Probucol

The hypocholesterolemic drug probucol was shown a decade ago to be an effective antioxidant and to protect LDL against oxidative modification in vitro (64). Studies in hypercholesterolemic rabbits indicate a protective effect against atherosclerosis that is unrelated to its ability to lower plasma cholesterol (65,66). In addition, a study by Carew, et al. showed that an analogue of probucol that has hypocholesterolemic properties but no antioxidant activity was found to be much less effective in preventing atherosclerosis in the Watanabe rabbit when compared with probucol (67). However, probucol possesses other properties that could account for the antiatherogenic responses observed. For example, it can increase the activity of plasma cholesteryl ester transferase (68), it inhibits the release of interleukin-1 (69), and it can alter the ability of macrophages to take up lipoproteins (70).

## IV.  ANTIOXIDANT DRUGS AND CLINICAL TRIALS

### A.  Cardiovascular Disease

Early observations of an association between diet and cardiovascular disease were made in 1934 (71). Since that time, several observational studies have reported an inverse relationship between dietary antioxidant intake and the incidence of cardiovascular disease (72–76). Very few of these studies made any adjustment for concomitant changes in risk factors such as smoking, exercise, blood pressure, or cholesterol level.

### 1.  Observational Studies

During the past decade, numerous epidemiological studies on antioxidant vitamins and cardiovascular disease have been published. The Nurses' Health Study addressed the association between vitamin E intake and the incidence of major coronary events in 87,245 females aged 34 to 59 years (77). The use of antioxidant vitamin supplements was recorded and dietary intake of nutrients was measured. A total of 552 major coronary events, 437 nonfatal myocardial infarctions, and 115 coronary deaths, were documented over an 8-year follow-up period. Adjusting for age and smoking status, the risk of a coronary event was significantly lower in the highest quintile of vitamin E intake as compared with those in the lowest quintile. The significant protective effect persisted after adjusting for obesity, exercise level, dietary intake, hypertension, hypercholesterolemia, diabetes, menopausal status, the use of estrogen-replacement therapy, aspirin, alcohol intake or multivitamins, $\beta$-carotene, or vitamin C. Apparent benefit, in the case of vitamin E, seemed attributable mainly to the use of supplements, because high intake from diet alone was not associated with a significant risk reduction. The use of vitamin E supplements for 2 or more years was associated with a decrease in risk of 41%. The final conclusion of the study was that, although the data do not prove a cause and effect relationship, the use of vitamin E supplements in middle-aged women is associated with a reduced risk of coronary heart disease.

The Health Professionals Follow-up Study, started in 1986, investigated 39,910 males, aged 40–75 years with no history of cardiovascular disease, diabetes, or hypercholesterolemia (78). The use of supplements was recorded and a diet history was obtained. During 4 years of follow-up, 667 coronary endpoints were documented; 360 bypass grafts or angioplasties, 201 nonfatal myocardial infarctions, and 106 fatal coronary events. The age-adjusted risk for coronary heart disease was significantly lower in the highest quintile for vitamin E intake. The maximal reduction in risk was seen among men consuming 100–249 mg vitamin E per day for 2 or more years with no further decrease at higher doses. Carotene intake was inversely associated with the risk of coronary disease among current smokers and former smokers, but no reduction of risk was observed among those who had never smoked. Interestingly, vitamin C was not associated with a lower risk. Again, although this study does not prove a cause and effect relationship, it provides further evidence associating vitamin E intake with a reduction in this disease.

Dietary $\beta$-carotene was associated with decreased cardiovascular mortality in a prospective cohort of 1299 elderly Massachusetts residents. There were 161 cardiovascular deaths (48 from myocardial infarction) during the 4.75-year follow-up period (79). The age- and sex-adjusted relative risk for cardiovascular death among those with the highest $\beta$-carotene intake was 0.54 (range, 0.34–0.87). The relative risk was 0.25 for fatal myocardial infarction.

The Edinburgh Artery Study was a cross-sectional survey of 1592 men and women aged 55–74 years carried out to determine the relationship between peripheral arterial disease, as measured the ankle brachial pressure index, and dietary factors (80). Dietary vitamin E intake, as assessed by a food frequency questionnaire, was significantly associated with an improved ankle brachial pressure index.

The only large cohort study not finding any association between vitamin E, in this case serum levels, and cardiovascular risk was the Basel Prospective Study, which enrolled 2975 healthy male pharmaceutical employees. Subjects were monitored for coronary death for a 7-year follow-up period.

Baseline cardiovascular risks, however, were not characterized and the study lacked power, because the mortality rate was less than 3% (81). This study, however, did show a lower risk (RR 0.65; $p<.02$) of mortality from ischemic heart disease in the group with the highest concentrations of carotene fraction.

In summary, the results of the most recent observational studies suggest that dietary antioxidant vitamin consumption is associated with a decreased incidence of coronary heart disease. The result of the Nurses' Health Study and the Health Professionals Follow-up Study suggest that the use of vitamin supplements may further reduce the risk of coronary heart disease. In addition, $\beta$-carotene seems to reduce the risk for coronary heart disease in patients who are heavy smokers. Observational studies, however, may confound vitamin intake with a "healthy" lifestyle, including general dietary habits, exercise, and smoking patterns rather than indicate a direct beneficial role from vitamins whether as dietary constituents or as supplements.

## 2.   Intervention Studies

A review of the experimental and epidemiological evidence for benefit from antioxidant vitamins in cardiovascular disease in 1991 led to the recommendation that clinical trials were timely (82). It is important to remember that the evidence was based largely on animal models. For the most part, such studies assessed the effect of antioxidants on the evolution of early atherosclerotic lesions (fatty streaks). Whether or not antioxidants have inhibitory effects on advanced atherosclerotic disease, plaque rupture, or thrombosis in such models remains to be determined.

This may be of relevance in the planning of a clinical trial. If the effects of antioxidants are limited to retarding the initiation of lesions, there may be no demonstrable effect on clinical events for some time. After a "long enough" treatment period, one would expect to see a reduction in event rates, but because it is not known how long it takes for clinically significant atherosclerotic disease to develop, it is impossible to determine accurately the duration of such a clinical trial. Similarly, it is difficult to estimate the sample size for such a study in a presently event-free population. The performance of such primary prevention studies in patients at risk, for example, those with hypercholesterolemia and perhaps hyperhemocysteinemia, may be expected to reduce the sample size. At present, data from large scale intervention studies on antioxidant vitamins and cardiovascular disease are not available, and only a limited number of small studies applying different doses of antioxidant supplements have been published. The studies can be subdivided into three groups: those focusing on surrogate risk factors such as LDL oxidizability, those involving clinical endpoints such as intermittent claudication and myocardial infarction, and those which include surrogates for atherogenesis, such as restenosis rates following percutaneous transluminal angioplasty.

Three recent studies demonstrated that the short-term (83) and long-term (84,85) administration of large doses of vitamin E strongly protects LDL against oxidative modification *ex vivo*. Treatment with 1000 IU α-tocopherol/day for 7 days resulted in an increased resistance of LDL to oxidation. The increase in resistance times highly correlated with LDL vitamin E content (83). Other studies using either 800 IU α-tocopherol/day or 1600 mg vitamin E/day for several months also reported increased protection of LDL, whereas 3 months of supplementation with 60 mg/day of β-carotene had no effect on LDL oxidizability.

One small, prospective randomized controlled trial of subjects with intermittent claudication showed that exercise capacity, as determined by a walking test, improved significantly with 600 mg vitamin E/day for 10 months therapy (86). A double-blind crossover trial of vitamin E found that daily doses of 400 IU α-tocopherol for 6 months did not improve symptoms in patients with stable angina pectoris (87). Supplementation also failed to improve significantly exercise performance or left ventricular function. However, this study only enrolled 52 subjects and the treatment period was brief.

Further evidence for a protective effect from β-carotene came from analysis of a subgroup of the Physicians Health Study (88). This study enrolled 22,071 American male physicians aged 40–84 years. Among the 333 men with angina and/or coronary revascularization who received 50 mg of β-carotene on alternate days, 44% had a reduction in all major coronary events defined as myocardial infarction, revascularization, or cardiac death. These subjects also had a 49% reduction in all vascular events, defined as stroke, myocardial infarction, revascularization, or cardiovascular death, after adjusting for age and aspirin intake. The beneficial effect did not appear until the second year of follow-up. This study was primarily undertaken to determine whether or not β-carotene would reduce the incidence of gastrointestinal cancer. A limitation to the study was that subjects were assigned rather than randomized to β-carotene treatment.

Two trials have investigated the efficacy of antioxidants in preventing the progression of coronary artery disease. In a double-blind, placebo-controlled trial, DeMaio et al. investigated the effects of α-tocopherol on restenosis following PTCA (89). The study randomized 115 subjects to receive 1200 IU α-tocopherol (n=52) or placebo (n=48). After 4 months of follow-up, subjects receiving vitamin E had a 34% incidence of restenosis compared with a 50% incidence int he placebo group. The 31% risk reduction did not reach statistical significance ($p<.06$), but the small numbers and the short duration of treatment/follow-up may limit the study's power to detect a difference between the groups. More recently, the Cambridge Heart Association Study (CHAOS) study tested the hypothesis that treatment with 400 or 800 IU of vitamin E for 7 months would reduce the risk of myocardial infarction in patients with angiographic evidence of coronary atherosclerosis (90). Two thousand and two patients were prestratified by planned therapy (angioplasty, bypass grafting) and by risk factors for coronary disease and then randomly assigned to a placebo or treatment group. The primary endpoints were a combination of cardiovascular death plus nonfatal myocardial infarction and nonfatal myocardial infarction alone. Vitamin E reduced these two endpoints significantly by 35 and 66%, respectively, but cardiovascular deaths alone tended to increase, although not significantly. An unusual feature of the study was that the first 546 patients in the vitamin E group received 800 IU/day, and thereafter, those assigned to the treatment group received 400 IU/day. The investigators indicate that they reduced the dose once they noted that they exceeded physiological plasma levels with the lower dose. The stated motive was that they did not want to interrupt recruitment due to limitation of drug supply. The two dosing groups were not distinguished in the analysis.

## 3. Conclusion

The observational studies described in the previous section have suggested that daily supplements of at least 100 IU of $\alpha$-tocopherol may be needed to decrease cardiovascular risk (91,92). Randomized trials of sufficient power and duration are underway to establish the efficacy of "high-dose" antioxidant supplementation in this setting. The Physicians Health Study, which has randomized subjects to receive 50 mg $\beta$-carotene on alternate days, should be reported this year. The Women's Health study is randomizing 40,000 healthy females aged 50 years and older to receive $\beta$-carotene, vitamin E, and low-dose aspirin in a factorial design. These two studies should provide data as to whether antioxidant vitamins can prevent coronary artery disease de novo. The Women's Antioxidant Cardiovascular Disease study will enroll 8000 nurses with existing cardiovascular disease to determine whether antioxidant supplementation, with daily doses of 20 mg of $\beta$-carotene, 400 IU of vitamin E, and 100 mg of vitamin C, is effective in secondary prevention.

## B. Cancer

Carcinogenesis is considered to be a multistage process. The mechanisms involved in the conversion of a normal cell into a malignant one are not fully understood. Carcinogenesis can be simplified as a process of initiation, promotion, and progression. Tumor initiation is caused by spontaneous or carcinogen-induced DNA damage. Two important initiators are mutagens, genotoxic prooxidants, and radiation. $\beta$-Carotene may have an effect at the initiation stage, through its ability to quench the active intermediates that interact with DNA. A recent study showed that plasma $\beta$-carotene levels inversely correlates with the frequency of micronuclei induced by radiation in human lymphocytes (93). Following 6 days of supplementation with 30 mg/day of $\beta$-carotene, the frequency of lymphocyte micronuclei following x-ray irradiation was significantly lower in the supplemented group.

Promotion is the process of growth and proliferation in the initiated abnormal cell. There are many different known promoters, and most produce reactive oxygen species as by-products. This provides further rationale for the use of $\beta$-carotene, because the most common reactive oxygen species produced is singlet oxygen.

### 1. Observational Studies

The antitumorigenic effect of antioxidants were first described in 1934 when wheat germ oil was found to prevent tar carcinoma in mice, with this effect being tentatively attributed to vitamin E in the oil (94). Subsequently, dietary vitamin E was shown to prevent subcutaneous sarcomas induced by 3-methylcholanthrene (95). The antioxidants vitamin E, selenium, and vitamin C applied to mouse skin also reduced tumor formation induced by 7,12-dimethylbenzanthracene (96,97). Several epidemiological studies indicate that a diet rich in vegetables and fruits lowers the incidence of cancer in humans (98). In a review of 172 published studies, it was reported that the quarter of the population with the lowest dietary intake of fruits and vegetables had twice the cancer rate than in the highest quartile. This held true for most types of cancer (lung, larynx, oral cavity, esophagus, stomach, colon, rectum, bladder, pancreas, cervix, and ovary) (99). Indeed, much of the cancer resulting in liver, colon, bladder, stomach, and lung have been attributed to oxidative stress resulting from infection or inflammation (100). A recent review by van Poppel reported that 11 of 15 studies carried out in different countries around the world reported a significant association of low carotenoid intake with the risk of cancer (101). These results have been confirmed by results of the Basel Prospective Study (102). After a 12-year follow-up of 2974 participants, 204 cases of cancer were observed. The relative risk of bronchial and stomach cancer was significantly increased in subjects with low $\beta$-carotene levels. The largest epidemiological study relating antioxidant status and mortality from various sites was published in 1992 (103). Fasting blood samples were obtained from 3225 randomly selected male and 3225 female subjects from 130 rural communes widely distributed in the populated areas of 24 provinces in China. Subjects were aged 35–64 years. The parameters measured included biochemical indicators of reactive oxygen species, antioxidant vitamin status, and several minerals (selenium, copper, and iron). The results of these tests were correlated with mortality rates by age and gender for each cancer cite, as published in the *Atlas of Cancer Mortality* in China (104). The results of regression analysis by gender and cancer site showed a significant inverse association of $\beta$-carotene intake with stomach cancer in males and females. The incidence of lung cancer was negatively associated with ascorbic acid in males.

In summary, a large number of observational studies have shown that dietary intake of antioxidant vitamins, in particular $\beta$-carotene, is associated with risk reduction in various cancer sites. The same caveat applies to these observations as to the results from the cardiovascular studies; that is, the reduced risk seen in the groups with high dietary vitamin intake may be in part a reflection of the overall dietary, exercise and smoking habits which are covariates with vitamin intake.

## 2. Intervention Studies

The endpoints of the interventional studies of antioxidants in cancer can be broadly divided into three groups: studies measuring early surrogate biomarkers for cancer risk (e.g., immunological response), studies investigating the clinical course of premalignant lesions (e.g., leukoplakia), and studies with true clinical endpoints of cancer (e.g., incidence and mortality).

Several studies, as reviewed by Bendich et al., have demonstrated that supplementation with $\beta$-carotene resulted in a beneficial effect on lymphocyte subpopulations in cancer patients (105). The vitamins most likely to improve several determinants of the immune response in elderly subjects were shown to be $\beta$-carotene and vitamins A, E, C, and $B_6$ (106).

Seven different clinical trials have reported substantial regression of oral leukoplakia following supplementation with $\beta$-carotene alone or in combination with vitamins E and C and that discontinuation of vitamin intake resulted in a rapid recurrence of the lesion (107).

The Linxian Dysplasia Trial investigated whether supplementation with multiple micronutrients (14 vitamins and 12 minerals) would reduce the incidence of esophageal and/or gastric cardia cancer in patients with established esophageal dysplasia. Three thousand and three hundred and eighteen patients were randomized to treatment groups for a 6-year period. The risk for total mortality was 7% lower in the supplemented group, the incidence of cancer was 4% lower, and the cumulative esophageal/gastric death rates were 8% lower. These figures, however, did not achieve statistical significance, and it was concluded that a longer period of follow-up might be more informative (108). The Linxian Nutrition Intervention Trial, designed to determine if dietary supplementation with vitamins and minerals reduces the incidence of cancer, studied 29,584 adults between the ages of 40 and 69 years (109). Subjects were randomly assigned to one of eight intervention groups. A total of 2127 deaths occurred among the participants during the 5-year intervention period. Cancer was the leading cause of death, with 32% of all deaths due to esophageal or gastric cancer. There was an 9% overall reduction in mortality in those subjects receiving $\beta$-carotene, vitamin E, and selenium ($p<.03$). The risk reduction started to be relevant 1–2 years following the start of the supplementation. The mortality from noncardiac stomach cancer was reduced by 41% ($p<.02$).

The Alpha-Tocopherol, Beta Carotene Cancer Prevention Study (ATBC) was a randomized double-blind, placebo-controlled primary prevention trial undertaken to determine whether supplementation with $\alpha$-tocopherol, $\beta$-carotene, or both would reduce the incidence of lung cancer in male smokers (110). A secondary outcome of interest was the incidence of other cancers. A total of 29,133 male smokers 50–69 years of age from southwestern Finland were randomly assigned to one of four treatment groups: 50 mg $\alpha$-tocopherol/day, 20 mg $\beta$-carotene/day, both $\alpha$-tocopherol and $\beta$-carotene, or placebo. Eight hundred and seventy-six new cases of lung cancer were diagnosed during the trial. There was no reduction in incidence observed among the men who received $\alpha$-tocopherol and, unexpectedly, a higher incidence of lung cancer was observed in those in the $\beta$-carotene group after 5–8 years of supplementation. It was noted that the men taking $\alpha$-tocopherol had a lower incidence of prostate cancer. This trial was the first to raise the possibility that $\beta$-carotene supplementation may actually have harmful as well as beneficial effects in cancer patients. The synthetic preparation of $\alpha$-tocopherol used in the study has a low bioavailability and the daily dose was just 50 mg. Median blood levels were increased by only 50%.

A more recent study, the Beta Carotene and Retinol Efficacy Trial (CARET), which studied men and women with a high risk of lung cancer, was recently terminated following analysis of preliminary data. The early results showed a 28% increase in the number of new cases of lung cancer and a 26% higher mortality from cardiovascular disease in the supplemented group when compared with placebo.

The results of the ATBC and CARET studies are in sharp contrast to those in the observational studies published during the last two decades, which report consistently a beneficial effect of high dietary $\beta$-carotene intake on the incidence of lung cancer. It is possible that in such a high-risk population of heavy smokers, the dose of $\beta$-carotene used in the ABTC study was too low and the follow-up period was too short. An alternative explanation might be that $\beta$-carotene is not the active cancer-inhibiting component of the fruits and vegetables identified as being protective in the observational studies. These same theories may also be applied to explain the lack of benefit seen in the vitamin E group. However, these results illustrate how the correlative data obtained from the observational studies can never establish causality.

Finally, several studies performed to test the ability of antioxidants to prevent colorectal adenomas have yielded inconsistent results (111–114). A randomized study of 143 patients with sporadic adenomas found no effect of supplemental vitamins C and E versus placebo on the rate of recurrence of adenomas over a 2-year period (113). However, an Italian study of 148 patients with adenomas showed a statistically significant reduction in the disease incidence in those randomized to receive vitamins A, C, and E compared with no treatment (114). The Poly Prevention study, started in 1984, randomized 864 patients to four treatment groups by a two-by-two factorial design to receive 25 mg $\beta$-carotene/day, 1 g vitamin C, and 400 mg vitamin E/day, $\beta$-carotene, vitamins E and C, or placebo (115). The primary endpoint for the study was the occurrence of new adenomas. Treatment was for 4 years with either $\beta$-carotene or vitamins C and E demonstrated no beneficial effects. Again, the lack of benefit of antioxidants in this study appears to conflict with the reduced risk suggested by the observational studies of invasive cancers of the colon and rectum.

## V.   SUMMARY

Oxygen free radicals have been implicated in a wide variety of disease processes. Targets for free radical attack include lipids, protein, and DNA. The role of oxidative stress in the evolution of disease is unclear, which is in part due to the limitation of current methodology to assess free radical generation *in vivo*. Oxidative stress is often inferred from measurements of oxidative damage or the extent of accumulation of oxidation products in tissues. More recently, however, the discovery of isoprostanes and other developments (116) has enabled assessment of free radical generation *in vivo*. Despite the suggestion from observational studies that antioxidant vitamins play a beneficial role in preventing cancer and cardiovascular disease, interventional data so far fail to confirm this effect. It may be that the anticarcinogenic effect seen with some diets is attributable to some active ingredient other than vitamins. Examples of such compounds might include flavonoids, phenols, indoles, and isothiocyanates. Morse et al. recently reviewed the published literature which implicates these compounds as having an antioxidant role in the inhibition of cancer (117). The results from the observational studies may, in fact, result from a healthier life style in those who consume antioxidants. They may also reflect a very prolonged antioxidant intake, whereas the intervention trials to date have been no longer than 8 years. There is no certainty that a trial of this, or lesser, duration will be sufficient to demonstrate an antioxidant effect on atherogenesis or carcinogenesis.

Apart from the duration of supplementation, a consensus of opinion has yet to be reached on the optimum dose of antioxidant vitamins required to demonstrate maximum effect. The intervention studies performed to date involved supplementation with a wide range of doses of vitamins E and C and β-carotene. It may be that adjustments to the dose of antioxidants are needed, based on endogenous vitamin levels. The observational studies found that subjects in the lowest quintile of antioxidant intake were at highest risk for cardiovascular disease. The ATBC study found an inverse relationship between baseline antioxidant levels and the incidence of subsequent lung cancers. These observations suggest that for a population-based sample, intervention may be most effective when targeted at subjects with the lowest endogenous antioxidant defense and/or dietary intake.

The conflicting nature of the results published to date reinforces the need to avoid making premature recommendations with respect to the benefits of antioxidant supplementation in the prevention and/or treatment of disease.

## ACKNOWLEDGMENT

Supported by grants NIH 5-M01.RR00040 and HL54500 for the National Institutes of Health.

## REFERENCES

1. Halliwell B. Free radicals and antioxidants. Nutrition Rev 1994; 52(8):253–265.
2. Pryor WA, Prier DG, Church DF. Electron spin resonance study of mainstream and side stream cigarette smoke: nature of the free radical in gas-phase smoke and in cigarette tar. Environ Health Perspect 1983; 47:345–355.
3. Singh A, Singh H. Time scale and nature of radiation biological damage: approaches to radiation protection and post irradiation therapy. Prog Biophys Mol Biol 1982; 39:69–107.
4. Bast A, Haenen GRMM, Doelman CJA. Oxidants and antioxidants: state of the art. Am J Med 1991; 91(suppl):3C, 2S–13S.
5. Fantone JC, Ward PA. Role of oxygen-derived free radicals and metabolites in leukocyte dependent inflammatory reactions. Am J Pathol 1982; 107:395–418.
6. Sies H (ed). Oxidative Stress. London: Academic Press, 1985.
7. Wayner DD, Burton GW, Ingold KU. The relative contribution of vitamin E, urate, ascorbate and proteins to the total peroxyl radical-trapping antioxidant activity of human blood plasma. Biochim Biophys Acta 1987; 924:408–419.

8.  Sies H. Oxidative stress: introductory remarks. In: Sies H, ed. Oxidative Stress. San Diego:Academic Press, 1991:XV.
9.  Halliwell B. Oxidants and human disease: some new concepts. FASEB J 1987; 1:358–364.
10. Davies KJA, Wiese AG, Sevanian A, Kim EH. Repair systems in oxidative stress. In: Finch CE and Johnson TE, eds, Molecular Biology of Aging. New York:Wiley-Liss, 1990:123.
11. Sies H. Biochemistry of oxidative stress. Angew Chem 1986; 25:1058.
12. Machlin LJ, Bendich A. Free radical tissue damage: protective role of antioxidant nutrients. FASEB J 1987; 1:441–445.
13. Halliwell B, Gutteridge JMC. Free radicals and antioxidant protection: mechanisms and significance in toxicology and disease. Hum Toxicol 1988; 7:7–13.
14. Fridovich I. Superoxide dismutases. Adv Enzymol 1974; 41:35–97.
15. Deisseroth A, Dounce AL. Catalase: physical and chemical properties, mechanism of catalysis and physiological role. Physiol Rev 1970; 50:319–3375.
16. Maddipati KR, Marnett LJ. Characterization of the major hydroperoxide-reducing activity of human plasma. Purification and properties of a selenium-dependent glutathione peroxidase. J Biol Chem 1987; 262:17398–17403.
17. Halliwell B, Gutteridge JMC. The antioxidants of human extracellular fluid. Arch Biochem Biophys 1990; 280:1–8.
18. Aruoma OI, Halliwell B, Gajewski E, Disdaroglu M. Copper-ion-dependent damage to the bases in DNA in the presence of hydrogen peroxide. Biochem J 1991; 273:601–604.
19. Giulivi C, Davies KJA. A novel antioxidant role for hemoglobin: the comproportionation of ferrylhemoglobin with oxyhemoglobin. J Biol Chem 1990; 265:19435–19460.
20. Grisham MB. Myoglobin cataysed hydrogen peroxide dependent arachidonic acid peroxidation. Free Radic Biol Med 1985; 1:227–232.
21. Niki E. Antioxidants in relation to lipid peroxidation. Chem Phys Lipid 1987; 44:227–253.
22. Rose RC, Bode AM. Biology of free radical scavengers: an evaluation of ascorbate. FASEB J 1993; 7:1135–1142.
23. Ames BN, Cathcart R, Schwiers E, Hochstein P. Uric acid provides an antioxidant defense in humans against oxidant and radical caused aging and cancer: a hypothesis. Proc Natl Acad Sci USA 1981; 78:6858–6862.
24. Stringer MD, Gorog PG, Freeman A, Kakkar VV. Lipid peroxides and atherosclerosis. Br Med J 1989; 298:281–284.
25. McCord JM. Oxygen derived free radicals in postischemic tissue injury. N Engl J Med 1985; 312:159–163.
26. Lunec J, Halloran SP, White AG, Dormandy TL. Free radical oxidation (peroxidation) products in serum and synovial fluid in rheumatoid arthritis. J Rheumatol 1981; 8:233–245.
27. Connors TA. In: Nigam SN, McBrien DCH, Slater TF, eds. Eicosanoids, Lipid Peroxidation and Cancer. Verlag, Springer- Berlin: 1989:143.
28. Thompson S, Smith MT. Measurement of the diene conjugated form of linoleic

acid in plasma by high performance liquid chromatography: a questionable non-invasive assay of free radical activity? Chem Biol Interact 189; 55:357–366.

29. Halliwell B, Gutteridge JMC. Lipid peroxidation oxygen radicals, cell damage, and antioxidant therapy. Lancet 1984; 1:1396–1397.

30. Haberland ME, Fogelman AM. The role of altered lipoproteins in the pathogenesis of atherosclerosis. Am Heart J 1987; 113:573–577.

31. Brown MS, Goldstein JL. Lipoprotein metabolism in the macrophage: implications for cholesterol deposition in atherosclerosis. Ann Rev Biochem 1983; 52:223–261.

32. Hoff HF, O'Neill J, Chisolm GM, et al. Modification of low density lipoprotein with 4-hydroxynonenal induces uptake by macrophages. Arteriosclerosis 1989; 9:538–549.

33. Qinn MT, Parthasarathy S, Fong LG, Steinberg D. Oxidatively modified low density lipoproteins: a potential role in recruitment and retention of monocyte/macrophages during atherogenesis. Proc Natl Acad Sci USA 1987; 84:2995–2998.

34. Quinn MT, Parthasarathy S, Steinberg D. Endothelial cell-derived chemotactic activity for mouse peritoneal macrophages and the effects of modified forms of low density lipoprotein. Proc Natl Acad Sci USA 1985; 82:5949–5953.

35. Halliwell B, Chirico S. Lipid peroxidation: its mechanism, measurement, and significance. Am J Clin Nutr 1993; 57(suppl):715S–725S.

36. Morrow JD, Hill KE, Burk RF, Nammour TM, Badr KF, Roberts LJ. A series of prostaglandin $F_2$-like compounds are produced in vivo in humans by a noncyclooxygenase, free radical-catalyzed mechanism. Proc Natl Acad Sci USA 1990; 87:9383–9387.

37. Morrow JD, Awad JA, Boss HJ, Blair IA, Roberts LF. Non-cyclooxygenase-derived prostanoids (F2-isoprostanes) are formed in situ on phospholipids. Proc Natl Acad Sci USA 1992; 89:10721–10725.

38. Morrow JD, Minton TA, Mukundan CR, et al. Free radical-induced generation of isoprostanes in vivo: evidence for the formation of D-ring and E-ring isoprostanes. J Biol Chem 1994; 269:4317–4325.

39. Pratico D, Lawson J, FitzGerald GA. Isothromboxane formation by human monocyte. Blood 1995; 86(suppl):509.

40. Delanty N, Reilly M, Pratico D, Fitzgerald DJ, Lawson JA, FitzGerald GA. 8-epi $PGF_2\alpha$: specific analysis of an isoeicosanoid as an index of oxidant stress in vivo. Br J Clin Pharm 1996; 42:15–19.

41. Wang Z, Ciabattoni G, Creminon C, Lawson JA, FitzGerald GA, Patrono C, MacLouf J. Immunoassay of urinary 8-epi $PGF_2\alpha$. J Pharm Exp Ther 1995; 275:94–100.

42. Reilly M, Delanty N, Lawson JA, FitzGerald GA. Modulation of oxidant stress in vivo in chronic cigarette smokers. Circulation 1996; 94:19–25.

43. Delanty N, Reilly M, Lawson JA, McCarthy J, Wood F, Fitzgerald DJ, FitzGerald GA. 8-epi $PGF_2\alpha$ generation during coronary reperfusion: a potential quantitative marker of oxidant stress in vivo. Circulation 1996. In press.

44. Pratico D, Iuliano J, Delanty N, Reilly M, Violi F, FitzGerald GA. Increased

levels of the isoprostane, 8-epi $PGF_2\alpha$, in atherosclerotic plaque and urine of patients with cerebrovascular disease. 1996; submitted.

45. Burton GW, Ingold KU. Vitamin E as an in vitro and in vivo antioxidant. Ann NY Acad Sci 1989; 570:7–22.

46. Gey KF. On the antioxidant hypothesis with regard to arteriosclerosis. Bibl Nutr Dieta 1986; 37:53–91.

47. Esterbauer H, Striegl G, Phul H, et al. The role of vitamin E and carotenoids in preventing oxidation of low density lipoproteins. Ann NY Acad Sci 1989; 570:254–267.

48. Van Gossum A, Kurian R, Whitwell J, Jeejeebhoy KN. Decrease in lipid peroxidation measured by breath pentane output in normals after oral supplementation with vitamin E. Clin Nutr 1988; 7:53–57.

49. Packer L, Maguire J, Melhorn R, Serbinova E, Kagan V. Mitochondria and microsomal membranes have a free radical reductase activity that prevents chromanoxyl radical accumulation. Biochem Biophys Res Commun 1989; 159:229–235.

50. Kayden HJ, Traber MGJ. Absorption, lipoprotein transport and regulation of plasma content of vitamin E in humans. J Lipid Res 1993; 34:343–358.

51. Esterbauer H, Gebicki J, Jurgens G. The role of lipid peroxidation and antioxidants in oxidative modifications of LDL. Free Radic Biol Med 1992; 13:341–390.

52. Reaven PD, Khouw A, Beltz WF, Parthasarathy S, Witztum JL. Effect of dietary antioxidant combinations in humans: protection of LDL by vitamin E but not by beta-carotene. Arterioscler Thromb 1993; 13:590–600.

53. Jialal I, Grundy SM. Effect of dietary supplementation with alpha-tocopherol on the oxidative modification of low density lipoprotein. J Lipid Res 1992; 33:899–906.

54. Jialal I, Grundy SM. Influence of antioxidant vitamins on LDL oxidation. Ann NY Acad Sci 1992; 669:237–248.

55. Esterbauer H, Dieber-Rotheneder M, Striegel M, Waeg G. Role of vitamin E in preventing the oxidation of low-density lipoprotein. Am J Clin Nutr 1991; 53:314S–321S.

56. Blackman C, White P, Tsou W, Finkel D. Peroxidation of plasma and platelet lipids in chronic cigarette smokers and insulin-dependent diabetics. Ann NY Acad Sci 1984; 435:385

57. Ferrari R, Curello S, Boffa GM, et al. Oxygen free radical-mediated heart injury in animal models and during bypass surgery in humans: effects of $\alpha$-tocopherol. Ann NY Acad Sci 1992; 570:237–253.

58. Liu SK, Dolensek EP, Tappe JP, Stover J, Adams CR. Cardiomyopathy associated with vitamin E deficiency in seven gelada baboons. J Am Vet Med Assoc 1984; 185:1347–1350.

59. Nelson JS. Pathology of vitamin E deficiency. In: Machlin L, ed. Vitamin E: A Comprehensive Treatise. New York:Dekker, 1980:397–428.

60. Niki E. Action of ascorbic acid as a scavenger of active and stable oxygen radicals. Am J Clin Nutr 1991; 54:1119S–24S.

61. Bendich A, Machlin LJ, Scandurra O, Burton GW, Wayner DDM. The antioxidant role of vitamin C. Adv Free Radic Biol Med 1986; 2:419–444.
62. Halliwell B. How to characterize a biological antioxidant. Free Radic Res Commun 1990; 9:1–32.
63. Levine M, Conry-Cantilena C, Wang Y, et al. Vitamin C pharmacokinetics in healthy volunteers: evidence for a recommended dietary allowance. Proc Natl Acad Sci USA 1996; 93:3704–3709.
64. Parthasarathy S, Young SG, Witzum JL, Pittman RC, Steinberg D. Probucol inhibit oxidative modification of low density lipoprotein. J Clin Invest 1986; 77:641–644.
65. Kita T, Nagano Y, Yokode M, Ishii K, Kume N, Ooshima A, Yoshica H, Kawai C. Probucol prevents the progression of atherosclerosis in the Watanabe heritable hyperlipidemic rabbit, an animal model for familial hypercholesterolemia. Proc Natl Acad Sci USA 1987; 84:5928–5931.
66. Daugherty A, Zweifel BS, Schonfeld G. Probucol attenuates the development of aortic atherosclerosis in cholesterol-fed rabbits. Br J Pharmacol 1989; 98: 612–618.
67. Carew TE, Schwenke DC, Steinberg D. Antiatherogenic effect of probucol unrelated to its hypercholesterolemic effect: evidence that antioxidants in vivo can selectively inhibit low density lipoprotein degradation in macrophage-rich fatty streaks and slow the progression of atherosclerosis in the Watanabe heritable hyperlipidemic rabbit. Proc Natl Acad Sci USA 1987; 84:7725–7729.
68. Francheschini G, Sirtori M, Vaccarino V, Gianfranceschi G,. Rezzonico L, Chiesa G, Sirtori CR. Mechanisms of HDL reduction after probucol: changes in HDL subfractions and increased reverse cholesteryl ester transfer. Arteriosclerosis 1989; 9:462–469.
69. Ku G, Doherty NS, Schmidt LF, Jackson RL, Dinerstein RJ. Ex vivo lipopolysaccharide-induced interleukin-1 secretion from murine peritoneal macrophages inhibited by probucol, a hypocholesterolemic agent with antioxidant properties. FASEB J 1990; 4:1645–1653.
70. Yamamoto A, Takaichi S, Hara H, Nishikawa O, Yokoyama S, Yamamura T, Yamaguchi T. Probucol prevents lipid storage in macrophages. Atherosclerosis 1986; 62:209–217.
71. Rouse IL, Armstrong BK, Beilin W, Vandongen R. Vegetarian diet, blood pressure and cardiovascular risk. Aust NZ J Med 1934; 14:439–443.
72. Acheson RM, Williams DRR. Does consumption of fruit and vegetables protect against stroke? Lancet 1983; 1:1191–1193.
73. Armstrong K, Mann JI, Adelstein AM, Ekin F. Commodity consumption and ischemic heart disease mortality, with special reference to dietary practices. J Chronic Dis 1975; 28:455–469.
74. Smith WCS, Tunstall-Pedoe H, Crombie IK, Tavendale R. Concomitants of excess coronary deaths: major risk factor and lifestyle findings from 10359 men and women in the Scottish Heart Health Study. Scott Med J 1989; 34:550–555.
75. Ginter E. Decline of coronary mortality in United States and vitamin C. Am J Clin Nutr 1979; 32:511–512.

76. Riemersma RA, Oliver M, Elton RA, et al. Plasma antioxidants and coronary heart disease: vitamins C and E and selenium. Eur J Clin Nutr 1990; 44: 143–150.

77. Stampfer MJ, Hennekens CH, Manson JE, Colditz GA, Rosner B, Willett WC. Vitamin E consumption and the risk of coronary disease in women. N Engl J Med 1993; 328:1444–1449.

78. Rimm EB, Stampfer MJ, Ascherio A, Giovannucii GA, Colditz GA, Willett WC. Vitamin E consumption and the risk of coronary artery disease in men. N Engl J Med 1993; 328:1450–1456.

79. Gaziano JM, Manson JE, Branch LG, Colditz GA, Willett WC, Buring JE. A prospective study of consumption of carotenoids in fruit and vegetables and decreased cardiovascular mortality in the elderly. Ann Epidemiol 1995; 5: 333–335.

80. Donnan PT, Thomson M, Fowkes FG, Precott RJ, Housley E. Diet as risk factor for peripheral arterial disease in the general population: the Edinburgh artery study. Am J Clin Nutr 1993; 57:917–921.

81. Gey KF, Stahelin HB, Eichholzer M. Poor plasma status of carotene and vitamin C is associated with higher mortality from ischemic heart disease and stroke: Basel Prospective Study. Clin Invest 1993; 71:3–6.

82. Steinberg D and Workshop Participants. Antioxidants in the prevention of human atherosclerosis. Summary of the proceedings of a National Heart, Lung and Blood Institute Workshop. Circulation 1992; 85:2338–2344.

83. Princen HMG, van Poppel G, Bogelzang C, Buytenhek R, Kok FJ. Supplementation with vitamin E but not beta-carotene in vivo protects low density lipoprotein from lipid peroxidation in vitro. Effect of cigarette smoking. Arterioscler Thromb 1992; 12:554–562.

84. Reaven PD, Khouw A, Beltz WF, Parthasarathy S, Witzum JL. Effect of dietary antioxidant combinations in humans. Arterioscler Thromb 1993; 13: 590–600.

85. Jialal I, Grundy SM. Effect of dietary supplementation with alpha-tocopherol on the oxidative modification of low density lipoprotein. J Lipid Res 1992; 33:899–906.

86. Haeger K. Long-time treatment of intermittent claudication with vitamin E. Am J Clin Nutr 1987; 45:1368–1377.

87. Gillilan RE, Mondell B, Warbasse JR. Quantitative evaluation of vitamin E in angina pectoris. Am Heart J 1977; 110:401–406.

88. Gaziano JM, Manson JE, Ridker PM, Buring JE, Hennekens CH. Beta carotene therapy for chronic stable angina. Circulation 1990; 82(suppl II):201.

89. DeMaio SJ, King SB, Lembo NJ, et al. Vitamin E supplementation, plasma lipids and incidence of restenosis after percutaneous transluminal coronary angioplasty (PTCA). J Am Coll Nutr 1992; 11:68–73.

90. Stephens NG, Parsons A, Schofield PM, Kelly F, Cheeseman K, Mitchinson MJ, Brown MJ. Randomised controlled trial of vitamin E in patients with coronary disease: Cambridge Heart Antioxidant Study (CHAOS). Lancet 1996; 347:781–786.

91. Stampfer MJ, Hennekens CH, Manson JE, Colditz GA, Rosner, Willett WC. Vitamin E consumption and the risk of coronary disease in women. N Engl J Med 1993; 328:1444–1448.

92. Rimm EB, Stampfer MJ, Ascherio A, Giovannucci E, Colditz GA, Willett WC. Vitamin E consumption and the risk of coronary heart disease. N Engl J Med 1993; 328:1450–1456.

93. Umegaki K, Ikegame S, Inoue K, Ichidawa T, Kobayashi S, Soeno N. Beta-carotene prevents x-ray induction of micronuclei in human lymphocytes. Am J Clin Nutr 1994; 59:409–412.

94. Jaffe W. The influence of wheat germ oil on the production of tumors in rats by methylcholanthrene. Proc Soc Exp Biol Med 1946; 111:714–715.

95. Haber SL, Wissler RW. Effect of vitamin E or carcinogenicity of methyl-cholanthrene. Proc Soc Biol Med 1962; 111:774–775.

96. Graham S. Results of case-control studies of diet and cancer in Buffalo. NY. Cancer Res 1983; 43:2409S–2413S.

97. Shamberger RJ. Relationship to selenium to cancer: inhibitory effect of selenium on carcinogenesis. J Natl Cancer Inst 1970; 44:931–936.

98. Hocman, G. Prevention of cancer: vegetables and plants. Comp Biochem Physiol 1989; 93B:201–212.

99. Ames BN, Shigenaga MK, Hagen TM. Oxidants, antioxidants and the degenerative diseases of aging. Proc Natl Acad Sci 1993; 90:7915–7922.

100. Ames BN. Dietary carcinogens and anticarcinogens: oxygen radicals and degenerative diseases. Science 1983; 221:1256–1264.

101. Poppel G. Carotenoids and cancer: an update with emphasis on human intervention studies. Eur J Cancer 1993; 29A:1335.

102. Eichholzer M, Staehlin HB, Grey KF. Inverse correlation between essential antioxidants in plasma and subsequent risk to develop cancer, ischemic heart disease and stroke respectively: 12-year follow-up of the Basel Prospective Study. Free Radic Aging 1992; 398.

103. Chen J, Geissler C, Papria BK, Li J, Campell TC. Antioxidant status and cancer mortality in China. Int J Epidemiol 1992; 21:625–635.

104. Li J-Y, Liu B-Q, Li G-Y. Atlas of cancer mortality in the People's Republic of China. Int J Epidemiol 1981; 10:127.

105. Bendich A. Carotenoids and immunity. Clin Appl Nutr 1991; 1:45.

106. Chandra RK. Effect of vitamin and trace-element supplementation on immune responses and infection in elderly subjects. Lancet 1992; 340:1124.

107. Garewal HS. Beta-carotene and vitamin E in oral cancer. J Cell Biochem 1993; 17F(suppl):262–269.

108. Li J-Y, Taylor PR, Li B, Dawsey S, Wang G-Q, Ershow AG, Guo W, Liu S-F, Yang CS, Sheng Q, Wang W, Mark SD, Zou X-N, Greenwald P, Wu Y-P, Blot WJ. Linxian Dysplasia Tial; multiple vitamin/mineral supplementation, cancer incidence and disease-specific mortality among adults with esophageal dysplasia. J Natl Cancer Inst 1993; 85:1492.

109. Blot WJ, Li J-Y, Taylor PR, Guo W, Dawsey S, Wang G-Q, Yang CS, Zheng S-F, Gail M, Li G-Y, Yu Y, Liu B-Q, Tangrea J, Sun Y-H, Fraumeni JF,

Zhang Y-H, Li B. Nutrition Intervention Trials, Linxian, China; supplementation with specific multiple vitamin/mineral combinations, cancer incidence and disease-specific mortality in the general population. J Natl Cancer Inst 1993; 85:1480–1482.

110. The Alpha-Tocopherol, Beta Carotene Cancer Prevention Study Group. The effect of vitamin E and beta carotene on the incidence of lung cancer and other cancers in male smokers. N Engl J Med 1994; 330:1029.

111. Bussey HJ, DeCosse J, Deschner EE, et al. A randomized trial of ascorbic acid in polyposis coli. Cancer 1982; 50:1434–1439.

112. DeCosse JJ, Miller HH, Lesser ML. Effect fiber and vitamins C and E on rectal polyps in patients with familial adenomatous polyposis. J Natl Cancer Inst 1989; 81:1290–1297.

113. McKeown-Eyssen B, Holloway C, Jazmaji V, Fright-See E, Dion P, Bruce WR. A randomized trial of vitamin C and E in the prevention of recurrence of colorectal polyps. Cancer Res 1988; 48:4701–4705.

114. Roncucci L, DiDonato P, Carati L, et al. Antioxidant vitamins or lactulose for the prevention of the recurrence of colorectal adenomas. Dis Colon Rectum 1993; 36:227–234.

115. Greenberg ER, Baron JA, Tosteson TD, et al. A clinical trial of antioxidant vitamins to prevent colorectal adenoma. N Engl J Med 1994; 331:141–147.

116. Loft S, Fischer-Nielsen A, Jeding IB, Vistisen K, Poulsen HE. 8-Hydroxydeoxyguanosine as a urinary biomarker of oxidative DNA damage. J Toxic Environ 1993; 40:391–404.

117. Morse MA, Stone GD. Cancer chemoprevention: prevention: principles and prospects. Carcinogenesis 1993; 14:1737–1746.

# 16

# Vasculoprotection by Estrogen Contributes to Gender Difference in Cardiovascular Diseases: Potential Mechanism and Role of Endothelium

**Katalin Kauser and Gabor M. Rubanyi**

*Berlex Biosciences, Inc., Richmond, California*

## I. INTRODUCTION

Cardiovascular morbidity and mortality statistics show that premenopausal women are protected against coronary heart disease compared with men of similar age (1). Gender difference has been observed in the prevalence of essential hypertension between premenopausal women and age-matched men (2). Indeed, ample clinical evidence suggest that male sex should be considered as a risk factor. Gender difference in cardiovascular diseases has been mainly attributed to the vasculoprotective effect of the female sexual steroid hormone, estrogen. Antiatherogenic properties of $17\beta$-estradiol have been demonstrated in experimental animal models (3,4) including subhuman primates (5,6) and humans (7–11).

Although $17\beta$-estradiol has a beneficial effect on plasma lipoprotein composition in both women and men, it has been reported that the cholesterol-lowering effect cannot fully account for all the benefits of estrogen on vascular lesion development (12). Hormones, in general, exert effects on target organs via their receptors. Several data demonstrate the presence of estrogen receptors in the cellular elements of the vascular wall (13,16). In search of understanding the key element in the gender difference of cardiovascular morbidity and mortality, experimental evidence has been accumulated suggesting direct effects of sexual steroid hormones on the vascular wall (17,18).

In this chapter, we review clinical and experimental evidence that the ovarian steroid hormone 17$\beta$-estradiol contributes to gender difference in the incidence and severity of hypertension and atherosclerosis. We also attempt to summarize present knowledge about the cellular mechanism of vasculoprotection by estrogen.

## II. HYPERTENSION

### A. Blood Pressure Regulation

#### 1. Gender Difference

Sexual dimorphism in the incidence and degree of high blood pressure have been reported both in humans (2) and in several forms of experimental hypertension, such as the spontaneously hypertensive rat (19), the deoxycorticosterone acetate salt rat (20), and the Dahl salt-sensitive rat (21). The mechanism of gender difference in hypertension is not known. Diminished endothelium-dependent relaxation has been demonstrated in all of the above-mentioned models of experimental hypertension (22,23) and also in patients with various forms of hypertension (24). Besides the effect of sexual steroid hormones, in some rat strains, a direct role of chromosomal loci has been suggested (25,26).

#### 2. Gonadectomy

Experiments examining gonadectomized and hormone-treated animals clearly indicate a role of sexual steroid hormones in the development of hypertension in spontaneously hypertensive rats (2,27,28). Female sexual steroid hormones have been shown to decrease blood pressure significantly (28). More recent studies have indicated that the male steroid hormone, testosterone, accelerates the development of hypertension in spontaneously hypertensive rats (29). The role of sexual steroid hormones on endothelial function has been demonstrated recently in association with the control of blood pressure in spontaneously hypertensive rats (30).

#### 3. Pregnancy

Pregnancy in rodents and humans is associated with a decrease in systemic vascular resistance (31,32). The blood pressure of spontaneously hypertensive rats is lowered significantly during pregnancy (33). It has been suggested that the increased release of endothelium-derived relaxing factor, nitric oxide (NO), plays a role in blood pressure regulation in vivo (34). It was also proposed that pregnancy is associated with enhanced NO activity in spontaneously hypertensive rats, which is likely to contribute to the observed hemodynamic changes (35).

## B. Gender Difference in Vascular Tone Regulation

Although the cause of high blood pressure is not clear yet, changes in the function and structure of blood vessels, augmented sympathoadrenergic activity, and elevated levels of circulating vasoconstrictor substances (e.g., renin, vasopressin, cathecholamine, endothelin) and the consequent increase in periferial vascular resistance have been implicated (36). Gender difference in vascular responsiveness have been observed in several experimental animal models. Male and female differences have been reported at the level of smooth muscle contractility (37,38), adrenergic receptor sensitivity (39), and the synthesis of vasoactive factors, such as arachidonic acid metabolites (40), endothelium-derived NO (41), and endothelium-derived contracting factor (30). In addition to changes in vascular smooth muscle and endothelial function, sexual steroid hormones can alter vascular resistance by other mechanisms as well (e.g., neuroendocrine function modulation, changes in circulating level of vasoconstrictors, such as renin, angiotensin, vasopressin, endothelin, catecholamines). However, these potential mechanisms are not discussed in this chapter.

### 1. Vascular Smooth Muscle Contractility

Vasopressin-induced vascular contraction is significantly augmented in rat aorta isolated from male animals compared with those isolated from female rats (38). It has been shown that pressor responsiveness to vasopressin in female animals is affected by the phase of the estrus cycle (38). The reactivity of isolated rat aortic segments to the thromboxane A2 analogue U-46619, has also been found to be greater in male than in female animals (42). Increased contractile sensitivity to endothelin-1 was also demonstrated in isolated aortas of male spontaneously hypertensive rats (43). Some of these variances in vascular contractility between the vessels of male and female animals could be explained by differences in the endothelium-dependent modulation of smooth muscle responses (40).

### 2. Endothelial Function

Under physiological conditions, the tone of peripheral blood vessels is controlled by a balance between endothelium-derived vasodilator (NO, prostacyclin, endothelium-derived hyperpolarizing factor [EDHF]) and vasoconstrictor factors (thromboxane, oxygen-derived free radicals, endothelin and endothelium-derived constrictor factor [EDCF]) (44,45).

*Endothelium-Dependent Vasorelaxation.* Vascular contractile responses are suppressed by the endothelium mainly via local synthesis and the release of NO (46). Studies in our laboratory revealed significant endothelium-dependent differences in contractile responses to phenylephrine between endothelium intact and denuded thoracic aortic rings isolated from male and female rats (Fig. 1A). To understand the mechanism underlying gender differences in response to phenylephrine, we have investigated whether these changes in vascular contraction are due to increased production of endothelial NO or due to differences in smooth muscle responsiveness either to the $\alpha$-adrenergic agonist or to NO (41). Our results demonstrated that the intact endothelium in female rats had a greater suppressing effect on smooth muscle contractility than in male rats (Fig. 1B). Differences in the sensitivity of vascular smooth muscle to NO was ruled out by obtaining overlapping dose-response curves to sodium nitroprusside in denuded aortic rings of male and female rats (Fig. 1C). Indeed, utilizing a perfusion-superfusion bioassay system, we demonstrated a significantly higher release of NO from female than from male rat aortas (Fig. 2). Our results, in good agreement with findings of Hayashi et al. (47) in isolated rabbit vascular tissues, demonstrate that gender differences in endothelium-dependent responses are due to a greater release of endothelium-derived NO in female animals.

This conclusion is supported by several reported findings. Increased endothelial NO production has been also demonstrated in pregnant and estradiol-treated ovariectomized ewes (48), in pregnant and estradiol-treated ovariectomized guinea pigs (49,50), and in cultured human umbilical vein endothelical cells (HUVECs) exposed to 17$\beta$-estradiol (51,52).

*Endothelium-Dependent Vasoconstriction.*    Impairment of endothelial function, characterized as a disturbance in the physiological balance between the production of endothelium-derived relaxing factors (EDRFs) and endothelium-derived vasoconstrictor substances (EDCFs), has been documented in several cardiovascular diseases (including hypertension) in animals and humans (for review see ref. 45). Endothelial dysfunction, defined by increased EDCF release, has been extensively studied in relationship to spontaneous hypertension (22). Based on experimental data obtained by studying spontaneously hypertensive rats, it has been proposed that EDCF is likely to be a cyclooxygenase product, prostaglandin $H_2$ (53), which increases blood vessel resistance by acting on thromboxane receptors of vascular smooth muscle leading to systemic hypertension (54). The causative relationship between enhanced vessel wall contractility due to EDCF release and the development of hypertension has not been clearly established. Some experimental evidence suggest that augmented EDCF release precedes the manifestation of high blood pressure (55).

Sexual dimorphism in the degree of endothelial dysfunction as a contributing factor to the severity of hypertension has recently been demonstrated in our laboratory (30). The purpose of our investigations was to characterize endothelial dysfunction in age-matched male and female spontaneously hy-

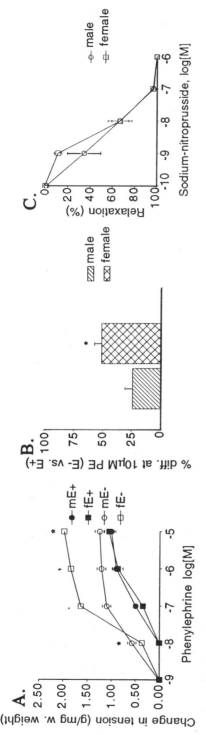

**Figure 1** (A) Phenylephrine dose-response curves ($10^{-9}$–$10^{-5}$ M) in intact (filled symbols) and deendothialized (open symbols) thoracic aortic rings isolated from male (circles) and female (squares) rats. Values represent means ± SEM of eight experiments. Rings isolated from female animals showed significantly ($p < .05$) greater response after endothelium removal than those isolated from males. (B) Endothelial modulation of contraction evoked by $10^{-5}$ M phenylephrine (PE) in thoracic aortic rings isolated from male (hatched bars) and female (cross-hatched bar) rats. Values represent means ± SEM of 8 experiments as a percentage of difference between contraction of endothelium-denuded (E−) and intact (E+) rings. Asterisk (*) indicates significantly ($p < .05$) greater suppression of the phenylephrine-induced contraction in aortic rings isolated from female rats than from male animals. (C) Sodium nitroprusside (SNP)–induced relaxation in deendothelialized thoracic aortic rings isolated from male (open circle) and female (open square) rats. Values represent means ± SEM of 8 experiments expressed as a percentage of relaxation of phenylephrine-contracted thoracic aortic rings. (Modified from ref. 41 with permission of the American Physiological Society.)

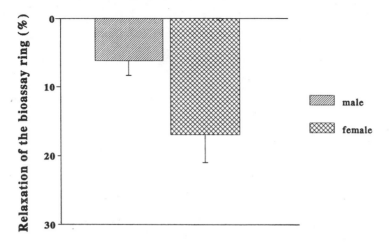

**Figure 2** Relaxation of the bioassay ring in the superfusion bioassay expressed as a percentage of phenylephrine contraction. Significantly ($p<.05$) greater relaxation of the same bioassay ring in response to the perfusate from female donor segment (cross-hatched bar) represents greater release of endothelium-derived NO from female rat thoracic aortas compared with donor segments from male animals (hatched bars). Values represent means $\pm$ SEM of 8 experiments. (Modified from ref. 41 with permission of the American Physiological Society.)

pertensive rats. These studies demonstrated significantly less pronounced endothelial dysfunction in female animals compared with males. Results of our experiments showed that the greater endothelium-dependent relaxation in the female spontaneously hypertensive rats is due to two components. One of them is the greater production of endothelium-derived NO in female animals (Fig. 3) similar to that found in normotensive rats (41) (see Figs. 1 and 2). Our experiments also unveiled significant gender difference in the release of EDCF between thoracic aortic rings isolated from male and female spontaneously hypertensive rats (Fig. 4); that is, endothelium-dependent contraction mediated by a cyclooxygenase metabolite in response to acetylcholine was absent in aortic rings obtained from female spontaneously hypertensive rats, and it was significantly lower than that observed in male rats in the presence of an NO synthase inhibitor.

## C.   Direct Vasodilation by 17$\beta$-Estradiol

Several studies reported rapid (nongenomic) vasodilator effects of 17$\beta$-estradiol in vitro (56,57). In the rabbit coronary artery, this relaxation was

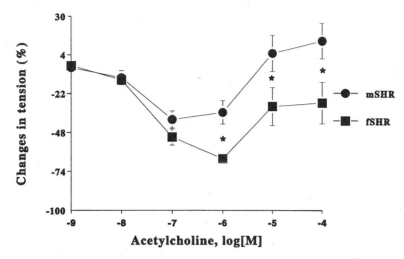

**Figure 3** Acetylcholine-induced endothelium-dependent relaxation in male (filled circle) and female (filled square) spontaneously hypertensive rats. Values represent means ± SEM of 10 experiments expressed as a percentage of phenylephrine contraction. Although endothelium-dependent relaxation appeared to be impaired in both sexes compared with normotensive controls (not shown), NO-mediated vasodilation was significantly (*$p < .05$) greater in thoracic aortic rings isolated from female rats. (Modified from ref. 30 with permission of the American Heart Association.)

shown to be endothelium independent (56). 17$\beta$-Estradiol inhibited contractions elicited by the activation of either receptor- or potential-operated $Ca^{2+}$ channels. Since calcium-dependent contraction was shifted to the right by 17$\beta$-estradiol, it was suggested that estrogen mimics the effect of $Ca^{2+}$ antagonists (56).

Exposure to estrogen caused a direct negative inotropic effect in perfused rabbit heart (58). A similar observation was made by Eckstein et al. (59) studying perfused working heart preparation isolated from male rats. In this species, the negative inotropic effect was accompanied by dose-dependent decreases in the heart rate in response to 17$\beta$-estradiol (59). A negative inotropic effect of estrogen has also been demonstrated in vitro on ventricular myocytes isolated from guinea pig (57).

Although micromolar concentrations of 17$\beta$-estradiol are needed to evoke direct vasodilation in most species studied, the calcium antagonistic properties of 17$\beta$-estradiol may have clinical significance contributing to vasculoprotection. Both animal (60) and clinical (61) studies demonstrated

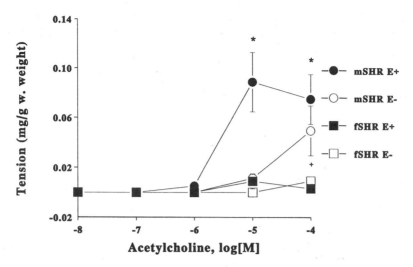

**Figure 4** Acetylcholine (ACh) dose-response curves ($10^{-8}$–$10^{-4}$ M) in intact (filled symbols) and deendothelialized (open symbols) quiescent thoracic aortic rings isolated from male (circles) and female (squares) spontaneously hypertensive rats. Values represent means ± SEM of 10 experiments. Intact rings isolated from male animals showed significantly (*$p<.05$) greater contraction to acetylcholine that those isolated from females. (Modified from ref. 30 with permission of the American Heart Association.)

the beneficial effects of $Ca^{2+}$ channel blockers on the development of hypertension and early atheromatous lesions.

## D.  Effect of 17β-Estradiol on Endothelium-Dependent Responses

The blood pressure of spontaneously hypertensive rats (SHRs) became significantly lower during pregnancy, correlating with improved endothelial function of aortic segments isolated from pregnant animals (35). Another study reported that 2 weeks' treatment of female SHRs with mestranol significantly enhanced endothelium-dependent relaxation (62).

We have also conducted studies to examine the effect of 17β-estradiol on blood pressure and endothelial function in male gonadectomized spontaneously hypertensive rats (30). Rats were divided into three experimental groups. In two groups, animals underwent gonadectomy and the third group of rats was sham operated. One week following surgery, rats in one of the gonadectomized groups received daily a 1-μg subcutaneous injection of 17β-estradiol. The systolic blood pressure was measured in conscious animals by

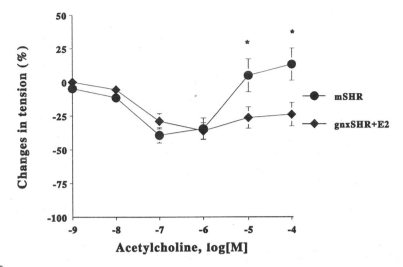

**Figure 5.** Endothelium-dependent relaxation induced by acetylcholine in isolated thoracic aortic rings of spontaneously hypertensive male (filled circle, mSHR) and 17β-estradiol–treated gonadectomized spontaneously hypertensive male rats (filled diamonds, gnxSHR+E2). Data are expressed as a percentage of changes in phenylephrine-evoked contraction ± SEM of 10 experiments. Two weeks of treatment with 17β-estradiol of gonadectomized male rats resulted in significant (*$p<.05$) improvement in the NO-mediated endothelium-dependent responses.

the tail-cuff method. Although no significant change was observed in systolic blood pressure, endothelial function became significantly "improved" by estrogen treatment in gonadectomized male spontaneously hypertensive rats compared with sham controls (Fig. 5). A possible explanation for the mechanism(s) responsible for the attenuating effect of 17β-estradiol on endothelial dysfunction includes an increase in endothelial nitric oxide production and the decreased production of EDCF. This hypothesis is supported by our earlier results demonstrating that female spontaneously hypertensive rats had higher endothelial NO generation and significantly lower EDCF production than age-matched males (see Figs. 3 and 4).

In conclusion, 17β-estradiol reduces vascular smooth muscle tone by at least four mechanisms in hypertension: (1) direct vasodilation, (2) decreased smooth muscle reactivity to vasoconstrictors, (3) increased production of endothelial NO, and (4) decreased production of EDCF. These vascular effects of estrogen (in combination with modulation of other neuroendocrine systems) may contribute to the lower incidence and less severity of hypertension in women.

## III.  ATHEROSCLEROSIS

### A.   Hormonal Influences on Atherosclerosis

1.  Epidemiology

*Gender Difference.*   It has long been known that premenopausal women are "relatively immune" to myocardial infarction and other clinical complications of cardiovascular diseases compared with men. After menopause, this "outstanding advantage of women" is lost (63). Some of the preponderance for coronary heart disease in men has been attributed to sex differences in cardiovascular risk factor levels, such as the lipid profile (64). The antiatherosclerotic serum lipoprotein, high-density lipoprotein (HDL), is lower in men than in women. Some reports indicate that puberty and increasing testosterone levels are associated with decreased levels of HDL (65). However, the effect of androgens on lipid levels is controversial, since several other studies reported a positive correlation between testosterone and HDL levels (66,67). Estrogen, on the other hand, induces favorable changes in the lipid profile (68): reducing total and LDL cholesterol and increasing HDL cholesterol levels.

Carroll et al. (69) reported that cardiac function is more frequently depressed in men than in women around 60 years of age. Left ventricular function is an important predictor of survival after balloon aortic valvuloplasty of patients with aortic stenosis. Female patients, owing to better left ventricular performance, have a greater chance of event-free survival (70).

It has been suggested that besides the beneficial effect of estrogen on serum lipids, regular menstrual blood loss also contributes to protection of women from coronary heart disease (71). The risk in men and postmenopausal women relates to accumulated iron, reflected by an increased ferritin level, contributing to elevated oxidant activity of iron-dependent enzymes (72).

The onset of atherosclerotic disease is delayed by 10–15 years in women compared with men. The rate of formation of atherosclerotic lesions in the aorta and coronary arteries accelerates at 25–30 years in men and 40–45 years in women, and in women, a greater proportion of atherosclerotic lesions are localized in the aorta (73).

*Hormone-Replacement Therapy.*   The protection of women from heart disease and stroke is lost after surgical or natural menopause. Several studies show that estrogen replacement has a potentially beneficial effect on cardiovascular risk factors (10). Case control and prospective cohort studies have demonstrated that morbidity and mortality due to coronary and cerebral vascular diseases decreased in postmenopausal women using hormone-replacement therapy (HRT) compared with those not treated with hormones. The treatment of postmenopausal women for cardiovascular disease prevention with estrogens is not yet widely accepted. The risks of HRT in women include the development of endometrial and breast cancer.

Addition of progestins to HRT seems to protect against endometrial and mammary carcinoma. However, concerns have emerged that added progestins may oppose the beneficial effects of estrogen on the cardiovascular system. Some progestins counterbalance the effect of estrogen on serum lipoproteins (74). Clinical reports with new, selective progestins, such as norgestimate, are encouraging in this regard (75).

The prevention of coronary artery disease by the administration of estrogen is likely, but ultimate proof of the benefit will be achieved only by larger, randomized long-term prospective clinical trials, such as the HERS (Heart Estrogen/progestin Replacement Study) and WHI (Women's Health Initiative) trials, which are currently underway (76).

## 2. Experimental Atherosclerosis

Like many other complex human diseases, atherosclerosis is also difficult to study experimentally owing to the lack of a "perfect" animal model. Most animals do not develop atherosclerosis spontaneously. Models most relevant to the human disease include hypercholesterolemic subhuman primates and the pig. High-cholesterol–fed rabbits and hamsters are more extensively used because of the favorable size of the animals. These animals (within the relative short time frame studied), however, do not exceed the "fatty streak" stage. Recently, genetically engineered mice strains were developed to study specific aspects of the pathophysiology of atherosclerosis. Among these the apolipoprotein(E) (apo[E])–deficient mouse was shown to develop a full range of lesions from fatty streaks to fibrous plaques (77). These animals have spontaneous hypercholesterolemia, and the aortic lesions can progress into the more advanced lesions containing smooth muscle cells, leukocytes, necrotic cores, and calcification in a relatively short period of time (78). Independent of lesion complexity, animal models in general are useful to systematically study the sequence of events occurring in the development of atherosclerosis.

*Gender Difference.* Evidence exists for sexual dimorphism in the rate of progression of atherosclerosis in some arteries of the cynomologus monkey (79). Atherosclerosis in male hyperlipidemic cynomologus monkeys leads to more pronounced reduction of the coronary artery diameter than in female monkeys. Oophorectomy (surgical menopause) abolishes gender difference in atherosclerotic lesion development in these monkeys (5). Sex-related differences in vascular contractility was also observed in Watanabe heritable hyperlipidemic (WHHL) rabbits (80).

Studies in our laboratory revealed substantial gender difference in atherosclerotic lesion development in high-cholesterol–fed golden Syrian hamsters
(81). Differences in the complexity of lesions between male and female animals became apparent after the third month of high-lipid diet. Subsequent
studies investigating endothelium-dependent responses of the isolated thoracic aortas demonstrated that endothelium dysfunction progressed parallel
to the lesion development over the duration of the study (Fig. 6). Female
hamsters exhibited significantly more pronounced acetylcholine-induced
endothelium-dependent relaxation at each time point investigated (81).

*Effect of 17β-Estradiol Treatment.*    The beneficial effect of estrogen on
atherosclerosis was first described in cholesterol-fed chicken (82), where
estrogen treatment inhibited atheroma development in the aorta and coronary arteries. Similar results were reported later by Subbiah et al. (83) in
white Carneau pigeons. In this model, estrogen was shown to increase the
activity of enzymes involved in the hydrolysis and esterification of lipids in
the arterial wall (83). In recent years, experimental evidence supporting
the antiatherosclerotic effect of estrogens has been accumulated studying
atherosclerosis in different animal species, including rabbits (4,84) and

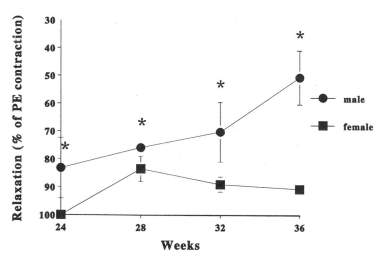

**Figure 6.**    Acetylcholine ($10^{-6}$ M) induced endothelium-dependent relaxation expressed as a percentage of phenylephrine (PE) induced contraction of isolated
thoracic aortic rings of high-cholesterol–fed male (filled circles) and female (filled
squares) hamsters at different time points after start of the high-cholesterol diet.
Asterisks (*) indicate statistically significant ($p<.05$) differences in endothelium-
dependent relaxation between male and female hamsters. Values represent mean
± SEM of four hamsters in each group.

monkeys (5). Williams at al. (6) demonstrated by angiographic studies that estrogen treatment, besides inhibiting atherosclerotic plaque formation, normalized pathological vasoconstrictor responses to acetylcholine in atherosclerotic coronary arteries in vivo.

Results from our laboratory demonstrated a correlation between the inhibitory effect of estrogen on plaque size and on endothelium-dependent vasorelaxation in thoracic aorta of cholesterol-fed rabbits (85). Ovariectomized New Zealand white rabbits were kept on a high-cholesterol (1%) diet and subsequently treated with different doses of 17β-estradiol. Endothelium-dependent vascular responses were measured in organ chambers using freshly isolated rings of the distal part of the thoracic aorta. The antiatherosclerotic effect of estrogen was determined by planimetric measurement of the plaque-covered surface area of the remaining, formalin fixed, oil-red-o–stained segment of the thoracic aorta, including the aortic arch. Our study revealed, that estrogen dose-dependently reduced plaque formation in the hyperlipidemic rabbit aorta (Fig. 7) and significantly and

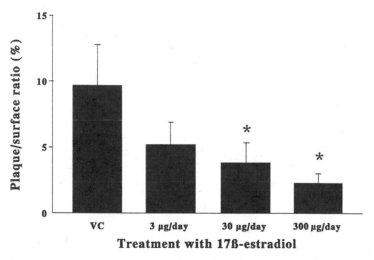

**Figure 7.** Plaque/surface ratio of ovariectomized, high-cholesterol–fed female New Zealand white rabbits after 8 weeks of high-cholesterol diet feeding. Atherosclerotic plaque areas of the thoracic aorta and the aortic arch were determined by planimetric measurement. Lesion areas are expressed as a percentage of the total aortic surface investigated. Values represent means ± SEM of 10 thoracic aorta in each treatment group. Rabbits on high-cholesterol diet were treated with vehicle or with different doses of 17β-estradiol. Asterisks (*) indicate significant reduction in the plaque/surface ratio by 17β-estradiol treatment compared with vehicle-treated high-cholesterol–fed controls.

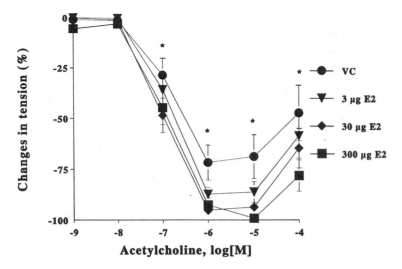

**Figure 8.** Acetylcholine-induced endothelium-dependent relaxation in ovariecto-mized, high-cholesterol–fed New Zealand white rabbits at the end of 8 weeks of high-lipid feeding. Values represent means ± SEM of 10 experiments expressed as a percentage of phenylephrine-induced contraction. Endothelium-dependent, NO-mediated relaxation was impaired in the vehicle-treated high-cholesterol–fed controls (filled circles) compared with rabbits on normal diet (not shown). 17β-Estradiol treatment of the ovariectomized, high-cholesterol–fed rabbits resulted in dose-dependent signifi-cant (*$p<.05$) improvement in the endothelium-dependent relaxation parallel to the observed decrease in the plaque covered areas in the thoracic aorta (see Fig. 7).

dose-dependently increased endothelium-dependent relaxation to acetyl-choline (Fig. 8). These data raised the possibility that elevation of endo-thelial nitric oxide production could, in part, mediate the antiatherosclerotic effects of estrogen.

## B.  Potential Mechanism of the Antiatherosclerotic Effect of Estrogen

Cardiovascular morbidity and mortality increases in women after meno-pause. Estrogen-replacement therapy has been established to relieve the symptoms associated with perimenopause (e.g., hot flushes, mood changes) and for the prevention of postmenopausal osteoporosis. In addition, most epidemiological studies demonstrate a beneficial effect of hormone replace-ment on cardiovascular diseases, such as coronary heart disease and stroke (10,11). Angiographic studies showed that estrogen-replacement therapy of postmenopausal women had a statistically significant protective effect against coronary atherosclerosis (86). Approximately one third of the cardioprotective effect is mediated through the beneficial effects of exogenous estrogens on the lipid profile, although the exact mechanism of the rest of the protection is still uncertain (5,12,85).

## 1. Serum and Vessel Wall Cholesterol

Earlier epidemiological studies suggested that an important part of the vasculoprotective effect of estrogen-replacement therapy involves an effect on the serum cholesterol level (86). Estrogens have favorable effects on the lipid profile: lowering the serum levels of total cholesterol and low-density lipoprotein (LDL) cholesterol and increasing the level of high-density lipoprotein (HDL) cholesterol (68). The predominant effect of estrogen on LDL cholesterol is mediated via the stimulation of LDL receptor expression in the liver (87). Changes in HDL cholesterol are due to the increased expression of apolipoprotein(AI) and the suppression of hepatic lipase activity (87).

High concentrations of plasma lipoprotein(a) (Lp[a]) is considered to be an independent risk factor for cardiovascular diseases (88). Recent studies described a reduction in Lp(a) levels in estrogen-treated male patients with prostate cancer (89) as well as in women on HRT (90).

Cholesterol esters are characteristic components of atherosclerotic lesions. Predilected areas of the aorta were shown to have a focally elevated concentration of undegraded LDL in rabbits (91). A greater LDL accumulation, an increased LDL degradation rate, and a high concentration of undegraded LDL have been reported in coronary arteries and in the bifurcation of the carotid arteries of ovariectomized cynomologus monkeys (92). In the same experiment, hormone replacement of the monkeys resulted in a marked reduction of LDL accumulation in the blood vessels without any effect on serum cholesterol (92).

In several studies, the inhibition of lesion development by $17\beta$-estradiol could not be completely explained by changes in serum cholesterol or lipoprotein composition (5,85). In these cases, it has been suggested that estrogen exerts its effect by acting directly on the cellular components of the atherosclerotic plaques.

## 2. Endothelial Cell Activation/Dysfunction

The endothelium plays a pivotal role in the maintenance of cardiovascular homeostasis by forming a barrier between tissues and the circulating blood and synthesizing biologically active substances, which modulate vascular tone and inhibit smooth muscle cell proliferation, platelet aggregation, and leukocyte adhesion. Impairment in these physiological functions of the endothelium (endothelial dysfunction) occurs early in the development of cardiovascular diseases (45).

Estrogen receptors were demonstrated in cultured endothelial cells by Colburn and Buonassisi (13). High-affinity, specific binding sites for estrogen were demonstrated by [³H]17β-estradiol binding to the cytosolic extracts of rabbit aortic endothelial cells. Estrogen receptors have also been shown in rat endothelial cells (93), and saturable estrogen binding was demonstrated in dog vascular tissues (14). The potential presence of estrogen receptor in the endothelial cells and numerous in vivo data demonstrating enhanced endothelium-dependent relaxation supports the hypothesis that estrogen may directly act on endothelial cells, maintaining its integrity and restoring its physiological function in atherosclerosis.

*Nitric Oxide.*    Endothelial synthesis of NO is catalyzed by the endothelial constitutive nitric oxide synthase (NOS III). NO can serve as a key antiatherogenic and vasculoprotective molecule owing to its inhibitory effects on vascular tone (46), vascular smooth muscle cell proliferation (94), monocyte adhesion (95), platelet activation (96), superoxide free radical generation (97), lipoprotein oxidation (98), and NF-κB activation (99). Therefore factors, which modulate the expression or activity of NOS III, can be important in modulating vascular lesion formation or vasospasm. Indeed, recent studies showed that chronic administration of $N^G$-L-arginine-methyl ester (L-NAME) accelerated aortic lesion formation in hypercholesterolemic rabbits (100), and that feeding with L-arginine (precursor of NO) had the opposite effect (101).

Gender difference in the basal release of endothelium-derived NO in rabbits and the attenuation of NO-mediated vascular reactivity by ovariectomy (47) suggest that aortic NO production is influenced by ovarian steroid hormones (102) in these animals. In support of these results, it has been shown earlier that 4 days' treatment of rabbits by estrogen enhanced endothelium-dependent relaxation to acetylcholine in isolated femoral arteries (103). Weiner et al. (49) reported that calcium-dependent NOS activity and NOS gene expression increased during pregnancy and after 17β-estradiol treatment in guinea pigs. However, the in vitro regulation of the NOS III gene by estrogen in cultured endothelial cells is controversial, such as in cultured bovine (52) and porcine (51) endothelial cells. In early passages of human aortic endothelial cells, physiological concentrations of 17β-estradiol caused a significant increase in calcium-dependent NO production parallel to increased NOS III protein levels (104). In contrast, 17β-estradiol had no effect in later passages of human umbilical endothelial cells even after transient transfections with the human estrogen receptor gene (105).

*Vascular Cell Adhesion Molecules.*    The earliest events in the development of atherosclerotic lesions is the increased adherence of circulating monocytes to the vascular endothelium. Endothelial leukocyte adhesion molecules such as vascular cell adhesion molecule-1 (VCAM-1), intercellular adhesion molecule-1 (ICAM-1), and endothelial-leukocyte adhesion molecule-1 (ELAM-1, or E-selectin) facilitate the recruitment of monocytes and lymphocytes to sites of lesion formation (106,107). ICAM-1 is constitutively expressed on the surface of vascular endothelium, whereas ELAM-1 and VCAM-1 are normally not detectable. In rabbit models of atherosclerosis, such as the diet-induced hypercholesterolemic rabbit and the Watanabe heritable hyperlipidemic rabbit, the increased expression of VCAM-1 has been demonstrated (107). Immunohistochemistry of human atherosclerotic arteries showed intense staining for ICAM-1 (108) and VCAM-1 (109).

Nakai et al. (110) demonstrated that 17$\beta$-estradiol suppressed the induction of VCAM-1 mRNA expression in HUVECs. Although the mechanism by which estrogen regulates VCAM-1 expression is not clarified yet, a potential involvement of the activation of NF-$\kappa$B or other $\kappa$B-specific protein has been suggested (110). However, other reports on in vitro VCAM-1 regulation by 17$\beta$-estradiol are controversial. For example, Cid et al. (111) found a significant increase of VCAM-1 expression in estrogen-treated HUVECs, whereas others found the opposite effect (110).

Soluble ICAM-1, but not soluble VCAM-1 or ELAM-1, levels correlated with the severity of cardiovascular diseases in patients, suggesting that increases in soluble adhesion molecules may be a useful index of endothelial cell activation in the clinical manifestations of atherosclerosis (112). In a double-blind crossover study including 33 young, healthy men, exogenous estrogen had no significant effect on the level of circulating soluble ELAM-1, ICAM-1, and VCAM-1 (113).

*NF-$\kappa$B Regulation.* Activation of the transcription factor nuclear factor kappa B (NF-$\kappa$B) was originally described and studied in leukocytes (114). Its importance, however, in vascular pathophysiology has also been recognized. NF-$\kappa$B may influence the progression of atherosclerosis by regulating genes involved in acute phase and inflammatory responses. NF-$\kappa$B activation has been shown to enhance the expression of proinflammatory mediators and adhesion molecules in macrophages, endothelial cells, and smooth muscle cells (115). Promoters of these genes contain consensus binding sites for NF-$\kappa$B (107,115).

Activation of NF-$\kappa$B involves phosphorylation of its inhibitor I$\kappa$Balpha, which results in rapid degradation of the inhibitory subunit (116). NF-$\kappa$B activation can be prevented by stabilization of the NF-$\kappa$B/I$\kappa$Balpha complex or inhibition of I$\kappa$Balpha phosphorylation or degradation. Antioxidants have been shown to stabilize the NF-$\kappa$B/I$\kappa$Balpha complex through scavenging reactive oxygen species, like superoxide anion, which may activate NF-κB (117). The inhibition of the endogenous endothelial production of NO by L-arginine analogues activated NF-κB, indicating a role of NO in the tonic inhibition of this transcription factor (99). The mechanism by which NO can prevent the activation of NF-κB probably involves the induction and stabilization of its inhibitor IκBalpha either through scavenging superoxide anions (97) or via direct interaction with protein kinases or phosphatases (99).

Recent studies by Register et al. (118) indicated that NF-κB activity of nuclear extracts isolated from the aortic arch of ovariectomized, cholesterol-fed female cynomologus monkeys were significantly greater than that in aortic tissue isolated from an estrogen-treated group. Estrogen may evoke its vasculoprotective effect by interfering with NF-κB activity, either directly or via increasing the release of a mediator, like NO.

## 3. Smooth Muscle Cell Proliferation

During the pathogenesis of atherosclerosis, the initial endothelial cell injury is rapidly followed by a number of events. One of these pathological processes is the migration and proliferation of medial smooth muscle cells in the neointima of vascular lesions. The proliferating, dedifferentiated smooth muscle cells are capable of migrating through the elastic lamina to the intimal layer. They continue to proliferate in the intima forming a thick neointimal layer (98).

Vascular smooth muscle cells possess estrogen receptors in vivo (15) as well as in vitro under defined culture conditions (119,120). Vascular smooth muscle cells in culture respond to physiological concentrations of 17β-estradiol. Estradiol significantly inhibited the proliferation of vascular smooth muscle isolated from porcine coronary arteries (119). Suppression of smooth muscle cell proliferation involved inhibition of DNA synthesis in the cells, which was confirmed by the measurement of radioactive thymidine incorporation. Others have shown that the c-*fos* proto-oncogene is induced in vascular smooth muscle cells by estrogen (120). The 5′ flanking region of c-*fos* contains an estrogen-response element, which binds the estrogen receptor (121). This observation suggests that estrogen can regulate the growth and differentiation of smooth muscle cells. This effect could potentially delay the development of vascular lesions, which involve smooth muscle proliferation, supporting the hypothesis that the antiproliferative effects of estrogen may be part of its antiatherosclerotic action. It is suggested that the direct effect of estrogen on smooth muscle cells is involved in the decrease of myointimal hyperplasia in an allograft model of accelerated atherosclerosis (122) and in neointimal thickening following balloon injury in the rat (123), cardiac transplant atherosclerosis in the rabbit (124), and explant culture of pig coronary arteries (119).

## 4. Macrophages

Besides endothelial and smooth muscle cells, estrogen receptors have been demonstrated in human blood mononuclear cells (125) and in macrophages (126). Macrophages are a dominant component of human atherosclerotic plaques and also in lesions found in high-lipid–fed animals. The earliest detectable lesion in the development of atherosclerosis is the fatty streak, consisting mostly of foam cells, that is, lipid-laden macrophages, within the intimal layer of the vascular wall. Macrophages are derived from circulating monocytes. They are recruited to the lesion by chemotactic stimuli, such as monocyte chemoattractant protein-1 (MCP-1) (127). During extravasation, monocytes first adhere to the endothelium. VCAM-1 plays an important role in this event by selectively promoting the adhesion via very late activation antigen-4 (VLA-4) expressed on mononuclear cells (109). Macrophages in the vascular wall accumulate lipids, such as cholesterol. Plasma LDL becomes oxidized in the intima (128). Oxidatively modified LDL, recognized and taken up by the scavenger receptor expressed on the foam cell surface, contributes to the maintenance of inflammation in the arterial wall (129).

It has been demonstrated that estrogen acts directly on foam cells by influencing lipoprotein metabolism or uptake by macrophages via regulating lipoprotein receptor expression or cholesterol esterase activity (130–132).

It is likely that part of the antiatherogenic effect of estrogen is due to the modulation of inflammatory responses in the vascular wall. Indeed, we have shown that $17\beta$-estradiol reduces interleukin-$1\beta$–induced excessive NO production in rat aortic rings in vitro and LPS-induced elevated blood NO level in ovariectomized rats in vivo (133). Physiological levels of $17\beta$-estradiol inhibit lipopolysaccharide (LPS)–induced expression of the murine homologue (JE) of MCP-1 in murine macrophage cell lines and isolated murine peritoneal macrophages (135).

Other studies suggest that the beneficial effects of estrogen may be related to its antioxidant properties. $17\beta$-Estradiol inhibited copper- and cell-mediated oxidative modification of LDL in vitro (136). Estrogen was also effective in protecting endothelial cells against the cytotoxic effects of oxidized LDL (137).

## IV. SUMMARY

The following effects of $17\beta$-estradiol on various components of the atherosclerotic lesion (in combination with beneficial effects on serum cholesterol) may contribute to the well-documented antiatherosclerotic action of the ovarian sex steroid: (1) decreased accumulation and/or retention of cholesterol in the vessel wall, (2) suppression of endothelial cell activation, (3) augmentation of constitutive NOS activity and suppression of excessive NO production by the inducible NOS, (4) inhibition of smooth muscle proliferation, (5) modulation of monocyte/macrophage function, (6) anti-oxidant activity, and (7) vasodilation.

Experimental studies revealed gender differences in endothelium-dependent responses in several animal species. Gender differences generally manifest in significantly greater endothelium-dependent relaxation, more endothelial NO production, and/or less endothelium-dependent contraction in female animals. In animal models of human cardiovascular diseases, such as atherosclerosis and hypertension, the activity of NO has been shown to be diminished. It is accepted that endothelial dysfunction owing to impaired NO production, substantially contributes to the development of cardiovascular diseases. Enhanced endothelial NO production in women correlates with epidemiological data demonstrating vasculoprotection against cardiovascular diseases in women compared with men.

Human statistics have already indicated the role of estrogen in the protection against coronary artery diseases by reporting progressive increase in risk for ischemic heart disease after menopause (9) and showing that estrogen-replacement therapy of postmenopausal women markedly reduces morbidity and mortality due to cardiovascular diseases (10). The vasculoprotective effect of $17\beta$-estradiol has been demonstrated in experimental atherosclerosis and hypertension. Estrogen treatment in these experimental models also resulted in improved endothelial function. Greater endothelium-dependent relaxation correlated with attenuated atherosclerotic plaque formation in hyperlipidemic rabbits and sexual dimorphism in endothelial dysfunction with lower blood pressure in female spontaneously hypertensive rats.

In conclusion, various evidence suggest that male gender can be considered a risk factor. Gender differences in endothelial function could explain the differential manifestation of cardiovascular diseases in men and women. Understanding the mechanism of sexual dimorphism in endothelial function may provide a key in developing treatments directed at restoration of physiological cardiovascular function.

## REFERENCES

1. Isles CG, Hole DJ, Hawthorne VM, Lever AF. Relation between coronary risk and coronary mortality in women of the Refew and Paisely Survey: comparison with men. Lancet 1992; 339:702–706.
2. von Eiff AW, Gogolin E, Jacobs U, Neus H. Ambulatory blood pressure in children followed for 3 years: influence of sex and family history on hypertension. Clin Exp Hypertens 1986; 8:577–581.

3. Kushwaha RS, Hazard WR. Exogenous estrogens attenuate dietary hyper-cholesterolemia and atherosclerosis in the rabbit. Metabolism 1981; 30:359.
4. Hough JL, Zilversmit DB. Effect of 17 beta estradiol on aortic cholesterol content and metabolism in cholesterol-fed rabbits. Arteriosclerosis 1986; 6:57–63.
5. Adams MR, Kaplan JF, Manuck SB, Koritnik DR, Parks JS, Wolfe MS, Clarkson T. Inhibition of coronary artery atherosclerosis by 17-beta estradiol in ovariectomized monkeys. Arteriosclerosis 1990; 10:1051–1057.
6. Williams JK, Adams MR, Klopfenstein HS. Estrogen modulates responses of atherosclerotic coronary arteries. Circulation 1990; 81:1680–1687.
7. Colditz GA, Willett WC, Stampfer MJ, Rosner B, Speizer FE, Hennekens CH. Menopause and the risk of coronary heart disease in women. N Engl J Med 1987; 316:1105–1110.
8. Ross RK, Paganini-Hill A, Mack TM, Henderson BE. Cardiovascular benefits of estrogen replacement therapy. Am J Obstet Gynecol 1989; 60:1301–1306.
9. Knopp RH. The effects of postmenopausal estrogen therapy on the incidence of atherosclerotic vascular disease. Obstet Gynecol 1988; 72:23S.
10. Stampfer MJ, Colditz GA, Willett WC, Manson JE, Rosner B, Speizer FE, Hennekens CH. Postmenopausal estrogen therapy and cardiovascular disease: ten-year follow-up from the Nurses' Health Study. N Engl J Med 1991; 325: 756–762.
11. Stampfer MJ. A review of the epidemiology of postmenopausal estrogens and the risk of coronary heart disease. In Sex Steroids and the Cardiovascular System. Berlin: Springer-Verlag, 1992:145–160.
12. Barrett-Connor E, Bush TL. Estrogen and coronary heart disease in women. JAMA 1991; 265:1861–1867.
13. Colburn P, Buonassisi V. Estrogen-binding sites in endothelial cell cultures. Science 1978; 201:817–819.
14. Horwitz KB, Horwitz CD. Canine vascular tissues are targets for androgens, estrogens, progestins and glucocorticoids. J Clin Invest 1982; 69:750–758.
15. Losordo DW, Kearney M, Kim EM, Jekanowski J, Isner JM. Variable expression of the estrogen receptor in the normal and atherosclerotic coronary arteries of premenopausal women. Circulation 1994; 89:1501–1510.
16. Rosano GM, Sarrel PM. Ovarian hormones and the cardiovascular system: recent findings. Cardiologica 1994; 39:275–279.
17. Gangar KF, Reid BA, Crook D, Hillard TC, Whitehead MI. Oestrogens and atherosclerotic vascular disease—local vascular factors. Baillieres Clin Endocrinol Metab 1993; 7:47–59.
18. Riedel M, Rafflenbeul W, Lichtlen P. Ovarian sex steroids and atherosclerosis. Clin Invest 1993; 71:406–412.
19. Iams SG, Wexler BC. Inhibition of the development of spontaneously hypertension in SH rats by gonadectomy or estradiol. J Lab Clin Med 1979; 10:608–616.
20. Crofton JT, Share L, Brooks DP. Gonadectomy abolishes the sexual dimorphism in DOCA-salt hypertension in rat. Clin Exp Hypertens 1989; 11: 1249–1261.

21. Dahl LK, Knudsen KD, Ohanian EV, Muirhead M, Tuthill R. Role of gonads in hypertension prone rats. J Exp Med 1975; 142:748–759.
22. Lüscher TF, Vanhoutte PM. Endothelium-dependent contractions to acetylcholine in the aorta of the spontaneously hypertensive rat. Hypertension 1986; 8:344–348.
23. Lüscher TF, Romero JC, Vanhoutte PM. Bioassay of endothelium-derived vasoactive substances in the aorta of normotensive and spontaneously hypertensive rats. J Hypertens 1987; 4(suppl 6):581–583.
24. Linder L, Kiowski W, Bühler FR, Lüscher TF. Indirect evidence for release of endothelium-derived relaxing factor in human forearm circulation in vivo. Circulation 1990; 81:1762–1767.
25. Yamori Y, Horie R, Nara Y, Kihara M, Igawa T, Kanage T, Mori K, Ikeda K. Genetic markers in spontaneously hypertensive rats. Clin Exp Hypertens 1981; 3:713–725.
26. Vincent M, Kaiser MA, Orea V, Lodwick D, Samani NJ. Hypertension in the spontaneously hypertensive rat and sex chromosomes. Hypertension 1994; 23:161–166.
27. Tanase H, Suzuki Y, Oohsima A, Yamori Y, Okamoto K. Genetic analysis of blood pressure in spontaneously hypertensive rats. Jpn Circ J 1970; 34:1197–1202.
28. Iams SG, Wexler BC. Retardation in the development of spontaneously hypertension in SH rats by gonadectomy. J Lab Clin Med 1977; 90:977–1003.
29. Ganten U, Schroder G, Witt M, Zimmerman F, Ganten D, Stock G. Sexual dimorphism of blood pressure in spontaneously hypertensive rats: effects of anti-androgen treatment. Hypertension 1989; 7:721–726.
30. Kauser K, Rubanyi GM. Gender difference in endothelial dysfunction in the aorta of spontaneously hypertensive rats. Hypertension 1995; 25:517–523.
31. de Swiet M. The physiology of normal pregnancy. In: Rubin PC, ed. Hypertension in Pregnancy. Handbook of Hypertension. Vol. 10 Amsterdam: Elsevier, 1988:1.
32. Blizard DA, Folk TG. Resource sharing in rat gestation: role of maternal cardiovascular hemodynamics. Am J Physiol 1990; 258:R1299–1307.
33. Ahokas RA, Sibai BM. The relationship between experimentally determined litter size and maternal blood pressure in spontaneously hypertensive rats. Am J Obstet Gynecol 1990; 162:841–847.
34. Rees DD, Palmer RMJ, Moncada S. Role of endothelium-derived nitric oxide in the regulation of blood pressure. Proc Natl Acad Scil USA 1989; 86:3375–3378.
35. Ahokas RA, Mercer BM, Sibai BM, Enhanced endothelium-derived relaxing factor activity in pregnant, spontaneously hypertensive rats. Am J Obstet Gynecol 1991; 165:801–807.
36. Folkow B. Intravascular pressure as a factor regulating the tone of the small vessels. Acta Physiol Scand 1949; 17:289–310.
37. Altura BM, Altura TT. Influence of sex hormones, oral contraceptives and pregnancy on vascular muscle and its reactivity. In: Carrier O, Shibata S, eds. Factors Influencing Vascular Reactivity. New York: Igaku-Shoin, 1977:221–254.

38. Stallone JN, Crofton JT, Share L. Sexual dimorphism in vasopressin-induced contraction of rat aorta. Am J Physiol 1991; 260:H453–458.
39. Colucci W, Gimbrone Jr. MA, McLaughlin MK, Halpern W, Alexander RW. Increased vascular catecholamine sensitivity and a adrenergic receptor affinity in female and estrogen-treated male rats. Circ Res 1982; 50:805–811.
40. Maddox YT, Falcon JG, Ridinger M, Cunard CM, Ramwell PW. Endothelium-dependent gender differences in the response of the rat aorta. J Pharmacol Exp Ther 1987; 240:392–395.
41. Kauser K, Rubanyi GM. Gender difference in bioassayable endothelium-derived nitric oxide release from isolated rat aortae. Am J Physiol 1994; 267:H2311–H2317.
42. Karanian JW, Moran FM, Ramey ER, Ramwell PW. Gender differences in prostaglandin receptors in the rat aorta. Br J Pharmacol 1981; 72:10–12.
43. Fortes ZB, Nigro D, Scivoletto R, Carvalho MHC. Influence of sex on the reactivity to endothelin-1 and noradrenaline in spontaneously hypertensive rats. Clin Exp Hypertens Theory Pract 1991; A13:807–816.
44. Rubanyi GM. Cardiovascular Significance of Endothelium-Derived Vasoactive Factors. New York: Futura, 1991.
45. Rubanyi GM. Role of endothelium in cardiovascular homeostasis and diseases. J Cardiovasc Pharamacol 1993; 22(suppl 4):S1–S13.
46. Furchgott RF, Zawadzki JV. The obligatory role of endothelial cells in the relaxation of arterial smooth muscle by acetylcholine. Nature 1980; 228:373–376.
47. Hayashi T, Fukuto JM, Ignarro LJ, Chaudhuri G. Basal release of nitric oxide from aortic rings is greater in female rabbits than in male rabbits: implications for atherosclerosis. Proc Natl Acad Sci USA 1992; 89:11259–11263.
48. Van Buren GA, Yang DS, Clark KE. Estrogen-induced uterine vasodilation is antagonized by L-nitroarginine methyl ester, an inhibitor of nitric oxide synthesis. Am J Obstet Gynecol 1992; 167:828–833.
49. Weiner CP, Knowles RG, Moncada S. Induction of nitric oxide synthases early in pregnancy. Am J Obstet Gynecol 1994; 171:838–843.
50. Weiner CP, Lizasoain I, Baylis SA, Knowles RG, Charles IG, Moncada S. Induction of calcium-dependent nitric oxide synthases by sex hormones. Proc Natl Acad Sci USA 1994; 91:5212–5216.
51. Schray-Utz B, Zeiher AM, Busse R. Expression of constitutive NO synthase in cultured endothelial cells is enhanced by 17 beta-estradiol. Circulation 1993; 88:1–80.
52. Sayegh HS, Ohara Y, Havas JP, Peterson TE, Dockery S, Harrison DG. Endothelial nitric oxide synthase regulation by estrogens. Circulation 1993; 88:1–80.
53. Kato T, Iwama Y, Okumura K, Hashimoto H, Ito T, Satake T. Prostaglandin H2 may be the endothelium-derived contracting factor released by acetylcholine in the aorta of the rat. Hypertension 1990; 15:475–481.
54. Auch-Schwelk W, Katusic ZS, Vanhoutte PM. Thromboxane A2 receptor antagonists inhibit endothelium-dependent contractions. Hypertension 1990; 15: 699–703.

55. Jameson M, Dai F-X, Lüscher T, Skopec J, Diederich A, Diederich D. Endothelium-derived contracting factors in resistance arteries of young spontaneously hypertensive rats before development of over hypertension. Hypertension 1993; 21:280–288.
56. Jiang C, Sarrel PM, Lindsay DC, Poole-Wilson PA, Collins P. Endothelium-independent relaxation of rabbit coronary artery by 17β-oestradiol in vitro. Br J Pharmacol 1991; 104:1033–1037.
57. Jiang C, Poole-Wilson PA, Sarrfel PM, Mochizuki S, Collins P, Macleon KT. effect of 17β-estradiol on contraction $Ca^{2+}$ current and intracellular free $Ca^{2+}$ in guinea-pig isolated cardiac myocytes. J Pharmacol 1992; 106:739–745.
58. Raddino R, Manca C, Poli E, Bologneis R, Visioli O. Effects of 17-beta-estradiol on the isolated rabbit heart. Arch Int Pharmacodyn 1986; 281:57–65.
59. Eckstein N, Nadler E, Barnea O, Shavit G, Ayalon D. Acute effects of 17β-estradiol on the rat heart. Am J Obstet Gynecol 1994; 171:844–888.
60. Henry PD, Bentley KI. Suppression of atherogenesis in cholesterol-fed rabbits treated with nifedipine. J Clin Invest 1981; 68:1366–1369.
61. Water D, Lesperance J, Francetich M, Causey D, Theroux P, Chiang Y-K, Hudon G, Lemarbre L, Reitman M, Joyal M, Gosselin G, Dyirda I, Macer J, Havel RJ. A controlled clinical trial to assess the effect of a calcium channel blocker on the progression of coronary atherosclerosis. Circulation 1990; 82: 1940–1953.
62. Williams SP, Shackelford DP, Iams SG, Mustafa SJ. Endothelium-dependent relaxation in estrogen-treated spontaneously hypertensive rats. Eur J Pharmacol 1988; 145:205–207.
63. Barr DP, Russ EM, Eder HA. Influence of estrogens on lipoproteins in atherosclerosis. Am J Med 1951; 11:480–485.
64. Khaw, K-T, Barett-Connor E. Endogenous sex hormones, high density lipoprotein cholesterol, and other lipoprotein fractions in men. Arterioscler Thromb 1991; 11:489–494.
65. Kirkland RT, Keenan BS, Probstfield JL, Patsch W, Lin T-L, Clayton GW, Insull W Jr. Decrease in plasma high-density lipoprotein cholesterol levels at puberty in boys with delayed adolescence. JAMA 1987; 257:502–507.
66. Dai WS, Gutai JP, Kuller LH, Laporte RE, Falvo-Gerard L, Caggiula A. Relation between high-density lipoprotein cholesterol and sex hormone concentrations in men. Am J Cardiol 1984; 53:1259–1263.
67. Duell PB, Bierman EL. The relationship between sex hormones and high-density lipoprotein cholesterol levels in healthy adult men. Arch Intern Med 1990; 150:2317–2320.
68. Walsh BW, Schiff I, Rosner B, Greenberg L, Ravnikar V, Sackhs FM. Effects of postmenopausal estrogen replacement on the concentrations and metabolism of plasma lipoproteins. N Engl J Med 1991; 325:1196–1204.
69. Carroll JD, Carroll EP, Feldman T, Ward DM, Lang RM, McGaughey D, Kary RB. Sex-associated differences in left ventricular function in aortic stenosis of the elderly. Circulation 1992; 86:1099–1107.
70. Kuntz RE, Tosteson NA, Berman AD, Goldman L, Gordon PC, Leonard

BM, McKay RG, Diver DJ, Safian RD. Predictors of event-free survival after balloon aortic valvuloplasty. N Engl J Med 1991; 325:17–23.

71. Sullivan JL. The iron paradigm of ischemic heart disease. Am Heart J 1981; 117:1177–1294.
72. Sullivan JL. Iron and the sex difference in heart disease risk. Lancet 1989; 1:1293–1294.
73. Kayan AR, Sternby NH, Uemura K, Vanecek R, Vihert HM, Lifsic HM, Matova EE, Zahor Z, Zdanov VS. Atherosclerosis of the aorta and coronary arteries in five towns. Bull WHO 1976; 53:485.
74. Gabmbrell RD Jr. Use of progestogens in postmenopausal women. Int J Fertil 1989; 34:315–321.
75. Bringer J. Norgestimate: a clinical overview of a new progestin. Am J Obstet Gynecol 1992; 166:1969–1977.
76. Knopp RH, Zhu Ziaodong, Bonet B. Effects of estrogens on lipoprotein metabolism and cardiovascular disease in women. Atherosclerosis 1994; 110 (suppl):S83–S91.
77. Nakashima Y, Plump AS, Raines EW, Breslow JL, Ross R. ApoE-deficient mice develop lesions of all phases of atherosclerosis throughout the arterial tree. Arterioscler Thromb 1994; 14:133–140.
78. Reddick RL, Zhang SH, Maeda N. Atherosclerosis in mice lacking Apo E evaluation of lesional development and progression. Arterioscler Thromb 1994; 14:141–147.
79. Wagner JD, St Clair RW, Schwenke DC, Shively CA, Adams MR, Clarkson TB. Regional differences in arterial low density lipoprotein metabolism in surgically postmenopausal cynomologus monkeys. Arterioscler Thromb 1992; 12:717–726.
80. Brizzolara AL, Tomlinson A, Aberdeen J, Gourdie RG, Burnstock G. Sex and age as factors influencing the vascular reactivity in Watanabe heritable hyperlipidaemic (WHHL) rabbits: a pharmacological and morphological study of the hepatic artery. J Cardiovasc Pharmacol 1992; 19:86–95.
81. Kauser K, Sonnenberg D, Henrichmann F, Werner M, Whitcomb J, Wilson K, Polokoff R, Vergona R, Rubanyi GM. Gender differences in vascular reactivity in high cholesterol fed hamsters. Atherosclerosis 1994; 109:328.
82. Pick R, Stamler J, Rodbard S, Katz LN. The inhibition of coronary atherosclerosis by estrogens in cholesterol-fed chicks. Circulation 1952; 6:276–280.
83. Subbiah MTR. Effect of estrogens on the activities of cholesteryl ester synthetase and cholesteryl ester hydrolases in pigeon aorta. Steroids 1977; 30:259–275.
84. Haarbo J, Leth-Espensen P, Stender S, Christiansen C. Estrogen monotherapy and combined estrogen-progestogen replacement therapy attenuate aortic accumulation of cholesterol in ovariectomized cholesterol-fed rabbits. J Clin Invest 1991; 87:1274.
85. Kauser K, Sonnenberg D, Mertens H, Werner M, Wilson K, Polokoff R, Vergona R, Rubanyi GM. Vasculoprotective effect of 17β-estradiol in high cholesterol fed, ovariectomized rabbits. FASEB J 1995; 9:I-A854.

86. Sullivan JM. Atherosclerosis and estrogen replacement therapy. Int J Fertil 1994; 39(suppl 1):28–35.
87. Kushwaha RS, McMahon CA, Mott GE, Carey KD, Reardon CA, Getz GS, McGill HC Jr. Influence of dietary lipids on hepatic mRNA levels of proteins regulating plasma lipoproteins in baboons with high and low levels of large high density lipoproteins. J Lipid Res 1991; 32:1929–1940.
88. Scanu AM, Lawn RM, Berk K. Lipoprotein(a) and atherosclerosis. Ann Intern Med 1991; 115:209–218.
89. Henriksson P, Angelin B, Berglund L. Hormonal regulation of serum Lp(a) levels. Opposite effects after *estrogen* treatment and ordhidectomy in males with prostatic carcinoma. J Clin Invest 1992; 89:1166–1171.
90. Kim CJ, Jang HC, Cho DM, Min YK. Effects of hormone replacement therapy on lipoprotein(a) and lipids in postmenopausal women. Arterioscler Thromb 1994; 14:275–281.
91. Schwenke DC. Selective increase in cholesterol at atherosclerosis-susceptible aortic sites after short-term cholesterol feeding. Arterioscler Thromb Vasc Biol 1995; 15:1928–1937.
92. Wagner JD, Clarkson TB, St Clair RW, Schwenke DC, Shively CA, Adams MR. Estrogen and progesterone replacement therapy reduces LDL accumulation in the coronary arteries of surgically postmenopausal cynomologus monkeys. J Clin Invest 1991; 88:1995–2002.
93. Lin AL, McGill HC, Shain SA. Hormone receptors of the baboon cardiovascular system. Circ Res 1982; 50:610–616.
94. Garg UC, Hassid A. Nitric oxide-generating vasodilators and 8-bromo-cyclic guanosine monophosphate inhibit mitogenesis and proliferation of cultured rat vascular smooth muscle cells. J Clin Invest 1989; 83:1774–1777.
95. Bath PM, Hassall DG, Gladwin AM, Palmer RM, Martin JF. Nitric oxide and prostacyclin. Divergence of inhibitory effects on monocyte chemotaxis and adhesion to endothelium in vitro. Arterioscler Thromb 1991; 11:254–260.
96. Radomski MW, Palmer RM, Moncada S. Endogenous nitric oxide inhibits human platelet adhesion to vascular endothelium. lancet 1987; 2:1057–1058.
97. Rubanyi GM, Vanhoutte PM. Oxygen-derived free radicals, endothelium, and responsiveness of vascular smooth muscle. Am J Physiol 1986; 250:H815–H821.
98. Kanner J, Harel S, Granit R. Nitric oxide, an inhibitor of lipid oxidation by lipoxygenase, cyclooxygenase and hemoglobin. Lipids 1992; 27:46–49.
99. Peng HB, Libby P, Liao JK. Induction and stabilization of I kappa B alpha by nitric oxide mediates inhibition of NF-kappa B. J Clin Invest 1995; 270:14214–14219.
100. Naruse KM, Shimizu M, Muramatsu M, Toki Y, Miyazaki Y, Okurama K, Hashimoto H, Ito T. Long-term inhibition of NO synthesis promotes atherosclerosis in the hypercholesterolemic rabbit thoracic aorta. Arterioscler Thromb 1994; 14:746–752.
101. Cooke JP, Singer AH, Tsao P, Zera P, Rowan RA, Billingham ME. Antiatherogenic effects of L-arginine in the hypercholesteremic rabbit. J Clin Invest 1992; 90:1168–1172.

102. Kauser K, Rubanyi GM. 17β-estradiol and endothelial nitric oxide synthase. Endothelium 1994; 2:203–208.
103. Gisclard V, Miller VM, Vanhouette PM. Effect of 17β-estradiol on endothelium-dependent responses in the rabbit. J Pharmacol Exp Ther 1988; 244:19–22.
104. Hishikawa K, Nakaki T, Marumo T, Suzuki H, Kato R, Saruta T. Upregulation of nitric oxide synthase by estradiol in human aortic endothelial cells. FEBS Lett 1995; 36:291–293.
105. Harrison DG, Venema RC, Arnal JF, Inoue N, Ohara Y, Sayegh H, Murphy TJ. The endothelial cell *nitric oxide* synthase: is it really constitutively expressed? Agents Actions 1995; 45(suppl):107–117.
106. Bevilacqua MP, Stengelin S, Gimbrone MAJ, Seed B. Endothelial leukocyte adhesion molecule 1: an inducible receptor for neutrophils related to complement regulatory proteins and lectins. Science 1989; 243:1160–1165.
107. Cybulsky MI, Gimbrone MA. Endothelial expression of a mononuclear leukocyte adhesion molecule during atherogenesis. Science 1991; 251:788–791.
108. Poston RN, Haskard DO, Coucher JR, Gall NP, Johnson-Tidey RR. Expression of intercellular adhesion molecule-1 in atherosclerotic plaques. Am J of Pathol 1992; 140:665–672.
109. Li H, Cybulsky MI, Gimbrone MJ, Libby P. An atherogenic diet rapidly induces VCAM-1, a cytokine-regulatable mono-nuclear leukocyte adhesion molecule, in rabbit aortic endothelium. Arterioscler Thromb 1993; 13:197–204.
110. Nakai K, Itoh C, Hotta K, Itoh T, Yoshizumi M, Hiramori I. Estradiol-17β regulates the induction of VCAM-1 expression interleukin-1β in human umbilical vein endothelial cells. Life Sci 1994; 54:221–227.
111. Cid MC, Kleinman HK, Grant DS, Schnager HW, Fauci AS, Hoffman GS. Estradiol enhances leukocyte binding to tumor necrosis factor (TNF)–stimulated endothelial cells via an increase in TNF-induced adhesion molecules E-selectin, intercellular adhesion molecule type 1, and vascular cell adhesion molecule type 1. J Clin Invest 1994; 93:17–25.
112. Blann AD, McCollum CN. Circulating Endothelial cell/leukocyte adhesion molecules in atherosclerosis. Thromb Haemost 1994; 72:151–154.
113. Jilma B, Eichler H-G, Breiteneder H, Wolzt M, Aringer M, Graninger W, Röhkrer C, Veitl M, Wagner O. Effects of 17β-estradiol on circulating adhesion molecules. J Clin Endocrinol Metabol 1994; 79:1619–1624.
114. Baeuerle PA, Henkel T. Function and activation of NF-kappa B in the immune system. Annu Rev Immunol 1994; 12:141–179.
115. Collins T, Read MA, Neish AS, Whitley MZ, Thanos D, Maniatis T. Transcriptional regulation of endothelial cell adhesion molecules: NF-κB and cytokine-inducible enhancers. FASEB J 1995; 9:899–909.
116. Palombella VJ, Rando OG, Goldberg AL, Maniatis T. The ubiquitin-proteasome pathway is required for processing the NF-kB1 precursor protein and the activation of NF-kB. Cell 1994; 78:773–785.
117. Schreck R, Rieber P, Baeuerle PA. Reactive oxygen intermediates as widely

used messengers in the activation of NF-κB transcription factor and HIV-1. EMBO J 1991; 10:2247–2258.

118. Register TC, Bora TA, Adams MR. Estrogen Inhibits Activation of Arterial NF-kB transcription Factor in Early Diet-Induced Atherogenesis. Scientific Conference on Hormonal, Metabolic and Cellular Influences on Cardiovascular Disease in Women, San Diego, Abstract No. 53, October 19–21, 1995.

119. Vargas R, Wroblewska B, Hatch J, Grojec M, Foegh M, Ramwell PW. Estradiol inhibition of thymidine uptake in explants of porcine left anterior descending coronary artery. Circulation 1990 82(suppl III)III-572.

120. Orimo A, Inoue S, Ouchi Y, Orimo H. Vascular smooth muscle cells possess estrogen receptor and respond to estrogen. Ann NY Acad Sci 1995; 748:592–594.

121. Weisz A, Rosales R. Identification of an estrogen response element upstream of the human c-fos gene that binds the estrogen receptor and the AP-1 transcription factor. Nucleic Acids Res 1990; 18:5097–5106.

122. Jacobsson J, Cheng L, Lyke K, Kuwahara M, Kagan E, Ramwell PW, Foegh ML. Effect of estradiol on accelerated atherosclerosis in rabbit heterotopic aortic allografts. J Heart Lung Transplant 1992; 11:1188–1193.

123. Chen S-J, Huaibin L, Durand J, Oparil S, Chen Y-F. Estrogen reduces myointimal proliferation after balloon injury of rat carotid artery. Circulation 1996; 93:577–584.

124. Kuwahara M, Jacobsson J, Kuwahara M, Kagan E, Ramwell PW, Foegh ML. Coronary artery ultrastructural changes in cardiac transplant atherosclerosis in the rabbit. Transplantation 1991; 52:759–765.

125. Weusten JJ, Blankenstein MA, Gmelig-Meyling FH, Scuurman HJ, Kater L, Thijssen JH. Presence of oestrogen receptors in human blood mononuclear cells and thymocytes. Acta Endocrinol 1986; 112:409.

126. Gulshan S, McCruden AB, Stimson WH. Oestrogen receptors in macrophages. Scand J Immunol 1990; 31:691.

127. Ylä-Herttuala S, Lipton BA, Rosenfeld ME, Säkioja T, Yoshimura T, Leonard EJ, Witztum JL, Steinberg D. Expression of monocyte chemoattractant protein 1 in macrophage-rich areas of human and rabbit atherosclerotic lesions. Proc Natl Acad Sci USA 1991; 88:5252–5256.

128. Steinberg D, Parthasarathy S, Carew T, Khoo JC, Witztum JL. Beyond cholesterol. Modifications of LDL that increase its atherogenicity. N Engl J Med 1989; 320:915.

129. Salonen JT, Yla-Herttuala S, Yamamoto R, Butler S, Korpela H, Salonen R, Nyyssonen K, Palinski W, Witztum JL. Autoantibodies against oxydized LDL and progression of carotid atherosclerosis. Lancet 1992; 339:883.

130. Huber LA, Scheffler E, Poll T, Ziegler R, Dresel HA. 17 Beta-estradiol inhibits LDL oxidation and cholesteryl ester formation in cultured macrophages. Free Radic Res Commun 1990; 8:167–173.

131. Haarbo J, Nielsen LB, Stender S, Christiansen C. Aortic permeability to LDL during estrogen therapy. Arterioscler Thromb 1994:14:243.

132. Tomita T, Sawamura F, Uetsuka R, Ikeda M, Tomita I. The regulation of

cholesteryl ester metabolism by 17 beta-estradiol in macrophages. Activation of neutral *cholesterol* esterase. Ann NY Acad Sci 1995; 748:637–639.

133. Kauser K, Sonnenberg D, Henrichmann F, Rubanyi GM. 17β-estradiol inhibits IL-1β-induced suppression of contractile activity in isolated rat thoracic aorta. Circulation 1994; 90:1–577.

134. Kauser K, Sonnenberg D, Tse J, Rubanyi GM. Effect of Ovariectomy and estrogen-substitution on endotoxin-induced nitric oxide production in rats. Endothelium 1995; 3:S82.

135. Frazier-Jessen MR, Kovacs EJ. Estrogen modulation of JE/monocyte chemoattractant protein-1 mRNA expression in murine macrophages. J Immunol 1995; 154:1838–1845.

136. Maziere C, Ronveaus MF, Salmon S, Santus R, Mazier JC. Estrogens inhibit copper and cell-mediated modification of low-density lipoprotein. Atherosclerosis 1991; 89:175–182.

137. Nègre-Salvayre A, Pieraggi M-T, Mabile L, Salvayre R. Protective effect of 17β-estradiol against the cytotoxicity of minimally oxidized LDL to cultured bovine aortic endothelial cells. Atherosclerosis 1993; 99:207–217.

# 17

# Lipoprotein(a): Insights from Transgenic Mice

**Steven D. Hughes and Edward M. Rubin**

*Lawrence Berkeley National Laboratory, University of California at Berkeley, Berkeley, California*

## I. INTRODUCTION

Despite more than 30 years of investigation since the discovery of lipoprotein(a) (Lp[a]) (1), many of the biological properties of this molecule, especially those relevant to its connection with vascular disease, have remained enigmatic. Lp(a), a macromolecular complex found in human plasma, is structurally distinct from low-density lipoproteins (LDL) by the addition of a single protein, apolipoprotein(a) (apo[a]). This hydrophilic glycoprotein is associated with the apolipoprotein B (apoB) moiety of LDL through a disulfide bond joining the carboxyl terminal region of both molecules (2,3).

Plasma concentrations of Lp(a) vary considerably among individual (from <1 to >100 mg/dl) and have been shown to be largely genetically determined (4,5). The highly polymorphic apo(a) locus has been estimated to contribute >90% of the variability among individuals (6). At least 34 alleles of apo(a) have been identified, which vary in their number of a tandemly repeated 5.5-kb sequence (7). This type of polymorphism determines the size of the apo(a) protein owing to the presence of an exon within each of these repeats, and it may also affect apo(a) synthesis. Plasma levels of Lp(a) show a strong inverse correlation with the molecular weight of apo(a) (8), and recent evidence suggests that this relationship is due to the proportionally lower secretory efficiency of larger apo(a) molecules

(9). Additional sequence polymorphisms have been identified throughout the apo(a) locus (10–12) both in coding and 5′ flanking regions, possibly giving rise to further heterogeneity in levels and properties of apo(a).

Evidence for the connection between Lp(a) and atherosclerosis is derived from clinical as well as laboratory observations. Numerous cross-sectional and prospective studies have been undertaken to determine the relative atherosclerosis risk associated with Lp(a). Many of these studies have identified a positive correlation between relatively high levels of Lp(a) (<25 mg/dl) and coronary vessel occlusion (13–17), although two recent studies have refuted the significance of the correlation (18,19). Immunochemical analyses of atherosclerotic lesions in human arterial samples (20) and bypass grafts (21) have demonstrated marked accumulation of Lp(a). In addition, several recent studies have provided extensive experimental evidence of apo(a)'s affinity for vessel wall components (22); a characteristic which is central to most hypotheses accounting for the atherogenicity of Lp(a). Of the numerous potential interactions of apo(a) with vascular endothelial cells, the most compelling was realized through the cloning and sequencing of the apo(a) cDNA (23). This information revealed a high degree of homology between apo(a) and plasminogen (PMG), a protease zymogen involved in fibrinolysis. Most notably, both apo(a) and PMG contain cysteine-rich structural motifs known as kringles. Apo(a) contains multiple kringle domains highly homologous (75–85%) to PMG kringle 4 followed by one kringle domain homologous to PMG kringle 5. It is the variable number of kringle 4–like repeats in different apo(a) alleles which leads to the size heterogeneity of apo(a). Apo(a) also contains a protease domain 88% homologous to that of PMG with a conserved serine protease triad, but it does not exhibit significant proteolytic activity and cannot be activated owing to the lack of a functional zymogen cleavage site. This extensive sequence similarity between apo(a) and PMG supports a yet to be fully tested hypothesis that Lp(a) functions as a proatherogenic molecule by competitive inhibition of PMG binding and activation at the cell surface, disrupting important regulatory processes dependent on plasmin activity (i.e., fibrinolysis) (20,24).

Despite a variety of tantalizing hints concerning Lp(a)'s possible biological activity, it has been difficult to obtain direct in vivo evidence for the majority of hypotheses addressing its pathophysiological mechanism. This is, in large part, a result of the limited availability of animal models in which to study apo(a) and Lp(a). Presently, the apo(a) gene has been found in only one nonprimate species, the European hedgehog. The lack of apo(a) and Lp(a) in animals more commonly used in medical research (e.g., rodents, rabbits) has limited our ability to test in vivo hypotheses concerning the role of these molecules in atherogenesis.

Owing to the development of transgenic and gene-targeting technologies, the mouse has increasingly been used as a model of human disease states. The relatively recent application of this technology to the genetics of atherosclerosis susceptibility required the development of experimental atherogenic diets tolerated by mice and reproducible methods to quantify atheroma formation (25). The assessment of atherogenesis in mice where various candidate genes have been overexpressed or inactivated has provided many new insights into genetic factors leading to atherosclerosis (26). Generation of transgenic mice containing the components of Lp(a), apo(a), and apo B has begun to provide important insights into apo(a) and Lp(a) function with regard to atherogenesis, Lp(a) assembly, regulation of apo(a) gene expression and plasma levels, and the impact on the vasculature in vivo.

## II. CREATION OF TRANSGENIC MICE EXPRESSING COMPONENTS OF HUMAN Lp(a)

### A. apo(a) cDNA Construct

Chiesa et al. were the first to describe transgenic mice which expressed human apo(a) (27). The transgene construct in these studies contained the mouse transferrin promoter linked to an apo(a) cDNA encoding 17 kringle 4–like repeats. The transgene was shown to be expressed primarily in the liver of the resulting animals, and plasma levels of apo(a) were approximately 5 mg/dl. Although the use of the transferrin promoter precluded the analysis of normal factors regulating expression of this gene, studies of apo(a) in the plasma of these animals have provided important insights into the assembly of Lp(a), the atherogenic properties of apo(a), and the effect of apo(a) on plasminogen activation.

### B. apo(a) Genomic Construct

More recently, Frazer et al. created four separate lines of transgenic mice using a 270-kb yeast artificial chromosome (YAC) containing the entire 110-kb human apo(a) gene surrounded by greater than 60 kb of 5′ and 3′ flanking DNA (28). (YACs are large-insert cloning vectors that exist extrachromosomally in yeast and are capable of propagating over 1 Mb of foreign DNA.) The intact transfer of the native human apo(a) to the germline of mice has provided a valuable resource for studying the regulation of apo(a) gene expression. The transgene represents a different apo(a) allele than the one which produced the apo(a) cDNA transgene described above. It contains 12 kringle 4–like repeats, and thus it produces a somewhat smaller form of apo(a). Plasma levels of apo(a) in the different lines of transgenic mice ranged from 10 to 75 mg/dl and were subject to gender-specific changes during sexual maturation, suggesting a significant regulatory role for sex hormones in expression of the transgene. An additional feature of these mice which may prove useful in the future is their expression of the apo(a)-related gene C. Although its significance is unknown, this neighbor of apo(a) is known to be expressed in human liver (29), and this is also its site of synthesis in the transgenic mice.

## C.  apoB

One of the surprising findings first observed in the apo(a) cDNA transgenics, also noted in the apo(a) YAC transgenics, was the failure of human apo(a) to form a covalent association with LDL containing murine apoB. Thus, apo(a) circulated as a free glycoprotein in the plasma of these animals. Formation of Lp(a) was demonstrated in the apo(a) cDNA mice by infusion of human LDL (27), suggesting that murine apo(B) lacks structural features required for its covalent association with apo(a).

The importance of apoB in determining LDL structure, as well as in the interaction with apo(a), has driven persistent attempts to create transgenic mice expressing human apoB. Owing to the large size of the apoB gene (>40 kb), initial attempts to produce human apoB transgenic mice utilized apoB minigene and cDNA constructs. Unfortunately, these failed to generate mice expressing significant levels of the transgene. The difficulty in expressing apoB cDNA transgenes suggests that flanking or intronic genomic DNA sequences are required for efficient expression of this gene. The recent availability of P1 phagemid cloning vectors has enabled two groups to independently produce transgenic mice from P1 clones containing the entire apoB gene along with more than 15 kb of 5' and 3' flanking DNA (30,31). (P1 phagemids are bacteriophage-based cloning vectors capable of extrachromosomal propagation of 80–90 kb DNA sequences in bacteria.) A surprising feature of these mice was the expression of the human apoB transgene exclusively in the liver despite the fact that both human and murine apoB are normally also expressed in the intestine. This finding suggests that regulatory elements involved in the intestinal expression of apoB may be located extremely distal to its coding sequences.

In mice, apoB-containing lipoproteins (primarily triglyceride-rich very low-density lipoprotein [VLDL]) are found at low levels relative to HDL. Transgenic mice expressing high levels of human apoB (plasma level = 70 mg/dl) were shown to have high levels of LDL even when fed a mouse chow diet low in fat and cholesterol (30,31). These LDL particles were smaller and contained proportionally more triglyceride than human LDL, but on feeding a high-fat diet, the particle composition was altered from a triglyceride-rich to a cholesterol-rich particle similar in size to human LDL (32). Thus, relative to normal mice, human apoB transgenic mice possess a lipoprotein which more closely approximates that of humans.

## D.  Mice Producing Lp(a)

Mice expressing human apoB were bred with mice expressing either the human apo(a) cDNA or the apo(a) YAC transgene. In both cases, the apo(a)/apoB combined transgenics contained significant plasma levels of lipid-associated apo(a). Characterization of lipoprotein particles in these animals revealed Lp(a) particles virtually identical to Lp(a) particles found in the plasma of humans (30,31). Thus, by combining the apo(a) and apoB transgenes, it is possible to recapitulate the naturally occurring human Lp(a) in the plasma of mice.

## III.  ASSEMBLY OF Lp(a)

## A.  Insights from apoB Mutagenesis Studies

Although the cysteine of apo(a) involved in the disulfide bond with apoB has been identified as Cys4057 (2,3), studies have suggested a number of cysteine residues of apoB which might form the disulfide linkage. Guevara and colleagues used fluorescent probes to label free cysteine residues in Lp(a), as well as molecular modeling of apo(a) kringles 4–9 with candidate regions of apoB (33) indirectly to identify two cysteines, 3734 and 4190, both within the carboxyl terminal region of apoB, as potentially participating in the formation of a disulfide bond between apoB and apo(a). Studies examining the ability of various naturally occurring truncations of apoB to form the covalent association with apo(a) (34) and truncations induced by mutagenesis of apoB transgenes in mice (35) have suggested that the Cys4326 of apoB is involved in the formation of the disulfide bond with apo(a). These two approaches are indirect means for studying the amino acids from apoB involved in the interactions with apo(a). They both rely on assumptions regarding the unknown secondary structure of apoB, which may lead to experimental artifacts in the labeling studies and may not be valid in the carboxyl terminal deletion mutants of apoB. Recently, two studies have directly identified the cysteine whose removal by site-specific mutagenesis precludes human apoB's ability to interact with human apo(a) in vivo. Using site-specific mutagenesis of the 90-kb apoB P1 phage, Callow and Rubin examined the ability of Cys3734 and Cys4326 to form a disulfide bond with apo(a) in vivo. This study clearly demonstrated the requirement of Cys4326 in human apoB for the assembly of Lp(a), whereas removal of Cys3734 had no effect on Lp(a) assembly (36). Parallel studies on apoB manipulated as a YAC clone (37) showed the mutagenesis of the same cysteine, Cys4326, abolished Lp(a) assembly. These studies have demonstrated the power of the transgenic mouse system specifically to dissect in vivo the assembly of Lp(a) in a manner relevant to its native condition, as well as provide new and valid targets for possible approaches to inhibit this interaction.

## IV.  ATHEROGENESIS

### A.   apo(a) Transgenic Mice

Despite their failure to form Lp(a) particles, analysis of mice expressing a human apo(a) transgene has provided important insights into the in vivo properties of apo(a). Although apo(a) is normally lacking in mice, the apo(a) transgenics have a significantly increased risk for diet-induced atherosclerosis compared with nontransgenic control animals (38). Analysis of fatty streak lesions that develop in the apo(a) transgenics revealed the presence of colocalizing immunoreactive apo(a), suggesting a causative relationship between apo(a) and the formation of these lesions. This finding was most unexpected owing to the fact that the majority of apo(a) in these animals is free in the plasma and not associated with murine apoB and LDL. Since both apo(a) transgenic and nontransgenic control animals have nearly identical lipoprotein profiles, atherosclerosis in the transgenic mice suggest that the apo(a) component is at least partially responsible for the atherogenic properties attributed to Lp(a).

Reproducible atheroma formation in apo(a) transgenic mice provided the opportunity to test the effect of other lipoproteins on apo(a)-induced atherogenesis in these mice. In a recent study, Lieu et al. examined the effect of increasing HDL levels due to overexpression of a human apoAI transgene. These studies confirmed that apo(a) transgenic mice were more susceptible to fatty streak lesion formation, and they also found that that increased HDL was able to mitigate this effect (39). It should be noted that a recent attempt to reproduce atherosclerosis studies in apo(a) transgenic mice found no significant increase in lesion formation associated with apo(a) expression (40). These contrasting effects of the same apo(a) transgene on atherosclerosis in several studies (32,38–40) may be attributable to different atherosclerosis-susceptibility loci segregating into the hybrid background of mice used in the different experiments. YAC apo(a) transgenic mice have much higher levels of apo(a) and were produced in a pure FVB background. Forthcoming analysis of atherosclerosis in the mice should help to resolve this issue.

## B. Combined apoB/apo(a) Transgenics

Callow et al. recently compared atherosclerosis in mice containing apo(a) versus Lp(a) (32). A low-expressing human apoB transgenic founder line (17 mg/dl) was chosen for these studies in order to minimize the effect of excess apoB contributing to non-Lp(a) atherogenic lipoproteins. Without the apo(a) transgene, this low-level apoB transgenic background demonstrated a similar lipoprotein profile and susceptibility to diet-induced atherosclerosis when compared with non-transgenic control mice. In contrast, extensive lesions were found in the apo(a) alone and the combined apo(a)/apoB transgenics. Quantitation of the lesions revealed a statistically significant twofold increase in the combined apo(a)/apoB transgenics compared with mice expressing apo(a) alone. Several possibilities exist as to how the linkage of apo(a) and apoB leads to increased lesion development. When cholesterol-rich particles are physically associated with apo(a), cholesterol may be targeted directly to sites where the atherogenic properties of apo(a) are also active, thereby combining two atherogenic processes at a single site in the vessel wall. Alternatively, the increased atherosclerosis could be due to higher apo(a) plasma levels in human apoB transgenic mice. Further studies of the combined apo(a)/apoB transgenic mice will be necessary to discriminate between these possibilities.

## C. Plasmin Activity and Vascular Smooth Muscle Cell Proliferation

The demonstration of apo(a) effects on vessel wall pathophysiology, independent of the LDL moiety of Lp(a), supports the hypothesis that apo(a) promotes atherosclerosis by inhibiting vascular cell surface plasmin generation. Apo(a) transgenic mice have provided a means to test this hypothesis in vivo. Grainger et al. have recently shown that plasmin activity was significantly reduced in the vessel wall of apo(a) transgenic mice compared with nontransgenic littermates (41). Consistent with this observation, Palabrica et al. (42) reported increased clot dissolution time of radiolabeled blood clots introduced into the apo(a) transgenic mice. Along with the reduced plasmin activity in the apo(a) transgenic mice, Grainger et al. also observed a decrease in the active form of transforming growth factor (TGF-$\beta$), a growth factor known to inhibit growth and migration of smooth muscle cells (43). The effect was especially pronounced in areas prone to lesion development in these animals. These in vivo studies support the initial work of this group done with cultured vascular smooth muscle cells, where the decline in active TGF-$\beta$ was associated with proliferation of these cells (44).

## D. Genetic Interventions to Inhibit Lp(a) Assembly in apo(a)/apoB Transgenic Mice

Mice containing the native Lp(a) particle also will provide an excellent model system for testing various strategies to prevent assembly of Lp(a) or otherwise reduce its concentration in the plasma. Studies in both human apoB/apo(a) transgenic mice (30,31,35) and in humans (45) have suggested the availability of apoB100 is an important determinant of Lp(a) concentrations. Thus, reduction of apoB100 plasma concentration may provide a novel approach for lowering levels of this atherogenic lipoprotein. ApoB100 levels are naturally regulated in mice by posttranscriptional editing of apoB mRNA in the liver. Human apoB mRNA in the transgenic mice is also subject to this editing mechanism (30,31), which results in the formation of a truncated form of apoB (apoB48) that is unable to form a covalent linkage with apo(a). To test the hypothesis that increased apoB mRNA editing can reduce plasma levels of Lp(a), human apoB/apo(a) transgenic mice were treated with a recombinant adenovirus directing expression of apoBEC-1, the cytidine deaminase component of the apoB mRNA editing complex (46), and the in vivo effects on apoB, apo(a), and Lp(a) levels were examined. Results of this study indicated that transfer of apoBEC-1 can increase hepatic apoB mRNA editing in human apoB/apo(a) transgenic mice, causing a significant reduction in plasma levels of Lp(a) (47).

## V. REGULATION OF EXPRESSION IN THE apo(a) GENE

### A. Sex Hormones

As previously mentioned, the lack of animal models available to study apo(a) expression in vivo has severely limited studies of apo(a) gene regulation. Sex steroids are among the most extensively studied possible regulators of the human apo(a) gene with most, but not all, human studies suggesting they actually lower plasma apo(a) levels (48–50). The effect of sex steroids on apo(a) expression has been examined in animals containing the YAC apo(a) transgene. A series of controlled studies on how apo(a) levels were influenced in male mice by castration and subsequent androgen replacement clearly demonstrated that apo(a) increased severalfold following orchiectomy (28). This increase in plasma levels following orchiectomy was shown to be the result of increased transcription of the apo(a) gene. In order to further evaluate the role of sex hormones in regulating apo(a) gene expression, orchiectomized animals were treated with exogenous testosterone and estrogen analogues. In both cases, the introduction of androgens and estrogens into these animals resulted in a decrease in apo(a) plasma levels, as well as a decrease in transcription of the apo(a) gene.

These results observed in the mouse were somewhat parallel to human studies. Plasma levels of Lp(a) have been shown to increase in men treated with orchiectomy for prostate cancer (49). The finding that the apo(a) levels are lowered in the castrated mice treated with estrogen is also consistent with findings of the same study, where males with prostatic cancer demonstrate a 50% decrease in Lp(a) concentration in response to estrogen therapy. Thus, it appears that both androgens and estrogens in the transgenic mice repressed plasma levels of apo(a) in a manner similar to that observed in humans. This important confirmation of the human data in the YAC apo(a) transgenic mice supports the use of these animals as a substrate for examining factors affecting regulation of the apo(a) gene.

## B. Acute Phase Inducers

Human studies, although disputed, have suggested that apo(a) plasma levels may rise in response to trauma and, therefore, apo(a) may be considered a positive acute phase reactant. Consistent with this hypothesis is the presence of multiple interleukin-6 (IL-6) response element consensus sequences in the promoter region of the apo(a) gene (51). (IL-6 is a potent acute phase inducer.) Myocardial infarctions and other types of tissue injury, such as chronic atherosclerotic heart disease, are postulated to generate an acute phase response characterized by changes in plasma levels of acute phase reactant proteins. The behavior of apo(a) as an acute phase reactant has been a subject of some controversy in the literature. Studies by Maeda et al. (52) reported that plasma Lp(a) levels increased following myocardial infarctions in a manner consistent with positive acute phase reactants, whereas a study by Slunga et al. (53) found no evidence for Lp(a) behaving as a positive acute phase reactant. The ability to examine the effects of treatment with acute phase inducers in transgenic mice containing apo(a) in its native regulatory environment allowed this issue to be addressed in a manner not feasible in human studies. Injection of acute phase inducers into the apo(a) YAC transgenic mice did not result in increases in apo(a) mRNA or plasma levels, as would be predicted if apo(a) were a positive acute phase reactant (28). These results suggest that the rise in Lp(a) serum levels that has been observed in some individuals following myocardial infarction is probably not due to apo(a) acting as a positive acute phase protein but may be a secondary effect of other changes.

## VI. SUMMARY AND FUTURE DIRECTIONS

Transgenic mice expressing apo(a) and apoB have proven to be valuable resources for studying the biological properties of Lp(a) and the regulation of its plasma concentration. Apo(a)/apoB transgenic mice have allowed a very careful dissection of the interaction between apoB and apo(a), information which may eventually facilitate development of small molecule inhibitors Lp(a) assembly. The measurement of atherosclerosis in mice expressing the transgenes alone and in combination has provided insight into the contribution of the two components of Lp(a) to its pathogenic mechanism. Studies utilizing the apo(a) YAC transgenic mice have extended results from studies in humans on the roles that sex hormones and acute phase inducers play in the regulation of the apo(a) gene. The data indicating that sex hormones decrease apo(a) plasma concentrations agree with their previous hypothesized role. In contrast, the finding that acute phase inducers do not increase apo(a) plasma levels contradicts what their effect was predicted to be based on correlative studies in humans. Thus, the apo(a) YAC transgenic mice have been useful to examine the regulation of this important human atherosclerosis gene and may serve in the future as an invaluable substrate in the development of therapeutic agents which decrease apo(a) gene expression. The cloning of various apo(a) alleles coupled with the use of transgenic technology may eventually help researchers identify features of specific apo(a) alleles which render them more atherogenic than others, helping to resolve some of the controversy concerning the role of this molecule in vascular disease.

## REFERENCES

1. Berg K. A new serum type system in man: the Lp system. Acta Pathol Microbiol Scand 1963; 59:369–382.
2. Brunner C, Kraft H-G, Utermann G, Muller H-J. Cys$^{4057}$ of apolipoprotein(a) is essential for lipoprotein(a) assembly. Proc Natl Acad Sci USA 1993; 90: 11643–11647.
3. Koschinsky ML, Cote GP, Gabel B, van der Hoek YY. Identification of the cysteine residue in apolipoprotein(a) that mediates extracellular coupling with apolipoprotein B-100. J Biol Chem 1993; 268:19819–19825.
4. Boerwinkle E, Menzel H G, Kraft H G, Utermann G. Genetics of the quantitative Lp(a) lipoprotein trait. III. Contribution of Lp(a) glycoprotein phenotypes to normal lipid variation. Hum Gen 1989; 82:73–78.
5. Utermann G. The mysteries of lipoprotein(a). Science 1989; 246:904–910.
6. Boerwinkle E, Leffert CC, Lin J, Lackner C, Chiesa G, Hobbs HH. Apolipoprotein(a) gene accounts for greater than 90% of the variation in plasma lipoprotein(a) concentrations. J Clin Invest 1992; 90:52–60.
7. Lackner C, Boerwinkle E, Leffert CC, Rahmig T, Hobbs HH. Molecular basis of apolipoprotein(a) isoform size heterogeneity as revealed by pulsed-field gel electrophoresis. J Clin Invest 1991; 87:2153–2161.
8. Utermann G, Kraft HG, Menzel HJ, Hopferwieser T, Seitz C. Genetics of the

quantitative Lp(a) lipoprotein trait. I. Relation to Lp(a) glycoprotein phenotypes to Lp(a) lipoprotein concentrations in plasma. Hum Gen 1988; 78:41–46.

9. White AL, Hixson JE, Rainwater DL, Lanford RE, Molecular basis for "Null" lipoprotein(a) phenotypes and the influence of apolipoprotein(a) size on plasma lipoprotein(a) level in the baboon. J Biol Chem 1993; 269:9060–9066.

10. Cohen JC, Chiesa G, Hobbs HH. Sequence polymorphisms in the apolipoprotein(a) gene. J Clin Invest 1993; 91:1630–1636.

11. Scanu AM, Pfaffinger D, Klezowitch O, Edelstein C. Genetically-determined polymorphism of kringle iv-37 of human apolipoprotein(a). Circulation 1994; 90:619–623.

12. Mooser V, et al. Sequence polymorphisms in the apo(a) gene associated with specific levels of Lp(a) in plasma. Hum Mol Genet 1995; 4:173–181.

13. Sandkamp M, Funke H, Schulte H, Kohler E. Assmann. G. Lipoprotein(a) is an independent risk factor for myocardial infarction at a young age. Clin Chem 1990; 36:20–23.

14. Rhoads GG, Dahlen G, Berg K, Morton NE, Dannenberg AL. Lp(a) lipoprotein as a risk factor for myocardial infarction. JAMA 1986; 256: 2540–2544.

15. Dahlen GH, Guyton JR, Attar J, Farmer JA, Kautz JA, Gotto AM. Association of levels of lipoprotein Lp(a) plasma lipids, and other lipoproteins with coronary artery disease documented by angiography. Circulation 1986; 74:758–765.

16. Cremer P, Nagel D, Labrot B, Mann H, Muche R, Elster H, Seidel D. Lipoprotein Lp(a) as predictor of myocardial infarction in comparison to fibrinogen, LDL cholesterol and other risk factors: results from the prospective Gottingen Risk Incidence and Prevalence Study (GRIPS). Eur J Clin Invest 1994; 24:444–453.

17. Schaefer EJ, Lamon-Fava S, Jenner JL, et al. Lipoprotein(a) levels and risk of coronary heart disease in men. JAMA 1994; 271:999–1003.

18. Ridker PM, Hennekens CH, Stampfer MJ. A prospective study of lipoprotein(a) and the risk of myocardial infarction. JAMA 1993; 270:2195–2199.

19. Alfthan G, Pekkanen J, Jauhiainen M, et al. Relation of serum homocysteine and lipoprotein(a) concentrations to atherosclerotic disease in a prospective Finnish population based study. Atherosclerosis 1994; 106:9–19.

20. Hajjar KA, Gavish D, Breslow JL, Nachman RL. Lipoprotein(a) modulation of the endothelial cell surface fibrinolysis and its potential role in atherosclerosis. Nature 1989; 339:303–305.

21. Cushing GL, et al. Quantification and localization of apolipoprotein(a) and B in coronary artery bypass vein grafts resected at re-operation. Arteriosclerosis 1989; 9:593–603.

22. Nachman RL. Thrombosis and atherogenesis: molecular connections. Blood 1992; 79:1897–1906.

23. McLean JW, Tomlinson JE, Kuang WJ, et al. cDNA sequence of human apolipoprotein(a) is homologous to plasminogen. Nature 1987; 330:132–137.

24. Miles LA, Fless GM, Levin EG, Scanu AM, Plow EF. A potential basis for the thrombotic risk associated with lipoprotein(a). Nature 1989; 339:301–303.

25. Paigen B, Morrow A, Holmes PA, Mitchell D, Williams RA. Quantitative assessment of atherosclerotic lesions in mice. Atherosclerosis 1987; 68:231–40.
26. Rubin EM, Smith DJ. Getting to the Heart of a polygenic disorder: atherosclerosis in mice. Trends Genet 1994; 19:199–203.
27. Chiesa G, Hobbs HH, Koschinsky ML, Lawn RM, Maika SD, Hammer RE. Reconstitution of lipoprotein(a) by infusion of human low density lipoprotein into transgenic mice expressing human apolipoprotein(a). J Biol Chem 1992; 267:24369–24374.
28. Frazer KA, Narla G, Zhang JL, Rubin EM, The apolipoprotein(a) gene is regulated by sex hormones and acute-phase inducers in YAC transgenic mice. Nat Genet 1995; 9:424–431.
29. Byrne CD, Schwartz K, Meer K, Cheng J–F, Lawn RM. The human apolipoprotein(a)/plasminogen gene cluster contains a novel homologue transcribed in liver. Arterioscler Thromb 1994; 14:534–541.
30. Callow MJ, Stoltzfus LJ, Lawn RM, Rubin EM. Expression of human apolipoprotein B and assembly of lipoprotein(a) in transgenic mice. Proc Natl Acad Sci USA 1994; 91:2130–2136.
31. Linton MF, Farese Jr RV, Chiesa G, et al. Transgenic mice expressing high plasma concentrations of human apolipoprotein B100 and lipoprotein(a). J Clin Invest 1993; 92: 3029–3037.
32. Callow MJ, Verstuyft J, Rubin EM. Atherogenesis in transgenic mice with human apolipoprotein(a), apolipoprotein B, and lipoprotein(a). J Clin Invest 1995; 96:1639–1646.
33. Guevara JJ, Jan AY, Yang CY, et al. Proposed mechanisms for binding of apo(a) kringle type 9 to apo B-100 in human lipoprotein(a). Biophys J 1993; 64:686–700.
34. Gabel B, Yao Z, McLeod RS, Young SG, Koschinsky ML. Carboxyl-terminal truncation of apolipoproteinB-100 inhibits lipoprotein(a) particle formation. FEBS Lett 1994; 350:77–81.
35. McCormick SPA, Linton MF, Hobbs HH, Taylor S, Curtiss LK, Young SG. Expression of human apolipoprotein B90 in transgenic mice. J Biol Chem 1994; 269:24284–24289.
36. Callow MJ, Rubin EM. Site-specific mutagenesis demonstrates that Cysteine 4326 of apolipoprotein B is required for covalent linkage with apolipoprotein(a) in vivo. J Biol Chem 1995; 270:23914–23917.
37. McCormick SPA, Ng JK, Taylor S, Flynn LM, Hammer RE, Young SG. Mutagenesis of the human apolipoprotein B gene in a yeast artificial chromosome reveals the site of attachment of apolipoprotein(a). Proceedings, National Academy of Science 1995; 92:10147–10151.
38. Lawn RM, Wade DP, Hammer RE, Chiesa G, Verstuyft JG, Rubin EM. Atherogenesis in transgenic mice expressing human apolipoprotein (a). Nature 1992; 360:670–672.
39. Liu AC, Lawn RM, Verstuyft JG, Rubin EM. Human apolipoprotein A–I prevents atherosclerosis associated with apolipoprotein(a) in transgenic mice. J Lipid Res 1994; 35:2263–2267.

40. Mancini FP, Mooser V, Murata J, Newland D, Hammer RE, Sanan DA, Hobbs HH. Metabolism and atherogenicity of apo(a) in transgenic mice. Atherosclerosis 1995; 10:884–887.
41. Grainger DJ, Kemp PR, Liu AC, Lawn RM, Metcalfe JC. Activation of transforming growth factor $\beta$ is inhibited in transgenic apolipoprotein(a) mice. Nature 1994; 370:460–462.
42. Palabrica TM, Liu AC, Aronovitz MJ, Furie B, Furie BC, Lawn RM. Influence of human apo(a) expression on fibrinolysis in vivo in transgenic mice. Circulation 1994; 90:623.
43. Kojima S, Harpel PC, Rifkin DB. Lipoprotein(a) inhibits the generation of transforming growth factor $\beta$: an endogenous inhibitor of smooth muscle cell migration. J Cell Biol 1991; 113:1439–1445.
44. Grainger DJ, Kirschenlohr HL, Metcalfe JC, Weissberg PL, Wade DP, Lawn RM. Proliferation of human smooth muscle cells promoted by lipoprotein(a). Science 1993; 260:1655–1658.
45. Menzel HJ, Dieplinger H, Lacknert C, et al. Abetalipoproteinemia with an apoB-100-lipoprotein(a) glycoprotein complex in plasma. J Biol Chem 1990; 265:981–986.
46. Teng B, Burant CF, Davidson NO. Molecular cloning of an apolipoprotein B messenger RNA editing protein. Science 1993; 260:1816–1819.
47. Hughes SD, Rouy D, Navaratnam N, Scott J, Rubin EM. Gene transfer of cytidine deaminase p27 lowers lipoprotein(a) in transgenic mice and induces apolipoprotein B editing in rabbits. Hum Gene Ther 1996; 7:39–49.
48. Haffner SM, Mykkanen L, Gruber KK, Rainwater DL, Laakso M. Lack of association between sex hormones and Lp(a) concentrations in American and Finnish men. Arterioscler Thromb 1994; 14:19–24.
49. Henriksson P, Angelin B, Berglund L. Hormonal regulation of Serum Lp(a) levels. J Clin Invest 1992; 89:1166–1171.
50. Soma MR, Meschia M, Bruschi F, Morrisett JD, Paoletti R, Fumagalli R, Crosignani P. Hormonal agents used in lowering lipoprotein(a). Chem Phy Lipids 1992; 67:3451–350.
51. Wade DP, et al, 5' control regions of the apolipoprotein(a) gene and members of the related plasminogen gene family. Proc Natl Acad Sci USA 1993; 90: 1369–1373.
52. Maeda S, Abe A, Seishima M, Makino K, Noma A, Kawade M. Transient changes of serum lipoprotein(a) as an acute phase protein. Atherosclerosis 1989; 78:145–150.
53. Slunga L, Johnson O, Dahlen GH, Eriksson S. Lipoprotein(a) and acute-phase proteins in acute myocardial infarction. Scand J Clin Lab Invest 1992; 52:95–101.

# 18

# Gene Therapy with Vascular Endothelial Growth Factor

**Jeffrey M. Isner**

*Tufts University School of Medicine and St. Elizabeth's Medical Center,
Boston, Massachusetts*

## I.  INTRODUCTION

The therapeutic implications of angiogenic cytokines were identified by the pioneering work of Folkman and colleagues over two decades ago (1). Their work documented the extent to which tumor development was dependent on neovascularization and suggested that this relationship might involve angiogenic growth factors which were specific for neoplasms. Beginning a little over a decade ago (2), a series of polypeptide growth factors were purified, sequenced, and demonstrated to be responsible for natural as well as pathological angiogenesis. At least eight such factors have now been cloned (3).

More recent investigations have established the feasibility of using recombinant formulations of such angiogenic growth factors to expedite and/or augment collateral artery development in animal models of myocardial and hindlimb ischemia. This novel strategy for the treatment of vascular insufficiency, depicted schematically for peripheral vascular disease in Figure 1, has been termed *therapeutic angiogenesis* (4). The angiogenic growth factors first employed for this purpose comprised members of the fibroblast growth factor (FGF) family. Baffour et al. administered basic FGF (bFGF) in daily intramuscular doses of 1 or 3 $\mu$g to rabbits with acute hindlimb ischemia; at the completion of 14 days of treatment, angiography and necropsy measurement of capillary density showed evidence of augmented

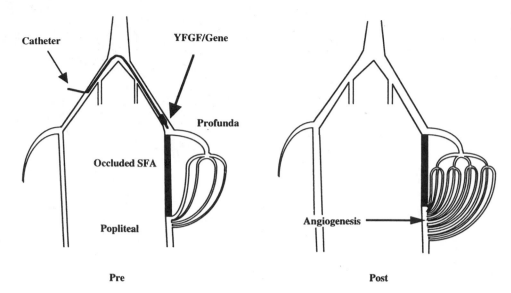

**Figure 1** Schematic depiction of strategy of therapeutic angiogenesis applied to lower extremity vascular insufficiency. Pretreatment (left): superficial femoral artery (SFA) of one leg is occluded. Percutaneous catheter techniques are employed to delivery your favorite growth factor (YFGF) or gene encoding that growth factor to the profunda artery which serves as stem artery for collateral vessels reconstituting the popliteal artery. Posttherapy (right): collateral network has increased to accommodate greater volume of blood transport to distal limb.

collateral vessels in the lower limb compared with controls (5). Pu et al. used acidic FGF (aFGF) to treat rabbits in which the acute effects of surgically induced hindlimb ischemia were allowed to subside for 10 days before beginning a 10-day course of daily 4-mg intramuscular injections; at the completion of 30 days follow-up, both angiographic and hemodynamic evidence of collateral development was superior to ischemic controls treated with saline (6). Yanagisawa-Miwa et al. likewise demonstrated the feasibility of bFGF for salvage of infarcted myocardium, but in this case, growth factor was administered intra-arterially at the time of coronary occlusion and followed 6 hr later by a second intra-arterial bolus (7).

We have used the same animal model developed by Pu et al. (6) to investigate the therapeutic potential of 45-kD dimeric glycoprotein, vascular endothelial growth factor (VEGF) isolated initially as a heparin binding factor secreted from bovine pituitary folliculo stellate cells (8). VEGF was also purified independently as a tumor-secreted factor that induced vascular permeability by the Miles assay (9,10), and thus its alternate designation, vascular permeability factor (VPF). Two features distinguish VEGF from other heparin binding, angiogenic growth factors. First, the $NH_2$ terminus of VEGF is preceded by a typical signal sequence; therefore, unlike bFGF, VEGF can be secreted by intact cells (11). Second, its high-affinity binding sites, shown to include the tyrosine kinase receptor *Flt-1* (12) and *Flk-1* /KDR (13,14) are present on endothelial cells but not other cell types; consequently, the mitogenic effects of VEGF—in contrast to acidic and basic FGF, both of which are known to be mitogenic for smooth muscle cells (15,16) and fibroblasts as well as endothelial cells—are limited to endothelial cells (8,17). (Interaction of VEGF with lower-affinity binding sites has been shown to induce mononuclear phagocyte chemotaxis) (18,19).

Evidence that VEGF stimulates angiogenesis in vivo had been developed in experiments performed on rat and rabbit cornea (20,21), the chorioallantoic membrane (8), and the rabbit bone graft model (21). We investigated the hypothesis that the angiogenic potential of VEGF was sufficient to constitute a therapeutic effect (22). The soluble 165–amino acid isoform of VEGF ($VEGF_{165}$) was administered as a single intra-arterial bolus to the internal iliac artery of rabbits in which the ipsilateral femoral artery was excised to induce severe, unilateral hindlimb ischemia. Doses of 500–1000 $\mu$g of VEGF produced statistically significant augmentation of angiographically visible collateral vessels and histologically identifiable capillaries; consequent amelioration of the hemodynamic deficit in the ischemic limb was significantly greater in animals receiving VEGF than in nontreated controls (calf blood pressure ratio=$0.75\pm0.14$ vs $0.48\pm0.19$, $p<.05$). Serial (baseline as well as 10 and 30 days post-VEGF) angiograms disclosed progressive linear extension of the collateral artery of origin (stem artery) to the distal point of parent-vessel (reentry artery) reconstitution in 7 of 9 VEGF-treated animals. Similar results were achieved in a separate series of experiments in which VEGF was administered by an intramuscular route daily for 10 days (23). More recent experiments established that site-specific angiogenesis may be achieved with systemic (i.e., intravenous) administration as well (24). These findings thus established proof of principle for the concept that the angiogenic activity of VEGF is sufficiently potent to achieve therapeutic benefit.

Although each of these studies documented an increase in the number of angiographically visible collaterals and increased capillary density in the muscles studied at necropsy, evidence regarding the physiological consequences of such anatomical improvement was initially limited to blood pressure measurements recorded in the ischemic versus the normal limb. Accordingly, we subsequently completed a series of studies in the ischemic hindlimb model in which an intra-arterial Doppler wire (25), sufficiently diminutive (0.018 in) to measure phasic blood flow velocity in the rabbit's internal iliac artery, was used to investigate resting and maximum flow following therapeutic angiogenesis with a single, intra-arterial bolus of $VEGF_{165}$. By 30 days post-$VEGF_{165}$, flow at rest as well as maximum flow velocity and maximum blood flow provoked by 2 mg papaverine were all significantly higher in the VEGF-treated group.

## II.  PRESERVATION OF ENDOTHELIUM–DEPENDENT VASOMOTOR TONE

Chronic perfusion through native coronary collaterals produces endothelial dysfunction in the recipient downstream, reconstituted vasculature (26). In vitro analyses indicated that collateral vessels themselves responded appropriately to endothelium-dependent agonists such as acetylcholine. In contrast, an abnormal response (reduced vasodilation to acetylcholine and ADP) was documented in microvessels (100–200 $\mu$m) perfused by mature collaterals as opposed to microvessels of the normal arterial circulation; the response of the microvessels perfused by mature collaterals to direct smooth muscle dilators (e.g., nitroglycerin) was not reduced (in fact was slightly enhanced). Sellke et al. (26) suggested that perfusion through coronary collaterals selectively alters the recipient, downstream arterial circulation, reducing endothelial cell membrane receptor affinity, number, or interaction with second-messenger systems in the recipient vessels. (The biosynthetic pathway, release, or degradation of endothelium-derived relaxing factor [EDRF] itself seemed not to be implicated owing to the fact that the response to the calcium ionophore A23187—which causes vasodilation by releasing EDRF through nonreceptor, non–second-messenger–mediated pathways—was preserved intact.) The basis for impaired endothelial regulation of collateral-dependent microvasculature remains enigmatic. It is possible that the collateral circulation fails to develop at a rate sufficiently rapid to prevent ischemic damage to endothelial cells (ECs) of the recipient downstream, reconstituted microvasculature. Alternatively, the receptor-mediated production or release of EDRF may be regulated by ambient blood pressure within the recipient vasculature; compromised blood pressure, with or without a pulsatile character, may further compromise deranged endothelium-dependent flow.

It is conceivable that augmented and/or expedited development of collaterals in response to administration of angiogenic growth factors may preserve, at least in part, endothelium-dependent modulation of distal vasomotor tone; if so, such a result would provide additional evidence for the functional utility of the collateral network resulting from therapeutic angiogenesis. To this point, Sellke et al. (27) have more recently reported preliminary findings suggesting that collateral arteries formed following administration of bFGF in an ameroid constrictor–induced coronary occlusive swine model do in fact, when harvested and studied ex vivo 5–8 weeks following constrictor placement, preserve endothelium-dependent relaxation in coronary microvessels subserved by the newly formed collaterals.

Our own studies performed in vivo using the intra-arterial Doppler flow guidewire have indicated that endothelium-dependent flow is markedly improved following therapeutic angiogenesis induced by VEGF (28). The response (increased flow) to endothelium-independent agonists (e.g., papaverine) is preserved both in ischemic limbs perfused by native collaterals as well as in ischemic limbs perfused by VEGF-induced collaterals; the magnitude of endothelium-independent response in VEGF-treated animals was, however, superior to that of nontreated ischemic controls.

## III. ARTERIAL GENE TRANSFER OF ANGIOGENIC CYTOKINES

More recently, we considered that one of the distinguishing features of VEGF mentioned above—the fact that the VEGF gene encodes a secretory signal sequence—might be exploited as part of a strategy designed to accomplish therapeutic angiogenesis by arterial gene transfer. We had previously observed that site-specific transfection of rabbit ear arteries with the plasmid pXGH5 encoding the gene for human growth hormone—a secreted protein—yields local levels of human growth hormone equivalent to what has been considered to be in a physiological range—despite the fact that immunohistochemical examination of the transfected tissue disclosed evidence of successful transfection in <1% of cells in the transfected arterial segment (29). Thus, gene products which are secreted may have profound biological effects even when the number of transduced cells remains low. In contrast, for genes such as bFGF which do not encode a secretory signal sequence, transfection of a much larger cell population might be required for that intracellular gene product to express its biological effects.

We therefore applied 400 $\mu$g of phVEGF$_{165}$, encoding the 165–amino acid isoform of VEGF, to the hydrogel layer coating the outside of an angioplasty balloon (30) and delivered the balloon catheter percutaneously to the iliac artery of rabbits in which the femoral artery had been excised to cause hindlimb ischemia (Fig. 2). Site-specific transfection of phVEGF$_{165}$ was confirmed by analysis of the transfected internal iliac arteries using reverse transcriptase-polymerase chain reaction (RT-PCR) (31) and then sequencing the RT-PCR product. Augmented development of collateral vessels was documented by serial angiograms in vivo and increased capillary density at necropsy. Consequent amelioration of the hemodynamic

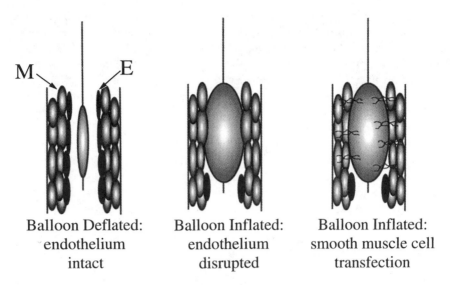

Balloon Deflated:     Balloon Inflated:     Balloon Inflated:
endothelium         endothelium     smooth muscle cell
intact              disrupted         transfection

**Figure 2** Schematic depiction of gene transfer using hydrogel polymer–coated angioplasty balloon. Balloon inflation leads to endothelial (E) denudation. Extensive endothelial disruption exposes smooth muscle cells of arterial media (M), which are then transfected on balloon inflation.

deficit in the ischemic limb was documented by improvement in the calf blood pressure ratio (ischemic/normal limb) to $0.70 \pm 0.08$ in the VEGF-transfected group versus $0.50 \pm 0.18$ in controls ($p < .05$). These findings thus established that site-specific arterial gene *transfer* can be used to achieve physiologically meaningful *therapeutic* modulation of vascular disorders, including therapeutic angiogenesis.

These potential options are made all the more intriguing by the isoform differences that characterize VEGF biology. At least four isoforms—VEGF$_{121}$, VEGF$_{165}$, VEGF$_{189}$, and VEGF$_{206}$—have been identified and shown to result from alternative splicing of the VEGF transcript (32). These isoforms all share the important biological property of mitogenicity for ECs, but they differ markedly in one important respect: The longer the isoform, the more basic amino acid residues, the greater is the avidity for cell-surface heparan sulfates and proteoglycans of the extracellular matrix. Consequently, despite the presence of a secretion signal, the longer isoforms are *not* freely secreted but remain almost completely bound to the cell surface or surrounding extracellular matrix. The 121 isoform, in contrast, is freely soluble. We are currently investigating the potential impact of this issue on the outcome of therapeutic angiogenesis.

## IV. CELLULAR PROLIFERATION FOLLOWING ANGIOGENIC CYTOKINES

The paradigm for new blood vessel growth, elegantly outlined by D'Amore and Thompson (33), suggests that the initiating feature of angiogenesis is the "activation" of ECs within a parent vessel, followed by disruption of the parent vessel's basement membrane, and subsequent migration of the ECs into the interstitial space, possibly in the direction of an ischemic stimulus. Concomitant and/or subsequent EC proliferation, intracellular-vacuolar lumen formation, pericyte "capping," and the production of a basement membrane complete the developmental sequence. It is intriguing to note that a very preliminary feature of this model—a feature which is viewed, in fact, as preliminary to mobilization of the ECs—includes "increased vascular permeability" (33); this, of course, was on of the initial properties identified for VEGF and accounts for its alternative nomenclature, "vascular permeability factor" (34–36). It also should be noted that this paradigm is typically applied to new capillary formation, or angiogenesis, a process that some have suggested may be distinct from the formation of larger blood vessels, or vasculogenesis (37).

The relative contribution of proliferation versus migration of ECs to angiogenesis is in fact controversial. Sholley et al. (38), using a model of inflammation-induced neovascularization of the rat cornea, demonstrated that initial vascular sprouting does not require EC proliferation. EC proliferation in this model was suppressed by x-irradiation with 2000 or 8000 rad prior to application of the inflammatory stimulus. In irradiated corneas displaying no cellular proliferation, vascular sprouting at 2 days was similar to that seen in contralateral shielded corneas. Although vascular ingrowth was subsequently blunted and ultimately ceased by 4–7 days, these experiments documented the critical, if not exclusive, roles of migration and redistribution of existing ECs in the commencement of neovascularization. Similar implications resulted from work by Nicosia et al. (39): Fibronectin was shown to promote, in a dose-dependent fashion, the elongation of microvessels which sprout from explants of rat aorta placed in serum-free collagen gel—despite the fact that neither DNA synthesis nor mitotic activity was increased in comparison with fibronectin-negative gels. Fibronectin was therefore inferred to promote angiogenesis in vitro by migratory recruitment of ECs.

In contrast to these in vivo inflammatory and in vitro organ culture models of neovascularization, angiogenesis which develops in response to experimental vascular obstruction, that is, collateral vessel development, has been shown by several previous investigators to involve proliferation of not only ECs but SMCs as well (40). Several important principles were suggested by these studies.

First, evidence of EC proliferation is nearly absent in normal arteries (41); a finding which is consistent with an estimated EC turnover time of "thousands of days" in quiescent microvasculature (3). Even a relatively low percentage of EC proliferation observed in response to arterial occlusion or exogenous growth factors may therefore represent considerable enhancement of EC proliferative activity, and, when considered in relation to a denominator of thousands of ECs, is clearly sufficient to provide the basis for new blood vessel formation. Second, peak EC proliferation which contributes to collateral development in the setting of vascular occlusion varies from 2.6 to 3.5% in the canine coronary circulation (41,42); from 5 to 6% in the rodent renal vasculature (43,44); and is <1% in swine coronaries (45). The contrasting rates of EC proliferation between the canine and swine coronary circulations are indeed representative of the contrasting propensity for collateral artery development in these two species. Third, proliferation of smooth muscle cells (SMCs), the additional requisite cell type for the formation of larger blood vessels ("vasculogenesis"), is an implicit component of neovascularization regardless of animal species or circulatory site. Schaper et al. in fact speculated nearly 25 years ago that, ". . . it is tempting to assume that EC proliferation not only serves the purpose of forming the endothelium of a finally larger artery but rather actively participates in the development of the tunica media" (46). Fourth, proliferative activity—for SMCs as well as ECs—is highest at the level of the smallest diameters of the collateral vessels; namely the so-called midzone collateral segments (41–43,46).

Limited investigation has been performed regarding the extent to which EC and/or SMC proliferation are altered by interventions designed to *augment* native collateral vessel development; that is, therapeutic angiogenesis (22). Graham et al. established arteriovenous fistulas at the popliteal level in a canine model of hindlimb ischemia, following which the vein proximal to the arteriovenous anastomosis was ligated; this so-called "arteriovenous reversal" was designed to augment perfusion to the distal limb in a retrograde manner (47). A consistent feature of this procedure (in humans [48] as well as animals) was the development of an extensive network of new vessels in the proximity of the arteriovenous anastomosis. A significant increase in the uptake of tritiated thymidine, administered 3 hr prior to death, was observed in those hindlimbs treated by arteriovenous reversal versus controls, and together with histological evidence of increased capillary density, this was interpreted as evidence for therapeutically augmented EC proliferation. More recently, Unger et al. (49) administered bromodeoxyuridine (BrdU) to dogs in which collateral artery development had been provoked by the application of an ameroid constrictor around the left circumflex coronary artery; following administration of bFGF directly into the circumflex distal to the constrictor, cellular proliferation was found to be increased in both collateral-dependent viable myocardium and infarcts. Based on morphology and location, cells immunopositive for BrdU were judged to consist predominantly of ECs.

We investigated the contribution and sequence of cellular proliferation to the natural process of collateral vessel development in a rabbit hindlimb model of lower extremity ischemia and determined the extent to which this is modified by therapeutic angiogenesis (50). Proliferative activity (BrdU index) among collateral arteries developing in the untreated, ischemic limbs of control animals varied from 0 to 3.3% in the stem segments; from 0 to 4.1% in the midzone segments; and from 0 to 3.6% in the reentry segments. Thus, regardless of anatomical site, EC proliferation varied between 0 and 4.1% per day, which is similar to the range reported previously by Pasyk et al. (42) and White et al. (45) for canine and swine coronary artery collaterals, respectively. EC proliferation among the controls failed to reach statistical significance for any individual collateral zone or time point. For SMCs, proliferative activity among the control animals was even lower in the stem and reentry zones; the degree of proliferative activity in the midzone was similar to that of ECs and thereby significantly greater than that of the stem and reentry zones. With regard to time course, however, no significant variation was observed.

Administration of VEGF was shown to augment EC proliferation in the midzone collateral vessels by roughly threefold compared with control animals; this difference was most profound—and statistically significant—at day 5 post-VEGF. The increase in EC proliferation observed at day 5 post-VEGF was followed by reduction of hemodynamic deficit in the ischemic limb by day 7, which is consistent with improved collateral artery development after VEGF therapy. In the stem arteries, EC proliferation was quite high (up to 11.4%) in selected cases, but it did not reach statistical significance for the treated group as a whole. At the level of the reentry arteries, EC proliferation among VEGF-treated animals was in no case >2.6%. Thus, a statistically significant increase in EC proliferation in response to VEGF versus controls was limited to the midzone collaterals. These findings suggest that the locus of augmented EC proliferation consequent to therapeutic angiogenesis is similar to that previously noted during naturally occurring collateral development (41); namely, the smallest diameter, or midzone, collateral vessels.

Despite the fact that the mitogenic effects of VEGF have been previously shown to be limited to ECs (8,17), the proliferative activity of SMCs in the midzone collaterals also increased by approximately threefold. The augmentation in midzone SMC proliferation was statistically significant compared with the degree of SMC proliferation observed in naturally occurring collateral artery and exceeds that reported in previous studies (41,-42,45) as well. Although VEGF has been shown to interact with lower-affinity binding sites to induce mononuclear phagocyte chemotaxis (18,19), higher-affinity binding sites presumed to mediate the mitogenic effects of VEGF are limited to ECs (8,17). Increased SMC proliferation observed in response to VEGF is therefore not likely to represent a direct effect of VEGF. Two indirect effects are possible. The ability to induce vascular permeability is a well-known feature of VEGF that is responsible in fact for its alternate designation as vascular permeability factor (VPF) (9,21,51). It is possible that extravasation of certain angiogenic growth factors from circulating blood might result in the activation of SMC proliferation. Alternatively, ECs stimulated by VEGF may secrete factor(s) that promote SMC proliferation. It has been previously shown, for example, that VEGF induces expression of tissue-type plasminogen activators (tPA)—a potent mitogen for cultured human SMCs (52)—in cultured bovine microvascular ECs (53). Platelet-derived growth factor (PDGF), a mitogen and chemoattractant for vascular SMCs (54) which is expressed by ECs (55–57), has been previously shown to be induced in human umbilical vein ECs by the addition of another angiogenic growth factor, acidic fibroblast growth factor (aFGF) (58); it is entirely possible that VEGF may have a similar effect.

## V.  DIRECT VERSUS INDIRECT CYTOKINES

Certain stimuli capable of inducing the development of neovessels in vivo, specifically certain cytokines (15,59,60) and hypoxia, fail to stimulate EC proliferation in vitro, suggesting a role for additional mediators and/or cell types. We considered whether these so-called *indirect* angiogenic growth factors might stimulate vascular SMCs to express genes encoding *direct* EC mitogens. Such a sequential cascade would provide a mechanism by which growth factors which are otherwise nonmitogenic or frankly inhibitory for EC proliferation in vitro could instead stimulate angiogenesis in vivo. We identified two principal candidates as potential mediators of this phenomenon: VEGF, a secreted angiogenic growth factor which, as discussed earlier, is exclusively mitogenic for ECs (11); and bFGF, a nonsecreted angiogenic polypeptide capable not only of inducing neovascularization but also known to stimulate SMC proliferation and hyperplasia (61,62).

Although plate-derived growth factor (PDGF) BB, for example, can directly stimulate proliferation of selected populations of microvascular ECs in vitro (63–65), ECs from most vascular districts do not respond to treatment with PDGF BB (66). Nonetheless, in vivo PDGF BB has been clearly demonstrated to induce supportive angiogenesis in both a wound-healing model (67) and chorioallantoic membrane assay (60). More recently, Sundberg et al. have observed that pericytes, a cell type structurally and functionally similar to vascular SMCs and often associated with ECs in the capillary sprouts that form during angiogenesis (68), express PDGF type B receptors in vivo (69). Furthermore, microvascular ECs isolated from rat epididymal fat pads and *not directly responsive* to PDGF BB stimulation when cocultured with myofibroblasts from the same tissue source form capillary chords in the presence of PDGF BB (70). The angiogenic action of PDGF BB documented in this way was attributed to the production of soluble EC mitogen(s) by myofibroblasts in response to stimulation with PDGF BB (70).

We demonstrated that the PDGF BB treatment of human vascular SMCs concurrently induces VEGF and bFGF mRNA species (71). This finding indicates that PDGF BB, a known mitogen for SMCs, could also stimulate SMCs to produce direct angiogenic factors and thereby promote angiogenesis.

The plurality of mechanisms that contribute to the angiogenic activity of transforming growth factor-$\beta$1 (TFG-$\beta$1) (59) has been the subject of intense investigation. Although clearly inhibiting growth and migration of subconfluent ECs in vitro (72), TGF-$\beta$1 facilitates capillary formation in vivo (59). Furthermore, TGF-$\beta$1 modulates the composition of the extracellular matrix (73) and may therefore act in part by locally creating a proangiogenic environment. Although TGF-$\beta$1 directly inhibits EC proliferation (72), it may nevertheless direct organization of ECs into tube-like structures depending on conditions of culture tested (74). TGF-$\beta$1 in high concentrations was found to inhibit the formation of capillary-like structures in an in vitro model of angiogenesis, whereas low doses were observed to potentiate VEGF- or bFGF-induced neovessel formation in the same assay system (72). This phenomenon was interpreted by Pepper et al. as an example of "contextual" angiogenesis to indicate that the angiogenic response to a given cytokine is dependent on the presence and concentration of other mediators in the pericellular environment of the target ECs. Finally, Winkles et al. have also observed the TGF-$\beta$1 stimulates bFGF expression by SMCs; thus supporting the notion that direct angiogenic mediators (75) might contribute in part to TGF-$\beta$1–induced angiogenesis. Our finding (71) that TGF-$\beta$1 stimulation induces VEGF as well as bFGF gene expression, in concert with the above-described mechanisms, suggests that *both* EC mitogens are likely instrumental for mediating the indirect angiogenic effects of TGF-$\beta$1 in vivo.

Hypoxia is generally considered to represent a fundamental stimulus for angiogenesis, although the mechanism(s) responsible for its angiogenic activity remain enigmatic. Increased expression of VEGF at the periphery of necrotic foci of certain neoplasms as well as hypoxia-stimulated induction of

VEGF in cultured cells from glial tumor and rat skeletal muscle have been reported previously (76). We investigated whether, in addition to VEGF, hypoxia might also regulate bFGF gene expression and found that low $O_2$ tension selectively modulates VEGF but not bFGF in vascular SMCs (71) and endothelial cells (77). This observation is intriguing in light of homology between a sequence in the VEGF promoter and a nucleotide sequence in the erythropoietin promoter identified as a binding site for an hypoxia-specific transcription factor (HIF-1). More recently, we have determined that conditioned media from hypoxic myoblasts and/or smooth muscle cells upregulates VEGF receptor (KDR expression) (78); in contrast, certain cytokines, for example, tumor necrosis factor–alpha (TNF-$\alpha$), downregulate KDR expression (B. Witzenbichler and J. Isner, unpublished data).

## VI.  SYNERGISM OF ANGIOGENIC CYTOKINES

Recent reports have demonstrated potent synergism between VEGF and bFGF for the development of microvessel-like structures in two different experimental models of in vitro angiogenesis (53,79). Our finding of the concurrent induction of VEGF and bFGF in human vascular SMCs suggests that such synergism may effectively operate under a variety of physiological or pathological conditions characterized by increased levels of either PDGF BB or TGF-$\beta$1. To our knowledge, this is the first report of concomitant regulation of VEGF and bFGF gene expression by otherwise normal human cells. This finding thus provides further support for Pepper's (72) concept of "contextual" angiogenesis.

Previous studies from several groups disclosed evidence for a synergistic effect of growth factors on angiogenesis in vitro. Pepper et al. (72) demonstrated that whereas endothelial cell migration and capillary lumen formation were inhibited by TGF-$\beta$1 alone, a lower concentration of TGF-$\beta$1 potentiated the effect of bFGF- and VEGF-induced migration. Furthermore, those same investigators (53) demonstrated that adding VEGF or bFGF to microvascular endothelial cells grown on the surface of three-dimensional collagen gels induced the cells to invade the underlying matrix and form capillary-like tubules. When these same two mitogens were added simultaneously, however, they induced an angiogenic response which was far greater than additive, and which occurred with greater rapidity than the response to either cytokine alone. Goto et al. (79) measured the combined effect of VEGF and bFGF on both the proliferative and morphological changes exhibited by bovine capillary endothelial cells cultured in a gel of type I collagen; when the two factors were added simultaneously, both the number of cells and the number of cord-like structures were greater than the sum of those stimulated with either growth factor alone.

Results of in vivo studies performed in our laboratory (80,81) are in agreement with these previous in vitro experiments. When the magnitude of collateral development in ischemic limbs of treated rabbits was compared with spontaneous collateral formation seen in control animals, coadministration of VEGF and bFGF produced an increase in vascularity that was greater than the sum of the effects observed with either growth factor alone for all indices studied.

Anatomical evidence of neovascularity was investigated at two levels. Necropsy examination documented an increase in vascularity at the capillary level, which is consistent with the classic definition of angiogenesis formulated by Klagsbrun and Folkman (82). We also assessed the diameter and number of angiographically visible collateral vessels by systematic quantification of the angiographic examinations. These analyses documented that the angiographic luminal diameter of the stem artery was significantly greater in the group treated with VEGF + bFGF than VEGF or bFGF alone. Although the angiographic score of VEGF, bFGF, and VEGF + bFGF was superior to that observed in controls, coadministration of these cytokines did not achieve the same magnitude of improvement over independent cytokine treatment in angiographic score demonstrated for the other indices cited above.

The potential therapeutic benefit of stimulating formation of larger, more "mature" collaterals is suggested by the physiological evidence of increased downstream perfusion documented on serial measurements of the lower limb blood pressure ratio. The dramatic increase in blood pressure ratio in the VEGF and bFGF group between day 0 and day 10 compared with that seen following administration of either growth factor alone is likely to be a consequence of better arterial reconstitution in the combined therapy group. This conclusion is further supported by recent findings in our laboratory in which the combination of VEGF + bFGF has been found to have a synergistic effect on maximum flow reserve in this same animal model compared with bFGF or VEGF alone (C. Bauters, unpublished observations). The physiological consequences of increased capillary density within the ischemic muscles were not assessed independently in the present study. It seems plausible, however, that such increased microvascular capacity should, for a similar level of blood flow, allow better oxygen extraction by the ischemic muscles and, consequently, better muscle performance.

The fundamental basis for the synergistic effect of VEGF and bFGF in vivo remains to be elucidated. Although VEGF is endothelial cell specific, bFGF is also a potent mitogen for a variety of other cell types, including SMCs. Wilting et al. (83), for example, compared the effects of VEGF and bFGF on in vivo angiogenesis in the chick chorioallantoic membrane and demonstrated that VEGF induced vigorous EC proliferation, whereas bFGF elicited primarily fibrocyte proliferation with only minor endothelial cell proliferation. A direct stimulation of SMCs by bFGF might be responsible for some of the in vivo effects we observed, such as the statistically significant increase in the angiographic luminal diameter of the stem artery.

Conversely, the increase in capillary density and capillary/muscle fiber ratio in the ischemic muscles is more likely to be a consequence of a synergistic effect on endothelial cells similar to that observed in the previously cited in vitro experiments. It is important in this regard to underscore the independent receptor systems responsible for signaling the mitogenic effects of VEGF and bFGF in endothelial cells. Two tyrosine kinases, the *fms*-like tyrosine kinase (*Flt-1*) (12) and the kinase domain region (KDR) (14) proteins, have been shown to bind VEGF with high affinity. An independent dual receptor system comprising cell surface heparan sulfate proteoglycans and high-affinity tyrosine kinase receptors modulates the activity of bFGF (84). Thus, amplification of the endothelial response to these mitogens is feasible based on their independent receptor systems alone.

Park et al. (85) have recently proposed another possible basis for synergism among angiogenic growth factors. They demonstrated that the 152–amino acid isoform of placenta growth factor (PlGF) potentiates the action of low, marginally efficacious concentrations of VEGF on EC growth in vitro; and in vivo potentiates Evans blue dye extravasation observed in a Miles assay. Although PlGF binds with high affinity to *Flt-1*, it does not bind to the KDR receptor. The latter receptor appears to account for most bioactivity induced by VEGF. These investigators thus suggested that potentiation in this case might be the result of the *Flt-1* receptor behaving as a "decoy"; that is, binding either ligand but having little or no transducing activity. PlGF might therefore act to release VEGF from *Flt-1* and increase its availability to the more relevant KDR receptor. Because PlGF failed to potential low doses of bFGF, these findings were interpreted to be specific for VEGF. Whether an as yet unidentified high-affinity receptor for VEGF/bFGF could similarly contribute to the synergism we observed remains to be investigated.

We assessed the extent of neointimal thickening in the internal iliac artery of animals receiving VEGF, bFGF, and VEGF + bFGF at day 30 and found no evident differences among the three experimental groups. Whereas VEGF is an endothelial cell–specific mitogen, Lindner et al. (61) have demonstrated that systemic administration of bFGF is a potent mitogen for SMCs in arteries denuded by a balloon catheter: Prolonged administration of bFGF ($12\mu$g/day for 2 weeks) after balloon denudation of the rat carotid artery caused an approximately twofold increase in intimal thickening. In the current study, the use of single-bolus administration, a lower does of bFGF (10 $\mu$g/rabbit), and no prior balloon denudation may explain the absence of neointimal thickening. In addition, a recently described protective effect of VEGF in diminishing intimal hyperplasia by expediting endothelial "repaving" after balloon injury (80) may further offset any potentially adverse effects of bFGF. These results suggest that it might be possible to determine a dosing regimen of angiogenic growth factors that will increase vascularity while causing minimal deleterious effects in terms of local progression of atherosclerosis.

## VII. SUMMARY

The therapeutic potential of angiogenic cytokines in patients with cardiovascular disease remains to be fully defined. Current clinical investigation (86) involving arterial gene transfer of VEGF for patients with peripheral artery disease is likely to be followed by trials of gene transfer or recombinant protein administration of other angiogenic cytokines for coronary and possibly cerebrovascular disease (87). Concurrent laboratory studies will hopefully clarify the manner in which the signal transduction pathways, receptor-ligand interactions, and multicytokine cascades can be modulated to optimize the host response.

Angiogenic cytokines constitute a potentially novel form of therapy for patients with cardiovascular disease. The feasibility of using recombinant formulations of angiogenic growth factors to expedite and/or augment collateral artery development in animal models of myocardial and hindlimb ischemia—therapeutic angiogenesis—has now been well established. These studies have suggested that two angiogenic growth factors in particular, basic fibroblast growth factor and vascular endothelial growth factor, are sufficiently potent to merit further investigation. More recently, experiments performed in our laboratory have indicated that in the case of VEGF, a secreted protein, similar results may be achieved by percutaneous arterial gene transfer. Further laboratory and clinical studies may yield promising insights into the fundamental basis for native as well as therapeutic angiogenesis and at the same time more explicitly define the manner in which therapeutic angiogenesis may be successfully incorporated into clinical practice.

## ACKNOWLEDGMENT

The contributions of Satoshi Takeshita, Takayuki Asahara, Yukio Tsurumi, Edi Brogi, Lu Zheng, Christophe Bauters, Marianne Kearney, Napoleone Ferrara, Stuart Bunting, and James Symes to the work described in this chapter are gratefully acknowledged.

# REFERENCES

1. Folkman J. Tumor angiogenesis: therapeutic implications. N Engl J Med 1971; 285:1182–1186.
2. Shing Y, Folkman J, Sullivan J, Butterfield R, Murray J, Klagsbrun M. Heparin-affinity purification of a tumor-derived capillary endothelial cell growth factor. Science 1984; 223:1296–1299.
3. Folkman J, Shing Y. Angiogenesis. J Biol Chem 1993; 267:10931–10934.
4. Hockel M, Schlenger K, Doctrow S, Kissel T, Vaupel P. Therapeutic angiogenesis. Arch Surg 1993; 128:423–429.
5. Baffour R, Berman J, Garb JL, Rhee S., Kaufman J, Friedmann P. Enhanced angiogenesis and growth of collaterals by in vivo administration of recombinant basic fibroblast growth factor in a rabbit model of acute lower limb ischemia: dose-response effect of basic fibroblast growth factor. J Vasc Surg 1992; 16:181–191.
6. Pu LQ, Sniderman AD, Brassard R, et al. Enhanced revascularization of the ischemic limb by means of angiogenic therapy. Circulation 1993; 88:208–215.
7. Yanagisawa-Miwa A, Uchida Y, Nakamura F, et al. Salvage of infarcted myocardium by angiogenic action of basic fibroblast growth factor. Science 1992; 257:1401–1403.
8. Ferrara N, Henzel WJ. Pituitary follicular cells secrete a novel heparin-binding growth factor specific for vascular endothelial cells. Biochem Biophys Res Commun 1989; 161:851–855.
9. Keck PJ, Hauser SD, Krivi G, et al. Vascular permeability factor, an endothelial cell mitogen related to PDGF. Science 1989; 246:1309–1342.
10. Connolly DR, Olander JV, Heuvelman D, et al. Human vascular permeability factor: isolation from U937 cells. J Biol Chem 1989; 264:20017–20024.
11. Leung DW, Cachianes G, Kuang WJ, Goeddel DV, Ferrara N. Vascular endothelial growth factor is a secreted angiogenic mitogen. Science 1989; 246:1306–1309.
12. deVries C, Escobedo JA, Ueno H, Houck K, Ferrara N, Williams LT. The *fms*-like tyrosine kinase, a receptor for vascular endothelial growth factor. Science 1992; 255:989–991.
13. Millauer B, Wizigmann-Voos S, Schnurch H, et al. High affinity VEGF binding and developmental expression suggest *Flk-1* as a major regulator of vasculogenesis and angiogenesis. Cell 1993; 72:835–846.
14. Terman BI, Dougher-Vermozen M, Carrion ME, et al. Identification of the KDR tyrosine kinase as a receptor for vascular endothelial growth factor. Biochem Biophys Res Commun 1992; 187:1579–1586.
15. Klagsbrun M, D'Amore PA. Regulators of angiogenesis. Annu Rev Physiol 1991; 53:217–239.
16. Reidy MA, Clowes AW, Schwartz SM. Endothelial regeneration V. inhibition of endothelial regrowth in arteries of rat and rabbit. Lab Invest 1983; 49: 569–575.
17. Conn G, Soderman D, Schaeffer M-T, Wile M, Hatcher VB, Thomas KA.

Purification of glycoprotein vascular endothelial cell mitogen from a rat glioma cell line. Proc Natl Acad Sci USA 1990; 87:1323–1327.

18. Shen H, Clauss M, Ryan J, et al. Characterization of vascular permeability factor/vascular endothelial growth factor receptors on mononuclear phagocytes. Blood 1993; 81:2767–2773.
19. Clauss M, Gerlach M, Gerlach H, et al. Vascular permeability factor: A tumor-derived polypeptide that induces endothelial cell and monocyte procoagulant activity, and promotes monocyte migration. J Exp Med 1990; 172:1535–1545.
20. Levy AP, Tamargo R, Brem H, Nathans D. An endothelial cell growth factor from the mouse neuroblastoma cell line NB41. Growth Factors 1989; 2:9–19.
21. Connolly DT, Hewelman DM, Nelson R, et al. Tumor vascular permeability factor stimulates endothelial cell growth and angiogenesis. J Clin Invest 1989; 84:1470–1478.
22. Takeshita S, Zheng LP, Brogi E, et al. Therapeutic angiogenesis: a single intraarterial bolus of vascular endothelial growth factor augments revascularization in a rabbit ischemic hind limb model. J Clin Invest 1994; 93:662–670.
23. Takeshita S, Pu LQ, Stein LA, et al. Intramuscular administration of vascular endothelial growth factor induces dose-dependent collateral artery augmentation in a rabbit model of chronic limb ischemia. Circulation 1994; 90 (Part 2):II-228–II-234.
24. Bauters C, Asahara T, Zheng LP, et al. Site-specific therapeutic angiogenesis following systemic administration of vascular endothelial growth factor. J Vasc Surg 1995; 21:314–325.
25. Bauters C, Asahara T, Zheng LP, et al. Physiologic assessment of augmented vascularity induced by VEGF in rabbit ischemic hindlimb. Am J Physiol 1994; 36:H1263–H1271.
26. Sellke FW, Quillen JE, Brooks LA, Harrison DG. Endothelial modulation of the coronary vasculature in vessels perfused via mature collaterals. Circulation 1990; 81:1938–1947.
27. Sellke FW, Harada K,Wang SY, et al. Basic Fibroblasts growth factor preserves endothelial function in the microcirculation perfused by collaterals (abstr.). Abstracts of the Scientific Conference on the Molecular Cellular Biology of the Vascular Wall, Boston, October 15–17, 1993.
28. Bauters C, Asahara T, Zheng LP, et al. Recovery of disturbed endothelium-dependent flow in the collateral-perfused rabbit ischemic hindlimb following administration of vascular endothelial growth factor. Circulation 1995; 91:2802–2809.
29. Losordo DW, Pickering JG, Takeshita S, et al. Use of the rabbit ear artery to serially assess foreign protein secretion after site-specific arterial gene transfer in vivo: Evidence that anatomic identification of successful gene transfer may underestimate the potential magnitude of transgene expression. Circulation 1994; 89:785–792.
30. Riessen R, Rahimizadeh H, Blessing E, Takeshita S, Barry JJ, Isner, JM.

Arterial gene transfer using pure DNA applied directly to a hydrogel-coated angioplasty balloon. Hum Gene Ther 1993; 4:749–758.

31. Isner JM, Walsh K, Symes J, et al. Arterial gene therapy for therapeutic angiogenesis in patients with peripheral artery disease. Circulation 1995; 91: 2687–2692.
32. Ferrara N, Houck KA, Jakeman LB, Winer J, Leung DW. The vascular endothelial growth factor family of polypeptides. J Cell Biochem 1991; 47: 211–218.
33. D'Amore PA, Thompson RW. Mechanisms of angiogenesis. Annu Rev Physiol 1987; 49:453–464.
34. Senger DR, Perruzzi CA, Feder J, Dvorak HF. A highly conserved vascular permeability factor secreted by a variety of human and rodent tumor cell lines. Cancer Res 1986; 46:5629–5632.
35. Senger DR, Galli SJ, Dvorak AM, Perruzzi CA, Harvey VS, Dvorak HF. Tumor cells secrete a vascular permeability factor that promotes accumulation of ascites fluid. Science 1983; 219:983–985.
36. Dvorak HF, Sioussat TM, Brown LF, et al. Distribution of vascular permeability factor (vascular endothelial growth factor) in tumors: concentration in tumor blood vessels. J Exp Med 1991; 174:1275–1278.
37. Schaper W. Coronary collateral development: concepts and hypothesis. In: Schaper W, Schaper J, eds. Collateral Circulation: Heart, Brain, Kidney, Limbs. Norwell, MA: Kluwer, 1993:41–64.
38. Sholley MM, Ferguson GP, Seibel HR, Montour JL, Wilson JD. Mechanisms of neovascularization: vascular sprouting can occur without proliferation of endothelial cells. Lab Invest 1984; 51:624–634.
39. Nicosia RF, Bonanno E, Smith M. Fibronectin promotes the elongation of microvessels during angiogenesis in vitro. J Cell Physiol 1993; 154:654–661.
40. Schaper J, Weibrauch D. Collateral vessel development in the porcine and canine heart. In: Schaper W, Schaper J, eds. Collateral Circulation: Heart, Brain, Kidney, Limbs. Norwell, MA: Kluwer, 1993:65–102.
41. Schaper W, de Brabander M, Lewi P. DNA synthesis and mitoses in coronary collateral vessels of the dog. Circ Res 1971; 28:671–679.
42. Pasyk S, Schaper W, Schaper J, Pasyk K, Miskiewicz G, Steinseifer B. DNA synthesis in coronary collaterals after coronary artery occlusion in conscious dog. Am J Physiol. 1982; 242:H1031–H1037.
43. Cowan DF, Hollenberg NK, Connelly CM, Williams DH, Abrams HL. Increased collateral arterial and venous endothelial cell turnover after renal artery stenosis in the dog. Invest Radiol 1978; 13:143–149.
44. Ilich N, Hollenberg NK, Williams DH, Abrams H. Time course of increased collateral arterial and venous endothelial cell turnover after renal artery stenosis in rat. Circ Res 1979; 45:579–582.
45. White FC, Carroll SM, Magnet A, Bloor CM. Coronary collateral development in swine after coronary artery occlusion. Circ Res 1992; 71:1490–1500.
46. Schaper W. Schaper J, Xhonneux R, Vandesteene R. The morphology of intercoronary anastomoses in chronic coronary artery occlusion. Cardiovasc Res 1969; 3:315–323.

47. Graham AM, Baffour R, Burdon T, et al. A demonstration of vascular proliferation in response to arteriovenous reversal in the ischemic canine hind limb. J Surg Res 1989; 47:341–347.
48. Symes JF, Graham AM, Stein L, Sniderman AD. Salvage of a severely ischemic limb by arteriovenous revascularization: a case report. Can J Surg 1984; 27:274–276.
49. Unger EF, Banai S, Shou M, et al. Basic fibroblast growth factor enhances myocardial collateral flow in a canine model. Am J Physiol 1994; 266: H1588–H1595.
50. Takeshita S, Rossow ST, Kearney M, et al. Time course of increased cellular proliferation in collateral arteries following administration of vascular endothelial growth factor in a rabbit model of lower limb vascular insufficiency. Am J Path 1995; 147:1649–1660.
51. Dvorak HF. Tumors: Wound that do not heal. Similarities between tumor stroma generation and wound healing. N Engl J Med 1986; 315:1650–1659.
52. Herbert JM, Lamarche I, Prabonnaud V, Dol F, Gauthier T. Tissue-type plasminogen activator is a potent mitogen for human aortic smooth muscle cells. J Biol Chem 1994; 269:3076–3080.
53. Pepper MS, Ferrara N, Orci L, Montesano R. Vascular endothelial growth factor (VEGF) induces plasminogen activators and plasminogen activator inhibitor type 1 in microvascular endothelial cells. Biochem Biophys Res Commun 1991; 189:824–831.
54. Ross R, Glomset B, Kariya B, Harker L. A platelet-dependent serum factor that stimulates the proliferation of arterial smooth muscle cells in vitro. Proc Natl Acad Sci USA 1974; 71:1207–1210.
55. Collins T, Ginsburg D, Boss JM, Orkin SH, Pober JS. Cultured human endothelial cells express platelet-derived growth factor B chain: cDNA cloning and structural analysis. Nature 1985; 316:748–750.
56. Collins T, Pober JS, Gimbrone MA Jr, Betsholtz C, Westermark B, Heldin C-H. Cultured human endothelial cells express platelet-derived factor A chain. Am J Pathol 1987; 126:7–12.
57. Zerwes H-G, Risau W. Polarized secretion of a platelet-derived growth factor–like chemotactic factor by endothelial cells in vitro. J Cell Biol 1987; 105:2037–2041.
58. Gay CG, Winkles JA. Heparin-binding growth factor-1 stimulation of human endothelial cells induces platelet-derived growth factor A-chain gene expression. J Biol Chem 1990; 265:3284–3292.
59. Roberts AB, Sporn MB, Assoian RK, et al. Transforming growth factor type-beta: rapid induction of fibrosis and angiogenesis in vivo and stimulation of collagen formation in vitro. Proc Natl Acad Sci USA 1986; 83:4167–4171.
60. Risau W, Drexler H, Mironov V, et al. Platelet-derived growth factor is angiogenic in vivo. Growth Factors 1993; 7:261–266.
61. Lindner V, Lappi DA, Baird RA, Majack RA, Reidy MA. Role of basic fibroblast growth factor in vascular lesion formation. Circ Res 1991; 68: 106–113.
62. Lindner V, Reidy MA. Expression of basic fibroblast growth factor and its

receptor by smooth muscle cells and endothelium in injured rat arteries. Circ Res 1993; 73:589–595.

63. Beitz JG, Kim IS, Calabresi P, Frackelton AR. Human microvascular endothelial cells express receptors for platelet-derived growth factor. Proc Natl Acad Sci USA 1991; 88:2021–2025

64. Smits A, Hermansson M, Nister M, Karnushina I, Heldin C-H, Oberg K. Rat brain capillary endothelial cells express functional PDGF B–type receptors. Growth Factors 1989; 2:1–8.

65. Bar RS, Boes M, Booth BA, Dake BL, Henley S, Hart MN. The effects of platelet-derived growth factor in cultured microvessel endothelial cells. Endocrinology 1989; 124:2021–225.

66. D'Amore P, Smith SR. Growth factor effects on cells of the vascular wall: a survey. Growth Factors 1993; 8:61–75.

67. Pierce GF, Tarpley JE, Yanagihara D, Mustoe TE, Fox GM, Thomason A. Platelet derived growth factor (BB homodimer), transforming growth factor-beta1, and basic fibroblast growth factor in dermal wound healing. Am J Pathol 1992; 140:1375–1388.

68. Sims DE. The perycite—a review. Tissue Cell 1986; 18:153–174.

69. Sundberg C, Ljungstrom M, Lindmark G, Gerdin B, Rubin K. Microvascular pericytes express platelet-derived growth factor-b receptors in human healing wounds and colorectal adenocarcinoma. Am J Pathol 1993; 143:1377–1388.

70. Sato N, Beitz JG, Kato J, et al. Platelet-derived growth factor indirectly stimulates angiogenesis in vitro. Am J Pathol 1993; 142:1119–1139.

71. Brogi E, Wu T, Namiki A, Isner JM. Indirect angiogenic cytokines upregulate VEGF and bFGF gene expression in vascular smooth muscle cells, whereas hypoxia upregulates VEGF expression only. Circulation 1994; 90: 649–652.

72. Pepper MS, Vassalli JD, Orci L, Montesano R. Biphasic effect of transforming growth factor-b1 on in vitro angiogenesis. Exp Cell Res 1993; 204:356–363.

73. Chen JK, Hoshi H, McKeehan WL. Transforming growth factor type b specifically stimulates synthesis of proteoglycans in human adult arterial smooth muscle cells. Proc Natl Acad Sci USA 1987; 84:5287–5291.

74. Madri JA, Pratt BM, Tucker AM. Phenotypic modulation of endothelial cells by transforming growth factor-b depends upon the composition and organization of the extracellular matrix. J Cell Biol 1993; 106:1375–1384.

75. Winkles JA, Gay CG. Serum, phorbol ester, and polypeptide mitogens increase class 1 and 2 heparin binding (acidic and basic fibroblast growth factor) gene expression in human vascular smooth muscle cells. Cell Growth Differ 1991; 2:531–540.

76. Shweiki D, Itin A, Soffer D, Keshet E. Vascular endothelial growth factor induced by hypoxia may mediate hypoxia-initiated angiogenesis. Science 1992; 359:843–845.

77. Namiki A, Brogi E, Kearney M et al. Hypoxia induces vascular endothelial growth factor in cultured human endothelial cells. J Biol Chem 1995; 270: 31189–31195.

78. Brogi E, Schatteman G, Wu T, et al. Hypoxia-induced paracrine regulation of VEGF receptor expression. J Clin Invest 1996; 97:469–476.
79. Goto F, Goto K, Weindel K, Folkman J. Synergistic effects of vascular endothelial growth factor and basic fibroblast growth factor on the proliferation of bovine capillary endothelial cells within collagen gels. Lab Invest 1993; 69:508–517.
80. Asahara T, Bauters C, Pastore CJ, et al. Local delivery of vascular endothelial growth factor accelerates reendothelialization and attenuates intimal hyperplasia in balloon-injured rat carotid artery. Circulation 1995; 91:2793–2801.
81. Asahara T, Bauters C, Pastore CJ, et al. Synergistic effect of vascular endothelial growth factor and basic fibroblast growth factor on angiogenesis in vivo. Circulation. 1995; 92:II-365–II-371.
82. Klagsbrun M, Folkman J. Angiogenesis. In: Sporn MB, Roberts AB, eds. Peptide Growth Factors and Their Receptors II. New York: Springer-Verlag, 1990:459–586.
83. Wilting J, Christ B, Bokeloh M, Weich HA. In vivo effects of vascular endothelial growth factor on the chicken chorioallantoic membrane. Cell Tissue Res 1993; 68:106–113.
84. Klagsbrun M, Baird A. A duel receptor system is required for basic fibroblast growth factor activity Cell 1991; 67:229–231.
85. Park JE, Chen HH, Winer J, Houck KA, Ferrara N. Placenta growth factor: potentiation of vascular endothelial growth factor bioactivity, in vitro and in vivo, and high affinity binding to *Flt-1* but not to *Flk-1*/KDR. J Biol Chem 1994; 269:25646–25654.
86. Isner JM, Feldman L. Gene therapy for arterial disease. Lancet 1994; 333: 1653–1654.
87. Fischer M, Meadows M-E, Do T, et al. Delayed treatment with intravenous basic fibroblast growth factor reduces infarct size following permanent cerebral ischemia in rats. J Cereb Blood Flow Metab. In press.

# 19

# Vascular Disease and the Prospect of Gene Therapy

**Heiko E. von der Leyen and Victor J. Dzau***

*Stanford University School of Medicine, Stanford, California*

*The recombinant DNA breakthrough has provided us with a new and powerful approach to the questions that have intrigued and plagued man for centuries. I, for one, would not shrink from that challenge.*    Paul Berg (1)

## I. INTRODUCTION

Based on cellular and molecular biology research, it is becoming increasingly clear that the heart and blood vessels are biologically active organs capable of synthesizing active molecules that participate in the regulation of cardiovascular function and structure and in the pathogenesis of cardiovascular disease. In this book, some of the most recent key advances in vascular biology, especially endothelial biology, are described. In addition, potential targets for pharmacological therapy are identified. In this chapter, we review the possibility of *cardiovascular gene therapy*. It was essential to create the "molecular" approach to cardiovascular disease. This therapeutic approach is based on (1) the elucidation of pathobiological processes, especially at the molecular and genetic level; (2) the development of animal models of diseases, including transgenic animals; (3) the in vivo transfer of genes and oligonucleotides; and (4) the development of genetic therapeutic strategies, including gene replacement, gene correction, or gene augmentation.

---

*Current affiliation:* Brigham and Women's Hospital and Harvard Medical School, Boston, Massachusetts.

## II.  GENE TRANSFER TECHNIQUES AND THEIR APPLICATION IN VASCULAR DISEASE

Genetic material can be delivered to the vasculature either by a direct in vivo, vector-based gene transfer or by an ex vivo, indirect cell-based gene transfer. Ex vivo gene transfer approaches require individualized recipient-related cell harvest, preparation of transduced cells, and reimplantation of genetically engineered cell material (2). In contrast, direct in vivo gene transfer approach circumvents these problems and is theoretically easier to handle. However, the success of this approach is dependent on the development of efficient gene transfer methods. Currently, several transduction systems have been employed (Table 1).

This chapter focuses on the methods available for the treatment of vascular diseases.

### A.  Virus-Mediated Gene Transfer

#### 1.  Retrovirus-Mediated Gene Transfer

Retroviral expression vectors are constructed by incorporating exogenous cDNA into the genome of the virus (3). The recombinant viral vector can deliver the inserted gene into actively dividing cells with high efficiency (4). A retroviral vector is constructed by several steps (5). First, in order to render the vector nonreplicating, the structural genes required for viral

**Table 1**  Experimental Gene Transfer Methods

*Virus mediated*
  retrovirus
  adenovirus
    adenoviral coat/
        transferrin-polylysin
    adenoassociated virus
*Lipid mediated*
  liposomes
  cationic lipids (Lipofectin)
*Fusigenic liposome mediated*
  Sendai virus (HVJ)–
  liposomes
*Other methods*
  microinjection
  microparticle bombardment
  myoblast implantation

replication are deleted from the retrovirus using appropriate restriction enzymes (although the packaging signals are left intact). Next, the exogenous gene of interest is inserted into the viral backbone by ligation. The recombinant retrovirus now contains the exogenous gene, regulatory sequences, and packaging signals but lacks the actual structural genes required to produce a complete virion. It requires a helper cell in order to produce infectious viral particles. The defective retroviral vector DNA is introduced into a packaging helper cell line that contains a second plasmid encoding the structural genes. When a retroviral vector, in which the structural genes are removed but the packaging signal remains intact, is introduced in such a "packaging cell line," the packaging signal is recognized by the structural proteins provided by the second plasmid, and a complete infectious virion is produced. The defective retroviral vector then infects a host organism. The genome from the retroviral vector becomes incorporated in the host genome, and the host cell can express the gene of interest (6). In case of the *single-gene vector,* the structural genes of the retrovirus are replaced by a single gene that is then transcribed under the control of the viral regulatory sequences contained in the long terminal repeat (LTR) (4,5,7). Nabel et al. (8,9) first demonstrated the feasibility of transfecting blood vessels with foreign DNA in vivo. Using a double-balloon catheter and direct infection with a murine amphotropic retroviral vector containing a recombinant β-galactosidase gene, these investigators showed in pig iliofemoral arteries that several cell types in the vessel wall were transduced, including endothelial and vascular smooth muscle cells. With a similar retroviral vector containing the β-galactosidase gene, Wilson et al. (2) reported that prosthetic vascular grafts seeded with genetically modified endothelial cells expressed β-galactosidase activity and protein up to 5 weeks as detected by enzymatic assay and in situ cytohistochemistry. Other studies demonstrated only low transfection efficiency using retroviral vectors (10,11). Possible explanations for inefficient retrovirus- mediated gene transfer include the requirement of actively dividing cells for integration and expression of the viral genome (12), the moderately high titers of infectious virions that can be propagated (13), and rapid inactivation by complement-mediated processes of retrovirus in primates in vivo (14–16). Since the retroviral vectors stably integrate into chromosomal DNA of the transfected cell, the potentially stable gene expression may result in insertional mutagenesis (4). It has been reported that monkeys developed malignant T-cell lymphomas after undergoing bone marrow transplantation with a gene transfer protocol in which a helper virus contaminated the retroviral vector preparation (17) Although having potential transfection efficiency in replicating cells, the retroviral method encounters several disadvantages: (1) a limitation of insert size, (2) stable transfection depends on actively dividing cells, (3) the possibility of side effects such as viral infection or activation of oncogenes, (4) the potential of an autoimmune response against the intrinsic retroviral antigens, and (5) mutagenesis by random integration, since retroviral gene transfer results in stable transformation of target cells (18). For efficient clinical application to in vivo gene therapy, retroviral vectors must be developed that achieve high titers, are prevented from in vivo degradation, and can be targeted tissue specifically (13). Pseudotyped retroviral vectors which represent progeny virions containing the genome of one virus encapsidated by the envelope protein of another virus have an extremely broad host range and can be concentrated to high titers (19). To target a specific cell type by a retroviral vector, Kasahara et al. (20) engineered a chimeric protein containing the polypeptide hormone erythropoietin and part of the *env* protein of the ecotropic Moloney murine leukemia virus into the recombinant virus. This murine virus became several times more infectious for murine cells bearing the erythropoietin receptor, and it also became infectious for human cells bearing the erythropoietin receptor. Other approaches to target a retroviral vector for infection of mammalian cells have been reported using the introduction of an integrin sequence into the retroviral envelope (21) or by using chimeric promoter/enhancer elements (22). Tissue-specific targeting by means of ligand-receptor interactions may have broad applications to a variety of gene-delivery systems.

## 2. Adenovirus-Mediated Gene Transfer

Adenoviral vectors have been shown to be useful vehicles for cardiovascular gene transfer. Adenoviruses are DNA viruses that can transfect nondividing cells and generally do not integrate into the host genome. Another DNA virus is the herpes simplex virus, which is a neurotropic virus with high transfection efficiency in neuronal cells and mammalian central nervous system (23). Two different methods using adenoviral gene transfer are currently under investigation: (1) a replication-deficient adenoviral vector similar to the retroviral approach and (2) coupling of adenoviral coat to transferrin-polylysine/DNA complexes. For the first approach, adenoviral vectors commonly used are based on serotype 5, with the majority of E1a and E1b deleted to provide a replication-deficient vector. The E3 region can be deleted to provide space for inserting plasmid DNA of up to 7.5 kb (24,25). Usually, an expression cassette containing essential viral elements, a promoter, and the exogeneous gene are inserted in the E1 position. The vectors are propagated in a helper cell line that expresses E1 protein for the production of the replication-deficient (E1−) virus in high titers for in vivo delivery. Adenoviral vectors enter mammalian cells by receptor-mediated endocytosis. The internalization process involves the binding of adenovirus with the $\alpha_2\beta_3$-integrin (26). Aortic smooth muscle cells (27) and cardiac myocytes (28) were successfully transfected using replication-defective adenovirus carrying the $\beta$-galactosidase or chloramphenicol acetyltransferase reporter gene, respectively. Effective in vivo transfection by direct infusion into vessels was demonstrated in vascular tissue with the expression of the transgene for at least 2 weeks (27,29–31) and in myocardial tissue by direct injection into the myocardium (28,32). Physiological levels of recombinant proteins have been secreted into the circulation after adenoviral infection of skeletal muscle (33). Limitations of the current (first generation) adenoviral vectors include transient gene expression, inflammatory reactions in organs expressing the transgene (34–36), and viral antigen–induced immunity potentially limiting the use of these vectors (37).

An alternative, adenovirus-mediated gene transfer approach is reported using an adenovirus-augmented, receptor-mediated gene-delivery system by coupling inactivated adenovirus to DNA/polylysine complexes (38). Replication-deficient or chemically inactivated adenovirus is coupled to polylysine either enzymatically through the action of transglutaminase or biochemically by biotinylating adenovirus and streptavidinylating the polylysine moiety. Combination complexes containing DNA, adenovirus-polylysine, and transferrin-polylysine have the capacity to transfer the reporter gene into adenovirus-receptor–rich and/or transferrin-receptor–rich cells. The adenovirus and transferrin complexes are colocalized in endosomes. The virus, because of its endosomolytic properties, is thought to destroy the integrity of the endosomal membrane and to effect the exit of the colocalized DNA into the cytoplasm and eventually to the nucleus (39). Using the endosome-disruptive activity of inactivated adenovirus particles, gene constructs (up to 48 kb) have been transfected with high efficiency in vitro (40) and efficient gene transfer was demonstrated in vivo to autologous rabbit jugular vein grafts (41). An interesting extension of the adenoviral vector system was reported recently (42). A recombinant virus was constructed in which the firefly luciferase gene (serving as a reporter gene) was driven by a thyroid hormone–retinoic acid response element linked to the herpes simplex virus thymidine kinase promoter. Using this construct in vivo, the reporter gene activity was stimulated by injection of triiodothyronine ($T_3$) showing the potential to regulate endogenously the expression of genes transferred for the purpose of therapy.

Adenoassociated virus (AAV) is a dependent human parvovirus capable of integration into host DNA. Transducing vectors based on AAV are able to transfer nonviral genes into mammalian cells and represent an alternative to the integrating retroviral vectors currently used (43). The feasibility of stable in vivo gene transfer was demonstrated with the cystic fibrosis transmembrane conductance regulator (44); however, the use of AAV as a transfection vector in vascular diseases remains to be elucidated.

## B.   Lipid-Mediated Gene Transfer

The encapsulation of DNA in artificial lipid membranes (liposomes) can facilitate its uptake and cellular transport. Cationic liposomes have been used extensively during the last 5 years for the cellular delivery of DNA (18,45) and antisense oligonucleotides (46,47). The activity of cationic liposomes is supposed to be mediated by (1) spontaneous capture of the negatively charged polynucleotides with cationic lipids by a condensation reaction, (2) increased cellular uptake due to interaction of positively charged complexes with negatively charged biological membranes, and (3) membrane fusion (or transient membrane destabilization) with the plasmalemma or the endosome to achieve delivery into the cytoplasma, thereby avoiding degradation in the lysosomal compartment (48,49). Recent data indicate that the movement of DNA from the cytoplasm to the nucleus may be one of the most important limitations to successful cationic lipid-mediated gene transfer (50). The same investigators indicate that, before transcription can occur, successful dissociation of DNA from the lipid complex appears to be an important variable for lipid-mediated gene transfer. Based on experimental observations, it is predicted that new cationic and neutral lipid molecules that are effective in facilitating the functional entry of DNA into living cells will have relatively small polar head groups and relatively bulky, disordered aliphatic regions, respectively (49). The expression of recombinant genes after cationic lipid-mediated gene transfer has been demonstrated in vivo in several animal models (9,10,51–53). Gene expression after liposome-mediated arterial gene transfer may be augmented in the presence of ongoing cellular proliferation (e.g., intimal proliferation after balloon injury) (54). Using a single intravenous injection of expression plasmid and cationic lipid complexes in adult mice, expression of the transgene was targeted to specific tissues and cell types depending on the promoter element used (55).

## C.   Fusigenic Liposome–Mediated Gene Transfer

### 1.   Sendai Virus (HVJ)–Liposome Technique

This method represents a combination of fusigenic proteins of the Sendai virus (hemagglutinating virus of Japan, [HVJ]) in conjunction with neutral liposomes. HVJ belongs to the paramyxovirus family, which has HN and F glycoproteins on its envelope (56). HN binds with glycol-type sialic acid and degrades the receptor by its own neuraminidase activity. F glycoprotein is cleaved to generate hydrophobic fusion peptide by proteases, and the activated F protein can interact directly with the cellular lipid bilayer and induces fusion. For preparation of HVJ-liposomes for gene transfer experiments, DNA is mixed with a nuclear protein (high-mobility group-1 [HMG-1]). The nuclear protein can bind DNA and delivers the DNA to nuclei, thereby enhancing the integration of the transfected DNA into the nucleus (57,58). Next, DNA/HMG-1 complexes are entrapped in dried neutral liposomes (containing phosphatidylserine, phosphatidylcholine, and cholesterol) and subsequently mixed with ultraviolet light–inactivated HVJ virus (purified Z strain). After purification and removal of unincorporated virus particles by sucrose density gradient centrifugation, HVJ-liposome complexes are ready for use in transfection experiments. An interesting feature of the HVJ-liposome–mediated gene transfer method consists of the fact that after fusion of the liposome complex with the cell membrane, the DNA is directly released into the cytosol without undergoing endocytosis, thereby reducing lysosomal destruction of the DNA construct and enhancing the nuclear uptake (59). Human angiotensin-converting enzyme (ACE) cDNA transfected into the rat carotid artery in organ culture yielded high ACE expression in the tunica media at 3 days after transfection (60). HVJ-liposome–mediated in vivo gene transfer of a SV40 large T-antigen cDNA expression vector in rat carotid arteries yielded up to 30% SV40 T-antigen–positive cells within the vascular wall without apparent toxic effects (61). The HVJ method has been successfully employed for gene transfer in vivo to many tissues, including liver (58), the kidney (62,63), and the vascular wall (64,65). Owing to the hemagglutinating activity of the Sendai virus, a nonspecific binding for red blood cells may be disadvantageous. To avoid this side effect, a vessel segment needs to be flushed with physiological saline solution before introduction of the HVJ-liposome transfection solution. The Sendai virus–liposome method is also suitable for transfer of antisense oligonucleotides. In vivo transfer of fluorescin-labeled (FITC) phosphorothioate oligonucleotides into injured rat carotid arteries using HVJ-liposomes resulted in widespread distribution of fluorescence in medial vascular cells, was localized primarily in cell nuclei, and persisted up to 2 weeks after transfection (65). The HVJ-liposome method appears to possess several advantages for in vivo gene transfer such as (1) efficiency independent of cell differentiation or replication; (2) safety (since the virus is inactivated before transfection, only the viral coat is used for delivery of the transgene); (3) simplicity of preparation; (4) brevity of incubation time (in vitro 40 min; in vivo 10–15 min); and (5) no limitation of inserted DNA size.

## D. Other Gene Transfer Methods

Microinjection has been successfully used to introduce purified recombinant proteins, neutralizing antibodies, and competitor oligonucleotides into cells (66,67). An intramuscular injection of plasmid DNA into skeletal muscle demonstrated the transient expression of a foreign gene in different skeletal myotubes (68). By extending direct gene injection to the heart muscle, the expression of a reporter gene was demonstrated for up to 4 weeks after the initial injection (69). Furthermore, expression of injected genes can be targeted to specific cell types in vivo (e.g., cardiac muscle cells) and can be modulated by the hormonal status of the animal (70).

As mentioned above, ex vivo gene transfer methods utilize the transfer of recombinant genes into the vessel wall by reimplanting cells that have been genetically modified to express new genetic material. Nabel et al. (8) first demonstrated a cell-based vascular gene transfer technique. Endothelial cells were harvested from the jugular vein of a pig, transfected ex vivo with a retroviral vector expressing $\beta$-galactosidase, and reimplanted on the surface of balloon-injured porcine iliofemoral arteries. Following establishment of flow, genetically modified cells could be detected up to 2–4 weeks following reimplantation. After successfully seeding 90% of the area of denuded rabbit carotid arteries with genetically engineered endothelial cells, Conte et al. (71) reported a high degree of variation in the persistence of seeded endothelial cells which were transfected with a recombinant retrovirus encoding $\beta$-galactosidase. In addition to endothelial cells, ex vivo–transfected smooth muscle cells have been introduced in the vasculature (72). Lynch et al. (73) reported the seeding of smooth muscle cells transfected with adenosine deaminase gene into endothelium-denuded blood vessels. Expression of human genes transfected by retroviral vectors into smooth muscle cells which were seeded into injured rat carotid arteries was demonstrated for over 1 year (74). Another application of ex vivo gene transfer is the engineering of vascular grafts seeded with endothelial cells previously transfected in a culture dish (2,75). Dichek and colleagues (76,77) focused on the development of a stent coated with genetically modified endothelial cells for the prevention of restenosis. They were able to detect small quantities of tissue type plasminogen activator (tPA) from stents seeded with genetically modified endothelial cells containing recombinant tPA. Seeding of vascular grafts with soluble vascular cell adhesion molecule (sVCAM) using adenoviral ex vivo gene transfer has been reported by Chen et al (78). The potential of this approach to prevent or slow progression of vein graft disease is not yet determined.

An efficient approach to deliver gene products systemically is given by the implantation of genetically modified myoblasts or fibroblasts to muscular tissue providing systemic delivery of hormones (79). The implantation of myoblasts transfected with human factor IX using a retroviral vector resulted in the secretion of the protein into the circulation for up to 1 month (80).

## III. GENE TRANSFER AND VASCULAR DISEASE

Currently, most studies dealing with genetic engineering in vascular disease are concentrated on the delivery of genetic material locally to the site of a disease. The development of catheter-based drug-delivery systems compatible with the incubation times necessary for efficient gene transfer but yet capable of maintaining tissue perfusion will be a prerequisite to elucidate the full potential of in vivo gene transfer (81). As described in the following sections, current in vivo models for studying gene expression are mainly focused on iliac and carotid arteries or, in a few examples, on coronary arteries. In extending the range of vascular gene delivery, recent reports describe adenovirus-mediated gene transfer in vivo to cerebral blood vessels (82) and pulmonary arteries (83). Vascular gene transfer includes the application of synthetic oligonucleotides or recombinant DNA for gene replacement, gene inhibition, or gene augmentation (Table 2).

## IV. GENETIC ENGINEERING USING SYNTHETIC OLIGONUCLEOTIDES

Antisense oligonucleotides can be employed as therapeutic agents which exert their molecular actions during different steps of DNA-RNA processing either at the translational or transcriptional level; for example, uncoiling of DNA, transcription of DNA, export of RNA, DNA splicing, RNA stability, or RNA translation. Oligonucleotides are most widely applied to inhibit gene expression as inhibitors of ribosomal translation, with the

**Table 2** Strategies for Genetic Engineering in Vascular Disease

| Oligonucleotide | Plasmid DNA |
| --- | --- |
| Intracellular | Intracellular (cytostatic/cytotoxic effect) |
| • antisense: inhibition of translation | • herpesvirus thymidine kinase |
|  | • Rb gene product |
| • decoy: inhibition of transcription | Extracellular (paracrine effect) |
|  | • nitric oxide synthase |

complementary or "antisense" base sequence targeted to a specific "sense" sequence in the mRNA (84,85). Interestingly, antisense mRNAs occur naturally as a cellular regulatory mechanism (86,87). Mechanisms of antisense inhibition include interference with ribosome binding and processing of mRNA, interference with mRNA conformation or mRNA splicing, and RNase-H activation of mRNA digestion (85,88). Antisense inhibition is usually targeted at the 5'-initiation codon. An antisense oligonucleotide consist of 15–20 bases, since this should approximate to only one unique target sequence in the human genome (89). Three features of nucleic acids are relevant for the use of antisense oligonucleotides as pharmacological agents (90): (1) coding properties for gene transfer or gene therapy, (2) binding and recognition properties of antisense, antigene, or sense-directed oligonucleotides leading to inhibition or modulation of expression, targeting mRNA double-stranded DNA with the formation of a triple helix, and nucleic acid binding proteins; and (3) catalytic properties of ribozymes against sequence-specific sites on mRNA. The instability of oligonucleotides has been a significant problem in their experimental use. By chemically modifying the phosphate backbone of the oligonucleotide (phosphorothioate or phosphoroamidate bonding), the stability of oligonucleotides against nucleolytic phosphodiesterases could be improved (85,91,92). Under some conditions, phosphorothioate analogues can exert nonsequence-specific antiviral activity (93). Antisense oliogonucleotides can exhibit sequence-specific effects in mimicing bacterial DNA and triggering rather than inhibiting a specific immune response (94). Furthermore, a stretch of four contiguous guanosine (4G) residues, which is present in antisense c-*myb* and c-*myc* oligonucleotides that were used in previous studies (95–97), may have nonspecific effects (98–100).

The uptake of modified oligonucleotides can be enhanced by complexing the oligonucleotide with cationic liposomes (47,101) or fusigenic liposomes (HVJ-liposomes) (64,65). HVJ-liposome complexes fuse directly to the plasma membrane at neutral pH and release DNA entrapped in the complexes directly into the cell bypassing receptor-mediated endocytosis. Oligonucleotides delivered by fusigenic liposomes showed a 10-fold higher incorporation into cells than DNA-liposomes alone (57,65).

In the area of vascular gene therapy, several groups have investigated the effects of antisense oligonucleotides on intimal hyperplasia after balloon injury (Table 3).

Simons et al. (96) first reported that the administration of antisense oligonucleotides against c-*myb* (150 μM) applied by pluronic gel to the adventitial layer of rat carotid arteries inhibited the development of neointimal hyperplasia in response to balloon injury. Data from our labora-

**Table 3** Application of Antisense
Oligonucleotides in Vascular Disease

| Target of antisense oligonucleotide | Reference |
| --- | --- |
| c-*myb* | 96 |
| cdc2/Proliferating | |
| cell nuclear antigen (PCNA) | 64 |
| | 102 |
| c-*myc* | 95 |
| | 97 |
| PCNA | 103 |
| Angiotensinogen | 104 |

tory demonstrated that a single HVJ-liposome–mediated administration of antisense oligonucleotides against proliferating cell nuclear antigen (PCNA) and cdc2 kinase (15 $\mu$M) inhibited neointimal formation after balloon injury at least up to 8 weeks after transfection (64) (Fig. 1). The combination of antisense cdc2 kinase and cdk2 kinase oligonucleotides also resulted in nearly complete inhibition of neointima formation (65). Bennett et al. (95) showed an inhibition of vascular smooth muscle cell proliferation by the administration of c-*myc* antisense oligonucleotides to the adventitial

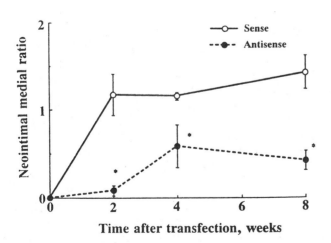

**Figure 1** Long-term effect of cdc2 kinase/PCNA antisense or sense oligonucleotide tretament on intimal/media area ratio after rat carotid balloon injury. * $p < .05$ versus sense treatment. (From ref 64.)

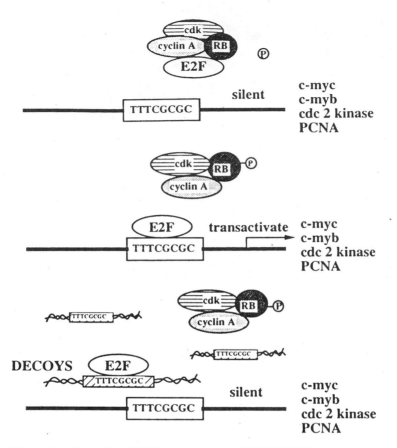

**Figure 2** Principle of E2F decoy strategy. TTTCGCGC, consensus sequence for the E2F binding site. In the quiescent cell state, E2F is complexed with Rb, cyclin A, and cdK (top). Phosphorylation of Rb releases free E2F, which binds to *cis* elements of the cell cycle–regulatory genes, resulting in the transactivation of these genes (middle). The E2F decoy *cis*-element double-stranded oligonucleotide binds to free E2F, preventing E2F-mediated transactivation of cell cycle–regulatory genes (bottom). (From ref. 107.)

surface of injured carotid arteries in a pluronic gel solution. Two other studies reported inhibition of neointima formation after the application of antisense oligonucleotides. Delivery of antisense PCNA oligonucleotides by pluronic gel (in a rat carotid model) and of antisense c-*myc* oligo-nucleotides by direct application through a porous balloon (in a porcine coronary artery model) resulted in significant inhibition of neointimal hyperplasia (97,103). Systemic effects have been reported using antisense oligonucleotides by inhibiting hypertension in spontaneously hypertensive rats by intracerebroventricular delivery of antisense oligonucleotides targeted against angiotensinogen mRNA (104).

Synthetic double-stranded oligonucleotides functioning as a transcriptional factor "decoy" can block the binding of nuclear factors to promoter regions of targeted genes, resulting in the inhibition of gene transactivation (105,106). This decoy strategy may be useful for treating a wide range of human diseases. Recently, our group showed that a single administration of E2F decoy (containing the E2F *cis* element) that binds the transcription factor E2F inhibits smooth muscle cell hyperplasia in a rat carotid balloon-injury model (107) (Fig. 2). The binding of E2F prevents it from transactivating the gene expression of cell cycle–regulatory proteins like PCNA, c-*myc*, and cdk2; thereby inhibiting vascular smooth muscle cell proliferation and subsequent neointima formation in vivo.

After vascular bypass surgery, vein graft remodeling results in a reduction of the high distensibility of the vein and decreases wall stress to a normal arterial level. This process involves the formation of a neointimal layer of smooth muscle cells that is highly susceptible to accelerated atherosclerosis (108). Thus, the efficacy of aortocoronary vein grafting is limited by early graft thrombosis and accelerated graft atherosclerosis. Our laboratory examined the effect of targeting antisense oligonucleotides against cell cycle–regulatory genes (cdc2 kinase/PCNA) in rabbit interposition vein graft in the carotid artery. Antisense treatment resulted in a complete inhibition of neointimal hyperplasia. In addition, in rabbits fed with a high-cholesterol diet, the occurrence of macrophage-laden atherosclerotic lesions was prevented (102) (Fig. 3). These findings established for the first time the feasibility of developing genetically engineered bioprostheses that are resistant to accelerated atherosclerosis and thus to graft failure.

## V. GENE TRANSFER FOR THE STUDY OF VASCULAR REMODELING

Cardiovascular molecular research has resulted in significant gains in the knowledge of disease processes at cellular as well as molecular levels. In vivo gene manipulation using gene transfer, antisense oligonucleotide application, or transgenic animals allows the study of the role of specific factors involved in a disease and led to the development of animal models of diseases. In particular, this technique is useful for the characterization of locally expressed genes in diseased blood vessels that have been postulated to play autocrine and/or paracrine roles in vascular pathophysiology.

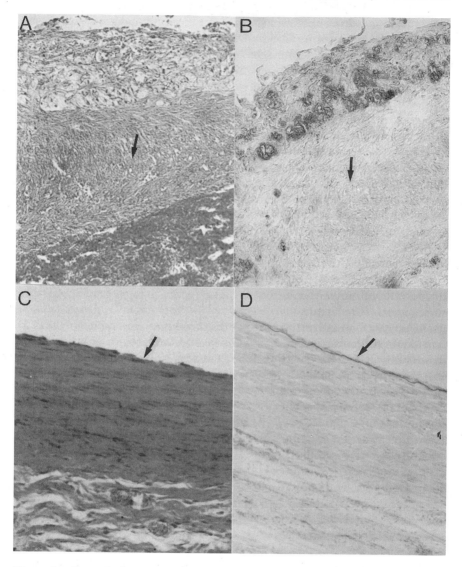

**Figure 3**   Control oligonucleotide-treated (A and B) and antisense oligonucleotide (against cdc2 kinase/PCNA)–treated vein grafts (C,D) in hypercholesterolemic rabbits, 6 weeks after surgery (×70). Five micrometer sections were stained with hematoxylin/van Gieson (A,C) and a monoclonal antibody against rabbit macrophages (B,D). Arrows indicate the location of the internal elastic lamina. (From ref. 102.)

**Table 4** Overexpression of Growth-Mediating Factors by Gene Transfer for the Study of Vascular Remodeling

| Transfected DNA | Reference |
| --- | --- |
| Fibroblast growth factor (FGF-1) | 52 |
| Transforming growth factor (TGF-$\beta_1$) | 109 |
| Platelet-derived growth factor (PDGF BB) | 51 |
| Angiotensin-converting enzyme (ACE) | 110 |
| Endothelial cell nitric oxide synthase (ecNOS) | 111 |

Table 4 summarizes recent applications of vivo gene transfer to study genes putatively involved in vascular diseases. These studies employed local overexpression of a specific gene (gene construct). During the last few years, several experimental studies were published which concentrated on the overexpression of pathobiological mediators in different animal models.

Using a retrovirus-mediated transfection method, Nabel et al. (52) overexpressed an expression vector encoding a secreted form of fibroblast growth factor-1 (FGF-1) in porcine arteries. FGF-1 expression was associated with intimal thickening of the transfected vessels together with neocapillary formation in the expanded intima. These findings suggest that FGF-1 induces intimal hyperplasia in the arterial wall in vivo and, through its ability to stimulate angiogenesis in the neointima, FGF-1 could stimulate neovascularization of atherosclerotic plaques. In the same porcine model, the overexpression of transforming growth factor-$\beta_1$ (TGF-$\beta_1$) in normal arteries resulted in substantial extracellular matrix production accompanied by intimal and medial hyperplasia (109). These findings showed that TGF-$\beta_1$ differentially modulates extracellular matrix production and cellular proliferation in the arterial wall and could play a reparative role in response to arterial injury. The increased extracellular matrix production that accompanied the intimal and medial hyperplasia was not observed following expression of other growth factor genes in the vessel wall, including genes for platelet-derived growth factor (PDGF BB) (51) or the secreted form of FGF-1 (52). Porcine arteries transfected with human PDGF B demonstrated intimal hyperplasia with increased numbers of intimal smooth muscle cells. However, an increased deposition of procollagen, as seen in TGF-$\beta_1$–transfected vessels, was not observed. By stimulating the formation of extracellular matrix, it is possible that TGF-$\beta_1$ could help to promote healing following vascular injury but limit the extensive cellular intimal hyperplasia which is observed with PDGF BB (109).

The pathogenesis of vascular diseases such as hypertension involves a process of vascular remodeling associated with increased vascular hypertrophy and the activation of the local angiotensin system (112). Angiotensin has been shown to stimulate vascular smooth muscle growth and proliferation, as well as collagen biosynthesis in vitro. Its in vivo role has been inferred from experiments using angiotensin-converting enzyme (ACE) inhibitors. Since these drugs produce hemodynamic effects, a direct role of local angiotensin in vascular remodeling has not been proven. To study the local effects of an autocrine/paracrine factor like angiotensin, Morishita et al. (110) overexpressed ACE within the vascular wall by using fusigenic liposomes (HVJ-liposomes) as delivery vehicle. Immunohistochemistry localized immunoreactive ACE activity in the medial vascular smooth muscle cells as well as in the intimal endothelial cells. The increase in vascular ACE activity was associated with increased DNA synthesis and vascular protein content via the local production and action of vascular angiotensin without changes in systemic blood pressure. Parallel to these biochemical changes, morphometric analysis documented a medial thickening of the ACE-transfected vessel segments with unchanged luminal diameters implicating a medial wall hypertrophy via local autocrine/paracrine angiotensin II production. Indeed, the vascular hypertrophic response to local ACE overexpression was inhibited by the angiotensin antagonist Dup 753. These experiments demonstrated that gene transfer techniques provide the unique opportunity to investigate autocrine/paracrine factors in vascular remodeling independently of systemic factors or hemodynamic stimuli.

Injury to the endothelium plays an essential role in the pathogenesis of vasculoproliferative disorders (113) and endothelium-derived relaxing factor/nitric oxide has an important regulatory function in maintaining vascular homeostasis (114). Vascular injury induces local expression of mitogens and chemotactic factors mediating neointimal lesion formation with subsequent vascular dysfunction. Nitric oxide has been shown to inhibit vascular smooth muscle cell proliferation and migration in vitro and has been postulated to be an important mediator in vascular remodeling. In a recent study, we showed that transfection of the cDNA encoding endothelial cell nitric oxide synthase (ecNOS) in injured carotid arteries inhibited neointimal hyperplasia after balloon injury (111) (Fig. 4). Thus,

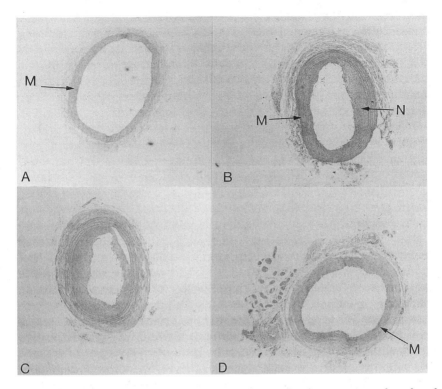

**Figure 4**  Inhibition of neointimal hyperplasia by in vivo gene transfer of endothelial cell nitric oxide synthase (ecNOS) in balloon-injured rat carotid arteries. (A) Normal artery. (B) Injured, untransfected artery. (C) Injured, control vector–transfected artery. (D) Injured, ecNOS-transfected. M; media; N; neointima. (From ref. 111.)

using in vivo gene transfer technology in a rat balloon-injury model, we could prove the concept that vascular-derived nitric oxide plays an important role in modulating vascular remodeling (see below).

## VI. THERAPEUTIC APPLICATIONS OF GENE THERAPY IN VASCULAR DISEASE

Potential applications in cardiovascular gene therapy include the treatment of vasculoproliferative disorders (restenosis, atherosclerosis, graft accelerated atherosclerosis, transplant vasculopathy), cardiac diseases (myocardial infarction, cardiac remodeling, cardiomyopathy), metabolic disorders (diabetes mellitus, hypercholesterolemia, hypertension), and

**Table 5**   Plasmid DNA Transfer and
Therapeutic Effects in Vessels

| Transfected DNA | Reference |
| --- | --- |
| Endothelial cell nitric oxide synthase (ecNOS) | 111 |
| Herpes simplex virus thymidine kinase (HSV-*tk*) | 115<br>116 |
| Constitutive active form of retinoblastoma (Rb) gene product | 117 |
| Vascular endothelial growth factor (VEGF) | 118 |
| *ras* Transdominant negative mutants | 119 |
| p21 | 120 |

kidney diseases (glomerulonephritis). Besides using synthetic oligonucleotides for inhibiting specific mRNA processing, plasmid DNA (gene
constructs) can be delivered into the vessel wall for therapeutic purposes.
Table 5 lists recent approaches using in vivo transfer of plasmid DNA to
treat neointimal hyperplasia after vascular injury.

We recently reported the construction of an expression vector containing the endothelial cell nitric oxide synthase (ecNOS) cDNA driven by a
$\beta$-actin promoter and cytomegalovirus (CMV) enhancer (111). To assess
the biological response to transfection of the ecNOS gene on vascular
lesion formation in vivo, we chose the well-characterized rat carotid artery balloon-injury model in which no significant regrowth of endothelium
is observed within 2–3 weeks after injury. Four complementary experimental methods were used to verify successful in vivo ecNOS gene transfer into the vessel wall: (1) transgene protein expression was documented
by Western blot, (2) localization of enzyme expression in the vessel wall
was verified by in situ histochemical staining using the NADPH-
diaphorase assay, (3) enzymatic activity of the transgene product was
confirmed by measurement of increased NO generation from transfected
vessel segments using the chemiluminescence method, and (4) biological
effectiveness of the transgene product was assessed by changes in vascular
reactivity induced by the increased local generation of NO; thereby potentially counterbalancing vasospasm induced by vascular injury. Thus, in
vivo transfection of ecNOS in balloon-injured rat carotid arteries not only
restored nitric oxide production within the vessel wall but also signifi-

cantly improved the vascular reactivity of the vessel. Furthermore, ecNOS transgene expression resulted in a 70% inhibition of neointima formation after balloon injury. This study documented the therapeutic effects utilizing direct in vivo gene transfer of a cDNA encoding a functional enzyme. Although the rat carotid model may not be a good model of human diseases, this study provides direct evidence that endothelium-derived NO is an important local inhibitor of neointimal hyperplasia in vivo. Since the regulation of vascular growth and migration in vivo involves a delicate balance of stimulatory versus inhibitory factors, the loss of endothelium-derived NO may play a fundamental role in the pathogenesis of vasculoproliferative diseases, including atherosclerosis. The overexpression of ecNOS may be useful for gene therapy of neointimal hyperplasia and associated local vasospasm after vascular injury.

Another therapeutic approach using gene transfer was reported recently using an adenoviral vector–mediated transfer of the herpesvirus thymidine kinase (HSV-*tk*) (115). After introduction of the vector into injured porcine arteries and vascular smooth muscle cells, respectively, the *tk* gene rendered the smooth muscle cells sensitive to the nucleoside analogue ganciclovir given immediately after balloon injury. After one course of ganciclovir treatment, intimal hyperplasia decreased by about 50%. Chang et al. (117) showed that localized arterial infection with a replication-defective adenovirus encoding a nonphosphorylatable, constitutively active form of the retinoblastoma gene product at the time of balloon angioplasty significantly reduced smooth muscle cell proliferation and neointima formation in both the rat carotid and porcine femoral artery models of restenosis. Similar results were obtained by adenovirus-mediated overexpression of human p21 in vivo (120). *ras* Proteins are key transducers of mitogenic signals from membrane to nucleus in many cells types. The local delivery of DNA vectors expressing *ras* transdominant negative mutants, which interfere with *ras* function, reduced neointimal lesion formation in a rat carotid artery balloon-injury model (119).

Angiogenic growth factors may be useful to expedite and/or augment collateral artery development in animal models of myocardial and hindlimb ischemia. Enhanced angiogenesis was demonstrated in the rabbit ischemic hindlimb following hydrogel polymer–mediated gene transfer of vascular endothelial growth factor (VEGF) (121), and improvement of resting and maximum flow was achieved that was comparable to a single administration of VEGF protein (118). Recently, a phase I study was initiated to study the effect of arterial gene transfer of VEGF using a hydrogel polymer–coated angioplasty balloon in patients with peripheral artery disease (122).

## VII. SUMMARY

In vivo gene transfer technology can be useful for the studies of vascular remodeling. The role of a specific autocrine or paracrine factor in the adaptation and pathobiology of the blood vessel can be investigated by the overexpression (gain of function) or the inhibition of expression (loss of function) of the gene. In vivo transfer of genetic materials may also be useful for gene therapy which has obvious potential as an approach for the treatment of vascular disease in the future.

## REFERENCES

1. Berg P. Dissections and reconstructions of genes and chromosomes. Science 1981; 213:296–303.
2. Wilson JM, Birinyi LK, Salomon RN, Libby P, Callow AD, Mulligan RC. Implantation of vascular grafts lined with genetically modified endothelial cells. Science 1989; 244:1344–1346.
3. Varmus H. Retroviruses. Science 1988; 240:1427–1435.
4. Cone RD, Mulligan RC. High-efficiency gene transfer into mammalian cells: generation of helper-free recombinant retrovirus with broad mammalian host range. Proc Natl Acad Sci USA 1984; 81:6349–6353.
5. Danos O, Mulligan RC Expression of retroviral trans-acting functions from complementary crippled genomes: A system for helper free packaging of retroviral vectors. J Cell Biochem 1988; 12:172–178.
6. Boris-Lawrie K, Temin HM. The retroviral vector. Replication cycle and safety considerations for retrovirus-mediated gene therapy. Ann NY Acad Sci 1994; 716:59–70.
7. Cepko CL, Roberts BE, Mulligan RC. Construction and applications of a highly transmissible murine retrovirus shuttle vector. Cell 1984; 37:1053–1062.
8. Nabel EG, Plautz G, Boyce FM, Stanley JC, Nabel GJ. Recombinant gene expression in vivo within endothelial cells of the arterial wall. Science 1989; 244:1342–1344.
9. Nabel EG, Plautz G, Nabel GJ. Site-specific gene expression in vivo by direct gene transfer into the arterial wall. Science 1990; 249:1285–1288.
10. Lim CS, Chapman GD, Gammon RS, Muhlestein JB, Bauman RP, Stack RS, Swain JL. Direct in vivo gene transfer into the coronary artery and peripheral vasculatures in the intact dog. Circulation 1991; 83:2007–2011.
11. Flugelman MY, Jaklitsch MT, Newman KD, Casscells W, Bratthauer GL, Dichek DA. Low level in vivo gene transfer into the arterial wall through a perforated balloon catheter. Circulation 1992; 85:1110–1117.
12. Miller DG, Adam MA, Miller AD. Gene transfer by retrovirus vectors occurs only in cells that are actively replicating at the time of transfection. Mol Cell Biol 1990; 10:4239–4242.

13. Friedmann T, Yee JK. Pseudotyped retroviral vectors for studies of human gene therapy. Nature Med 1995; 1:275–277.

14. Cooper NR, Jensen FC, Welsh RM, Oldstone MBA. Lysis of RNA tumor viruses by human serum: direct antibody-independent triggering of the classical complement pathway. J Exp Med 1976; 144:970–984.

15. Cornetta K, Moen RC, Culver K, Morgan RA, McLachlin JR, Sturm S, Selegue J, London W, Blaese RM, Anderson WF. Amphotropic murine leukemia retrovirus is not an acute pathogen for primates. Hum Gene Ther 1990; 1:15–30.

16. Takeuchi Y, Cosset FLC, Lachmann PJ, Okada H, Weiss RA, Collins MKL. Type C retrovirus inactivation by human complement is determined by both the viral genome and the producer cell. J Virol 1994; 68:8001–8007.

17. Donahue RE, Kessler SW, Bodine D, McDonagh K, Dunbar C, Goodman S, Agricola B, Byrne E, Raffeld M, Moen R. Helper virus induced T cell lymphoma in nonhuman primates after retroviral mediated gene transfer. J Exp Med 1992; 176:1125–1135.

18. Felgner PL, Rhodes G. Gene therapeutics. Nature 1991; 349:351–352.

19. Burns JC, Friedmann T, Driever W, Burrascano M, Yee JK. Vesicular stomatitis virus G glycoprotein pseudotyped retroviral vectors: concentration to very high titer and efficient gene transfer into mammalian and non-mammalian cells. Proc Natl Acad Sci USA 1993; 90:8033–8037.

20. Kasahara N, Dozy AM, Kan YW. Tissue-specific targeting of retroviral vectors through ligand-receptor interactions. Science 1994; 266:1373–1376.

21. Valsesia-Wittmann S, Drynda A, Deleage G, Aumailley M, Heard JM, Danos O, Verdier G, Cosset FL. Modifications in the binding domain of avain retrovirus envelope protein to redirect the host range of retroviral vectors. J Virol 1994; 68:4609–4619.

22. Couture LA, Mullen CA, Morgan RA. Retroviral vectors containing chimeric promoter/enhancer elements exibit cell-type-specific gene expression. Hum Gene Ther 1994; 5:667–677.

23. Andersen JK, Garber DA, Meaney CA, Breakefield XO. Gene transfer into mammalian central nervous system using herpes virus vectors: extended expression of bacterial lacZ in neurons using the neuron-specific enolase promoter. Hum Gene Ther 1992; 3:487–499.

24. Berkner KL. Expression of heterologous sequences in adenoviral vectors. Curr Top Microbiol Immunol. 1992; 158:39–66.

25. Brody SL, Crystal RG. Adenovirus-mediated in vivo gene transfer. Ann New York Acad Sci 1994; 716:90–101.

26. Wickman TJ, Mathias P, Cheresh DA, Nemerow GR. Integrins $\alpha v \beta 3$ and $\alpha v \beta 5$ promote adenovirus internalization but not virus attachment. Cell 1983; 73: 309–319.

27. Guzman RJ, Lemarchand P, Crystal RG, Epstein SE, Finkel T. Efficient and selective adenovirus-mediated gene transfer into vascular neointima. Circulation 1993; 88:2838–2848.

28. Kass-Eisler A, Falck-Pedersen E, Alvira M, Rivera J, Buttrick PM, Witten-

berg BA, Cipriani L, Leinwand LA. Quantitative determination of adeno-virus-mediated gene delivery to rat cardiac myocytes in vitro and in vivo. Proc Natl Acad Sci USA 1993; 90:11498–11502.

29. Barr J, Kalynych AM, Tripathy SK, Kozarsky K, Wilson JM, Leiden JM. Efficient catheter-mediated gene transfer into the heart using replication-defective adenovirus. Gene Ther 1994; 1:51–58.

30. Lemarchand P, Jones M, Yamada I, Crystal RG. In vivo gene transfer and expression in normal uninjured blood vessels using replication-deficient recombinant adenovirus vectors. Circ Res 1993; 72:1132–1138.

31. Losordo DW, Pickering JG, Takeshita S, Leclerc G, Gal D, Weir L, Kearney M, Jekanowski J, Isner JM. Use of the rabbit ear artery to serially assess foreign secretion after site-specific arterial gene transfer in vivo. Circulation 1994; 89:785–792.

32. Guzman RJ, Lemarchand P, Crystal RG, Epstein SE, Finkel T. Efficient gene transfer into myocardium by direct injection of adenovirus vectors. Circ Res 1993; 73:1202–1207.

33. Tripathy SK, Goldwasser E, Lu MM, Barr E, Leiden JM. Stable delivery of physiological levels of recombinant erythropoietin to the systemic circulation by intramuscular injection of replication-defective adenovirus. Proc Natl Acad Sci USA 1994; 91:11557–11561.

34. Engelhardt JF, Simon RH, Yang Y, Zepeda M, Weber-Pendleton S, Grossman M, Wilson JM. Adenovirus-mediated transfer of CFTR gene to lung of nonhuman primates: biological efficacy study. Hum Gene Ther 1993; 4:759–769.

35. Gerard RD, Herz J. Adenovirus-mediated low density lipoprotein receptor gene transfer accelerates cholesterol clearence in normal mice. Proc Natl Acad Sci USA 1993; 90:2812–2816.

36. Simon RH, Engelhardt JF, Yang Y, Zepeda M, Weber-Pendleton S, Grossman M, Wilson JM. Adenovirus-mediated gene transfer of CFTR gene to lung of nonhuman primates: toxicity study. Hum Gene Ther 1993; 4:771–780.

37. Quantin B, Perricaudet LD, Tajbakhsh S, Mandel JL. Adenovirus as an expression vector in muscle cells in vivo. Proc Natl Acad Sci USA 1994; 89:2581–2584.

38. Wagner E, Zatloukal K, Cotten M, Kirlappos H, Mechtler K, Curiel DT, Birnstiel ML. Coupling of adenovirus to transferrin-polylysine/DNA complexes greatly enhances receptor-mediated gene delivery and expression of transfected genes. Proc Natl Acad Sci USA 1992; 89:6099–6103.

39. Curiel DT, Agarwal S, Wagner E, Cotten M. Adenovirus enhancement of transferrin-polylysine-mediated gene delivery. Proc Natl Acad Sci USA 1991; 88:8850–8854.

40. Cotten M, Wagner E, Zatloukal K, Phillips S, Curiel DT, Birnstiel ML. High-efficiency receptor-mediated delivery of small and large (48 kilobase) gene constructs using the endosome-disruption activity of defective or chemically inactivated adenovirus particles. Proc Natl Acad Sci USA 1992; 89:6094–6098.

41. Kupfer JM, Ruan XM, Liu G, Matloff J, Forrester J, Chaux A. High-efficiency gene transfer to autologous rabbit jugular vein grafts using adenovirus-transferrin/polylysine-DNA complexes. Hum Gene Ther 1994; 5:1437–1443.

42. Hayashi Y, DePaoli AM, Burant CF, Refetoff S. Expression of a thyroid hormone–sensitive recombinant gene introduced into adult mice livers by replication-defective adenovirus can be regulated by endogenous thyroid hormone receptor. J Biol Chem 1994; 269:23872–23875.
43. Muzyczka N. Use of adeno-associated virus as a general transduction vector for mammalian cells. Curr Top Microbiol Immunol 1992; 158:97–129.
44. Flotte TR, Afione SA, Conrad C, McGrath SA, Solow R, Oka H, Zeitlin PL, Guggino WB, Carter BJ. Stable in vivo expression of the cystic fibrosis transmembrane regulator with an adeno-associated virus vector. Proc Natl Acad Sci USA 1993; 90:10613–10617.
45. Felgner PL, Gader TR, Holm M, Roman R, Chan HW, Wenz M, Northrop JP, Ringold GM, Danielsen M. Lipofectin: a highly efficient, lipid mediated DNA-transfection procedure. Proc Natl Acad Sci USA 1987; 84:7413–7417.
46. Chiang MY, Chan H, Zounes MA, Freier SM, Lima WF, Bennett CF. Antisense oligonucleotides inhibit intercellular adhesion molecule 1 expression by two distinct mechanisms. J Biol Chem 1991; 266:18162–18171.
47. Bennett CF, Chiang MY, Chan H, Shoemaker JE, Mirabelli CK. Cationic lipids improve antisense oligonucleotide uptake and prevent degradation in cultured cells and in human serum. Mol Pharmacol 1992; 41:1023–1033.
48. Düzgünes N, Goldstein JA, Friend DS, Felgner PL. Fusion of liposomes containing a novel cationic lipid, $N$-[2,3-(dioleyloxy)propyl]-$N,N,N$-trimethyl-ammonium: induction by multivalent anions and asymmetric fusion with acidic phospholipid vesicles. Biochemistry 1989; 28:9179–9184.
49. Felgner JH, Kumar R, Sridhar CN, Wheeler CJ, Tsai YJ, Border R, Ramsey P, Martin M, Felgner PL Enhanced gene delivery and mechanism studies with a novel series of cationic lipid formulations. J Biol Chem 1994; 269:2550–2561.
50. Zabner J, Fasbender AJ, Moninger T, Poellinger KA, Welsh MJ. Cellular and molecular barriers to gene transfer by a cationic lipid. J Biol Chem 1995; 270:18997–19007.
51. Nabel EG, Yang Z, Liptay S, San H, Gordon D, Haudenschild CC, Nabel GJ. Recombinant platelet-derived growth factor B gene expression in porcine arteries induce intimal hyperplasia in vivo. J Clin Invest 1993; 91:1822–1829.
52. Nabel EG, Yang Z, Plautz G, Forough R, Zhan X, Haudenschild C, Maciag T, Nabel GJ. Recombinant fibroblast growth factor-1 promotes intimal hyperplasia and angiogenesis in arteries in vivo. Nature 1993; 362:844–846.
53. Leclerc G, Gal D, Takeshita S, Nikol S, Weir L, Isner JM. Percutaneous arterial gene transfer in a rabbit model: efficiency in normal and balloon-dilated atherosclerotic arteries. J Clin Invest 1992; 90:936–944.
54. Takeshita S, Gal D, Leclerc G, Pickering JG, Riessen R, Weir L, Isner JM. Increased gene expression after liposome-mediated arterial gene transfer associated with intimal smooth muscle cell proliferation. J Clin Invest 1994; 93:652–661.
55. Zhu N, Liggitt D, Liu Y, Debs R. Systemic gene expression after intravenous DNA delivery into adult mice. Science 1993; 261:209–211.
56. Okada Y. Sendai virus-induced cell fusion. Methods Enzymol 1993; 221:18–41.

528 von der Leyen and Dzau

57. Kaneda Y, Morishita R, Tomita N. Increased expression of DNA cointroduced with nuclear protein in adult rat liver. J Mol Med 1995; 73:289–297.
58. Kaneda Y, Iwai K, Uchida T. Increased expression of DNA cointroduced with nuclear protein in adult rat liver. Science 1989; 243:375–378.
59. Okada Y, Koseki I, Kim J, Hashimotot T, Kanno Y, Matsui Y. Modification of cell membranes with viral envelopes during fusion of cells with HVJ (Sendai virus). Exp Cell Res 1975; 93:368–378.
60. Morishita R, Gibbons GH, Kaneda Y, Ogihara T, Dzau VJ. Novel in vitro gene transfer method for study of local modulators in vascular smooth muscle cells. Hypertension 1993; 21:894–899.
61. Morishita R, Gibbons GH, Kaneda Y, Ogihara T, Dzau VJ. Novel and effective gene transfer technique for study of vascular renin angiotensin system. J Clin Invest 1993; 91:2580–2585.
62. Tomita N, Higaki J, Morishita R, Kato K, Mikami H, Kaneda Y, Ogihara T. Direct in vivo gene introduction into rat kidney. Biochem Biophys Res Commun 1992; 186:129–134.
63. Isaka Y, Fujiwara Y, Ueda N, Kaneda Y, Kamada T, Imai E. Glomerulosclerosis induced by in vivo transfection of transforming growth factor-$\beta$ or platelet-derived growth factor gene into the rat kidney. J Clin Invest 1993; 92:2597–2601.
64. Morishita R, Gibbons GH, Ellison KE, Nakajima M, Zhang L, Kaneda Y, Ogihara T, Dzau VJ. Single intraluminal delivery of antisense cdc2 kinase and proliferating-cell nuclear antigen oligonucleotides results in chronic inhibition of neointimal hyperplasia. Proc Natl Acad Sci USA 1993; 90:8474–8478.
65. Morishita R, Gibbons GH, Ellison KE, Nakajima M, von der Leyen H, Zhang L, Kaneda Y, Dzau VJ. Intimal hyperplasia after vascular injury is inhibited by antisense cdk 2 kinase oligonucleotides. J Clin Invest 1994; 93:1458–1464.
66. Capecchi M. High efficiency transformation by direct microinjection of DNA into mammalian cells. Cell 1980; 22:479–488.
67. Adams BA, Tanabe T, Mikami A, Numa S, Beam KG. Intramembrane charged movement restored in dysgenic skeletal muscle by injection of dihydropyridine receptor cDNAs. Nature 1990; 345:569–572.
68. Wolff JA, Malone RW, Williams P, Chong W, Ascadi G, Jani A, Felgner PL. Direct gene transfer into mouse muscle in vivo. Science 1990; 247:1465–1468.
69. Lin H, Parmacek MS, Morle G, Bolling S, Leiden JM. Expression of recombinant gene in myocardium in vivo after direct injection of DNA. Circulation 1990; 82:2217–2221.
70. Kitsis RN, Buttrick PM, McNally EM, Kaplan ML, Leinwand LA. Hormonal modulation of a gene injected into rat heart in vivo. Proc Natl Acad Sci USA 1991; 88:4138–4142.
71. Conte MS, Birinyi LK, Miyata T, Fallon JT, Gold HK, Whittemore AD, Mulligan RC. Efficient repopulation of denuded rabbit arteries with autologous genetically modified endothelial cells. Circulation 1994; 89:2161–2169.
72. Plautz G, Nabel EG, Nabel GJ. Introduction of vascular smooth muscle cells expressing recombinant genes in vivo. Circulation 1991; 83:578–583.

73. Lynch CM, Clowes MM, Osborne RA, Clowes AW, Miller AD. Long-term expression of human adenosine deaminase in vascular smooth muscle cells of rats: a model for gene therapy. Proc Natl Acad Sci USA 1992; 89:1139–1142.
74. Clowes MM, Lynch CM, Miller AD, Miller DG, Osborne WR, Clowes AW. Long-term biological response of injured rat carotid artery seeded with smooth muscle cells expressing retrovirally introduced human genes. J Clin Invest 1994; 93:644–651.
75. Dichek DA, Neville RF, Zwiebel JA, Freeman SM, Leon MB, Anderson WF. Seeding of intravascular stents with genetically engineered endothelial cells. Circulation 1989; 80:1347–1353.
76. Dichek DA, Nussbaum O, Degen SJF, Anderson WF. Enhancement of the fibrinolytic activity of sheep endothelial cells by retroviral vector–mediated gene transfer. Blood 1991; 77:533–541.
77. Shayani V, Newman KD, Dichek DA. Optimization of recombinant t-PA secretion from seeded vascular grafts. J Surg Res 1994; 57:495–504.
78. Chen S, Wilson JM, Muller DWM. Adenovirus-mediated gene transfer of soluble vascular cell adhesion molecule to porcine interposition vein grafts. Circulation 1994; 89:1922–1928.
79. Barr E, Leiden JM. Systemic delivery of recombinant proteins by genetically modified myoblasts. Science 1991; 254:1507–1509.
80. Yao SN, Kurachi K. Expression of human factor IX in mice after injection of genetically modified myoblasts. Proc Natl Acad Sci USA 1992; 89:3357–3361.
81. Riessen R, Issner JM. Prospects for site-specific delivery of pharmacologic and molecular therapies. J Am Coll Cardiol 1994; 23:1234–1244.
82. Ooboshi H, Welsh MJ, Rios CD, Davidson BL, Heistad DD. Adenovirus-mediated gene transfer in vivo to cerebral blood vessels and perivascular tissue. Circ Res 1995; 77:7–13.
83. Schachtner SK, Rome JJ, Hoyt RF, Newman KD, Virmani R, Dichek DA. In vivo adenovirus-mediated gene transfer via the pulmonary artery of rats. Circ Res 1995; 76:701–709.
84. Zamecnik PC, Stephenson ML. Inhibition of Rous sarcoma virus replication and cell transformation by a specific oligodeoxynucleotide. Proc Natl Acad Sci USA 1978; 75:280–284.
85. Cohen JS. Oligonucleotide therapeutics. Trends Biotechnol. 1992; 10:87–91.
86. Inouye M. Antisense RNA: its functions and applications in gene regulation—review. Gene 1988; 72:25–34.
87. Krystal GW, Armstrong BC, Battey JF. N-myc mRNA forms an RNA-RNA duplex with endogenous antisense transcripts. Mol Cell Biol 1990; 10:4180–4191.
88. Colman A. Antisense strategies in cell and developmental biology. J Cell Sci 1990; 97:399–409.
89. Stein CA, Cheng YC. Antisense oligonucleotides as therapeutic agents—is the bullet really magical? Science 1993; 261:1004–1012.
90. Bricca G. Sense, antisense, nonsense: where's the right way? J Mol Med 1995; 73:417–419.

91. Uhlmann E, Peyman A. Antisense oligonucleotides: a new therapeutic principle. Chem Rev 1990; 90:544–552.
92. Crooke ST. Progress toward oligonucleotide therapeutics: pharmacodynamic properties. FASEB J 1993; 7:533–539.
93. Matsukura M, Shinozuka K, Zon G, Mitsuya H, Reitz M, Cohen JS, Broder S. Phosphorothioate analogs of oligodeoxynucleotides: inhibitors of replication and cytopathic effects of human immunodeficiency virus. Proc Natl Acad Sci USA 1987; 84:7706–7710.
94. Krieg AM, Yi A, Matson S, Waldschmidt T, Bishop GA, Teasdale R, Koretzky GA, Klinman DM. CpG motifs in bacterial DNA trigger direct B-cell activation. Nature 1995; 374:546–549.
95. Bennett MR, Anglin S, McEwan JR, Jagoe R, Newby AC, Evan GI. Inhibition of vascular smooth muscle cell proliferation in vitro and in vivo by C-*myc* antisense oligonucleotides. J Clin Invest 1994; 93:820–828.
96. Simons M, Edelman ER, DeKeyser JL, Langer R, Rosenberg RD. Antisense c-*myb* oligonucleotides inhibit intimal arterial smooth muscle cell accumulation in vivo. Nature 1992; 359:67–70.
97. Shi Y, Fard A, Galeo A, Hutchinson HG, Vermani P, Dodge GR, Hall DJ, Shaheen F, Zalewski A. Transcatheter delivery of c-myc antisense oligomers reduces neointimal formation in a porcine model of coronary artery balloon injury. Circulation 1994; 90:944–951.
98. Yaswen P, Stampfer MR, Ghosh K, Cohen JS. Effects of sequence of thioated oligonucleotides on cultured human mammary epithelial cells. Antisense Res Dev 1993; 3:67–77.
99. Villa AE, Guzman LA, Poptic EJ, Labhasetwar V, D'Souza S, Farrell CL, Plow EF, Levy RJ, DiCarleto PE, Topol EJ. Effects of antisense c-*myb* oligonucleotides on vascular smooth muscle cell proliferation and response to vessel wall injury. Circ Res 1995; 76:505–513.
100. Burgess TL, Fisher EF, Ross SL, Bready JV, Qian Y, Bayewitch LA, Cohen AM, Herrera CJ, Hu S, Kramer TB, Lott FD, Martin FH, Pierce GF, Simonet L, Farrell CL. The antiproliferative activity of c-myb and c-myc antisense oligonucleotides in smooth muscle cells is caused by nonantisense mechanism. Proc Natl Acad Sci USA 1995; 92:4051–4055.
101. Loke S, Stein C, Zhang X, Avigan M, Cohen J, Neckers LM. Delivery of c-myc antisense phosphorothioate oligodeoxynucleotides to hemopoietic cells in culture by liposome fusion: specific reduction in c-myc protein expression correlates with inhibition of cell growth and DNA synthesis. Curr Top Microbiol Immunol 1988; 141:282–289.
102. Mann MJ, Gibbons GH, Kernoff RS, Diet FD, Tsao PS, Cooke JP, Kaneda YM, Dzau VJ. Genetic engineering of vein grafts resistant to atherosclerosis. Proc Natl Acad Sci USA 1995; 92:4502–4506.
103. Simons M, Edelman ER, Rosenberg RD. Antisense proliferating cell nuclear antigen oligonucleotides inhibit intimal hyperplasia in a rat carotid artery injury model. J Clin Invest 1994; 93:2351–2356.
104. Wielbo D, Sernia C, Gyurko R, Phillips MI. Antisense inhibition of hypertension in the spontaneously hypertensive rat. Hypertension 1995; 25:314–319.

105. Bielinska A, Schivdasani RA, Zhang L, Nabel GJ. Regulation of gene expression with double-stranded phosphothioate oligonucleotides. Science 1990; 250:997–1000.
106. Sullenger BA, Gallardo HF, Ungers GE, Gilboa E. Overexpression of TAR sequences renders cells resistant to human immunodeficiency virus replication. Cell 1990; 63:601–608.
107. Morishita R, Gibbons GH, Horiuchi M, Ellison KE, Nakajima M, Zhang L, Kaneda Y, Ogihara T, Dzau VJ. A novel molecular strategy using cis element "decoy" of E2F binding site inhibits smooth muscle proliferation in vivo. Proc Natl Acad Sci USA 1995; 92:5855–5859.
108. Cox JL, Chiasson DA, Gotlieb AI. Stranger in a strange land: the pathogenesis of saphenous vein graft stenosis with emphasis on structural and functional differences between veins and arteries. Prog Cardiovasc Dis 1991; 34:45–68.
109. Nabel EG, Shum L, Pompili VJ, Yang Z, San H, Shu HB, Liptay S, Gold L, Gordon D, Derynck R, Nabel GJ. Direct transfer of transforming growth factor $\beta$1 gene into arteries stimulates fibrocellular hyperplasia. Proc Natl Acad Sci USA 1993; 90:10578–10763.
110. Morishita R, Gibbons GH, Ellison KE, Lee W, Zhang L, Yu H, Kaneda Y, Ogihara T, Dzau VJ. Evidence for direct local effect of angiotensin in vascular hypertrophy. In vivo gene transfer of angiotensin converting enzyme. J Clin Invest 1994; 94:978–984.
111. von der Leyen HE, Gibbons GH, Morishita R, Lewis NP, Zhang L, Nakajima M, Kaneda Y, Cooke JP, Dzau VJ. Gene therapy inhibiting neointimal vascular lesion: in vivo gene transfer of endothelial-cell nitric oxide synthase gene. Proc Natl Acad Sci USA 1995; 92:1137–1141.
112. Dzau VJ. The role of mechanical and humoral factors in growth regulation of vascular smooth muscle and cardiac myocytes. Curr Opin Nephrol Hypertens 1993; 2:27–32.
113. Ross R. The pathogenesis of atherosclerosis: A perspective for the 1990s. Nature 1993; 362:801–809.
114. Vane JR, Änggård EE, Botting RM. Regulatory functions of the endothelium. N Engl J Med 1990; 323:27–36.
115. Ohno T, Gordon D, San H, Pompili VJ, Imperiale MJ, Nabel GJ, Nabel EG. Gene therapy for vascular smooth muscle cell proliferation after arterial injury. Science 1994; 265:781–784.
116. Guzman RJ, Hirschowitz EA, Brody SL, Crystal RG, Epstein SE, Finkel T. In vivo suppression of injury-induced vascular smooth muscle cell accumulation using adenovirus-mediated transfer of the herpes simplex virus thymidine kinase gene. Proc Natl Acad Sci USA 1994; 91:10732–10736.
117. Chang MW, Barr E, Seltzer J, Jiang Y, Nabel GJ, Nabel EG, Parmacek MS, Leiden JM. Cytostatic gene therapy for vascular proliferative disorders with a constitutively active form of the retinoblastoma gene product. Science 1995; 267:518–522.
118. Takeshita S, Bauters C, Asahara T, Zheng L, Rossow ST, Kearney M, Barry JJ, Ferrara N, Symes JF, Isner JM. Physiologic assessment of angiogenesis by

arterial gene therapy with vascular endothelial growth factor (abstr). Circulation 1994; 90:I-90.

119. Indolfi C, Avvedimento EV, Rapacciuolo A, Lorenzo ED, Esposito G, Stabile E, Feliciello A, Mele E, Giuliano P, Condorelli G, Chiariello M. Inhibition of cellular *ras* prevents smooth muscle cell proliferation after vascular injury in vivo. Nature Med 1995; 1:541–545.

120. Chang MW, Barr E, Lu MM, Barton K, Leiden JM. Adenovirus-mediated over-expression of the cyclin/cyclin-dependent kinase inhibitor, p21 inhibits vascular smooth muscle cell proliferation and neointima formation in the rat carotid artery model of balloon angioplasty. J Clin Invest 1995; 96:2260–2268.

121. Takeshita S, Zheng LP, Asahara T, Riessen R, Brogi E, Ferrara N, Symes JF, Isner JM. In vivo evidence of enhanced angiogenesis following direct arterial gene transfer of the plasmid encoding vascular endothelial growth factor (abstr). Circulation 1993; 88:I-476.

122. Isner JM, Walsh K, Symes J, Pieczek A, Takeshita S, Lowry J, Rossow S, Rosenfield K, Weir L, Brogi E, Schainfeld R. Arterial gene therapy for therapeutic angiogenesis in patients with peripheral artery disease. Circulation 1995; 91:2687–2692.

# Index

# About the Editors

GABOR M. RUBANYI is Director of Vascular and Endothelial Research at Berlex Biosciences, Richmond, California. Previously, he was Director of the Institute of Pharmacology and Chairman of the Corporate Steering Committee on Molecular Biology and Biotechnology at Schering AG, Research Center, Berlin, Germany (1990–1992); Director of Pharmacology at Berlex Laboratories, Cedar Knolls, New Jersey (1987–1990); and Associate Professor and Associate Consultant at the Mayo Clinic Medical School, Rochester, Minnesota. The coeditor, with Una S. Ryan, of *Endothelial Regulation of Vascular Tone* (Marcel Dekker, Inc.) and the author or coauthor of 15 books and over 325 research articles and reviews, he serves on the editorial boards of several biomedical journals and is a member of numerous American and international scientific societies. He is the Founder and Editor-in-Chief of the biomedical journal *Endothelium* and the Founder and main organizer of the International Symposium Series on Endothelium-Derived Bioactive Factors. His pioneering work on the nature and characterization of endothelium-derived relaxing and contracting factors contributed in a significant way to our present knowledge about endothelial control of vascular function in health and disease. Dr. Rubanyi received the M.D. degree (1971) from Semmelweis Medical University, Budapest, Hungary, and the Ph.D. degree (1980) from the Hungarian Academy of Sciences.

VICTOR J. DZAU is Hersey Professor of the Theory and Practice of Medicine, Harvard Medical School, Boston, Massachusetts; and Chairman of the Department of Medicine and Director of Research at Brigham and Women's Hospital, Boston, Massachusetts. He is the coeditor of six books and the author or coauthor of over 400 professional papers and book chapters that reflect his research interests in vascular biology; the molecular and cellular biology, genetics, and gene therapy of cardiovascular disease; congestive heart failure; hypertension; and the pathophysiology and therapy of vascular disease. Dr. Dzau is a Fellow of the American Heart Association and the American College of Cardiology, a founding member of the Society of Vascular Medicine and Biology, and a member of numerous other organizations. He serves on the editorial boards of several important journals, including *Trends in Cardiovascular Medicine, Cardiovascular Pharmacology,* and *Circulation.* Dr. Dzau received the M.D. degree (1972) from McGill University, Montreal, Canada.